D1591951

PEDIATRIC PRACTICE

Gastroenterology

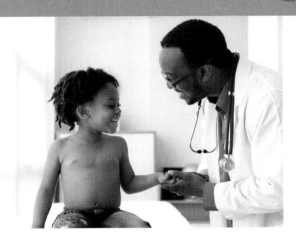

NOTICE

Medicine is an ever-changing science. As new research and clinical experience broaden our knowledge, changes in treatment and drug therapy are required. The authors and the publisher of this work have checked with sources believed to be reliable in their efforts to provide information that is complete and generally in accord with the standards accepted at the time of publication. However, in view of the possibility of human error or changes in medical sciences, neither the editors nor the publisher nor any other party who has been involved in the preparation or publication of this work warrants that the information contained herein is in every respect accurate or complete, and they disclaim all responsibility for any errors or omissions or for the results obtained from use of the information contained in this work. Readers are encouraged to confirm the information contained herein with other sources. For example and in particular, readers are advised to check the product information sheet included in the package of each drug they plan to administer to be certain that the information contained in this work is accurate and that changes have not been made in the recommended dose or in the contraindications for administration. This recommendation is of particular importance in connection with new or infrequently used drugs.

PEDIATRIC PRACTICE

Gastroenterology

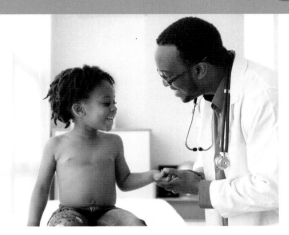

EDITOR

Warren P. Bishop, MD
Professor of Pediatrics
Carver College of Medicine
University of Iowa
Director, Division of Gastroenterology
University of Iowa Children's Hospital
Iowa City, Iowa

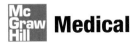 **Medical**

New York Chicago San Francisco Lisbon London Madrid Mexico City
Milan New Delhi San Juan Seoul Singapore Sydney Toronto

Pediatric Practice: Gastroenterology

Copyright © 2010 by The McGraw-Hill Companies, Inc. all rights reserved. Printed in China. Except as permitted under the United States Copyright Act fo 1976, no part of this publication may be reproduced or distributed in any form or by any means, or stored in a data base or retrieval system, without the prior written permission of the publisher.

1 2 3 4 5 6 7 8 9 10 CTP/CTP 14 13 12 11 10

ISBN 978-0-07-163379-6
MHID 0-07-163379-0

This book was set in Minon by Thomson Digital.
The editors were Alyssa Fried and Regina Y. Brown.
The production supervisor was Sherri Souffrance.
The cover designer was David Dell'Accio.
China Translation & Printing Services, Ltd. was printer and binder.

This book was printed on acid-free paper.

Library of Congress Cataloging-in-Publication Data

Pediatric practice. Gastroenterology / [edited by] Warren P. Bishop.
      p. ; cm.
  Other title: Gastroenterology
  Includes bibliographical references.
  ISBN-13: 978-0-07-163379-6 (pbk. : alk. paper)
  ISBN-10: 0-07-163379-0 (pbk. : alk. paper)
1. Pediatric gastroenterology. 2. Children—Diseases. I. Bishop, Warren P. II.
Title: Gastroenterology.
  [DNLM: 1. Gastrointestinal Diseases. 2. Adolescent. 3. Child. 4. Infant. 5. Liver Diseases.
  6. Pancreatic Diseases. WS 310 P3718 2010]
RJ446.P45 2010
618.92'33—dc22
                                    2010006300

McGraw-Hill books are available at special quantity discounts to use as premiums and sales promotions, or for use in corporate training programs. To contact a representative please e-mail us at bulksales@mcgraw-hill.com.

This book is dedicated to the memory of my parents and to my wife and life-long partner, Gail Bishop. My mother and father provided me with a love of reading and learning, and gave me innumerable opportunities throughout my growing years. None of this would have been possible without that great start in life.

My last 30-plus years have been spent in partnership with my wife. We struggled happily through our years as students and trainees together, followed by many rewarding years of challenges and advancement. Her success as a scientist has inspired me, and her love and support as a partner have made my career possible.

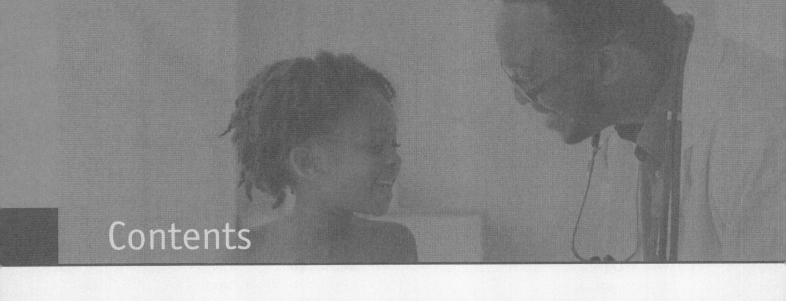

Contents

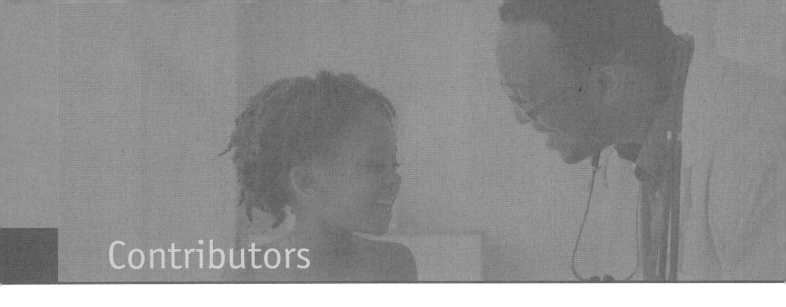

Contributors

Robert D. Baker, MD, PhD
Professor
Department of Pediatrics
University at Buffalo
The State University of New York
Buffalo, New York

Susan S. Baker, MD, PhD
Professor
Department of Pediatrics
University at Buffalo
The State University of New York
Buffalo, New York

Sanjoy Banerjee, MD, MPH
Assistant Professor of Pediatrics
The University of Toledo Health Science Campus
Pediatric Gastroenterologist
Toledo Children's Hospital/Promedica
  Physician Group
Toledo, Ohio

Warren P. Bishop, MD
Professor and Director
Division of Gastroenterology
Department of Pediatrics
University of Iowa
Carver College of Medicine
Lowa City, Iowa

Tyler M. Burpee, MD
Assistant Professor
Department of Pediatrics
University of Washington School of Medicine
Seattle, Washington

Eric Chiou, MD
Fellow
Department of Gastroenterology and Nutrition
Center for Motility and Functional Gastrointestinal
  Disorders
Children's Hospital Boston
Boston, Massachusetts

Dawn R. Ebach, MD
Clinical Assistant Professor
Department of Pediatrics
University of Iowa
Iowa City, Iowa

Steven T. Elliott, MD
Research Fellow
Department of Surgery
Children's National Medical Center
Washington, District of Columbia

Surgery Resident
Department of Surgery
University of California Davis Medical Center
Sacramento, California

Karan McBride Emerick, MD, MSCI
Associate Professor
Department of Pediatrics
University of Connecticut School of Medicine
Hartford, Connecticut

Thomas Flass, MD
Fellow
Department of Gastroenterology,
  Hepatology, and Nutrition
The Children's Hospital
Aurora, Colorado

Benjamin D. Gold, MD, FACG, FAAP
Adjunct Professor
Department of Pediatrics
Emory University School of Medicine
Atlanta, Georgia

Barbara A. Haber, MD
Associate Professor
Department of Pediatrics
The Children's Hospital of Philadelphia
Philadelphia, Philadelphia

Eyad Hanna, MD
Clinical Assistant Professor
Department of Pediatric Gastroenterology
  and Hepatology
University of Iowa
Iowa City, Iowa

Edward J. Hoffenberg, MD
Professor of Pediatrics
University of Colorado School of Medicine
Director, Program for Pediatric Inflammatory
  Bowel Diseases
The Children's Hospital
13123 East 16th Avenue
Aurora, Colorado 80045

Subra Kugathasan, MD
Professor
Department of Pediatrics
Emory University
Atlanta, Georgia

Melissa Leyva-Vega, MD
Fellow
Division of Gastroenterology, Hepatology,
  and Nutrition
The Children's Hospital of Philadelphia
Philadelphia, Philadelphia

B U.K. Li, MD
Professor
Division of Pediatric Gastroenterology, Hepatology
  and Nutrition
Department of Pediatrics
The Medical College of Wisconsin
Milwaukee, Wisconsin

Chris A. Liacouras, MD
Professor of Pediatrics
Department of Gastroenterology,
  Hepatology, and Nutrition
University of Pennsylvania School of Medicine
Philadelphia, Philadelphia

Jenifer R. Lightdale, MD, MPH
Assistant Professor
Department of Pediatrics
Harvard Medical School
Boston, Massachusetts

Mark E. Lowe, MD, PhD
Professor
Department of Pediatrics
University of Pittsburgh
Pittsburgh, Philadelphia

Michael A. Manfredi, MD
Instructor
Department of Pediatrics
Harvard Medical School
Boston, Massachusetts

Jonathan E. Markowitz, MD, MSCE
Associate Professor
Department of Clinical Pediatrics
University of South Carolina School of
  Medicine, Greenville
Greenville, South Carolina

John Meehan, MD
Associate Professor
Department of Surgery
Division of Pediatric Surgery
University of Washington
Seattle, Washington

Elizabeth Mileti, DO
Clinical Fellow
Department of Pediatric Gastroenterology,
  Hepatology and Nutrition
University of California, San Francisco
San Francisco, California

Hayat Mousa, MD, FAAP
Associate Professor
Medical Director of the Motility Center
Department of Pediatrics
Division of Pediatric Gastroenterology
Ohio State University
Columbus, Ohio

Karen F. Murray, MD
Professor
Department of Pediatrics
Division of Gastroenterology, Hepatology,
  and Nutrition
University of Washington School of Medicine
Seattle, Washington

Richard J. Noel, MD, PhD
Assistant Professor
Department of Pediatrics
Medical College of Wisconsin
Milwaukee, Wisconsin

Samuel Nurko, MD, MPH
Associate Professor
Department of Pediatrics
Harvard Medical School
Division of Gastroenterology
Children's Hospital Boston
Boston, Massachusetts

Judith A. O'Connor, MD, MS
Associate Professor
University of Arkansas for Medical Sciences
Section of Gastroenterology, Nutrition & Hepatology
Department of Pediatrics
Arkansas Children's Hospital
1 Children's Way
Little Rock, Arkansas 72202

Bharani Pandrangi, MD
Fellow
Department of Pediatric Gastroenterology
University of Iowa
Iowa City, Iowa

Dinesh S. Pashankar, MD, MRCP
Associate Professor
Department of Pediatrics
Yale University School of Medicine
New Haven, Connecticut

Uma Padhye Phatak, MD
Fellow
Department of Pediatric Gastroenterology
Yale University School of Medicine
New Haven, Connecticut

Graeme Pitcher, MBBCh, FCS(SA)
Clinical Associate Professor
Division of Pediatric Surgery
University of Iowa
Iowa City, Iowa

Riad M. Rahhal, MD
Assistant Professor
Department of Pediatrics
University of Iowa
Iowa City, Iowa

Jose R. Romero, MD, FAAP
Horace C. Cabe Endowed Professor of Pediatrics
University of Arkansas for Medical Sciences
Section Chief, Pediatric Infectious Diseases
Arkansas Children's Hospital
1 Children's Way
Little Rock, Arkansas 72202

Rachel Rosen, MD, MPH
Assistant Professor
Department of Pediatrics
Harvard Medical School
Center for Motility and Functional Gastrointestinal
  Disorders
Children's Hospital Boston
Boston, Massachusetts

Philip Rosenthal, MD
Professor of Pediatrics and Surgery
Department of Pediatrics
University of California, San Francisco
San Francisco, California

Anthony D. Sandler, MBChB, FACS, FAAP
Diane and Norman Bernstein Chair,
  Professor, and Chief
Department of Pediatric Surgery
Children's National Medical Center
George Washington University Medical Center
Washington, District of Columbia

Yutaka Sato, MD
Professor
Department of Radiology
University of Iowa
Iowa City, Iowa

Rebecca Scherr, MD
Fellow
Department of Pediatric Gastroenterology
Emory University
Atlanta, Georgia

Ross W. Shepherd, MD, FRACP
Professor
Department of Pediatrics
Washington University School of Medicine
St. Louis, Missouri

Joel Shilyansky, MD, FACS, FAAP
Associate Professor
Department of Surgery
University of Iowa
Carver College of Medicine
Iowa City, Iowa

Achint K. Singh, MD
Fellow
Department of Radiology
University of Iowa
Iowa City, Iowa

Jeffrey H. Teckman, MD
Associate Professor
Department of Pediatrics and Biochemistry
  and Molecular Biology
St. Louis University School of Medicine
St. Louis, Missouri

Yumirle P. Turmelle, MD
Assistant Professor
Department of Pediatrics
Washington University School of Medicine
St. Louis, Missouri

Aliye Uc, MD
Associate Professor of Pediatrics
Associate Professor of Radiation Oncology
Carver College of Medicine
University of Iowa
University of Iowa Children's Hospital
200 Hawkins Drive, 2868 JPP
Iowa City, Iowa

Narayanan Venkatasubramani, MD, MRCP, MBBS
Assistant Professor
Division of Pediatric Gastroenterology,
  Hepatology and Nutrition
Department of Pediatrics
The Medical College of Wisconsin
Milwaukee, Wisconsin

Preface

This textbook was conceived as a resource for all healthcare professionals who care for children. At its conception, the target audience was to consist of primary care physicians, but it will clearly be equally valuable to medical students, residents in family medicine, pediatrics, and surgery, specialists in many fields who may be confronted with a child experiencing gastrointestinal symptoms, and a variety of allied health professionals.

We have endeavored to supply a concise, illustrated, and current reference on gastrointestinal and liver disorders designed for all physicians who care for children. Many colorful illustrations are designed to enhance readability and improve understanding of complex topics. The first section deals with evaluation of common symptoms emphasizing the differential diagnosis and evaluation of the symptoms, as well as treatment of common causes. Disease chapters follow a similar practical approach, and are supplemented by several chapters on diagnostic modalities. Each chapter contains a list of references for the use of the reader in further exploration of selected topics. This is a book that is dense with practical information. It is beautifully illustrated, readable, portable, and, most importantly, highly informative and up-to-date.

Warren P. Bishop

Acknowledgments

This book would never have occurred without the support of many colleagues who trained me, especially Dr. Martin H. Ulshen, who was my mentor during fellowship training at the University of North Carolina and a role model for my career. Dr. Colin Rudolph has generously encouraged me in the writing of this book, and his example as a successful editor of a major textbook of pediatrics and a leader of a large academic gastroenterology group has been inspirational. The many fine chapter contributors have my gratitude for their hard work, dedication to providing a quality product, and their cheerful cooperation with the sometimes arduous editorial process. The North American Society of Pediatric Gastroenterology and Nutrition has been an enormous benefit to my career, providing networking, education, innumerable role models, and career growth opportunities. All of the authors of this book are members of that fine organization, which tirelessly advocates for the advancement of children's healthcare. Finally, I wish to thank my editor at McGraw Hill, Alyssa Fried, who has been a tireless cheerleader, advocate, and friend. She has been indispensable in the production of the book.

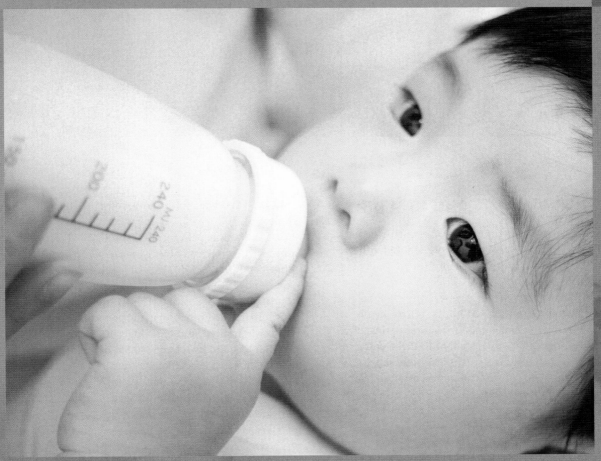

Symptoms and Assessment

CHAPTER 1

Abdominal Pain

Sanjoy Banerjee

DEFINITION AND EPIDEMIOLOGY

Abdominal pain is a common complaint in pediatric population, often resulting in unscheduled office or emergency room visits. This symptom can be acute, recurrent, or chronic.

Acute abdominal pain generally refers to pain that has been present for <24 hours. When the presentation is acute, the challenge for the evaluating physician is to differentiate potentially life-threatening and serious medical conditions from benign self-limited ones. The frequency of surgical intervention in patients presenting with acute abdominal pain is around 1%,[1] but the possibility of overlooking a serious organic etiology is a cause of concern to evaluating physicians and families.

Children are considered to have *recurrent* or *chronic abdominal pain* if they have experienced at least three bouts of abdominal pain, severe enough to affect activities, over a period of at least 3 months. Though this definition was initially used by Apley and Nash[2] as the entry criteria for their descriptive study, it later became a term to describe all children with abdominal pain without known organic etiology. *Recurrent abdominal pain* (RAP) should be used as a description rather than as a diagnosis. RAP may occur in functional abdominal pain (FAP; see below), but this pattern of discomfort can also occur with organic disease.[3] *Functional gastrointestinal disorders* (FGID) include a combination of chronic and/or recurrent symptoms not explained by known biochemical or structural abnormalities. According to Rome III criteria, symptoms must occur at least once per week for at least 2 months before making a diagnosis of FGID.[4] In a study of 227 patients with recurrent and chronic abdominal pain, only 76 (33%) were found to have well-defined organic etiologies.[5]

Abdominal pain accounts for 2–4% of all pediatric office visits.[6] In a study by Hyams et al., 13% of middle-school students and 17% of high-school students experienced weekly abdominal pain. In that study, approximately 8% students saw their physician for abdominal pain evaluation in the previous year.[7] In Apley and Nash original study involving 1000 children in primary and secondary schools, 10.8% of children had RAP, with a female preponderance (female to male ratio of 1.3:1).[2] In that survey, the age distribution was also examined. Ten to 12% of males aged 5–10 years had RAP, followed by decline in prevalence and a later peak at age 14 years. Females showed a sharp rise in prevalence after age 8 years and by age 9 years 25% of this group experienced RAP. The long-term outcome of patients with FGID is not known, but studies indicate patients with history of chronic abdominal pain that began in childhood and treated by a subspecialist are more likely to have lifelong psychiatric problems and migraine headaches.[3] Genetic factors and early life events may have a role in the pathogenesis of chronic abdominal pain.

Family History

There is a higher prevalence of alcoholism, psychiatric disorders, somatization disorders, migraine, and chronic pain symptoms among family members. Familial clustering is often seen in patients with FGID. Subjects with FGID, in a study by Locke et al., had an increased risk of reporting a first-degree relative with abdominal pain and/or bowel disturbance.[8] Possible explanations of familial clustering could include both environmental and/or genetic factors.

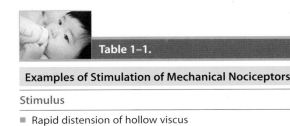

Table 1–1.

Examples of Stimulation of Mechanical Nociceptors

Stimulus	Event
■ Rapid distension of hollow viscus	Intestinal obstruction
■ Smooth muscle contractions	Biliary, renal "colic"
■ Rapid stretching of capsule of solid organ	Hepatic congestion
■ Torsion of the mesentery	Cecal volvulus
■ Traction on mesentery or mesenteric vessels	Retroperitoneal mass

Primary causes of visceral abdominal pain are distension and excessively strong contractions of the musculature of the digestive tract. Hypersensitivity of the mechanoreceptors that detect stretch and contractile force leads to increased nociceptive afferent stimuli, as seen in patients with functional gastrointestinal disorder.

Early Life Events

Noxious stimuli experienced during the neonatal period, when nociceptive neuronal circuits are formed, may result in decreased pain thresholds later in life. Respiratory distress, neonatal infections, colic, neonatal surgeries, or congenital hydronephrosis is reported in approximately 20% patients with chronic abdominal pain.[9]

PATHOGENESIS

Pain originating in the gut is initiated by stimulation of receptors (nociceptors) sensitive to specific mechanical and chemical stimuli. Stretch and the contractile force are the principal mechanical stimuli. Other stimuli, even crushing, cutting, or tearing of the viscera, do not cause pain. *Mechanical nociceptors* are located in the muscularis layers, between the muscularis layer and submucosa of hollow viscera, in the serosa of solid organs, and in the mesentery. Various intra-abdominal processes cause pain by stimulating these mechanical nociceptors (Table 1–1). *Chemical nociceptors* are present within the mucosa and submucosa of the gut. Various triggers such as inflammation, tissue ischemia and necrosis, and radiation injury stimulate these receptors via injury-associated release of mediators, such as prostaglandins, leukotrienes, bradykinin, serotonin, substance P, calcitonin gene-related peptide, histamine, and H^+ and K^+ ions.[10] These substances and mast cell proteases such as $5\text{-}HT_3$ receptors have the potential of elevating the sensitivity of intestinal sensory nerves. Postinfectious irritable bowel syndrome (IBS) develops in a significant percentage of individuals after an acute bout of infectious enteritis. It is unclear if this is the result of exposure of neural and glial elements of the enteric nervous system to the elevated levels of these inflammatory mediators.

Afferent nociceptive sensory neurons are either slow, unmyelinated C fibers or fast, myelinated A-δ fibers. The C fibers are located in visceral peritoneum, mesentery, and viscera. Signals transmitted by these fibers result in dull, poorly localized pain. Because pain fibers from abdominal organs communicate bilaterally with more than one adjacent spinal level, visceral pain is often felt in midline as a poorly localized sensation. The location of abdominal pain is determined by the developmental origin of the affected viscera (Table 1–2). A-δ fibers are found in the somatic structure surrounding the viscera: the abdominal wall, retroperitoneal skeletal muscles, and parietal peritoneum. These fibers have small receptive fields and nociceptive signals through these fibers result in sharp, well-localized sensations.

Patterns of Pain

Understanding the types of pain fibers and their distribution is important to understanding clinical phenomena. *Visceral pain* from most of the gut is poorly localized and difficult to characterize due to activation

Table 1–2.

Visceral Pain Perception and Embryological Origin of Organ

Embryological origin	Pain localization
Foregut: stomach, liver, biliary system, pancreas, spleen, duodenum	Epigastrium
Midgut: jejunum, ileum, appendix, and colon to the level of midtransverse colon	Periumbilical
Hindgut: distal transverse, splenic flexure, descending, and sigmoid colon	Hypogastrium, lower midline

Patterns of visceral pain. Visceral pain is felt in the midline in the epigastric, periumbilical, or hypogastric areas, and this pattern reflects the ontogenic origin of the involved organs from the foregut, midgut, or hindgut, respectively.

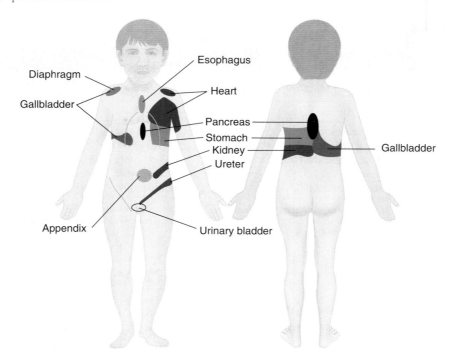

FIGURE 1–1 ■ Patterns of referred pain. The diagram shows important skin areas of referred visceral pain. Adapted from reference 19

of unmyelinated C fibers reporting to several spinal levels at once. A good example of this is the pain associated with Crohn's disease of the small intestine. *Somatoparietal pain* results from stimulation of the parietal peritoneum, and is more intense and somewhat better localized than visceral sensation. *Somatic pain* occurs when somatic structures, innervated by A-δ fibers, are injured or inflamed. In some cases, as in acute appendicitis, pain begins as poorly localized, dull periumbilical discomfort due to inflammation of the inner layers of the appendix, and then becomes progressively more severe and better localized with subsequent inflammation of first the parietal peritoneum and then the adjacent abdominal wall. *Referred pain* is felt in a body area that has its somatic innervation from the same spinal segments receiving visceral pain fibers from the diseased organ. It is usually well localized, as in left shoulder pain from myocardial infarction. Common patterns of referred pain in acute abdominal processes are shown in Figure 1–1.

Pain Perception

Afferent nerves mediating painful stimuli from abdominal viscera follow the distribution of the autonomic nervous system and have cell bodies in dorsal root ganglia. Although nociceptive fibers run together with the sympathetic fibers through sympathetic ganglia (celiac, superior mesenteric, and inferior mesenteric ganglia), they are not part of the sympathetic nervous system. The sympathetic nervous system does not convey pain, but may participate in the sensitization of peripheral nociceptors. The autonomic nervous system plays a role in pain modulation and the associated behavioral and emotional responses to pain. Secondary autonomic effects such as sweating, perspiration, and pallor often accompany visceral pain. The emotional aspects of pain are interpreted in the limbic system and frontal cortex through projection from the brain stem (reticular formation nucleus). Thus, it is important to conceptualize pain as a function of two phenomena: one providing the sensory information from afferent nociceptors and the other modulating the sensation and producing emotional, cognitive, physiological, and behavioral responses.

The functional connections between the brain and the spinal cord result in both inhibitory and excitatory modifications of afferent pain impulses. There are inhibitory mechanisms at the level of the spinal cord (inhibitory interneurons of substantia gelatinosa). Inhibitory neurons originating in mesencephalon, periventricular gray matter, and caudate nucleus participate in descending inhibition, and have dampening effect on pain.[11] Pain can be defined as *nociceptive* when it results from stimulation of peripheral nociceptors by mechanical or chemical stimuli (stretch, local injury, or inflammation). Changes in the pain pathway can result in *neuropathic* pain from aberrant signaling or alteration in inhibitory central processes. Neuropathic pain can happen without stimulation of peripheral nociceptors.

The pathophysiology of chronic, recurrent abdominal pain is not completely understood. There is a

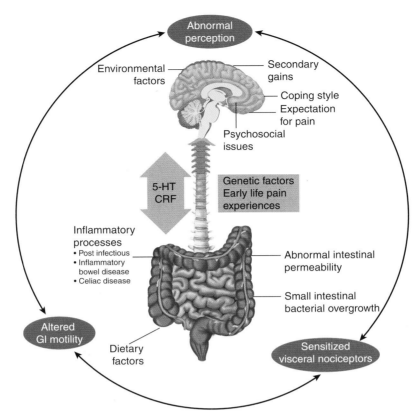

FIGURE 1–2 ■ Biopsychosocial model of chronic abdominal pain. Nociceptive input to the brain comes from sensitized enteric nervous system. Genetic, developmental, environmental, and psychological factors, and coping skills modify the pain experience. 5-HT = 5-hydroxytryptamine; CRF = corticotrophin-releasing factor. Image courtesy of Sumit Banerjee, Toledo, Ohio. Adapted from reference 10.

complex interplay of psychosocial and physiological factors that leads to disturbed gastrointestinal function. Physiological alterations can happen at the level of gut nociceptors, spinal afferents, central autonomic relay system, or pain centers in the brain. Failure of central down-regulation and pain amplification by psychosocial factors lead to *visceral hypersensitivity*. Key mediators of gut function, such as serotonin (5-HT) and corticotropin-releasing factor (CRF), may modulate input from central nervous system along the *brain gut axis*, and cause altered intestinal motility and visceral hypersensitivity.[11,12] Important psychosocial factors contributing to pain are lack of a social support system, anxiety-provoking events, a dysfunctional or abusive relationship, family attitude toward illness, and lack of coping skills. Pathophysiological mechanisms implicated in chronic, recurrent abdominal pain are summarized in Figure 1–2.

CLINICAL PRESENTATIONS

General Approach to Pain

The evaluating physician's role is to establish an accurate diagnosis in an expeditious manner. The immediate goal is to identify life-threatening emergencies that require urgent interventions. The most important component of the evaluation process is a carefully taken history and a detailed physical examination. Selective use of appropriate radiological and laboratory investigations may be required to establish a specific diagnosis. Both the evaluating physician and the caregivers, however, must realize that the diagnosis may remain uncertain despite a thorough initial evaluation. In the absence of an obvious indication for surgery, patients with concerning acute symptoms should be observed in the hospital or emergency department with serial abdominal examinations to clarify any diagnostic uncertainty. Infants and younger pediatric patients are especially challenging, as they are unable to describe or localize pain. Pain is often inferred based on inconsolability or crying with abdominal palpation. A school-age child can usually characterize the location, intensity, and temporal progression of pain with reasonable accuracy.

Acute Abdominal Pain

History

Important details of the history include pattern of onset, progression, location, intensity and character, aggravating and alleviating factors of abdominal pain, and associated symptoms. Key historical variables include age and gender

Table 1–3.

Presenting History of Common Causes of Acute Abdominal Pain

Condition:	Onset	Location	Radiation	Associated symptoms and review of systems
Appendicitis	Gradual	Periumbilical early; RLQ late	RLQ	Fever, nausea, vomiting
Pancreatitis	Rapid	Epigastric, back	Mid-back	Fever, nausea, vomiting
Cholecystitis	Rapid	RUQ	Right scapula	Nausea, vomiting, fever
Small bowel obstruction	Gradual	Periumbilical	None	Bilious emesis (high obstruction), feculent emesis (distal obstruction), h/o trauma, prior abdominal surgery (adhesions)
Gastroenteritis	Gradual	Periumbilical	None	Fever, diarrhea ± bloody stool, vomiting
Pelvic inflammatory disease	Gradual	Pelvic or LQ	Upper thigh	Fever, dysuria, vaginal discharge
Perforated peptic ulcer	Sudden	Epigastric	Mid-back	Fever nausea,
Ruptured ectopic pregnancy	Sudden	Pelvic or LQ	None	Lightheaded, vaginal bleeding

Patterns of common causes of acute abdominal pain. LQ = lower quadrant; RLQ = right lower quadrant; RUQ = right upper quadrant.

of the patient, history of abdominal trauma or prior abdominal surgery, and a thorough review of system. Common causes of acute abdominal pain have characteristic presentations and knowledge of these characteristics is essential for an expeditious diagnosis (Table 1–3).

Physical examination

Careful systemic and abdominal examinations are essential for accurate diagnosis. Physical examination findings must be interpreted by taking the patient's history and age into account. Examination of external genitalia, anus, and rectum is recommended as part of evaluation for abdominal pain. Pelvic examination is important in sexually active female patients. Key elements of the physical examination are as follows:

■ *Appearance*: Appearance, hydration status, facial expression, breathing pattern, position in bed, and degree of discomfort should be carefully assessed. A child reluctant to move or in a fetal position is likely to have peritonitis. Patients with pure visceral pain, as in biliary colic or bowel obstruction, change position frequently, often writhing in pain.
■ *Vital signs*: Vital signs are useful in assessing hypovolemia and provide useful clues for diagnosis. Patients with fever and acute abdominal pain may have acute gastroenteritis, pneumonia, pyelonephritis, pharyngitis, acute cholecystitis, appendicitis, or an intra-abdominal abscess. Tachypnea may indicate pneumonia. An acidotic breathing pattern is seen when

there is metabolic acidosis as in diabetic ketoacidosis, gastroenteritis with dehydration, peritonitis, and intestinal obstruction. Hypotension suggests intravascular volume loss (acute gastroenteritis and abdominal trauma with intra-abdominal hemorrhage), or third-space loss (volvulus, intussusception, and peritonitis).
■ *Abdominal examination*: Abdominal examination is often difficult to perform in a crying, uncooperative sick infant or child. Young patients are best examined in their position of comfort, usually in the lap of a parent. The abdomen should be examined before other anxiety-provoking examinations (e.g., examination of throat and ear). The examining physician must make efforts to determine the degree of abdominal tenderness and its location. Severe, diffuse tenderness with abdominal wall rigidity is indicative of peritonitis. Reproducible focal tenderness is indicative of intra-abdominal inflammatory process, as with McBurney's point tenderness in appendicitis, epigastric tenderness in acute pancreatitis, and right upper quadrant tenderness with acute cholecystitis. Abdominal distension is seen with intestinal obstruction or abdominal mass. Other inspection findings may include ecchymoses (abdominal trauma), scars (prior abdominal surgery and associated adhesions), hernias, and visible intestinal peristalsis (intestinal obstruction or gastroenteritis).
■ *Extra-abdominal findings*: Important diagnostic clues are often obtained from extra-abdominal findings. A characteristic rash is seen in Henoch–Schönlein

purpura or scarlet fever. Jaundice is observed in hepatitis, gallbladder disease, or hemolytic anemia. Evidence of trauma elsewhere may be associated with occult visceral injury.

Chronic or Recurrent Abdominal Pain

History

- If possible, interrogate the patient directly, using developmentally appropriate techniques.
- Ask the patient to localize the pain area with his or her own hand. Poorly localized pain suggests visceral or functional etiology.
- Obtain information about the quality, intensity, duration, and timing of the pain. Ask about other associated symptoms, including vomiting, diarrhea, constipation, fever, rectal bleeding, weight loss, joint symptoms, oral ulcers, dysuria, hematuria, or perianal discharge. These symptoms often indicate an organic disease.
- Enquire about aggravating and relieving factors of the pain, relationship to diet, activity, posture, or psychosocial stressors.
- Assess the impact of chronic pain on daily functioning. Is the pain debilitating? Has it become the central focus of the patient's life? What is the impact of pain on school attendance or sports participation?
- Enquire about the possibility of sexual or physical abuse, unresolved grief or losses, or depression.
- Ask about therapeutic attempts made to relieve abdominal symptoms and their efficacy. Specifically, enquire about the use of nonsteroidal anti-inflammatory drugs, narcotics, or laxatives.

There is no literature showing that pain frequency, location, timing (postprandial and nocturnal awakening), severity, and impact on quality of life are able to distinguish between patients with organic and functional disorders. There are also insufficient data to determine whether the presence of associated symptoms such as headache, anorexia, joint pain, vomiting, nausea, flatulence, and altered bowel pattern helps in distinguishing between organic and functional disorders. The presence of alarm symptoms such as involuntary weight loss, slowing of linear growth, severe vomiting, gastrointestinal blood loss, chronic severe diarrhea, unexplained fever, localized right upper or lower quadrant pain, and family history of inflammatory bowel disease suggests a higher probability of organic disease.

Physical examination

- Carefully note facial expression, body posture, breathing pattern, and interaction of the patient with the accompanying family members.
- Presence of pallor, growth retardation, acute weight loss, clubbing, jaundice, peripheral edema, or significant lymphadenopathy may indicate organic etiology.
- It is uncommon to find signs of autonomic arousal—diaphoresis, tachycardia, or elevated blood pressure—in absence of acute organic causes of abdominal pain.
- Carnett's test distinguishes abdominal wall pain from visceral pain. The pain from palpation at the site of maximal tenderness increases in abdominal wall pain with raising the head and contracting the rectus abdominis muscle, whereas in visceral pain it decreases.
- The "closed-eyes" sign is often seen in patients with FAP. These patients will wince with their eyes closed when the abdomen is palpated, whereas those with organic etiology keep their eyes open, fearfully anticipating pain with abdominal palpation.
- Inspect the abdomen for scars (indicative of prior surgery), distension, visible peristalsis, dilated vessels, or striae. It is important to examine the perianal area and hernial orifices, and perform digital rectal examination.
- Reexamination of the patient during acute exacerbation of abdominal pain will often provide important clinical information.

DIFFERENTIAL DIAGNOSIS

Acute Abdominal Pain

Acute abdominal pain generally refers to pain that has been present for <24 hours. The most common causes of the acute abdomen are listed in Tables 1–4 and 1–5. A detailed

Table 1–4.

Abdominal Causes of Acute Abdomen

Gastrointestinal	Acute cholangitis
Appendicitis	Acute hepatitis
Trauma	Hepatic abscess
Incarcerated hernia	Splenic rupture
Intussusception	**Abdominal wall**
Volvulus	Rectus abdominis
Intestinal obstruction	hematoma
Meckel diverticulitis	**Renal/urologic**
Necrotizing enterocolitis	Acute pyelonephritis
Intestinal perforation	Nephrolithiasis
Inflammatory bowel disease	Testicular torsion
Acute gastroenteritis	**Pelvic**
Constipation	Ovarian torsion
Spontaneous bacterial peritonitis	Ruptured ovarian cyst
Pancreatic, splenic, hepatobiliary	Pelvic inflammatory
Acute pancreatitis	disease
Acute cholecystitis	Ectopic pregnancy

Adapted from reference 10.

Table 1–5.

Extra-abdominal Causes of Acute Abdomen

Cardiac	Neurologic
Myocarditis	Abdominal epilepsy
Pericarditis	Abdominal migraine
Endocarditis	Herpes zoster
Congestive heart failure	Nerve root compression
Thoracic	Radiculitis
Lower lobe pneumonia	**Toxins/drug-related**
Pneumothorax	Lead poisoning
Hematologic	Hypersensitivity reactions
Sickle cell crisis	Narcotic withdrawal
Acute leukemia	**Miscellaneous**
Henoch–Schönlein purpura	Familial Mediterranean
Vaso-occlusive crisis	fever
Metabolic	
Diabetic ketoacidosis	
Acute adrenal insufficiency	
Acute porphyria	

Adapted from reference 10.

description of these disorders is beyond the scope of this chapter. A brief discussion of the common causes follows.

Acute appendicitis

*P*ain followed by *a*norexia, *n*ausea, and *t*emperature elevation (mnemonic PANT) describes classic progression of symptoms in appendicitis. Appendicitis is a clinical diagnosis, supported by appropriately selected radiological and laboratory studies. Patients with classic history and physical findings do not require additional studies, and urgent surgical intervention is appropriate. White blood cell count of >20,000 per mm³ is seen in perforated appendicitis, or appendiceal abscess. The appendix is visualized as a round structure of ≥7 mm in diameter with the anechoic lumen surrounded by hyperechoic and thickened wall (>2 mm) is the classic ultrasonographic finding. The pooled sensitivities and specificities from one meta-analysis describing use of ultrasonography in 9356 children were 88% and 94%, respectively.[5] Helical computed tomography (CT) of the appendix is a useful adjunct in selected patients and is a reliable method for differentiating periappendicular phlegmon from abscess. The sensitivity and specificity of CT for diagnosing appendicitis are >90% and 85–90%, respectively.[13]

Small bowel obstruction

In pediatric patients, common causes of bowel obstruction are intussusception, intestinal atresia, meconium ileus, postoperative adhesions, malrotation with midgut volvulus, and incarcerated inguinal hernia. Intestinal atresia and meconium ileus present in the newborn period. Distal intestinal obstruction syndrome (DIOS), sometimes called "meconium ileus equivalent," is seen in older children with cystic fibrosis. They present with ileal obstruction caused by thickened stool. Early diagnosis is essential in all cases of small bowel obstruction to avoid bowel ischemia. High intestinal obstruction is characterized by frequent bilious emesis and epigastric pain. Cramping, periumbilical or lower abdominal pain with infrequent feculent emesis is typical of distal intestinal obstruction. Radiological features of small bowel obstruction are dilated loops of small bowel, with air–fluid levels and decompressed distal bowel. Ultrasonography is useful for diagnosis of ileocolic intussusception, with sensitivity approaching 100%. Ultrasonographic findings suggestive of volvulus are dilated duodenum, an abnormal position of the superior mesenteric vein, and a "whirlpool" sign of volvulus caused by the vessels twisting around the base of the mesenteric pedicle. Abdominal CT and enteroclysis often help with diagnosing and locating the site of obstruction in patients with strictures, adhesions, or other focal lesions. A contrast (air or barium) enema is useful for diagnosis and treatment of intussusception.

Hepatobiliary disorders

Viral hepatitis, cholecystitis, cholangitis, gallbladder hydrops, choledocholithiasis, and perihepatitis (Fitz-Hugh–Curtis syndrome) present with acute right upper quadrant or epigastric abdominal pain. Patients with choledochal cyst experience recurrent bouts of biliary obstruction, right upper quadrant pain, and a palpable right upper quadrant mass. The pain associated with acute cholecystitis and biliary pain caused by bile stones ("biliary colic") are almost indistinguishable. Patients experience dull, persistent right upper quadrant or epigastric pain with radiation to the right scapula. Biliary colic pain usually resolves within 6 hours of onset, but that of acute cholecystitis is more persistent and is typically accompanied by low-grade fever, nausea, vomiting, right upper quadrant tenderness with guarding, and positive Murphy's sign—the patient stops inhaling as the inflamed gallbladder touches the palpating finger placed below the right costal margin. Laboratory abnormalities include mild elevation of white blood cells, serum total bilirubin, and alkaline phosphatase. More remarkable liver test abnormalities are seen in choledocholithisais, Mirrizzi's syndrome (compression of hepatic duct by gallstone in the neck of the gallbladder), and acute hepatitis. Cholangitis is characterized by a fever, chills, rigor, right upper quadrant tenderness, jaundice, and leukocytosis. Gallbladder hydrops can be seen with Kawasaki disease, Henoch–Schoenlein purpura, and scarlet fever. Fitz-Hugh–Curtis syndrome has been associated with pelvic inflammatory disease caused by *Neisseria gonorrhoeae* and *Chlamydia trachomatis*. Abdominal ultrasonography

Table 1–6.

Etiology of Abdominal Wall Pain

Condition	Features	Diagnosis
Abdominal wall hematoma	Trauma, laparoscopic procedure	Abdominal US, abdominal CT
Hernia	Protuberance in abdominal wall, decreasing in size with supine position	Abdominal US or CT, herniography
Abdominal muscle tear	Occurs in athletes	History and examination
Herpes zoster	Vesicles, pain, hyperesthesia along a dermatome	History and examination
Spinal nerve irritation	Disorders of thoracic spine	Spinal CT or MRI
Rectus nerve entrapment	Pain along the lateral edge of rectus sheath worsening with muscle contraction	Pain relief with local anesthetic
Thoracic lateral cutaneous nerve entrapment	Occurs spontaneously following surgery	History and examination
Ilioinguinal and ilio-hypogastric nerve entrapment	Lower abdominal pain after inguinal herniorrhaphy	History and examination
Slipping rib syndrome	Subluxation of 8–10th ribs causing sharp upper abdominal pain	Hooking maneuver to pull lower ribs anteriorly will reproduce pain

CT = computed tomography; MRI = magnetic resonance imaging; Adapted from reference 19.
US = ultrasound.

and hepatobiliary scintography are useful in initial evaluation of patients with hepatobiliary disorders.

Acute pancreatitis

Pancreatitis is characterized by acute-onset epigastric and upper abdominal pain, increasing rapidly in severity. The pain sometimes radiates to the back or the left scapula. Fever, nausea, anorexia, and vomiting are associated symptoms. Flank (Grey-Turner's sign) or periumbilical (Cullen's sign) ecchymoses are seen in the setting of hemorrhagic pancreatic necrosis. Elevation of serum amylase and lipase occurs within few hours of pain. A sentinel loop or a "cut-off sign," indicating focal ileus, may be seen on abdominal radiographs. Abdominal ultrasound is a useful diagnostic tool for identifying choledocholithiasis as the cause for pancreatitis. Abdominal CT is indicated in severe or complicated pancreatitis.

Chronic Abdominal Pain

Patients fall under two broad groups: (a) abdominal pain due to an organic etiology and (b) patients with FGID without identifiable biochemical or structural abnormalities. If enough tests are done, there is a considerable chance of discovering some abnormality. However, that abnormality may not be the explanation of the patient's symptoms. On the other hand, as our understanding of neurobiology of pain, gut microbiology, and gastrointestinal inflammation improves, there may eventually be an organic explanation for some patients with functional complaints.

Carnett's sign helps in distinguishing *abdominal wall pain* from visceral pain. The diagnosis of abdominal wall pain is also suggested when the pain is superficial, localized to a small area, or associated with dysesthesia in the involved area. Table 1–6 lists possible etiology of abdominal wall pain. More commonly identified organic causes of chronic abdominal pain are mentioned in Table 1–7. There are rare disorders affecting the visceral

Table 1–7.

Organic Causes of Chronic Abdominal Pain

Gastrointestinal	Hepatobiliary/pancreatic
Inflammatory bowel disease	Cholelithiasis
Celiac disease	Cholecystitis
Intermittent volvulus	Chronic or recurrent acute pancreatitis
Recurrent intussusception	
Chronic constipation	Sphincter of Oddi dysfunction
Esophagitis (reflux, eosinophilic, infectious)	Biliary dyskinesia
	Chronic hepatitis
Gastritis (peptic, eosinophilic, infectious)	**Renal/urologic**
	Nephrolithiasis
Peptic ulcer	Hydronephrosis, ureteropelvic junction obstruction
Hernia (internal, diaphragmatic, umbilical, inguinal)	Recurrent cystitis/ pyelonephritis
Carbohydrate malabsorption	**Pelvic**
Intestinal foreign body	Hematocolpos
Parasitic infection	Mittelschmerz
Tumor	Endometriosis

Adapted from references 10, 19.

Table 1–8.

Obscure Causes of Abdominal Pain

Etiology	Confirmatory tests
Compressive radiculopathy	CT or MRI
Lead poisoning	Elevated serum lead levels
Hereditary Mediterranean fever	Family history, MEFV gene mutation
Acute intermittent porphyria	Elevated urine porphobilinogen
Hereditary angioneurotic edema	Low levels of complement C1 inhibitor and complement C4
Narcotic withdrawal	History of narcotic use
Abdominal vasculitides	Angiography, clinical features of systemic disorders such as polyareteritis nodosa, lupus, etc.
Abdominal epilepsy	Electroencephalography
Abdominal migraine	Diagnosis of exclusion

CT = computed tomography; MRI = magnetic resonance imaging. Adapted from reference 19.

nerves rather than the abdominal organs, such as acute intermittent porphyria, lead or arsenic poisoning, and radiculopathies. Rare and obscure causes of chronic or intermittent abdominal pain are listed in Table 1–8. FAP is the most common cause of chronic or RAP in children. It is not a diagnosis of exclusion and can be diagnosed correctly, utilizing symptom-based criteria, without resorting to a battery of tests. These patients do not have any alarm symptoms or signs, the physical examination is normal, and stool tests are negative for occult blood. Rome III criteria for children aged 4–18 years are used for establishing the diagnosis of FGID associated with pain (Table 1–9).[4]

The following is a brief description of childhood FAP disorders.

Functional dyspepsia

A diagnosis of functional dyspepsia is made when symptoms of persistent or RAP *centered in the upper abdomen* occur at least once per week for at least 2 months before diagnosis. The pain is not relieved by defecation or associated with change in stool frequency or consistency. There is no evidence of any inflammatory, anatomic, metabolic, or neoplastic process. The prevalence of dyspepsia among children 4–18 years referred to tertiary care clinics in North America was between 12.5% and 15.9%.[14] Dyspeptic symptoms often follow a viral illness. Delayed gastric emptying, abnormal gastric myoelectrical activity, altered antroduodenal motility, and reduced gastric volume response to feeding have been described in children with functional dyspepsia. Dyspeptic children with bloat-

ing may have rapid gastric emptying with slow bowel transit.[4] Esophagogastroduodenoscopy is indicated in the presence of dysphagia, when symptoms persist despite the use of acid-reducing medications, or become recurrent on cessation of such medications, and for confirmation of *Helicobacter pylori*-associated disease.

Irritable bowel syndrome

A diagnosis of IBS is made when abdominal discomfort or pain occurring at least once per week for at least 2 months before diagnosis is associated with two or more of the following at least 25% of the time: (a) improvement with defecation; (b) onset associated with a change in stool frequency; and (c) onset associated with a change in stool form. In addition, there must be no inflammatory, anatomic, metabolic, or neoplastic abnormalities that may explain the symptoms. Other symptoms that support the diagnosis of IBS are (1) four or more stools per day and two or less stools per week, (2) lumpy/hard or loose/watery stool, (3) straining, urgency, or feeling of incomplete evacuation with stool passage, (4) presence of mucus in stool, and (5) bloating or feeling of abdominal distension. In Western countries, 6% of middle-school students and 14% of high-school students have IBS. Genetic predisposition, stressful events early in life, and ineffective coping mechanisms are often present in these patients. Various antecedents, including inflammation, intestinal trauma, allergy, or infection, could induce visceral hypersensitivity and/or altered gut motility.[4] Patients with normal physical examination and growth and no alarm signals do not require invasive testing for initial evaluation.

Abdominal migraine

These patients have two or more paroxysmal episodes of intense, acute periumbilical pain lasting for 1 hour or more in the preceding 12 months before diagnosis. The pain interferes with normal activities and is associated with two or more of the following: anorexia, nausea, vomiting, photophobia, and pallor. Patients remain symptom-free for weeks to months in between the paroxysmal episodes. There must be no evidence of any inflammatory, anatomic, metabolic, or neoplastic process that may explain the patient's symptoms. This disorder is present in 1–4% of children and is more common in girls than boys (3:2), with a mean age of onset at 7 years and peak at 10–12 years. Abdominal migraine, cyclic vomiting syndrome, and migraine headache are all probably manifestations of a single disorder. Abnormal visual-evoked responses, abnormalities in hypothalamic–pituitary–adrenal axis, and autonomic dysfunction have been described. When appropriate, diagnostic evaluation is done to rule out obstructive processes of urologic or digestive system, biliary disorders, recurrent pancreatitis, intracranial lesions,

Table 1–9.

Rome III Criteria for Functional Bowel Disorders Associated with Abdominal Pain or Discomfort in Children

Functional dyspepsia: Must include *all* of the following (criteria fulfilled at least once per week for at least 2 months before diagnosis):
- Persistent or recurrent pain or discomfort centered in the upper abdomen (above the umbilicus)
- Not relieved by defecation or associated with onset of a change in stool frequency or stool form
- No evidence of an inflammatory, anatomic, metabolic, or neoplastic process that explains the subject's symptoms

Irritable bowel syndrome: Must include *all* of the following (criteria fulfilled at least once per week for at least 2 months before diagnosis):
- Abdominal discomfort (an uncomfortable sensation not described as pain) or pain associated with two or more of the following at least 25% of the time: (a) improved with defecation; (b) onset associated with a change in frequency of stool (four or more stools per day and two or less stools per week); (c) onset associated with a change in form (appearance) of stool
- No evidence of an inflammatory, anatomic, metabolic, or neoplastic process that explains the subject's symptoms

Childhood functional abdominal pain: Must include *all* of the following (criteria fulfilled at least once per week for at least 2 months before diagnosis):
- Episodic or continuous abdominal pain
- Insufficient criteria for other functional gastrointestinal disorders
- No evidence of an inflammatory, anatomic, metabolic, or neoplastic process that explains the subject's symptoms

Childhood functional abdominal pain syndrome: Must include childhood functional abdominal pain at least 25% of the time and one or more of the following (criteria fulfilled at least once per week for at least 2 months before diagnosis):
- Some loss of daily functioning
- Additional somatic symptoms such as headache, limb pain, or difficulty sleeping

Abdominal migraine: Must include *all* of the following (criteria fulfilled two or more times in the preceding 12 months):
- Paroxysmal episodes of intense, acute periumbilical pain that last for 1 hour or more
- Intervening periods of usual health lasting weeks to months
- The pain interferes with normal activities
- The pain is associated with two or more of the following: (a) anorexia; (b) nausea; (c) vomiting; (d) headache; (e) photophobia; (f) pallor
- No evidence of an inflammatory, anatomic, metabolic, or neoplastic process that explains the subject's symptoms

familial Mediterranean fever, and metabolic disorders such as acute intermittent porphyria.[4]

Childhood functional abdominal pain

FAP is diagnosed when episodic or continuous abdominal pain is present at least once per week for at least 2 months before diagnosis. These patients do not satisfy criteria for other FGID. There is also no evidence of any underlying inflammatory, anatomic, metabolic, or neoplastic process. A diagnosis of functional abdominal pain syndrome (FAPS) is made when abdominal pain is associated with loss of daily functioning or other somatic symptoms such as headache, limb pain, or sleeping difficulty. In contrast to children with IBS, visceral hypersensitivity of the rectum has not been shown in children with FAPS. This, of course, does not preclude the possibility of a more proximally located visceral hypersensitivity. These patients may have lower pressure pain threshold but this theory is yet to be validated. Symptoms of anxiety, depression, and somatization are often present in children with FAPS and their parents.[4]

Readers should realize that establishing a working diagnosis of FGID and initiation of conservative management does not preclude the need for ongoing monitoring, careful follow-up, and focused diagnostic work-ups when indicated.

DIAGNOSIS

Acute Abdominal Pain

History and physical examination should determine the selection of laboratory and radiographic studies. Observation and repeat examination at appropriate intervals, without any studies, may be sufficient in a well-appearing child with abdominal pain and normal physical examination. Specific laboratory studies (Table 1–10) and radiographic evaluation (Table 1–11) help in formulating an accurate diagnosis and in assessing physiological status of the patient. A complete blood count with white blood cell differential and a urinalysis

Table 1–10.

Laboratory Tests in Patients with Acute Abdominal Pain

All patients	Complete blood count, urinalysis
Postmenarchal female	Urine pregnancy test
Upper abdominal pain	Liver biochemical test, serum amylase, serum lipase
Abdominal pain and pharyngitis	Throat swab for rapid screen and/or culture for group A β-hemolytic streptococcus
Sick-appearing, dehydrated	Serum electrolytes, blood urea nitrogen, creatinine, glucose
Febrile patients, immunocompromised patients	Blood culture and/or urine culture
Bloody stool	Stool culture ± *C. difficile* toxin

Suggested laboratory studies to evaluate patients with acute abdominal pain. History and physical examination findings determine selection of appropriate laboratory studies.

Table 1–11.

Radiological Imaging in Patients with Acute Abdominal Pain

Study	Conditions
Abdominal plain films	Small bowel obstruction, intestinal perforation, ingested foreign body
Ultrasonography	Gallstones, cholecystitis, ovarian torsion, ectopic pregnancy, tubo-ovarian abscess, testicular torsion, ileocolic intussusception, testicular torsion
Focused abdominal ultrasonography for trauma (FAST)	Abdominal trauma (hemoperitoneum)
Upper gastrointestinal contrast series	Midgut volvulus
Contrast (air or barium) enema	Intussusception
Computed tomography with contrast	Appendicitis, pancreatitis, intra-abdominal abscess, intra-abdominal mass, trauma
Noncontrast helical computed tomography	Urolithiasis
Chest radiograph	Lower lobe pneumonia, cardiomegaly (pericarditis, myocarditis), pneumoperitoneum

Suggested radiological studies to evaluate patients with acute abdominal pain. History and physical examination findings determine selection of appropriate radiographic studies.

are generally indicated in all patients with acute abdominal pain. Measurement of serum electrolytes, blood urea nitrogen, creatinine, and glucose levels helps in assessing patient's fluid balance, acid–base status, renal function, and physiological state. An algorithmic approach for evaluation of a patient presenting with acute abdominal pain is shown in Figures 1–3 and 1–4.

Chronic Abdominal Pain

Diagnostic evaluation of the patient with chronic abdominal pain is individualized based on history and physical examination findings. No study has evaluated the utility of common laboratory tests (complete blood count, erythrocyte sedimentation rate, serum electrolytes, blood urea nitrogen, creatinine, liver enzymes, serum albumin,

urine analysis, stool ova, and parasite analysis) in distinguishing between organic and FAP. Abnormal laboratory tests for a common intestinal disorder, such as lactose malabsorption or *H. pylori* infection, may co-exist with abdominal pain but do not necessarily establish a causal relationship between them. Pediatric patients with *H. pylori* infection are not more likely to have abdominal pain than those without *H. pylori* infection. Similarly, treatment of lactose malabsorption does not always result in clinical improvement. Lactose malabsorption may be a trigger that unmasks visceral hypersensitivity; it may be caused by another condition such as celiac disease, or may simply co-exist with IBS. Similarly, there is very little evidence that routine use of abdominal ultrasonography in the absence of alarm symptoms has a significant yield of organic disease.

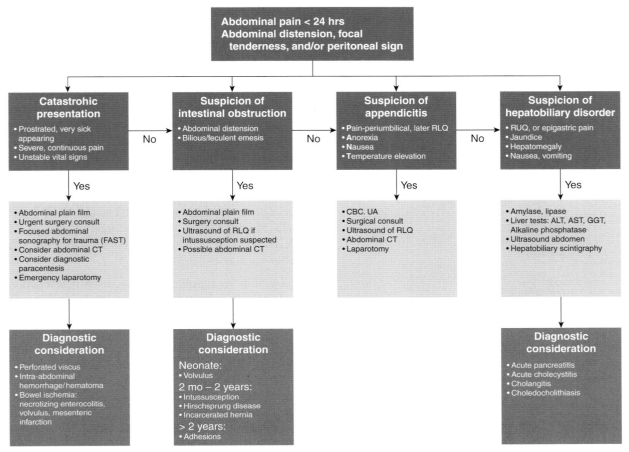

FIGURE 1–3 ■ Algorithmic approach to the patient with acute abdominal pain with catastrophic presentation, evidence of intestinal obstruction, localized abdominal tenderness, or suspicion of hepatobiliary disorder. CBC = complete blood count; UA = urinalysis; CT = computed tomography; RUQ = right upper quadrant; RLQ = right lower quadrant; ALT = alanine aminotransferase; AST = aspartate aminotransferase; GGT = γ-glutamyltransferase.

Diagnostic tests are sometimes indicated in patients with severe debilitating abdominal pain with impairment of functioning to reassure the patient, parents, or referring physician that an organic problem is not present. An algorithmic approach for evaluation of patients presenting with chronic or RAP is summarized in Figure 1–5.Commonly ordered studies are summarized in Table 1–12.

Invasive tests

There is no role for routine use of *capsule endoscopy* for the evaluation of patients with chronic abdominal pain. *Upper endoscopy* is indicated in patients with significant dysphagia, when dyspeptic symptoms persist despite the use of acid-reducing medications or become recurrent on cessation of such medications, hematemesis, and evaluation for Crohn's disease, for confirmation of *H. pylori*-associated disease, and for confirmation of celiac disease. Patients with RAP may require *colonoscopy* in the presence of gastrointestinal bleeding, profuse diar-

rhea, iron deficiency anemia, involuntary weight loss or deceleration of growth, elevated sedimentation rate or C-reactive protein, extraintestinal symptoms suggestive of inflammatory bowel disease (fever, rash, arthralgia, recurrent aphthous ulceration, and severe fatigue), localized right lower quadrant pain, and perianal fistula.

TREATMENT

Acute Abdominal Pain

Most children with acute abdominal pain have viral gastroenteritis or other minor illnesses. Children who are sick-appearing and immunocompromised, and have history of abdominal trauma, signs of bowel obstruction, or evidence of peritoneal irritation require prompt intervention and treatment. Initial resuscitation measures include correction of hypoxemia, replacement of intravascular volume loss, and correction of metabolic abnormalities. Empiric broad-spectrum antibiotics

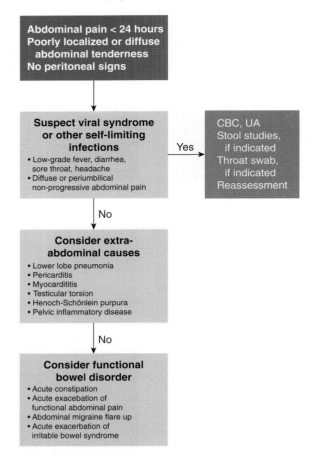

FIGURE 1–4 ■ Algorithmic approach to the patient with acute abdominal pain without peritoneal sign, localized pain, intestinal obstruction, or catastrophic presentation. CBC = complete blood count; UA = urinalysis.

are often indicated in immunocompromised patients and when there is clinical suspicion of a serious intra-abdominal infection. Gastric decompression with nasogastric suction is necessary when there is bowel obstruction. Analgesics should be used in patients with moderate-to-severe abdominal pain, preferably after a surgeon has been able to evaluate the patient. Management strategies for patients with acute abdominal pain are summarized in Figures 1–3 and 1–4.

Chronic Abdominal Pain

If an organic etiology of chronic abdominal pain is identified, disease-specific therapeutic measures are instituted. Physicians often feel challenged and frustrated while caring for patients with FAP. If the patient shows poor response to treatment, it is often perceived as a personal failure on the part of the treating physician. This sense of failure and frustration is exacerbated by a diagnosis that seems uncertain and has no obvious structural basis. It is extremely important for the treating physician to understand the following:

- FGID are a positive diagnosis, based on clinical criteria (Table 1–13).
- These syndromes are chronic, and the goal of treatment is resumption of normal functioning—not complete eradication of abdominal pain. The physician should reduce expectations for cure and focus on function.
- The patient and his or her family must understand that they bear significant responsibility for disease management. This is facilitated by the physician's empathy, support, guidance, and a hopeful attitude.

Evaluation of the patient presenting with chronic abdominal pain is done in the context of the *biopsychosocial model* of care. Psychological factors alone do not help to distinguish between organic and FGID. Nevertheless, it is important to identify and address the following factors:

- Establish an appropriate physician–patient relationship. An effective physician–patient relationship is the most important part of the disease management. It is important to validate the symptoms by acknowledging the pain and its impact on the quality of life. Providing a physiological explanation helps to clarify that the symptoms are not imagined. It is also helpful to provide clear age-appropriate examples of conditions associated with hyperalgesia such as chronic headache without intracranial pathology, or abnormal sensation at the site of a healing scar. Examples of interaction between the brain and the gut should be mentioned. A good example is diarrhea or vomiting occurring during stressful situations such as sports competition or school examinations. Identification of the patient's (and the family's) worries, concerns, and expectations helps physicians to understand the symptoms within a biopsychosocial context. Finally, patients and their family members need reassurance that the symptoms are not caused by a serious disease and do not require extremes of investigation and intervention.
- Set reasonable therapeutic goals. Therapeutic goals should be established early in the course of treatment. The goals are regular school attendance, resumption of normal activities, including participation in extracurricular activities, and reduction in the stress of a chronic disease. Obstacles to school attendance (adverse school environment, negative peer interactions, unreasonable academic expectations, and fear of a pain episode at school) must be identified and addressed. It is important to discuss the possibility of secondary gains perpetuating the pain behavior. For example, pleasurable activities such as watching television should not be allowed if the patient is sick enough to miss school. It is helpful to maintain a diary detailing the circumstances of pain episodes, aggravating factors, and the emotional and

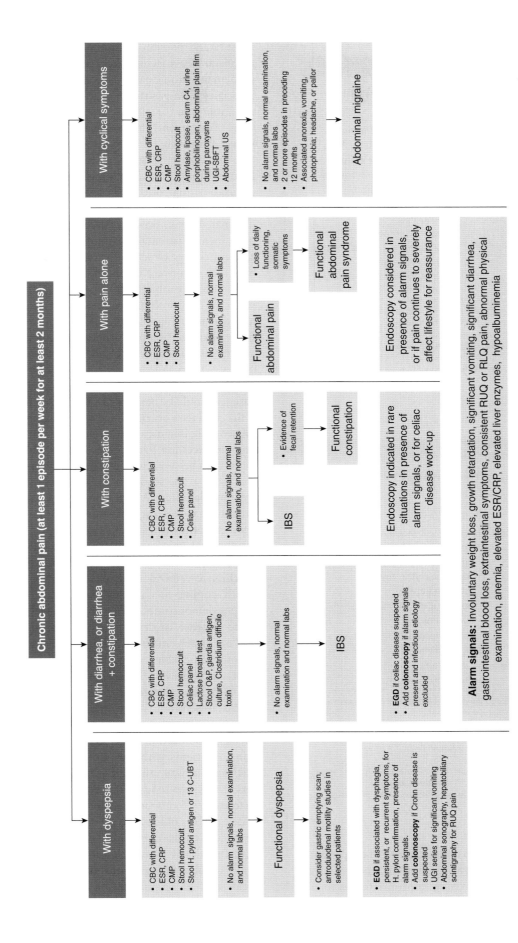

FIGURE 1–5 ■ Suggested algorithm for the evaluation of chronic abdominal pain. CBC = complete blood count; CRP = C-reactive protein; EGD = esophagogastroduodenoscopy; ESR = erythrocyte sedimentation rate; H. pylori = *Helicobacter pylori*; IBS = irritable bowel syndrome; O&P = ova and parasite; RLQ = right lower quadrant; RUQ = right upper quadrant; breath test; UBT = urea breath test; UGI-SBFT = upper gastrointestinal small bowel follow-through; US = ultrasound.

Table 1–12.

Laboratory and Imaging Studies in Patients with Chronic Abdominal Pain

All patients	CBC, CMP, ESR, UA, IgA tissue transglutaminase
Diarrhea	Stool O&P, *C. difficile* culture, lactose breath hydrogen test
RUQ, or RLQ pain, cyclic symptoms, abdominal mass	Abdominal ultrasound, abdominal and pelvic CT with contrast, UGI-SBFT
Dyspepsia, vomiting	UGI, gastric emptying scintigraphy, 13C-UBT or stool for *H. pylori* antigen Hepatobiliary scintigraphy with CCK

Suggested laboratory and imaging studies in patients with chronic abdominal pain based on clinical presentation. CBC = complete blood count; CCK = cholecystokinin; CMP = comprehensive metabolic panel; ESR = erythrocyte sedimentation rate; O&P = ova and parasite; RLQ = right lower quadrant; RUQ = right upper quadrant; UA = urine analysis; UBT = urea breath test; UGI-SBFT = upper gastrointestinal small bowel follow-through.

Table 1–13.

Pharmacotherapy for Functional Gastrointestinal Disorders

Diagnosis	drugs
Functional dyspepsia	H2 blockers: famotidine, ranitidine PPI: esomeprazole, lansoprazole, omeprazole, pantoprazole Prokinetics: erythromycin, metoclopramide
IBS	peppermint oil*, dicyclomine, hyoscyamine
FAP(S)	TCA: amitriptyline#, desipramine SNRI: duloxetine, venlafaxine
Abdominal migraine	cyproheptadine, pizotifen, propranolol, sumatriptan

There are no well-validated published controlled trials on efficacy and their doses of these pharmacological agents in pediatric patients with functional gastrointestinal disorders. FAP(S) = functional abdominal pain (syndrome); H2 = histamine 2; IBS = irritable bowel syndrome; PPI = proton pump inhibitor; SNRI = serotonin–norepinephrine reuptake inhibitor; TCA = tricyclic antidepressant.
*Peppermint oil enteric-coated capsule (187 mg) dose: 30–45 kg, one capsule three times daily; >45 kg, two capsules three times daily.
#Suggested dose of amitriptyline: 0.25 mg/kg/day and slowly titrated up to 1 mg/kg/day.

cognitive responses. An understanding of the patient's style of coping, severity of symptoms, and degree of disability helps in devising appropriate treatment strategies.

■ Identify and modify triggers of pain. It is important to identify and possibly reverse physiological and psychosocial stress factors that trigger, exacerbate, and perpetuate chronic pain. Dyspeptic symptoms may be associated with gastroesophageal reflux, delayed gastric emptying, or altered gastrointestinal motility. Other concurrent physiological processes that may trigger pain include celiac disease, constipation, lactose intolerance, *H. pylori* gastritis, aerophagia, spicy food, or exposure to various medications. Chronic use of laxatives, narcotic medications, and nonsteroidal anti-inflammatory drugs must be identified and eliminated when present. Psychosocial stress factors often include parental separation, death in the family, a recent change of school or residence, family members with significant handicap or illness, altered peer interactions, problems at school, or breakup of a romantic relationship. Identification of these stressors helps in reducing environmental reinforcement of pain behavior. Parents, teachers, and other caregivers are advised to support the child rather than focusing exclusively on the pain. A reasonable timeline for completion of schoolwork accrued during school absence should be negotiated with the school officials. If the child feels overwhelmed with the completion of missed assignments, a reduction of the workload may become necessary. The school officials must respond to the pain behavior with empathy and work with the child so that the school attendance or class activities are not disrupted. A child missing school often is caught in a vicious cycle of anxiety regarding accumulated schoolwork, anticipation of pain, reduced threshold of pain due to anxiety, and increased distress. A rapid return to school is extremely important. Psychiatric referral must be done if maladaptive family-coping mechanisms are identified or the patient demonstrates symptoms of anxiety disorder, panic disorder, or depression. Disease exacerbations that are clearly attributable to psychological distress are often amenable to psychological interventions. In cases unresponsive to these common-sense approaches, use of "central analgesics" (tricyclic antidepressants (TCAs) or serotonin–norepinephrine reuptake inhibitors (SNRIs)) may be considered.

■ Dietary modifications. The role of dietary modification in patients with chronic abdominal pain and FGIDs is not well validated. If there are obvious triggers such as spicy foods, caffeine, carbonated beverages, lactose, fatty foods, and gas-forming foods (legumes and vegetables of the cabbage family), attempts could be made to reduce or eliminate their intake. In patients with functional dyspepsia and postprandial symptoms, a trial of frequent small meals or eating low-fat meals may be helpful. Increasing fiber intake may benefit patients with both diarrhea-predominant and constipation-predominant IBS and FAP. The recommended amount of daily fiber intake (in grams) is estimated in children by adding 5 to the patient's age. Patients with excessive flatulence may benefit from avoidance of sorbitol containing chewing gum, carbonated beverages, legumes, and foods of the cabbage family. A sudden increase in daily fiber intake may lead to increased colonic gas production, abdominal distension, and worsening abdominal pain.

■ Pharmacotherapy. Published controlled trials regarding the efficacy of pharmacological agents for management of FGIDs are rare. Evidence of efficacy to be greater than placebo has been shown for famotidine for functional dyspepsia, pizotifen for abdominal migraine, and peppermint for IBS. Sedatives and anxiolytics are generally not effective, carry the risk of causing sedation and addiction, and have been shown to have no effect on bowel and sensory symptoms in human control subjects. In patients with functional dyspepsia, antisecretory medications such as H2 blockers or proton pump inhibitors and prokinetic agents (metoclopramide, erythromycin, and domperidone and cisapride where available) are often offered. The use of these therapeutic modalities has not been validated by controlled trials, and treatment should not be prolonged in the absence of improvement.

Antidepressants such as TCAs (e.g., desipramine, nortriptyline, and amitriptyline) and SNRIs (e.g., duloxetine and venlafaxine) have effects on central and peripheral nervous systems, and are useful for treating chronic pain syndromes because of their combined noradrenergic and serotonergic effects. The clinical benefit could also be due to anticholinergic effects, slowing of gastrointestinal transit, fundic relaxation, restoration of normal sleep pattern, treatment of comorbid depression, and analgesic effects on receptors throughout the pain transmission system. Physicians must emphasize that these medications are "central analgesics," have independent effects on pain, and can be used in lower dosages than are used to treat depression. To assure daily use and adherence, patients and families need to be informed that these medications are not addicting and can be stopped when needed without major withdrawal effects.

Amitriptyline has been studied in pediatric patients, but without any placebo-controlled evidence. A starting dose of 0.25 mg/kg/day, titrated to a maximum of 1 mg/kg/day over 8–10 weeks, is generally recommended for amitriptyline therapy. In older patients, alternate medications include desipramine (25–75 mg/day) or duloxetine (30 mg/day). There are anecdotal reports of other medications, including phenytoin, carbamezepine, gabapentin, pregabalin, lamotrigine, topiramate, zonisamide, and levetiracetam, benefiting

patients with visceral pain. These agents probably act by depressing abnormal neuronal discharges and raise the inappropriately lowered pain threshold of sensitized neurons. These agents must be used with caution because the pediatric experience is limited and the visceral pain indication is off-label.

Similarly, no controlled trial has been conducted in the pediatric population to study the efficacy of *anticholinergic agents* such as dicyclomine (bentyl) and hyoscyamine (Levbid and Levsin). However, these agents are commonly prescribed. The presumed clinical benefit is from smooth muscle relaxation due to blockage of muscarinic effects of acetylcholine on gastrointestinal tract. Patients must be cautioned about blurred vision, drowsiness, dry mouth, tachycardia, constipation, and urinary retention when these agents are used.

Peppermint oil is an antispasmodic agent that relaxes intestinal smooth muscle by decreasing calcium influx into the smooth muscle cells. Enteric-coated peppermint oil capsules (Colpermin) had a greater efficacy than placebo in reducing functional pain in a randomized double-blind controlled trial consisting of pediatric patients with IBS. There are no evidence-based data on the efficacy of antidiarrheal agents such as *loperamide* and *diphenoxylate*, and bile salt binding agent cholestyramine in patients with diarrhea-predominant IBS.

Polyethylene glycol 3350 is useful in treating constipation in patients with constipation-predominant IBS. Fiber supplements such as psyllium, methylcellulose, polycarbophil, wheat dextrin, and inulin are effective in treating symptoms of both diarrhea and constipation. Prophylactic agents that are used for abdominal migraine are pizotifen, propranolol, cyproheptadine, and sumatriptan.[4,15,16]

■ Psychological treatment. Psychological treatments such as *hypnotherapy* and *cognitive–behavioral therapy* (CBT) have been shown to be effective in treating somatic symptoms of adult patients with FGIDs. There are also emerging data from randomized trials about the effectiveness of these interventions among children and adolescents with FAP or IBS. These techniques promote the patient's ability to self-manage symptoms. Goals of CBT are to identify maladaptive thoughts, perceptions, and behaviors, improve coping and functioning, improve communication and problem solving, and develop ways to improve symptom control. These goals are achieved by modifying dysfunctional cognition, abnormal behavior, and erroneous assumptions or beliefs. *Stress management and relaxation techniques* such as progressive muscle relaxation and controlled breathing can be used to alter pain perception by counteracting physiological effects of stress and anxiety. "Gut-directed" hypnotherapy

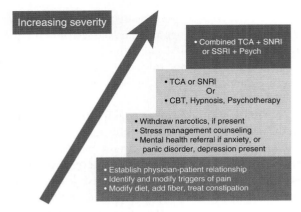

FIGURE 1–6 ■ Treatment algorithm for functional abdominal pain syndrome (FAPS). Multicomponent treatment of FAPS begins with establishment of effective physician–patient relationship. Behavioral and pharmacological treatments are added on the basis of the severity of the symptoms and impairment of daily functioning. CBT = cognitive–behavioral therapy; SNRI = serotonin–norepinephrine reuptake inhibitor; SSRI = selective serotonin reuptake inhibitor; TCA = tricyclic antidepressant.

and guided imagery focus attention away from the somatic symptoms, modify sensory experience, enhance feelings of mastery/self-control, and reduce distress. *Biofeedback* uses a computer-generated visual or auditory indicator of muscle tension, skin temperature, or heart rate and allows the patient to validate the physiological changes induced by controlled breathing, relaxation, or hypnotic techniques.[16,17] The referring physician's role is to help the patient and his family understand the value of these psychological treatments as part of their overall care.

The multicomponent treatment of patients with FAP is summarized in Figure 1–6. Patients with severe symptoms will need combined pharmacological and behavioral intervention.

PROGNOSIS AND CLINICAL COURSE

Most patients do well after the diagnosis of FAP, with subsequent follow-up rarely identifying an organic disorder. Once the child and parents are reassured that the origin of the pain is not organic and the diagnosis of FAP is accepted, symptom resolution or improvement occurs in 30–50% of patients by 2–6 weeks after diagnosis. Approximately one-third of children with FAP will continue to experience abdominal pain, or develop symptoms of chronic headache, backache, and menstrual irregularities as adults. Adverse prognostic factors described by Apley and Hale are male sex, age of onset at <6 years, a strong history of a "painful family," and symptom duration of >6 months prior to the diagnosis of FAP.[18]

REFERENCES

1. Scholer SJ, Pituch K, Orr DP, Dittus RS. Clinical outcomes of children with acute abdominal pain. *Pediatrics.* 1996;98(4):680–685.
2. Apley J, Nash N. Recurrent abdominal pains: a field survey of 1,000 school children. *Arch Dis Child.* 1958;33(168):165–170.
3. Di Lorenzo C, Colletti RB, Lehmann HP, et al. Chronic abdominal pain in children: a technical report of the American Academy of Pediatrics and the North American Society for Pediatric Gastroenterology, Hepatology and Nutrition. *J Pediatr Gastroenterol Nutr.* 2005;40(3):249–260.
4. Rasquin A, Di Lorenzo C, Forbes D, et al. Childhood functional gastrointestinal disorders: child/adolescent. *Gastroenterology.* 2006;130(5):1527–1537.
5. Hyams JS, Treem WR, Justinich CJ, et al. Characterization of symptoms in children with recurrent abdominal pain: resemblance to irritable bowel syndrome. *J Pediatr Gastroenterol Nutr.* 1995;20(2):209–214.
6. Starfield B, Hoekelman R, McCormick M, et al. Who provides health care to children and adolescents in the United States? *Pediatrics.* 1984;74(6):991–997.
7. Hyams JS, Burke G, Davis PM, et al. Abdominal pain and irritable bowel syndrome in adolescents: a community-based study. *J Pediatr.* 1996;129(2):220–226.
8. Locke GR III, Zinsmeister AR, Talley NJ, et al. Familial association in adults with functional bowel disorders. *Mayo Clin Proc.* 2000;75(9):907–912.
9. Miranda A. Early life events and the development of visceral hyperalgesia. *J Pediatr Gastroenterol.* 2008;47(5):682–684.
10. Glasgow RE, Mulvihill SJ. Acute abdominal pain. In: Feldman F, Friedman LS, Brandt LJ, eds. *Gastrointestinal and Liver Disease: Pathophysiology, Diagnosis, Management.* Philadelphia: Elsevier; 2006:87.
11. Wood JD. Functional abdominal pain: the basic science. *J Pediatr Gastroenterol Nutr.* 2008;47(5):688–693.
12. Drossman DA, Camilleri M, Mayer EA, Whitehead WE. AGA technical review on irritable bowel syndrome. *Gastroenterology.* 2002;123(6):2108–2131.
13. Doria AS, Moineddin R, Kellenberger CJ, et al. US or CT for diagnosis of appendicitis in children and adults? A meta-analysis. *Radiology.* 2006;241(1):83–94.
14. Caplan A, Walker L, Rasquin A. Validation of pediatric Rome II criteria for functional gastrointestinal disorders using the questionnaire on pediatric gastrointestinal symptoms. *J Pediatr Gastroenterol Nutr.* 2005;41(3):305–316.
15. LeBel AA. Pharmacology. *J Pediatr Gastroenterol Nutr.* 2008;47(5):703–705.
16. Drossman DA. Severe and refractory chronic abdominal pain: treatment strategies. *Clin Gastroenterol Hepatol.* 2008;6(9):978–982.
17. Bursch B. Psychological/cognitive behavioral treatment of childhood functional abdominal pain and irritable bowel syndrome. *J Pediatr Gastroenterol Nutr.* 2008;47(5):706–707.
18. Apley J, Hale B. Children with recurrent abdominal pain: how do they grow up? *BMJ.* 1973;3(5870):7–9.
19. Pasricha PJ. Approach to the patient with abdominal pain. In: Yamada T, Alpers DH, Kaplowitz N, et al., eds. *Textbook of Gastroenterology.* Philadelphia: Lippincott Williams & Wilkins; 2003:781.

CHAPTER 2

Vomiting

Narayanan Venkatasubramani and B.U.K. Li

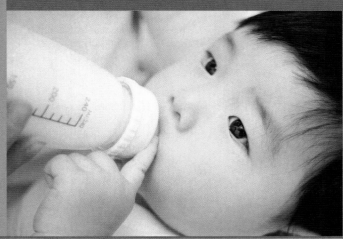

DEFINITIONS AND EPIDEMIOLOGY

Vomiting is the *forceful* retrograde expulsion of gastric contents through the mouth consequent to the coordinated contraction of diaphragm, abdominal, and respiratory muscles. It is associated with a characteristic autonomic response, including pallor, lethargy, hypersalivation, and tachycardia. This differentiates vomiting from *regurgitation*, which is an *effortless* involuntary reflux of undigested gastric contents and is not associated with abdominal/diaphragmatic contractions or autonomic responses. *Nausea* is the subjective unpleasant sensation of impending vomiting that precedes but is not always associated with vomiting. Emesis is a term that can be used to describe any expulsion of gastric contents, and is useful to the physician when describing symptoms that have not yet been fit into the more exact categories of vomiting or regurgitation. *Rumination* is voluntary reflux of gastric contents within the first hour after eating and is associated with chewing and reswallowing of undigested food. *Retching* or "dry heaves" is the activated emetic reflux without vomiting, due to vomiting motion against a closed glottis (Table 2–1). Vomiting should also be differentiated from coughing or spitting of mucus from the lungs.

Vomiting is a non-specific symptom caused by disorders affecting a wide range of organs. It can represent a mild self-limited illness (gastroenteritis), or occur as the result of severe life-threatening conditions (midgut volvulus). Vomiting is a common complaint among children who visit the pediatrician and the emergency department. Primary etiologies originate from the gastrointestinal tract, and are further divided into emergent disorders such as intussception and non-emergent causes such as viral gastroenteritis. Secondary causes involve etiologies that originate outside the gastrointestinal tract (Figure 2–1). Many of the secondary causes need immediate intervention, including cerebellar tumors, acute hydronephrosis from ureteropelvic junction (UPJ) obstruction, and adrenal failure.

Table 2–1.

Translation of Different Descriptions	
Vomiting	Forceful expulsion of stomach contents associated with pallor and is associated with contraction of the abdominal and chest wall musculature
Nausea	The unpleasant feeling of the need to vomit but does not always lead to vomiting
Regurgitation	Undigested food returning to the esophagus and mouth and is not associated with pallor or autonomic signs
Rumination	Deliberate but effortless regurgitation of undigested food within minutes to hour after eating and is associated with chewing and swallowing of regurgitated food
Retching	Spasmodic respiratory movements against a closed glottis with contractions of the abdominal musculature without expulsion of any gastric contents, referred to as "dry heaves"

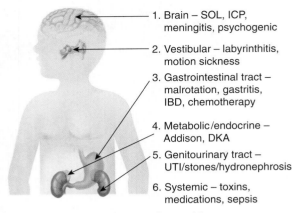

1. Brain – SOL, ICP, meningitis, psychogenic
2. Vestibular – labyrinthitis, motion sickness
3. Gastrointestinal tract – malrotation, gastritis, IBD, chemotherapy
4. Metabolic/endocrine – Addison, DKA
5. Genitourinary tract – UTI/stones/hydronephrosis
6. Systemic – toxins, medications, sepsis

FIGURE 2–1 ■ Organ systems causing vomiting.

In this chapter, we discuss a practical approach to a child who presents with vomiting.

PATHOGENESIS

Understanding the different neuroendocrine pathways and the neurotransmitters that mediate vomiting is useful in understanding the treatment of this symptom. Stimulation of the brain stem *vomiting center* is the final common result of many possible initiating events. The vomiting center is a complex of central nervous system nuclei, including the nucleus tractus solitarus (NTS), the parvicellular reticular formation, and the Bötzinger complex situated in the medulla oblongata.[1] The vomiting center is stimulated through four access points:

- area postrema (chemoreceptor trigger zone (CTZ));
- hypothalamus;
- vestibular region;
- gastrointestinal tract.

The *area postrema* is a circumventricular organ located in the floor of fourth ventricle and is located outside the blood brain barrier, allowing it to sense circulating substances easily. This area, also known as the CTZ, has numerous D_2, $5HT_3$, opiod, ACh, and substance P chemoreceptors that when stimulated by uremic toxins and emetic drugs (apomorphine) lead to vomiting.

The *hypothalamus* is stimulated by anxiety, stress, fear, and odors, leading to the release of GABA and corticotrophin-releasing factor that in turn leads to activation of vomiting center.

When activated by motion or inflammation (labyrinthitis), the eighth cranial nerve stimulates the vomiting center through the *vestibular system* by releasing acetylcholine and histamine.

Mucosal irritation (toxins or food poisoning) or distension of the *gastrointestinal tract* leads to stimulation of vomiting center via the vagal ($5HT_3$) and enteric nervous system afferents.

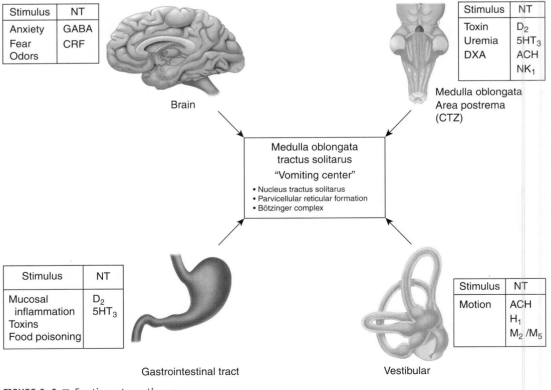

Stimulus	NT
Anxiety	GABA
Fear	CRF
Odors	

Brain

Stimulus	NT
Toxin	D_2
Uremia	$5HT_3$
DXA	ACH
	NK_1

Medulla oblongata
Area postrema
(CTZ)

Medulla oblongata
tractus solitarus
"Vomiting center"
- Nucleus tractus solitarus
- Parvicellular reticular formation
- Bötzinger complex

Stimulus	NT
Mucosal inflammation	D_2
	$5HT_3$
Toxins	
Food poisoning	

Gastrointestinal tract

Stimulus	NT
Motion	ACH
	H_1
	M_2/M_5

Vestibular

FIGURE 2–2 ■ Emetic center pathways.

Vomiting is a highly coordinated sequence of physiologic events as shown in Figure 2–2. Stimulation of vomiting center initiates a programmed emetic response that causes descent of the diaphragm and contraction of the intercostal muscles against the closed glottis. Finally, increase in intra-abdominal pressure from the contraction of abdominal muscles and elevation of diaphragm results in forceful expulsion of gastric contents into lower esophagus, and beyond.

CLINICAL PRESENTATION

The diagnostic approach to a patient begins by defining the symptoms and addressing the following questions:

- Is the child adequately hydrated?
- Is the emesis vomiting or regurgitation?
- What is the temporal pattern of vomiting?
- Are there any red flag symptoms or signs that require further evaluation?
- Are there any associated symptoms and signs?

The initial encounter with the patient should focus on assessing the degree of dehydration and managing the patient accordingly. Dehydration is classified as mild, moderate, or severe based on the child's appearance, urine output, skin turgor, mucous membranes, tears, capillary refill time, heart rate, and blood pressure.

Once the patient is stable, a detailed history and examination will often differentiate vomiting from regurgitation as shown in Table 2–2.[2] This difference is key to the identification of gastroesophageal reflux (regurgitation) and especially critical preoperatively identifying those at risk for post-Nissen retching syndrome.[3] Once the diagnosis of vomiting is established, the long list of differential diagnosis outlined in Table 2–3 can be narrowed down by obtaining the age and temporal pattern of vomiting (acute, chronic, or cyclic). Further questions should be elicited carefully to look for red flag symptoms and signs such as weight loss, bilious or bloody emesis, etc., as shown in Table 2–4. Other associated symptoms and signs also provide vital information such as contents of vomitus, dysphagia, and the relationship to meals (Table 2–5). The two most important parameters that are helpful in narrowing the differential diagnosis of vomiting are age of the patient and the pattern of vomiting.

Acute Vomiting

Self-limiting infections and food poisoning are the most common causes of acute vomiting.[4] It is important to assess the degree of dehydration as accurately as possible. Dehydration is classified as mild (3–5% body weight loss), moderate (5–10%), and severe (>10%) based on signs and symptoms as outlined in Table 2–6. The four most useful clinical signs in assessing dehydration are general appearance, eyes, tears, and mucous membranes.[5] Patients with moderate to severe dehydration may need intravenous fluid replacement. Children presenting with vomiting accompanied by abdominal distension, bilious vomiting, or severe abdominal pain need an abdominal X-ray series and prompt surgical consultation. In infants presenting with vomiting, sepsis, urinary tract infections, meningitis, and child abuse all need to be considered in the differential diagnosis. Hypertrophic pyloric stenosis commonly presents between 3 and 8 weeks of life with projectile, nonbilious emesis. An ultrasound of the pylorus demonstrates an elongated channel in an infant (Figure 2–3). In adolescents presenting with vomiting, pregnancy, drug abuse, and eating disorders need to be considered.

The location of abdominal pain may help to differentiate the potential causes of vomiting. The most common causes of *epigastric pain* associated with vomiting are eosinophilic esophagitis (EoE), gastritis, and *Helicobacter pylori* associated with peptic ulcer disease.[6] Sending the stool for *H. pylori* and a 2–4-week trial of proton pump inhibitors (PPI) may be helpful.[7] If the symptoms persist, endoscopy may be warranted. Esophageal furrows, edema, and white exudate are commonly seen in patients with EoE (see Figure 17–2).

 Table 2–2.

Features Differentiating Vomiting from Regurgitation

Feature	Regurgitation	Vomiting
Event	Effortless expulsion	Forceful expulsion of gastric contents
Prodrome	None	Pallor, salivation, tachycardia + retching
Cause(s)	Gastroesophageal reflux, rumination	Many disorders
Complications	Uncommon	Esophagitis, hematemesis
Implications	Few	Post-Nissen retching syndrome

Table 2–3.

Differential Diagnosis of Vomiting by Age and Pathology

Gastrointestinal Tract	Neonate	Infant	Childhood	Adolescent
Luminal (within the lumen)	Gastroesophageal reflux Esophageal atresia Antral web Malrotation with volvulus Incarcerated inguinal hernia	Gastroesophageal reflux Pyloric stenosis Intussception Malrotation with volvulus Incarcerated inguinal hernia	Malrotation with volvulus Intussception Incarcerated inguinal hernia	Malrotation with volvulus Superior mesenteric artery syndrome
Mucosal inflammation (intestinal surface)	Gastroesophageal reflux disease Formula protein allergy Necrotizing enterocolitis	Gastroesophageal reflux disease Formula protein allergy Gastroenteritis	Gastroenteritis Eosinophilic esophagitis (EoE) *H. pylori* gastritis Peptic ulcer disease	Gastroenteritis EoE Peptic ulcer disease Inflammatory bowel disease Appendicitis
Muscle/nerve (GI wall)	Achalasia Hirschsprung's disease Feeding intolerance (cardiac, renal, pulmonary)	Pseudo-obstruction	Gastroparesis Cyclic vomiting syndrome (CVS)	Gastroparesis CVS Rumination Irritable bowel syndrome
Hepatobiliary/pancreas	Hepatitis	Hepatitis	Hepatitis Pancreatitis	Gallstones Pancreatitis Pancreas divisum
Genitourinary system	Sepsis/UTI	UTI, hydronephrosis	Hydronephrosis RTA	Renal failure
CNS/vestibular	Posthemorrhagic hydrocephalus Chiari malformation	Subdural hemorrhage (SDH) Hydrocephalus	Space-occupying lesion (SOL) SDH Chiari malformation	Bulimia/psychogenic Drug abuse Motion sickness Ménière's disease
Metabolic/endocrine	Congenital adrenal hyperplasia Inborn errors of metabolism (galactosemia, organic academia, urea cycle defects)	Addison's disease Fatty acid oxidation disorder	Addison's disease DKA Fatty acid oxidation disorder	Pregnancy Addison's disease Porphyria Drug abuse Diabetes mellitus

Abbreviations: UTI = urinary tract infection; EoE = eosinophilic esophagitis.

Table 2–4.

Red Flags that Need Further Evaluation in Children with Vomiting

Symptoms	Causes
Projectile	Pyloric stenosis, gastric outlet obstruction, malrotation
Bilious	Obstruction distal to the ampulla of Vater, cyclic vomiting syndrome
Blood	Prolapse gastropathy, peptic injury, esophageal varices
Severe or persistent abdominal pain	Intussception, pancreatitis, peptic ulcer, cholelithiasis, appendicitis
Headache, neck pain, weakness	Space-occupying lesion, Chiari malformation, migraine
Polydipsia	Diabetic ketoacidosis
Dysuria	Urinary tract infection, renal stones

Signs	
Bulging anterior fontanelle (infants)	Meningitis, hydrocephalus, subdural hemorrhage (child abuse)
Nuchal rigidity	Meningitis, intracranial hemorrhage
Papilledema	Increased intracranial pressure (pseudotumor cerebri)
Hyperreflexia or hypertonia	Metabolic problems, upper motor lesion

Table 2–5.

Differential Diagnosis, Approach, and Key Elements in History in Children with Vomiting

	Differential Diagnosis	Management
Pattern		
Abrupt	Gastroenteritis (fever, diarrhea, sick contacts)	Stool rotazyme, culture and sensitivity, ova and parasites
	Pancreatitis (epigastric pain following URI, trauma)	Amylase, lipase, CT abdomen
	Cholelithiasis/hepatitis (RUQ pain radiating to back, fever, jaundice—Murphy's sign)	ALT, GGT, ultrasound abdomen
	Intestinal obstruction (bilious vomiting)	KUB, UGI, surgical consultation
Contents		
Bilious	Malrotation with volvulus (abdominal distension, hyperactive bowel sounds)	KUB, surgical consultation
	Intussception	Ultrasound abdomen
	Hirschsprung's (failure to pass meconium within 48 hours of birth)	Unprepped barium enema, rectal biopsy, surgical consultation
Blood	Prolapse gastropathy	EGD
	Mallory–Weiss tear (heartburn)	EGD
	Gastritis (epigastric abdominal pain)	EGD
	H. pylori	Stool for *H. pylori*, EGD
Undigested food	Achalasia (nighttime coughing, dysphagia)	UGI, motility study
	Gastroparesis (postviral, post-Nissen)	Gastric emptying scan
Timing		
Early morning	↑ Intracranial pressure (SOL, SDH)—headache, blurred vision	MRI/CT brain
	Sinusitis (postnasal drip)	CT sinus
	Pregnancy (LMP)	HCG
	Cyclic vomiting syndrome (stereotypical pattern, normal between episodes)	GI referral
After starvation/illness	Inborn errors of metabolism (FTT, lethargy, seizures)	Metabolic specialist referral
After meals	Peptic ulcer (epigastric pain)	PPI trial for 2 weeks, EGD
	Gastroparesis	Gastric emptying scan
	Eating disorder (food stashing)	Counseling
	Rumination (within 1 hour of eating)	Diaphragmatic breathing
Post-tussive	Asthma, allergy, foreign body	CXR, albuterol
Weight loss	Superior mesenteric artery (SMA) syndrome	UGI, nasojejunal feeding
	Inflammatory bowel disease	Endoscopy
Urinary symptoms	UTI, hydronephrosis	Urine culture and ultrasound
Vertigo, tinnitus	Vestibular disease	ENT referral
Previous surgery	Adhesions	UGI/SBF, surgical consultation

Abbreviations: ALT = alanine aminotransferase; GGT = gamma-glutamyl transpeptidase; SOL = space-occupying lesion; SDH = subdural hemorrhage; FTT = failure to thrive; EGD = esophagogastroduodenoscoy; PPI = proton pump inhibitor.

This is in contrast to distal esophageal erosions seen in patients with severe gastroesophageal reflux disease (GERD). Patients with pancreatitis present with epigastric to left-quadrant abdominal pain radiating to the back. *Right lower quadrant pain* suggests appendicitis or mesenteric lymphadenitis following a viral infection. *Intestinal obstruction* presents with bilious emesis, cramping abdominal pain, abdominal distension, and hyperactive bowel sounds. A characteristic upper gastrointestinal radiograph demonstrates malrotation, with absence of the ligament Treitz (duodenal–jejunal junction) normally found to the left of the midline (Figure 2–4). Hirschsprung's disease should be considered in the differential diagnosis in infants presenting with vomiting, constipation, and abdominal distension, especially with a history of failure to pass meconium within 48 hours of birth. An unprepped barium enema showing the transition zone in an infant with Hirschsprung's disease is shown in see Figure 19–6A. If the patient is well hydrated and there are no red flag symptoms as outlined in Table 2–4, patient can be safely discharged home. If the child presents with

Table 2–6.

Degree of Dehydration Based on Percent Body Weight Lost in Infants and Children

Findings	Mild (<5%)	Moderate (5–10%)	Severe (>10%)
Urine output	Normal	Reduced	No urine output for 12 hours
Appearance	Alert	Irritable	Lethargic
Fontanelle	Normal	Depressed	Markedly depressed
Tears	Present	Decreased tears	No tears
Eyes	Normal	Slightly sunken	Markedly sunken
Mucous membranes	Moist or slightly dry	Very dry	Parched
Skin turgor	Instant recoil	<2 seconds	>2 seconds
Capillary refill time	<2 seconds	Prolonged	Markedly prolonged
Pulse rate	Normal	Tachycardia	Marked tachycardia
Blood pressure	Normal	Normal or low	Low
Respiration	Normal	Rapid	Rapid and deep

moderate to severe abdominal pain, with or without jaundice, complete blood count (CBC), liver transaminases, lipase, urinalysis, and imaging studies may be needed to rule out pancreatitis, cholelithiasis, and other causes of visceral pain. Acute episodes of cyclic vomiting syndrome (CVS) may mimic gastroenteritis, but CVS patients tend to look more ill, because of the associated severe pallor and lethargy that can mimic shock or semi-coma.

Recurrent Vomiting

The patterns of recurrent vomiting are further divided into chronic and cyclic types.[8] Table 2–7 outlines the differences between the acute, chronic, and cyclic patterns of vomiting.[9] Chronic recurrent vomiting is characterized by continuous, low-frequency, daily episodes

of mild to moderate vomiting compared to the cyclic vomiting pattern, in which severe vomiting episodes are separated by weeks of normal health in between. The differential diagnosis of recurrent vomiting is shown in Table 2–8.

An astute clinician recognizes that chronic or cyclic patterns of vomiting can arise not only from the GI tract, but also from extra-intestinal sites including the genitourinary system, central nervous system, infections, metabolic disorders, and endocrine problems (such as Addison's disease).[10,11] An abdominal ultrasound abdomen for UPJ obstruction and brain MRI for Chiari malformation should be obtained in children presenting with cyclic pattern of vomiting (Figures 2–5 and 2–6).[11] It is important to rule out the

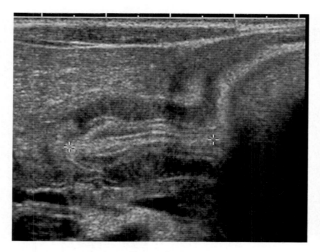

FIGURE 2–3 ■ Ultrasound shows the elongated pyloric channel in an infant with pyloric stenosis.

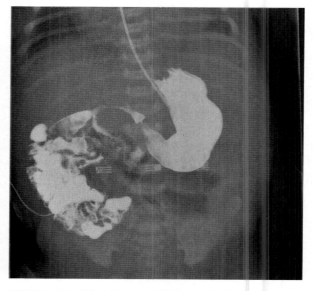

FIGURE 2–4 ■ Malrotation—an UGI shows the ligament of Treitz on the right side of the midline.

Table 2–7.

Features Distinguishing Acute, Recurrent–Chronic, and Recurrent–Cyclic or Episodic Patterns of Vomiting

Clinical Feature	Acute	Recurrent, Chronic	Recurrent, Cyclic or Episodic
Epidemiology	Most common	Two-thirds of recurrent vomiting patterns	One-third of recurrent vomiting patterns
Vomiting pace	Moderate–severe	Mild ~1–2 emeses/hour at peak	Severe ~6 emeses/hour at peak
Stereotype	—	None	98% have similar duration and symptoms, one-half with regular cycles (e.g., 4 weeks apart), and one-half with irregular episodes
Symptoms	Fever, vomiting, diarrhea	Vomiting, abdominal pain	Pallor, listlessness, nausea, abdominal pain, photophobia
Complications	Dehydration	Uncommon	Dehydration, hematemesis
Family	Sick household contacts	14% positive migraine headaches	72–83% positive migraine headaches
Causes	Viral gastroenteritis	Reflux, gastritis, duodenitis	Cyclic vomiting syndrome (88%)

Reproduced with permission from Kleinman, Goulet, Mieli-Vergani, Sanderson, Sherman, Shneider (eds): Walker's Pediatric Gastrointestinal Disease, Fifth Edition, © 2008

Table 2–8.

Causes of Acute, Chronic, and Cyclic Patterns of Vomiting

Causes	Acute	Chronic	Cyclic
Infection	Gastroenteritis, Sinusitis, Otitis media, Pharyngitis, Hepatitis	H. pylori gastritis, Chronic sinusitis, Giardiasis	Cyclic neutropenia, PFAFA
GI	Peptic ulcer, Pancreatitis	Gastritis, Celiac disease, Gastroparesis, Achalasia, Gallbladder dyskinesia, Crohn's disease	Malrotation with volvulus, Adhesions
Surgical	Malrotation with volvulus, Intussception, Appendicitis, Postoperative adhesions	Partial small bowel obstruction	Adhesions
CNS	Intracranial mass, Toxic ingestion, Migraine	Migraine, Space-occupying lesion	Cyclic vomiting syndrome
Endocrine/metabolic	Diabetic ketoacidosis, Addison's disease	Inborn errors of metabolism	Addison's disease, Fatty acid oxidation disorder, Familial Mediterranean fever (FMF)
GU	Urinary tract infection		Acute hydronephrosis secondary to UPJ obstruction
Miscellaneous	Pregnancy, psychogenic, drug abuse	Vestibular causes	

Abbreviations: PFAFA = periodic fever, apthous stomatitis, pharyngitis, cervical adenitis; UPJ = uretero-pelvic junction.

serious causes of vomiting, such as midgut volvulus, intussception, and adrenal crisis, before treating the patient symptoms with anti-emetics. Examination is directed toward assessing the patient's hydration and other organ systems as depicted in Figure 2–5. Investigations that may be required include CBC,

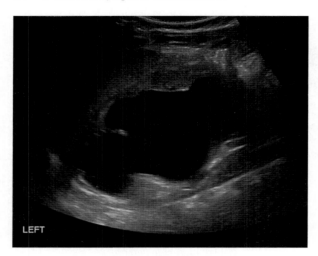

FIGURE 2–5 ■ UPJ obstruction—an ultrasound demonstrates acute hydronephrosis secondary to uretero-pelvic obstruction (UPJ) in an infant with vomiting.

electrolytes, blood urea nitrogen (BUN), creatinine, hepatic transaminases, amylase, lipase, and a KUB. Other investigations that need be ordered based on the clinical presentation are listed in Table 2–9. Hospital admission may be needed if the patient requires intravenous fluids for dehydration, fails to urinate for >12 hours, is found to have metabolic acidosis (anion gap >18 mEq/L), or is suspected to have metabolic or surgical problems. An algorithm showing the clinical approach to patients with vomiting is shown in Figure 2–7.[12]

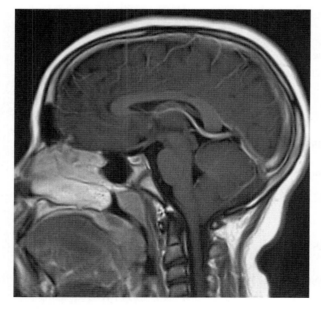

FIGURE 2–6 ■ Chiari malformation—MRI brain shows the herniation of cerebellar tonsils through the foramen magnum in a child with vomiting.

DIFFERENTIAL DIAGNOSIS

Gastroesophageal Reflux versus Gastroesophageal Reflux Disease

Gastroesophageal reflux is very common in neonates and infants and is described as effortless reflux of gastric contents into the esophagus in an otherwise healthy infant. No intervention is needed apart from parental education, reassurance, frequent burping, positioning, and thickening the formula with rice cereal. A 2-week limited trial of hydrolyzed formula is considered if the patient is irritable or has streaks of blood in the stool. H_2 receptor antagonists and PPI are usually not indicated unless there are signs of GERD, defined as gastroesophageal reflux associated with complications such as failure to thrive, esophagitis, hematemesis, apnea, or recurrent lower respiratory issues. Further evaluation by UGI and EGD is indicated if there are signs of GERD and gastrointestinal obstruction or if symptoms persist after 18 months of age (Figure 2–8).

Gastroparesis

The typical history is an adolescent patient with postprandial fullness, epigastric pain, early satiety, vomiting, and weight loss following a bout of viral gastroenteritis. It is important to exclude anatomical and mucosal causes of gastrointestinal obstruction before labeling the patients as gastroparesis. Other diseases that cause gastroparesis include diabetes mellitus, hypothyroidism, and motility disorders. Gastric retention of >60% at 2 hours and >10% at 4 hours with low-fat, egg-white meal gastric emptying study confirms the diagnosis. A 2-week trial of erythromycin may be helpful.[13] If there is no response, nasojejunal feeding or use of botox injection into the pylorus may be of temporary help as reported in a few case reports.

Superior Mesenteric Artery (SMA) Syndrome

The typical scenario is a 10-year-old patient with weight loss, abdominal pain, and bilious vomiting after spinal surgery. With weight loss, the fat pad between the SMA and duodenum is lost, leading to compression of the third portion of duodenum by SMA, thereby causing bilious emesis. Diagnosis is UGI with an abrupt cut off at the third portion of the duodenum. Treatment is increasing the weight of the child by giving nasojejunal feedings along with monitoring for refeeding syndrome.

Motion Sickness

Motion sickness is a common symptom that occurs while traveling in car, ship, or airplane. It is

Table 2–9.

Diagnostic Findings in Children with Vomiting

Labs	Abnormality	Diagnosis
CBC	Microcytic hypochromic anemia	Celiac disease, Crohn's disease, *H. pylori*, PUD
	↑ WBC	Infection, IBD
	Eosinophilia	Eosinophilic esophagitis (50% of patients)
Electrolytes	↓Cl⁻, ↓ K⁺, ↓ H⁺	Pyloric stenosis
	↓ Na⁺, ↑ K⁺	Congenital adrenal hyperplasia, Addison's disease
	↑ Cl⁻, ↑ H⁺	Renal tubular acidosis
	Increased anion gap	DKA, organic acidemia
BUN/creatinine	↑ BUN, creatinine	Dehydration, renal failure
Liver function tests	↑ ALT, bilirubin	Hepatitis, cholelithiasis, biliary obstruction
Lipase	Elevated	Pancreatitis
UGI	Ligament of Treitz located right of midline	Malrotation
	Delayed gastric emptying/filling defect	Antral web, pyloric stenosis
CT/MRI brain	Midline shift, mass	Space-occupying lesion, brain stem tumor, Chiari malformation, sinusitis
Ultrasound abdomen	Gallstones, pyloric channel	Cholelithiasis, pyloric stenosis
Endoscopy	Mucosal inflammation	Gastritis, peptic ulcer, *H. pylori*

Abbreviations: BUN = blood urea nitrogen; PUD = peptic ulcer disease; DKA = diabetic ketoacidosis.

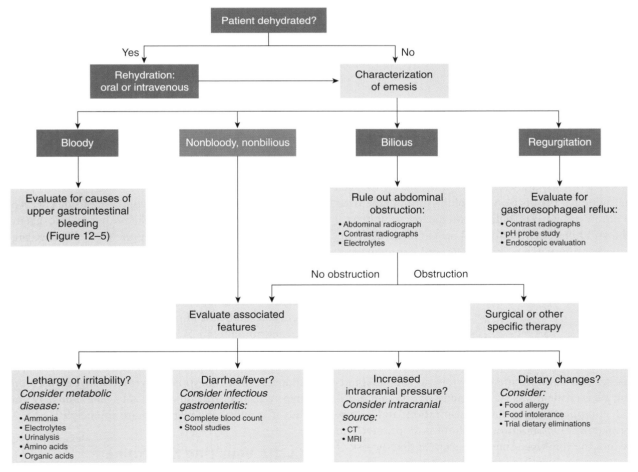

FIGURE 2–7 ■ Algorithm for vomiting in children. Used with permission from Rudolph et al. *Rudolph's Fundamentals of Pediatrics*, 3rd ed. © 2002 The McGraw-Hill Companies, Inc.

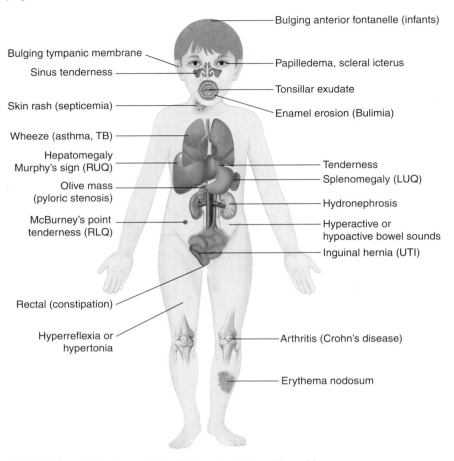

Bulging anterior fontanelle (infants)

Bulging tympanic membrane
Sinus tenderness

Papilledema, scleral icterus

Skin rash (septicemia)

Tonsillar exudate

Enamel erosion (Bulimia)

Wheeze (asthma, TB)

Hepatomegaly
Murphy's sign (RUQ)

Tenderness
Splenomegaly (LUQ)

Olive mass
(pyloric stenosis)

Hydronephrosis

McBurney's point
tenderness (RLQ)

Hyperactive or
hypoactive bowel sounds

Inguinal hernia (UTI)

Rectal (constipation)

Hyperreflexia or
hypertonia

Arthritis (Crohn's disease)

Erythema nodosum

FIGURE 2–8 ■ Pertinent examination findings in patients with vomiting.

characterized by nausea and dizziness preceding the vomiting, and is secondary to conflicting signals received by the brain from the visual and vestibular systems. The incidence peaks in childhood and often resolves by early adolescence. Simple treatments, such as looking at the horizon or looking through the front window of car, are helpful. Medications that have shown to be somewhat helpful are diphenhydramine, scopolamine patches, meclizine, and promethazine. Although motion sickness improves by early adolescence, it may forewarn the development of subsequent migraine headaches.

Postoperative Vomiting

Approximately 30% of postoperative patients develop nausea and vomiting after surgery. Postoperative vomiting affects patient satisfaction, medical costs, and medical complications including aspiration and suture breakdown. Ondansetron is helpful postoperatively to reduce the vomiting. Apfel et al. showed that the risk of postoperative vomiting decreased by 26% with the use of ondansetron, dexamethasone, and droperidol in high-risk patients.[14] These at-risk patients include female sex, previous history of postoperative vomiting, motion sickness, and use of opiods.

Chemotherapy-induced Vomiting

Nausea and vomiting are the commonest side effects of anti-cancer medications. Chemotherapeutic agents cause vomiting by stimulating the CTZ. Effective prevention of vomiting can be achieved by the combined use of three medications—ondansetron, dexamethasone, and aprepitant.[15] Ondansetron prevents early phase (<24 hours) of vomiting, whereas aprepitant prevents the late phase of postchemotherapy-induced nausea and vomiting (>24 hours). It is important to exclude other causes of vomiting in patients receiving chemotherapy, including brain metastasis, radiotherapy-induced small intestinal stricture, analgesic use, and hypercalcemia. Benzodiazepines to relieve anxiety and use of hypnosis and relaxation are also helpful.

Cyclic Vomiting Syndrome

CVS is the main cause of the cyclic pattern of recurrent vomiting. It is thought to be a childhood variant of

Table 2–10.

Criteria for CVS in Children

All of the following criteria must be met to meet the
consensus definition of CVS:
- At least five attacks in any interval, or a minimum of three attacks during a 6-month period
- Episodic attacks of intense nausea and vomiting lasting 1 hour to 10 days and occurring at least 1 week apart
- Stereotypical pattern and symptoms in the individual patient
- Vomiting during attacks occurs at least four times per hour for at least 1 week apart
- Return to baseline health between episodes
- Not attributed to another disorder

Adapted from NASPGHAN clinical guidelines, NASPGHAN consensus statement on the diagnosis and management of cyclic vomiting syndrome. J Pediatr Gastroenterol Nutr. 2008;47:379.

migraine diathesis and is characterized by recurrent, sudden, stereotypical, episodes of intense nausea and vomiting that last a few hours to days with normal interval in between. Although primarily recognized in children between 2 and 10 years of age, it also can begin in adolescents and adults. CVS is frequently misdiagnosed in emergency departments as acute viral gastroenteritis and food poisoning; however, patients with CVS are more ill both qualitatively (pallor and listlessness) and quantitatively (more likely to require IV rehydration). CVS is currently defined by fulfilling the consensus diagnostic criteria as outlined in Table 2–10.[16] The key to diagnosis of CVS is recognition of the repeated vomiting episodes, especially episodes starting early in the morning and with negative radiographic, laboratory, and endoscopic evaluations. However, 50% CVS episodes are sporadic. Precipitants include infection, excitement, and stress. Approximately one-third of patients with CVS develop typical migraine headaches by age 9.5 years and it is projected that 50% will develop migraines by age 15 years.[17] The treatment in CVS is largely empiric and involves: (a) lifestyle changes, (b) prophylactic antimigraine and/or anticonvulsant therapy, (c) abortive antimigraine therapy (triptans), and (d) supportive and symptomatic treatment during episodes. Patients and families are often greatly relieved when the physician identifies CVS as diagnosis and can reassure them that it is not life-threatening disease.

COMPLICATIONS

The most common complication encountered with severe vomiting is dehydration and metabolic acidosis. However, patients with pyloric stenosis develop hypokalemic, hypochloremic metabolic alkalosis secondary to loss of H^+ and Cl^- ions from the stomach associated with emesis. When the vomiting becomes severe and repetitive, repeated retrograde prolapse of gastric fundus through the gastroesophageal junction leads to either a submucosal hemorrhage in the herniated part of the fundus (prolapse gastropathy) and/or a mechanically induced laceration at the gastroesophageal junction (Mallory–Weiss tear). Both present usually with streaks of blood or occasionally massive hematemesis after forceful retching or vomiting. Complications associated with chronic vomiting from reflux esophagitis include stricture formation and Barrett's esophagus. Other complications reported with vomiting are dental enamel erosion, especially in patients with eating disorders, aspiration pneumonia in developmentally delayed children, and mid-esophageal strictures in untreated EoE.

TREATMENT

Acute Vomiting

Most cases of vomiting are uncomplicated and self-limited and no investigations or treatments are required, apart from maintaining hydration and preventing metabolic disturbances. Parents are instructed to give clear fluids or oral rehydration solutions slowly in small frequent aliquots. If the patient tolerates oral rehydration, resuming formula or breast feeding or a low-fat, high-carbohydrate diet after 8 hours works most of the time. If the child has persistent emesis (>12 hours in a neonate, >24 hours in children younger than 2 years of age, or >48 hours in older children), pharmacological treatment is directed to symptom improvement to prevent dehydration or metabolic derangements. Antiemetics should not be used in infants, suspected surgical conditions, or patients with alarm symptoms. Commonly used anti-emetics such as ondansetron ($5HT_3$ antagonist) have been shown to reduce the need for intravenous rehydration. In a trial involving 215 children aged 6 months to 10 years at the emergency department, a single dose of ondansetron improved the oral intake and decreased the frequency of vomiting in patients with gastroenteritis.[18,19] The use of metoclopramide has been tempered by the recent FDA black box warning of irreversible tardive dyskinesia associated with long-term use.

Chronic Vomiting

Counseling and cognitive behavioral therapy are needed in patient with rumination, eating disorders, and functional dyspepsia. In patients with chronic vomiting or red flags, it is important to do screening investigations including CBC, electrolytes, liver function tests, BUN, creatinine, amylase, lipase, and an UGI. If the cause is not identified, it is appropriate to refer the patient to a pediatric gastroenterologist for further evaluation. Endoscopic evaluation may be needed to rule out mucosal (*H. pylori*) infection or allergic inflammation (EoE). Table 2–11 shows the commonly used anti-emetics for different conditions. Prokinetics such as oral erythromycin 2 mg/kg every 8 hours for 2 weeks are used in patients with gastroparesis. If symptoms persist, referral to a pediatric gastroenterologist for further intervention includes botox injection into the pylorus or for nasojejunal tube

feeding. Antihistamines are useful in patients with motion sickness and mild chemotherapy-induced vomiting.

Cyclic Vomiting

The NASPGHAN consensus statement recommends prophylactic use of cyproheptadine (<5 years of age), amitriptyline (>5 years), and propranolol as second line in children with CVS. Nasal triptans (e.g., sumatriptan) are useful in some to abort the cyclic vomiting episodes given early on. Anticonvulsants useful in preventing episodes include topiramate and phenobarbital. If episodes occur despite preventive therapy, the

Table 2–11.

Conditions and Commonly Used Anti-emetics

Conditions	Medications	Receptor Blockade	Comment
Cyclic vomiting syndrome	Prophylaxis: <5 years – Cyproheptadine 0.25–0.5 mg/kg/day divided tid – Propranolol 0.25–0.5 mg/kg/day divided bid or tid	H_1 $\beta_1\ \beta_2$	↑ Weight gain Sedation Hypotension Monitor pulse
	Prophylaxis: >5 years – Amitryptiline 0.25–0.5 mg/kg/qhs, ↑ weekly by 5–10 mg until 1–1.5 mg/kg	$5HT_2$	Sedation
	– Propranolol 0.25–0.5 mg/kg/day divide bid or tid	$\beta_1\ \beta_2$	QTc prolongation Constipation Lethargy
	Abortive: >12 years, sumatriptan 0.4 mg/kg up to maximum 20 mg/dose	$5\text{-}HT_{1D}$	Neck pain
	Supportive: intravenous fluids D10 + 1/2 normal saline – 1.5 maintenance		
	Ondansetron 0.3–0.4 mg/kg/dose every 4–6 hours	$5\text{-}HT_3$	Headache
	Lorazepam 0.05–0.1 mg/kg/dose every 6 hours	GABA	Respiratory depression
	Diphenhydramine 1–1.25 mg/kg/dose every 6 hours	H_1	Sedation
Motion sickness	Scopolamine 1/4–1/2 patch behind the ear every 72 hours	M_1	Dry mouth Sedation
	Promethazine oral/rectal—0.5 mg/kg every 12 hours	H_1	Blurred vision Respiratory depression Sedation
Postoperative chemotherapy	Ondansetron	$5\text{-}HT_3$	Headache
	Dexamethasone	Unknown	Adrenal suppression
	Aprepitant: day 1—125 mg; days 2 and 3—80 mg	NK_1	Fatigue, diarrhea
Abdominal migraine	Hyoscyamine sublingual 0.125 mg qid prn	Histamine	Anti-cholinergic effects
	Dicyclomine oral 5–10 mg/dose tid	Serotonin	
Functional nausea	Ginger 250 mg tid Amitriptyline 0.25–0.5 mg/kg/qhs	Unknown ↑ Synaptic norepinephrine	Platelet aggregation Sedation Monitor QTc

combination of intravenous fluids, anti-emetics (e.g., ondansetron), and sedation (e.g., diphenhydramine or lorazepam) may ameliorate the episode severity. Other complementary treatment options used by the parents include ginger, acupuncture P6 point, hypnotherapy, and chiropractors.

ACKNOWLEDGMENT

We greatly appreciate the help of Dr. Sara Arnold, MD, Medical College of Wisconsin, for allowing us to use the radiology pictures.

REFERENCES

1. Ganong W. *Review of Medical Physiology*. 22nd ed. McGraw-Hill Medical; 2005:232.

2. Kleinman RE, Goulet OJ, Sanderson I, et al. *Pediatric Gastrointestinal Disease*. BC Decker Inc.; 2008:128.

3. Richards CA, Milla PJ, Andrews PL, Spitz L. Retching and vomiting in neurologically impaired children after fundoplication: predictive preoperative factors. *J Pediatr Surg*. 2001;36(9):1401–1404.

4. Granum PE, Lund T. Bacillus cereus and its food poisoning toxins. *FEMS Microbiol Lett*. 1997;157(2):223–228.

5. Friedman JN, Goldman RD, Srivastava R, Parkin PC. Development of a clinical dehydration scale for use in children between 1 and 36 months of age. *J Pediatr*. 2004;145(2):201–207.

6. Spergel JM, Brown-Whitehorn TF, Beausoleil JL, et al. 14 years of eosinophilic esophagitis: clinical features and prognosis. *J Pediatr Gastroenterol Nutr*. 2009;48(1):30–36.

7. Guarner J, Kalach N, Elitsur Y, Koletzko S. *Helicobacter pylori* diagnostic tests in children: review of the literature from 1999 to 2009. *Eur J Pediatr*. 2009: vol. 169(1):15-25.

8. Li BU. Cyclic vomiting: the pattern and syndrome paradigm. *J Pediatr Gastroenterol Nutr*. 1995;21(suppl 1):S6–S10.

9. Kleinman RE, Goulet OJ, Sanderson I, et al. *Pediatric Gastrointestinal Disease*. BC Decker Inc.; Hamilton, Ontario, Canada. 2008:129.

10. Li BU, Murray RD, Heitlinger LA, Robbins JL, Hayes JR. Heterogeneity of diagnoses presenting as cyclic vomiting. *Pediatrics*. 1998;102(3 Pt 1):583–587.

11. Tsai JD, Huang FY, Lin CC, et al. Intermittent hydronephrosis secondary to ureteropelvic junction obstruction: clinical and imaging features. *Pediatrics*. 2006;117(1):139–146.

12. Rudolph CD. *Rudolph's Pediatrics*. 21st ed. McGraw-Hill; 2002:1351–1353.

13. Haans JJ, Masclee AA. Review article: the diagnosis and management of gastroparesis. *Aliment Pharmacol Ther*. 2007;26(suppl 2):37–46.

14. Apfel CC, Korttila K, Abdalla M, et al. A factorial trial of six interventions for the prevention of postoperative nausea and vomiting. *N Engl J Med*. 2004;350(24):2441–2451.

15. Kris MG, Hesketh PJ, Somerfield MR, et al. American Society of Clinical Oncology guideline for antiemetics in oncology: update 2006. *J Clin Oncol*. 2006;24(18):2932–2947.

16. Li BU, Lefevre F, Chelimsky GG, et al. North American Society for Pediatric Gastroenterology, Hepatology, and Nutrition consensus statement on the diagnosis and management of cyclic vomiting syndrome. *J Pediatr Gastroenterol Nutr*. 2008;47(3):379–393.

17. Li BU, Balint JP. Cyclic vomiting syndrome: evolution in our understanding of a brain–gut disorder. *Adv Pediatr*. 2000;47:117–160.

18. Freedman SB, Adler M, Seshadri R, Powell EC. Oral ondansetron for gastroenteritis in a pediatric emergency department. *N Engl J Med*. 2006;354(16):1698.

19. Alhashimi D, Alhashimi H, Fedorowicz Z. Antiemetics for reducing vomiting related to acute gastroenteritis in children and adolescents. *Cochrane Database Syst Rev*. 2006 Oct 18;(4):CD005506.

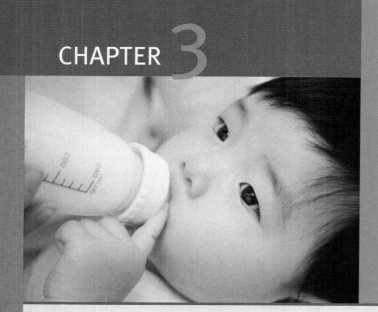

CHAPTER 3

Feeding and Swallowing Disorders

Richard J. Noel

DEFINITIONS AND EPIDEMIOLOGY

Pediatric feeding disorders may be defined as problems with the developmentally appropriate intake of food. This broad category includes difficulties that objectively result in nutritional or medical risk (e.g., refusal of dietary protein leading to protein energy malnutrition), as well as those perceived as problematic by the child's family that result in stressful mealtimes without objective medical consequence. These do not include eating disorders (i.e., anorexia and bulimia) or obesity. Pediatric feeding disorders may be associated with medical disease (often gastrointestinal), malnutrition or failure to gain weight, developmental delays affecting skill acquisition, and interpersonal disorders. Feeding problems have been characterized simply along axes of ability and desire,[1] by biophysical etiology,[2] or by criteria that focus on interpersonal relationships.[3] Children with feeding disorders are best assessed and managed by interdisciplinary teams that address all sides of the problem, given that distinct facets of the disorder require individual expert assessment and intervention.

Feeding disorders occur in children with an incidence as high as 25% in normal children,[4] with a higher incidence in those with neurologic disability.[5–7] While children with feeding disorders require evaluation by a gastroenterologist due to the high coincidence with gastrointestinal disorders,[1,8] skill acquisition and behavioral components are often present and require behavioral evaluation and management beyond what a gastroenterologist may provide.[9]

An individual patient's feeding disorder is unique. Environmental and family social-dynamic issues are different for each individual with the same underlying

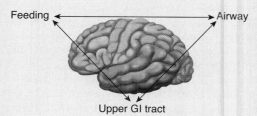

FIGURE 3–1 ■ Interplay between airway, gastrointestinal tract, and feeding ability. Feeding ability has a reciprocal relationship with the airway and the upper gastrointestinal tract, where one affects the others. In the background, the central nervous plays a role, in regard to both the motor and sensory function and the higher order personality and social dynamic issues.

pathology (e.g. hypoplastic left heart syndrome). Furthermore, feeding, the airway, and the upper gastrointestinal tract exist in a reciprocal relationship system where problems with one of these components may produce problems in the others (Figure 3–1); such may be seen in an infant with pulmonary disease, where cough and tachypnea may aggravate reflux and feeding problems, respectively. Additionally, the central nervous system, with respect both to basic motor and sensory function and to its higher order processes such as personality development, exists in the background of this relationship and can both contribute to, and be affected by, problems of the airway, upper GI tract, and feeding ability (Figure 3–1).

PATHOGENESIS

Achievement of normal feeding is a function of skill acquisition as permitted by the child's internal and external environments. The progression of feeding that

Table 3–1.			
Innervation of Swallowing			
		Touch	Taste
Oral phase			
Afferent	Trigeminal (V)	Oral cavity, anterior 2/3 of tongue	None
	Facial (VII)	None	Anterior 2/3 of tongue
	Glossopharyngeal (IX)	Posterior 1/3 of tongue	Posterior 1/3 of tongue
Efferent	Trigeminal (V)	Muscles of mastication	
	Facial (VII)	Lips and face	
	Vagus (X)	Tongue	
	Hypoglossal (XII)		
	C1 and C2		
Pharyngeal phase			
Afferent	Glossopharyngeal (IX)	Pharynx	
	Vagus (X)	Larynx and esophagus	
Efferent	Trigeminal (V)	Tensor veli palatini	
	Glossopharyngeal (IX)	Palate, pharynx, larynx	
	Vagus (X)		
	Trigeminal (V)	Hyoid and laryngeal movement	
	Facial (VII)		
	C1 and C2		

Cranial nerves V, VII, IX, X, and XII and cervical spinal nerves 1 and 2 provide all motor and sensory information for the oral and the pharyngeal phases of swallowing.

occurs over infancy is governed by neuromuscular and anatomic maturation that limit the manner of feeding at any specific age.[10] A newborn is limited by neurologic immaturity and unique anatomy that helps isolate the oral cavity from the airway. These limitations prevent the processing of solids, but maximize the efficiency of suckling from a nipple. As the infant grows, the oral cavity enlarges and neuromuscular maturation occurs, manifested as lateral motion of the tongue, as well as improved head and truncal stability that allows the introduction of smooth solids. As the oral cavity grows, the larynx descends, and teeth appear, which together with further skill acquisition allow the introduction of more complex solids and table foods into the diet by 1 year of age. A strong element of social bonding drives the progression across feeding milestones, and infants learn to respond to positive reinforcement. Early exposure to various tastes may also play a role in flavor programming and the later acceptance of a varied diet.[11]

Swallowing is a complex behavior that requires coordination of cranial nerves (V, VII, IX, X, and XII), cervical nerves (1 and 2), and corresponding sensory and motor endpoints to coordinate the oral and pharyngeal phases (Table 3–1). Similar to data on abnormal visual cortex development associated with early onset blindness,[12] children who miss developmental "critical periods" in infancy often fail to progress across feeding milestones, presumably due to abnormal cortical development allowing coordination of swallowing function. Such a patient typically would not progress across textures and may be subject to developing profound feeding disorders with possible social and/or medical consequences.

Interruption of this graded exposure and corresponding development occurs in many infants and children with congenital or transient disease states that interfere with progression of feeding skills. An infant with complex congenital heart disease may not be well enough to take initial oral feedings for several months after birth, resulting in a situation where graded food exposures have not occurred. This directly impairs neuromuscular development, not to mention the social bonding that typically occurs with feeding. Recognition of such a feeding disorder is the first step in properly addressing it and establishing realistic and developmentally appropriate expectations.

CLINICAL PRESENTATION

In the clinical setting, a feeding disorder may present as a nutritional consequence of an inadequate diet (e.g., poor weight gain and protein energy malnutrition), a medical consequence of prior or active disease (e.g., obstructive lung disease, eosinophilic esophagitis, seizures, and heart failure), a consequence of dysphagia (e.g., choking, aspiration pneumonia, or failure to advance across textures), or a psychodynamic problem (e.g., tantrums, disruptive mealtime behaviors, unmet parental expectations, and feeding schedule that result in grazing). Most patients with feeding problems exhibit a complex, mixed presentation of several such issues. Such inherent complexity benefits from a multidisciplinary approach that utilizes specialists to assess each facet of the feeding disorder, including a gastroenterologist, a nurse, a dietitian, a speech and language pathologist, an occupational therapist, and a behavioral psychologist.

The phases of normal feeding must each be carefully evaluated to understand the nature of the problem.[2] These include the *pre-oral phase* during which foods are identified, selected, and then placed within the oral cavity. The *oral phase* follows, processing the alimentary bolus by chewing with subsequent transit to the pharynx. The *pharyngeal phase* coordinates the passage of the bolus into the esophagus with ongoing respiration. The *esophageal phase* requires orderly transit, with peristaltic contractions moving the bolus into the stomach. The *gastrointestinal* phase involves temporary storage of the meal within the stomach, which enlarges to accommodate the meal and gradually releases it into the intestine in a manner that maximizes nutrient digestion and absorption.

It is easy to see how perturbation of any of these phases may result in a feeding disorder. The problem may be clear and limited, such as the ineffective esophageal phase of a patient with achalasia. Conversely, the problem may be more complex, as in an ineffective pre-oral phase of an infant with blindness, a depressed mother, or other sensory or environmental deprivation.

Families may not understand the underlying complexity of feeding disorders and may simply want things to be better. In particular, parents may not understand that they may have contributed to developing and/or sustaining the feeding disorder. It is critical for the clinician to probe the parents' understanding of the feeding disorder by simply asking, "What problem may I help you with?" It is also critical to understand the parents' beliefs about the underlying cause by following up the question, "Why do you think this is happening?" Failure to begin the work-up with these two simple questions may establish unrealistic expectations that will limit the progress that can be made over time. The family of a child who has already had a comprehensive multidisciplinary assessment that was negative may still believe a medical etiology is being missed. They may not be ready to address underlying interpersonal issues that are the likely etiology. Failure to both *acknowledge* and *move beyond* a family's initial perceptions will result in inability to establish the trust required to guide the family through management of a feeding disorder.

It is common for children with feeding disorders to have had previous extensive medical evaluations, often at different institutions. Review of these medical records should be done prior to the clinic evaluation, sometimes with a limited telephone conversation with the family. This may be helpful in deciding which diagnostic elements may be required, including videofluoroscopic swallow study (VSS), EGD, meal observations, or consultation and assessment with other subspecialists who are not routinely part of the team, such as neurology, genetics, or otolaryngology.

DIAGNOSIS

Diagnosis of a feeding disorder must include diagnosis of underlying and comorbid disorders. The former may include almost any pediatric disorder; the latter may include failure to gain weight, gastroesophageal reflux disease (GERD), and dysphagia. Conceptually, the physician leading the team must simultaneously evaluate three major issues: nutrition, upper GI tract dysfunction, and dysphagia (Figure 3–2).

Failure to Gain Weight

Although families seek help with a feeding disorder, they must realize the growth is always a higher priority than feeding dysfunction. Furthermore, it may be impossible to teach a child to eat in a background of marginal nutrition, as an underweight child may not respond to appetite manipulation and is likely to lose weight without generating an adequate hunger drive. Detailed dietary analysis by a dietitian is critical toward determining if gaps exist between caloric intake and requirements.[13] Failure to gain weight in a setting of apparently appropriate caloric intake requires medical evaluation toward identifying problems with caloric retention, maldigestion, malabsorption, or increased caloric demands.

Gastroesophageal Reflux

Gastroesophageal reflux (GER) is a common comorbidity in children with feeding disorders (see Chapter 12).[8] When coupled with dysphagia and

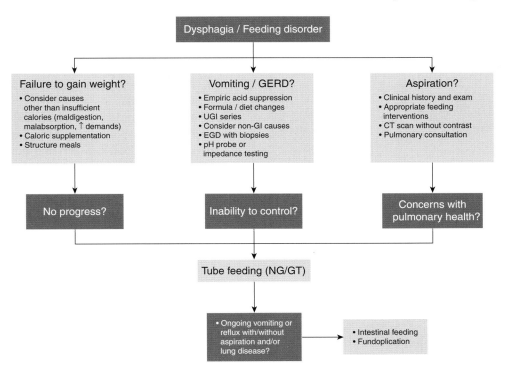

FIGURE 3–2 ■ Conceptual algorithm for management of feeding disorder with or without dysphagia. Three important questions for the gastroenterologist to consider are detailed in the diagram. Failure to gain weight may be assessed through traditional assessments of caloric retention, maldigestion, malabsorption, or increased caloric demands. Use of caloric supplementation and/or structuring of meals to foster appetite may be considered. Vomiting and GERD may require acid suppression, management of dietary protein intolerance, fluoroscopic studies, assessment of non-GI causes (e.g., brain MRI and renal ultrasound), pH probe testing, or impedance testing. Aspiration requires careful documentation of pulmonary health history, limiting oral feedings per findings from swallowing evaluations, possible imaging of the chest, and pulmonary consultation. Failure of controlling any of the above may require institution of nasogastric (NG) tube or gastrostomy tube (GT) feedings. Failure to control symptoms may indicate need to jejunal feeding via nasojejunal (NJ) tube, placement of gastrojejunostomy (GJ) tube feeding, or thoughtful consideration of a fundoplication.

aspiration, GER may also contribute to severe respiratory disease, particularly in children with neurologic impairment.[14] When clinically indicated, it may be important to perform endoscopy to specifically rule out eosinophilic esophagitis (see Chapter 17) that may mimic GER disease and may present solely with a feeding disorder.[15,16] The question of whether a fundoplication may be indicated must be considered carefully, especially in children with neurologic disability. In this population, post-operative retching and feeding intolerance may markedly complicate post-operative function.[17] Fundoplication-associated dumping syndrome may also complicate what can be done with regard to normal future feeding. Furthermore, neurologic disability is a statistical predictor of operative mortality and may explain why fewer fundoplications have been performed in this population over time.[18] If an upper gastrointestinal X-ray series is performed in a patient with a fundoplication and a gastrostomy tube, it is critical that some contrast be swallowed or instilled

through the esophagus in a manner that can assess esophageal emptying and transit across the fundoplication.

Dysphagia (Swallowing Problem)

Understanding the skill limitations of a child with feeding disorder is critical toward formulation of a developmentally appropriate plan of therapy. Swallowing problems are assessed by clinical, fluoroscopic, and/or endoscopic examination and require collaboration with a speech and language pathologist and/or an otolaryngologist. Possible evaluations include clinical evaluation of a meal,[19] VSS (Figure 3–3),[20] or the flexible endoscopic evaluation of swallow (FEES).[21] Evaluations based on ultrasonography[22] and scintigraphy[23] have been described, but have not proved useful toward developing a therapeutic regimen to improve the skill. Although VSS is thought to be the "gold standard" toward finding tracheal aspiration, one must be aware

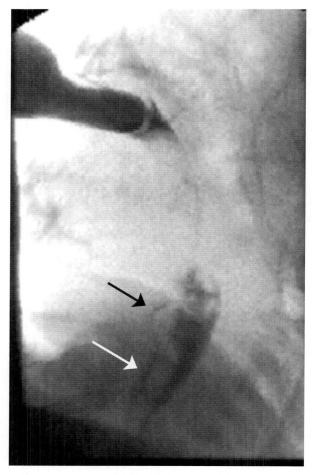

FIGURE 3–3 ■ Still image of a videofluoroscopic swallow study (VSS). The lateral image of an infant feeding barium-containing formula from a nipple bottle. The image shows laryngeal penetration (black arrow) where contrast is seen below the level of the vocal cords. Tracheal aspiration (white arrow) is noted inferior to the larynx and anterior to the contrast-filled esophagus.

of an overall lack of standardization in interpretation, as demonstrated by a high degree of inter-rater reliability on most facets of swallowing.[24] The FEES study is best performed when patients have a significant problem with secretions or when an airway abnormality is strongly suspected. FEES studies may also be performed with additional sensory testing (FEES/ST) where the laryngeal mucosa is assessed for mechanoreceptor response to an air-pulse stimulus in the course of a laryngoscopy; this type of study may be useful when a sensory neurologic etiology is suspected.[25] Dysphagia is particularly concerning when it is associated with silent aspiration, given that aspiration may result in recurrent pneumonia and may also impact pulmonary development that occurs for at least 18 months after birth.[26,27] The child with feeding disorder and silent aspiration requires a thoughtful approach based on clinical management, given that there is a

deficit of available literature on the topic.[28] A compromise between the need to develop feeding skills and the need to prevent damage to developing alveolar respiratory units may be achieved by restricting oral feedings within safe limits, based on the above studies, and providing the remainder of the diet via a gastrostomy tube. These limits should be individualized and must consider body positioning, food texture, onset of fatigue, pacing of food delivery, and duration of the meal, as guided by a speech and language pathologist. Surveillance of lung disease, even in the asymptomatic at-risk child, may be performed at intervals by computed tomography studies. These may identify subclinical pulmonary pathology[29] and guide oral feeding by early identification of complications.

Behavioral Factors

A pediatric psychologist should assess a children with feeding disorders, given the aforementioned influence of behavioral factors on underlying medical etiologies.[9] Assessment includes an interview, observation of feeding, and assessment on a variety of validated clinical instruments.[30,31]

Medical Subspecialty Consultation

Medical evaluation may encompass issues beyond those within a gastroenterologist's expertise. Airway issues are common in children with feeding disorders, in particular, those with dysphagia. Microlaryngoscopy and bronchoscopy may be indicated to formally assess the airway anatomy and function. Genetics consultation may be indicated when metabolic etiologies are considered or when physical findings suggest a genetic syndrome; microarray screening is now widely available for near-whole genome screening. Neurology consultation may be indicated for the assessment of abnormal neurologic findings, particularly when the patient has a history of abnormal brain and/or spine imaging, or when seizures may be associated with feeding disorders. Physical medicine and rehabilitation specialists are critical toward the management of muscle tone issues and provide guidance regarding acquisition of supportive equipment, such as feeding chairs. These specialists may also work in conjunction with orthopedic surgeons who perform operative repair of scoliosis with subsequent improvement of posture, ventilation, and ultimately feeding. Neuropsychologists or developmental pediatricians may be required to perform neuropsychologic assessment to formally estimate development across a variety of parameters at almost any age. Psychiatrists may be required to assess patients for the management of anxiety, mood, or hyperactivity disorders.

TREATMENT

Treatment for children with feeding disorders should address all relevant facets of the problem. An interdisciplinary approach greatly facilitates treatment, given that individual components of a feeding disorder are likely to be intertwined. The initial multidisciplinary evaluation will have identified a problem list for the child that, in turn, should dictate a specific set of therapies that ideally should resolve the feeding disorder.

Weight Gain and Nutrition

In all children, growth is of paramount importance and should always be among the most important assessments made on a regular basis.[13] The majority of children with failure to gain weight simply lack adequate nutrient intake. This may be commonly seen in children with a "grazing" feeding schedule, as well as in those with a lifestyle that includes many different, and typically inconsistent, caretakers. Children who graze ultimately do not take in sufficient calories to grow, given that they are never truly hungry and for that reason seldom eat larger, high-calorie meals. Among the first interventions that may be made by a physician is the restructuring of meals, typically into three meals and two intervening snacks for a toddler. These are spread out across the day to allow development of normal cycling of hunger and satiety. If this is not sufficient, a dietitian can suggest ways of increasing the caloric content of the diet. Cyproheptadine, used off-label, as an appetite stimulant (0.1 mg/kg/dose BID) may be a useful adjunct to a structured, high-calorie diet; the drug may have to be cycled given that the appetite stimulant effect wanes over time with constant use. Anecdotally, the medication has been useful when used for 2–3 weeks of each month, taking the remainder of the month as a "drug holiday." This approach also allows recurrent monitoring for a tangible benefit every time it is restarted and still generates an overall gain in hunger drive and willingness to feed.

Failure to achieve sustained growth through the above-noted means may require supplemental tube feeding, even in cases that appear to be primarily behavioral. Families may find the use of a nasogastric, or more likely gastrostomy, feeding tube difficult to accept, given that they seek resolution of a feeding problem and not escalation of medical care. They should understand that behavioral interventions are possible only for children who have a structured eating schedule. If this is not possible via oral feeding, full or partial tube feeding allows for establishment of a normal feeding routine and decompression of anxiety and stress associated with feedings, ideally improving nutrition while alleviating family discord. The family should understand that tube feeding is likely to be temporary with removal of the tube on achieving the feeding goals that where originally sought.

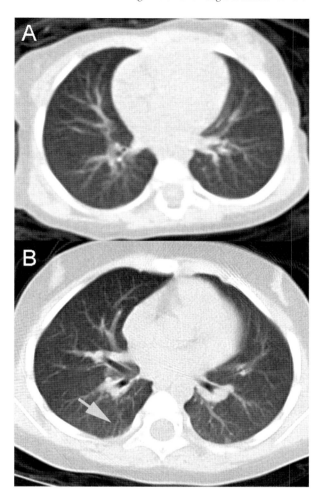

FIGURE 3–4 ■ CT scanning of chest as a screen for lung disease in a setting of dysphagia with silent aspiration. CT scans of the chest of two children with similar encephalopathy, normal chest physical exam, and dysphagia with silent aspiration. Patient A had unremarkable CT scanning. Patient B had small infiltrates (arrow) throughout the chest.

Dysphagia and Skill Development

If a child's feeding disorder has an element of dysphagia, the child's developmental skills dictate the potential maximal ability. For that reason, a family should understand that the goal of treatment for a given child is not "normal feeding," but "developmentally appropriate feeding." When dysphagia is complicated by silent aspiration, the historical approach was to place a gastrostomy and cease oral feedings in order to decrease the risk of recurrent pneumonia. The conundrum becomes one of balancing future acquisition of feeding skills against the risk of recurrent lung infections. Radiographic assessment with CT scan of the chest has been shown to identify lung pathology when it is in early, subclinical stages. Figure 3–4 shows CT scans from two children with static encephalopathy, silent aspiration on VSS, and normal chest physical examination. Child "A" has an unremarkable scan and may likely proceed with ongoing feeding in a manner deemed most effective by a speech and language pathologist with regard to texture, positioning, pacing, and fatigue. Conversely child "B" has subtle pulmonary infiltrates (arrow) and would merit more careful supervision along a slower course toward oral feeding. Assessments of this type are under ongoing evaluation.

Components of Behavioral Management

Behavioral management plays a very significant role in the treatment of children with feeding disorders. Behavioral strategies are typically employed to motivate a child with a feeding disorder to work to the full extent of his/her ability. For example, a child who associates feeding with aversive events (e.g., gagging, choking, and vomiting), and who has severe tantrums and aggressive behaviors when presented with foods, is in a relatively short period of time transformed into a child who willingly feeds. Behavioral treatment strategies are highly effective and empirically supported,[32] but require training and effort from both the patient/family and the therapy provider. To ensure lasting treatment effects, pediatric psychologists (psychologists especially trained to work with families of children with medical conditions) not only modify the child's behaviors, but must also change the family's style of responses that may have unknowingly reinforced the problem behaviors. Clinicians are advised to consult with professionals who have received training in the use of these assessment and treatment techniques, as no two cases are identical and goals may have to evolve as treatment progresses.

Behavioral treatment planning is used to combine the common treatment strategies to help the family achieve the desired feeding goal. Behavior therapy is most commonly used to (1) increase oral intake to promote growth, (2) increase the repertoire of foods to minimize the risks of nutrition deficiencies, (3) decrease/extinguish problem behaviors at meals (e.g., aggression and tantrums), and (4) increase positive feeding behaviors. Generally, the treatment plan will combine differential reinforcement, stimulus control, and appetite manipulation to achieve these goals. Ideally, caregivers are taught how to use each of these strategies and are given ample opportunity to continue to consult with the provider who developed the treatment plan. Families should be advised that consistent and immediate application of these techniques will help the family to realize treatment gains in the shortest period of time.

Differential reinforcement techniques are useful in helping a child to discriminate desired feeding behaviors, which will be reinforced, from undesirable behaviors, which will be ignored or punished. Typically, rewards include caregiver praise and attention, access to toys, or provision of a preferred food. Extinction techniques (withholding reinforcement) are generally used for nonaggressive refusals (whining and negotiating), whereas punishments are used only for aggressive behaviors that do not respond well to extinction efforts. When differential reinforcement techniques are applied and consistently utilized after desirable behaviors are observed, the child rapidly learns how to behave, strengthening the child's appropriate mealtime behaviors.

Stimulus control procedures systematically expose the child to new and nonpreferred foods and prevent the undesired behavior from occurring (e.g., preventing a child from fleeing the table). With repeated exposures the child comes to realize that the food is safe resulting in the extinction of the response. Often, exposures to foods are completed is small systematic steps called shaping. Shaping is a useful behavioral tool for the outpatient setting as families can gradually achieve a larger goal over time without undue stress on the child or the family system. For example, a transition from smooth to textured foods can occur with the gradual mixing of dissolvable crumbs into the smooth food. On occasion, negative reinforcement (taking away an aversive stimulus) may be used by trained personnel. An example may include contingency contacting where the spoon is held at the lips of a child who habitually turns away from the utensil; eventually the child will learn that accepting the spoon is the means of removing this unwanted exposure.

Appetite manipulation is one of the most effective techniques for modifying feeding behaviors. Essentially, appetite manipulation capitalizes on the internal experience of hunger and satiation of hunger from eating. Scheduled meals and restricting access to preferred foods contingent on successfully reaching a feeding goal are powerful methods to motivate a child to work toward specific feeding goals. Appetite manipulation, allowing a child to undergo the natural consequences of eating, achieving satiety, and experiencing the food,[33] provides positive reinforcement above and beyond any other reward methods or techniques to establish compliance. In the outpatient setting, appetite can be manipulated primarily by removing grazing on calories in between scheduled meals and snacks and using time limits on meals. If a meal or snack is "failed" by poor behavior, the parent must be willing to end the meal and have the child await the next snack or meal when they will likely find their child more motivated to eat and participate with the treatment plan. As described above, cyproheptadine may also be a helpful adjunct. Megestrol has also been

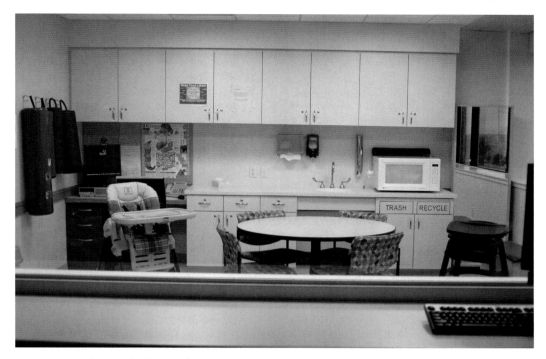

FIGURE 3–5 ■ Photograph of a clinic feeding room at the Children's Hospital of Wisconsin. The feeding room includes suitable tables and chairs for children of all ages. The room is viewed through a two-way mirror separating it from a viewing room where parents can observe a session with a psychologist or a speech and language pathologist. When the parent is feeding, he or she may also be coached remotely from this room via a wireless speaker earpiece.

utilized for appetite stimulation in children with feeding disorders.[34]

Generally, behavioral techniques are used in combination and are first employed in an outpatient setting. At times, outpatient strategies plateau or are unfeasible due to either medical complexity or a requirement for greater environmental control; in these situations inpatient treatment is the only opportunity. When these strategies prove insufficient in the outpatient setting, inpatient treatment allows a tighter control of appetite by limiting the child to three meals. Importantly, this should only be performed in an inpatient setting where weight, hydration, and glycemia/ketosis may be monitored. Occasionally, children may present with a primary psychiatric diagnosis that limits the effectiveness of behavioral strategies. In these cases clinicians may require psychiatric consultation to consider the use of psychotropic medications.

In both outpatient and inpatient settings, therapeutic interventions are best conducted in specialized feeding rooms (Figure 3–5) that typically have a two-way mirror through which people may observe the session without distracting the child and feeding provider. When a specialist is feeding, parents may be in the observation room with additional personnel receiving specialized instruction with the goal of continuing the treatment at home. When the parent is feeding, a treatment specialist can remotely coach the parent via a wireless earpiece.

SUMMARY

Treatment of feeding disorders is uniquely complex, as it often bridges cutting-edge medicine with the intricacies of higher order personality and social dynamics, all with the worthy goal of maximizing children's potential to feed themselves. Physicians treating feeding disorders must realize that all their medical knowledge encompasses only one facet of the required skill-set—the remainder lies with professionals that include dietitians, speech and language pathologists, occupational therapists, and behavioral psychologists. A team approach, utilizing all of these professionals, is critical to achieve the desired results.

REFERENCES

1. Manikam R, Perman JA. Pediatric feeding disorders. *J Clin Gastroenterol*. 2000;30(1):34–46.
2. Rudolph CD. Feeding disorders in infants and children. *J Pediatr*. 1994;125(6 Pt 2):S116–S124.
3. Davies WH, Satter E, Berlin KS, et al. Reconceptualizing feeding and feeding disorders in interpersonal context: the case for a relational disorder. *J Fam Psychol*. 2006;20(3):409–417.
4. Lindberg L, Bohlin G, Hagekull B. Early feeding problems in a normal population. *Int J Eat Disord*. 1991;10(4):395–405.
5. Thommessen M, Heiberg A, Kase BF, Larsen S, Riis G. Feeding problems, height and weight in different groups

of disabled children. *Acta Paediatr Scand.* 1991;80(5): 527–533.

6. Thommessen M, Kase BF, Heiberg A. Growth and nutrition in 10 girls with Rett syndrome. *Acta Paediatr.* 1992;81(9):686–690.

7. Dahl M, Thommessen M, Rasmussen M, Selberg T. Feeding and nutritional characteristics in children with moderate or severe cerebral palsy. *Acta Paediatr.* 1996;85(6): 697–701.

8. Field D, Garland M, Williams K. Correlates of specific childhood feeding problems. *J Paediatr Child Health.* 2003;39(4):299–304.

9. Burklow KA, Phelps AN, Schultz JR, McConnell K, Rudolph C. Classifying complex pediatric feeding disorders. *J Pediatr Gastroenterol Nutr.* 1998;27(2):143–147.

10. Arvedson JC, Brodsky L. *Pediatric Swallowing and Feeding; Assessment and Management.* 2nd ed. Canada: Singular Publishing Group; 2002.

11. Beauchamp GK, Mennella JA. Early flavor learning and its impact on later feeding behavior. *J Pediatr Gastroenterol Nutr.* 2009;48(suppl 1):S25–S30.

12. Jiang J, Zhu W, Shi F, et al. Thick visual cortex in the early blind. *J Neurosci.* 2009;29(7):2205–2211.

13. Kirby M, Noel RJ. Nutrition and gastrointestinal tract assessment and management of children with dysphagia. *Semin Speech Lang.* 2007;28(3):180–189.

14. Morton RE, Wheatley R, Minford J. Respiratory tract infections due to direct and reflux aspiration in children with severe neurodisability. *Dev Med Child Neurol.* 1999;41(5):329–334.

15. Pentiuk SP, Miller CK, Kaul A. Eosinophilic esophagitis in infants and toddlers. *Dysphagia.* 2007;22(1):44–48.

16. Noel RJ, Putnam PE, Rothenberg ME. Eosinophilic esophagitis. *N Engl J Med.* 2004;351(9):940–941.

17. Richards CA, Milla PJ, Andrews PL, Spitz L. Retching and vomiting in neurologically impaired children after fundoplication: predictive preoperative factors. *J Pediatr Surg.* 2001;36(9):1401–1404.

18. Lasser MS, Liao JG, Burd RS. National trends in the use of antireflux procedures for children. *Pediatrics.* 2006;118(5):1828–1835.

19. DeMatteo C, Matovich D, Hjartarson A. Comparison of clinical and videofluoroscopic evaluation of children with feeding and swallowing difficulties. *Dev Med Child Neurol.* 2005;47(3):149–157.

20. O'Donoghue S, Bagnall A. Videofluoroscopic evaluation in the assessment of swallowing disorders in paediatric and adult populations. *Folia Phoniatr Logop.* 1999;51 (4–5):158–171.

21. Willging JP. Endoscopic evaluation of swallowing in children. *Int J Pediatr Otorhinolaryngol.* 1995;32(suppl): S107–S108.

22. Bosma JF, Hepburn LG, Josell SD, Baker K. Ultrasound demonstration of tongue motions during suckle feeding. *Dev Med Child Neurol.* 1990;32(3):223–229.

23. Suiter DM, Leder SB, Karas DE. The 3-ounce (90-cc) water swallow challenge: a screening test for children with suspected oropharyngeal dysphagia. *Otolaryngol Head Neck Surg.* 2009;140(2):187–190.

24. Stoeckli SJ, Huisman TA, Seifert B, Martin-Harris BJ. Interrater reliability of videofluoroscopic swallow evaluation. *Dysphagia.* 2003;18(1):53–57.

25. Willging JP, Thompson DM. Pediatric FEESST: fiberoptic endoscopic evaluation of swallowing with sensory testing. *Curr Gastroenterol Rep.* 2005;7(3):240–243.

26. Owayed AF, Campbell DM, Wang EE. Underlying causes of recurrent pneumonia in children. *Arch Pediatr Adolesc Med.* 2000;154(2):190–194.

27. Thurlbeck WM. Postnatal human lung growth. *Thorax.* 1982;37(8):564–571.

28. Weir K, McMahon S, Chang AB. Restriction of oral intake of water for aspiration lung disease in children. *Cochrane Database Syst Rev.* 2005;4:CD005303.

29. Brody AS, Klein JS, Molina PL, Quan J, Bean JA, Wilmott RW. High-resolution computed tomography in young patients with cystic fibrosis: distribution of abnormalities and correlation with pulmonary function tests. *J Pediatr.* 2004;145(1):32–38.

30. Linscheid T, Budd K, Rasnake L. Pediatric feeding problems. In: Roberts M, ed. *Handbook of Pediatric Psychology.* 3rd ed. New York: Guilford Press; 2003:481–498.

31. Davies WH, Ackerman LK, Davies CM, Vannatta K, Noll RB. About your child's eating: factor structure and psychometric properties of a feeding relationship measure. *Eat Behav.* 2007;8(4):457–463.

32. Silverman A. Feeding and vomiting problems in pediatric populations. In: Roberts M, Steele R, eds. *Handbook of Pediatric Psychology.* 4th ed. Guilford Publications; 2009.

33. Linscheid TR. Behavioral treatments for pediatric feeding disorders. *Behav Modif.* 2006;30(1):6–23.

34. Davis AM, Bruce AS, Mangiaracina C, Schulz T, Hyman P. Moving from tube to oral feeding in medically fragile nonverbal toddlers. *J Pediatr Gastroenterol Nutr.* 2009;49(2):233–236.

CHAPTER 4

Diarrhea

Dawn R. Ebach

DEFINITIONS AND EPIDEMIOLOGY

Diarrhea is defined as a change in bowel movement pattern resulting in an increase in stool volume and/or frequency, usually with loose to watery stool consistency. Acute and chronic diarrhea are defined based on duration of symptoms. Acute diarrhea lasts <14 days, whereas chronic diarrhea persists for longer. In general, to be considered diarrhea, three or more stools are passed per day. Patients with chronic diarrhea may have periods of loose or frequent stools with normal bowel movements in between episodes. Diarrhea can also be defined based on stool volume; however, measuring this accurately is often difficult. Normal stool volume is about 5–10 g of stool/kg body weight/day for infants and about 100–200 g of stool/day in children and adults. A 24-hour stool volume of >10 g/kg in infants and >200 g in children and adults is considered diarrhea. Acute diarrhea is common. It is most often secondary to viral infections. Other causes of acute diarrhea include toxin-induced diarrhea and antibiotic-associated diarrhea. Infectious diarrhea is most often found in children under age 5 years with a rate of about one to three episodes per year. Causes of chronic diarrhea are more diverse and range from functional disorders such as Toddler's diarrhea and irritable bowel syndrome (IBS) to disorders that may impact overall health such as inflammatory bowel disease or celiac disease.

PATHOGENESIS

Diarrhea occurs due to a derangement in small bowel, colonic, or pancreatic function. Besides the classification of acute and chronic, diarrhea may be divided further by pathophysiologic mechanism (Figure 4–1; Table 4–1).[1] The small bowel both secretes and absorbs water and electrolytes, as well as absorbs nutrients. Imbalance between secretion and absorption can lead to diarrhea. The primary function of the colon is to absorb fluid and electrolytes as well as storage of its contents until it can be expelled. The colon absorbs fluid and

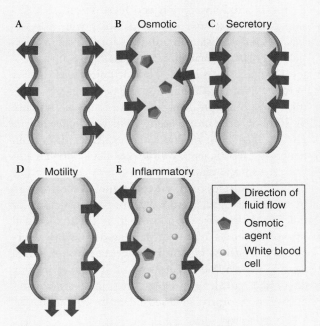

FIGURE 4–1 ■ (A) Normal intestine. Overall effect is absorption of fluid. (B) Osmotic diarrhea—osmotic agents draw fluid into the intestinal lumen. (C) Secretory diarrhea—increased fluid into the intestinal lumen, usually secondary to opening of channels by toxins or hormones. (D) Motility—increased rate of transit reduces absorption. (E) Inflammatory—decreased absorption of water, electrolytes, and nutrients.

Table 4–1.

Categories of Diarrhea

	Osmotic	Secretory	Motility	Inflammatory
Problem	Maldigestion	↑ Secretion with ↓ absorption	↓ Transit time	Inflammation leading to ↓ colonic absorption and ↑ motility
Stool characteristics	Watery ↓ pH ↑ osmolality $(>2(Na^+ + K^+))$ Improves with fasting	Watery Normal osmolality $(=2(Na^+ + K^+))$ Persists with fasting	Loose to normal, often worse after eating	Blood and/or white blood cells present
Examples	Lactose intolerance Lactulose, sorbitol, or magnesium ingestion	Cholera Congenital Cl^- diarrhea Enterotoxigenic *E. coli*	Irritable bowel syndrome Hyperthyroidism	*Salmonella* *Shigella* Ulcerative colitis

electrolytes. Disruption of the colon's function leads to frequent, loose, and occasionally bloody stools. The motor function of the intestines regulates forward propulsion of its contents. Abnormalities in this motility may also lead to diarrhea.

Osmotic diarrhea (Figure 4–1b; Table 4–1) occurs when increased solute load in the bowel lumen leads to decreased fluid absorption and increased fluid secretion.[2] Stools are loose and often foul-smelling. Bloating, abdominal distention, and gas are also characteristic. Carbohydrate malabsorption, such as from lactose intolerance, is an example of osmotic diarrhea. Another example occurs with ingestion of poorly absorbed solutes, including non-digestible sugars such as lactulose or sorbitol, or osmotic laxatives such as polyethylene glycol and milk of magnesia. Fat malabsorption from pancreatic insufficiency or bile acid depletion can also lead to osmotic diarrhea. When poorly absorbed fats and carbohydrates reach the colon, they are hydrolyzed by colonic bacteria, producing short-chain fatty acids that further increase the solute load. Injury to the small intestine mucosa results in decreased absorptive surface area and loss of brush border digestive enzymes, causing generalized malabsorption. Examples include decreased gut length from surgical excision and decreased absorptive area secondary to severe celiac or Crohn's disease.

Osmotic diarrhea subsides with fasting, which eliminates the osmotic load. This can be a useful diagnostic test for malabsorptive diarrhea in the hospitalized patient receiving intravenous fluids. Stool studies are also helpful, revealing an acidic pH due to fermentation, with increased osmotic gap. The osmotic gap is calculated after measuring stool sodium and potassium using the following formula:

$$290 - 2(Na^+ + K^+)$$

Because of the relatively free movement of water across the intestinal mucosa, all stools can be assumed to have an osmolarity equivalent to serum (290). The sum of sodium and potassium must be multiplied by 2 to account for their accompanying anions. An osmotic gap >50 is consistent with the presence of other unmeasured solutes in the stool, indicating that the diarrhea is osmotic in nature.

Secretory diarrhea (Figure 4–1c; Table 4–1) is caused by derangements in mechanisms regulating fluid and electrolyte movement in the small bowel mucosa, leading to active secretion of electrolytes, with passive loss of water.[3] This is characterized by chloride and bicarbonate secretion and inhibition of sodium and chloride absorption. Disorders caused by bacterial toxins, such as cholera (*Vibrio cholerae*) and traveler's diarrhea (enterotoxigenic *Escherichia coli*), are classic examples. Secretory diarrhea can also result from secretagogues produced by tumors; Zollinger–Ellison syndrome (gastrin) and vasoactive intestinal peptide (VIP)-secreting tumors, or VIPomas, are rare examples of this in children. Regardless of cause, secretory diarrhea is characterized by high-volume, frequent watery stools, which persist despite fasting. Stool osmolality is similar to plasma osmolality, with no osmotic gap present.[2]

Inflammatory diarrhea, typically seen with bacterial infection and inflammatory bowel disease (Figure 4–1e; Table 4–1), is caused by disruptions in the epithelial function of the bowel.[3] Bacterial toxins can alter ion transport, leading to increased secretion. In addition, some bacteria can invade the mucosa, directly disrupting function. Injury to the epithelial barrier, including the tight junctions, alters electrochemical gradients. Activated macrophages secrete cytokines such as tumor necrosis factor and interleukins such as IL-2 that increase intestinal permeability. Inflammation-associated diarrhea is aggravated by the release of various secretagogues, including cytokines, prostaglandins, histamine, and leukotrienes. Brush border and enterocyte injury (or death) from inflammation also contributes to diarrhea. In inflammatory diarrhea, the intestinal mucosa is thickened, hyperemic, and edematous. Stools may contain red or white blood cells. There is frequently loss of serum proteins into the stool. A component of osmotic diarrhea may also be present in inflammatory diarrhea secondary to malabsorption.

Motility disorders can cause diarrhea (Figure 4–1d; Table 4–1). Increased transit time decreases the ability of the colon to absorb fluid.[4] Increased motility may be secondary to increased secretion of serotonin, histamine, or other mediators. IBS and hyperthyroidism are examples of diarrhea secondary to increased motility. Decreased motility causes stasis, which leads to small bowel bacterial overgrowth and inflammatory diarrhea.

The above categorizations of diarrhea are helpful in narrowing down cause. However, it is important to keep in mind that many causes of diarrhea will have one or more characteristics. For example, patients with Crohn's disease often have osmotic diarrhea secondary to malabsorption, but will also have a secretory component secondary to inflammation. In this situation, fasting results in diminished stool output without complete resolution of diarrhea.

CLINICAL PRESENTATION

Children with acute diarrhea may present to their health care provider because of frequent passage of stool, abdominal pain, poor oral intake, fever, irritability, or dehydration. The clinical history should include the onset, duration, nature, and severity of symptoms. Assessment of hydration status is the most important aspect of the physical exam.

Patients with chronic diarrhea will present to their provider for concerns of ongoing frequent stools, abdominal pain, blood in stool, bloating and gassiness, or growth failure. History should include onset and duration of symptoms including if symptoms are intermittent. Stool frequency, consistency, and visual presence of blood should be determined. Any modify-

ing factors such as association with diet or stress should also be elicited. Nocturnal defecation is concerning for colonic inflammation and makes functional diarrhea (IBS or toddler's diarrhea) less likely. The presence of abdominal pain including timing, severity, and location can be an important clue to diagnosis. Extraintestinal manifestations such as a skin rash or joint pain that can be associated with celiac disease or inflammatory bowel disease should be inquired about. The *past medical history* may reveal a history of bowel surgery that may raise suspicion for malabsorption due to short bowel syndrome. Surgery may also lead to intestinal strictures, adhesions, or loss of the ileocecal valve, any of which may predispose to small bowel bacterial overgrowth. Medication and supplement history should be obtained. Some medications (orlistat) cause malabsorptive diarrhea, and laxative use must be ruled out. Ingestion of non-absorbable sugars such as "sugar-free" candy or gum or excessive juice intake can precipitate abdominal cramping, gas, and diarrhea. *Family history* can also be helpful, particularly history of inflammatory bowel disease or celiac disease in a first- or second-degree relative. *Social history* should include recent travel and exposures such as animal or sick contacts. Attendance at daycare increases the risk for infectious diarrhea.

Physical exam should begin with evaluation of growth parameters. Patients with lactose intolerance and IBS usually do not have weight loss or decrease in growth percentiles. However, patients with celiac disease, Crohn's disease, or pancreatic insufficiency may experience growth failure. Decreased subcutaneous tissue and loose skin are also signs of weight loss and possible malabsorptive disorders. Thyroid mass or fullness with or without proptosis, along with brisk reflexes and tachycardia, is suggestive of hyperthyroidism. Evaluate for abdominal distention, location of tenderness, and fullness. Tenderness and fullness in the right lower quadrant is concerning for Crohn's disease. Digital clubbing may be a sign of chronic disease such as Crohn's disease, celiac disease, or cystic fibrosis. Edema is suggestive of a protein losing enteropathy that may be secondary to inflammatory bowel disease or lymphangiectasia. Perianal exam may reveal skin tags, fissures, or fistulas that are suggestive of Crohn's disease. Skin exam may reveal dermatitis herpetiformis (celiac disease), erythema nodosum (IBD), or pyoderma gangrenosum (IBD). Perianal rash may be present secondary to prolonged diarrhea, but also may be suggestive of carbohydrate malabsorption as stool often is acidic. A combination of perianal and perioral rash may be a sign of acrodermatitis enteropathica. Additionally, signs of malnutrition should be noted such as sparse, brittle hair, cheilosis, or smooth tongue.

DIFFERENTIAL DIAGNOSIS

Acute Diarrhea

The most common causes of acute diarrhea are infectious agents (Table 4–2). Rotavirus is the most common cause of severe acute diarrhea and accounts for about 40% of hospitalizations due to diarrhea in children under age 5 years.[5] It is spread from person to person by the fecal–oral route and is most common during the winter months. The illness usually begins with fever and vomiting followed by frequent, loose, foul-smelling diarrhea that can last as long as 10 days. Malnourished patients or those with immunodeficiency can develop chronic diarrhea. Dehydration is common. Rotavirus can be detected by antigen or PCR testing of the stool.[6] An oral vaccine for the most common serotypes is now available and has been found to decrease hospitalizations and emergency room visits for acute diarrhea by 95%.[7]

Calciviruses (Norwalk virus and norovirus) are responsible for outbreaks of gastrointestinal illnesses, spread by the fecal–oral route, often via contaminated food or water. Outbreaks occur in confined environments such as cruise ships or daycare centers. The illness usually lasts 2–3 days. Symptoms include fever, abdominal cramping, diarrhea, and vomiting.[6] Astrovirus is another common cause of viral gastroenteritis that is transmitted via the fecal–oral route. Astroviral diarrhea tends to be less severe than rotavirus or norovirus.[6] Hepatitis A can present with acute diarrhea, with or without jaundice. It is often a foodborne illness, but can also be transmitted via close contacts.[8]

Bacterial causes of diarrhea may present similarly to viral-induced diarrhea, but invasive or toxigenic bacteria may cause bloody stools, and more prominent fever and abdominal pain. Abdominal pain can be quite severe and may be mistaken for appendicitis. *Salmonella* and *Campylobacter* are the most frequently isolated bacterial causes of diarrhea.

Campylobacter species can be found in contaminated poultry or other farm animals. It can precipitate immunoreactive complications such as Guillain–Barre' syndrome, reactive arthritis, or Reiter's syndrome.[9]

Salmonella species can be contracted from animals such as poultry and reptiles who are carriers. It is also associated with the ingestion of poultry, eggs, and dairy; however, outbreaks from other contaminated foods such as peanuts and produce have occurred. It is most commonly seen during the summer and fall.[9] Prolonged excretion of *Salmonella* in the stool can occur. Invasive infections such as osteomyelitis and meningitis can occur in young infants or immunocompromised patients.[8]

Patients infected with *Shigella* often have high fevers in addition to abdominal pain and diarrhea that may or may not be bloody. Only a small number of organisms are required to initiate infection that is most often spread from person to person but may also be contracted from contaminated food or water.[8] Infection with *Shigella* can be complicated by hemolytic uremic syndrome, Reiter's syndrome, or toxic megacolon.[9]

Yersinia enterocolitica infectious diarrhea is less common than other bacterial causes of diarrhea. It is transmitted by contaminated food, especially pork products such as chitterlings (pork intestines).[8] It mimics appendicitis in about 40% of patients. *Yersinia* can lead to a migratory arthritis, Reiter's syndrome, and erythema nodosum.[9]

Contaminated food or water is the source of *E. coli*. There are five subtypes of *E. coli*. *Shiga toxin-producing E. coli* is the most common cause of bloody

Table 4–2.		
Infectious Diarrhea		
Viral	**Bacterial**	**Parasitic**
Astrovirus	*Aeromonas*	*Cryptosporidium*
Calcivirus (Norwalk)	*Campylobacter* species	*Cyclospora*
Cytomegalovirus	*Clostridium difficile*	*Entamoeba histolytica*
Enteric adenoviruses	*Escherichia coli*	*Giardia lamblia*
Hepatitis A	*Listeria monocytogenes*	*Isospora belli*
HIV	*Mycobacterium*	Microsporidia
Rotavirus	*Salmonella* species	*Taenia*
	Shigella species	*Trichinella*
	Vibrio species	
	Yersinia enterocolitica	

diarrhea. Fever is either not present or minimal, and patients often present with severe abdominal pain and high white blood cell count. It has been associated with hemolytic uremic syndrome and thrombotic thrombo-cytopenic purpura. It can occur in outbreaks usually associated with contaminated food (undercooked beef or unpasteurized apple cider) or animal exposures (such as petting zoos). *Enterotoxigenic E. coli* is a cause of "traveler's diarrhea" and causes 1–5 days of loose stools and abdominal cramping. *Enteropathogenic, enteroinvasive E. coli and enteroaggregative E. coli* are seen mostly in undeveloped countries. Enteropathogenic *E. coli* causes watery diarrhea. Enteroinvasive *E. coli* causes dysentery and enteroaggregative *E. coli* is usually watery but may contain blood.[9]

Foodborne bacterial toxins are another cause of acute diarrhea. *Staphyloccocus* species cause a foodborne illness that is characterized by an abrupt onset of vomiting, abdominal pain, and diarrhea. It lasts 1–2 days and is usually caused by foods that are not kept warm or cold enough to inhibit staphylococcal growth. Illness usually occurs within 2–4 hours after ingestion. *Bacillus cereus* produces several toxins. Emetogenic toxins produce vomiting and abdominal pain; enterotoxins result in diarrhea in about one-third of patients. Symptoms depend on the toxin types being produced and usually last <24 hours.[8]

Parasite infection is another cause of acute diarrhea, but may also cause chronic diarrhea in young or immunocompromised children. The two most common offenders are *Giardia intestinalis* and *Cryptosporidium*.[10] *Giardia* (Figure 4–2) is the most common parasite and children between ages 1 and 9 years are the most common age group affected. Children may have an acute illness with diarrhea, abdominal pain, and bloating or may be completely asymptomatic. Severely affected children have decreased appetite and weight loss. Risks for transmission include waterborne exposure such as recreational water use or exposure to infected children in a daycare setting.

Cryptosporidium has been the culprit in several recent outbreaks associated with recreational water use in pools and water parks. The oocyte of this organism is resistant to chlorine. Transmission may also occur from person to person with outbreaks occurring in daycares. Symptoms are similar to *giardiasis*; however, fever and vomiting are more frequently seen with *Cryptosporidium*. Asymptomatic infection may also occur.[10]

The use of antibiotics can change the intestinal microbiota, with altered ecology leading to diarrhea by several mechanisms Diarrhea may occur secondary to overgrowth of antibiotic-resistant pathogenic bacteria, such as *Clostridium difficile*, and by decreased population of normal commensal bacterial. Because the normal flora serves to ferment undigested materials arriving in the colon, loss of this population increases colonic osmotic load. Reduction of normal colonic fermentation also causes decreased production of short-chain fatty acids, which are an important source of energy for colonocytes, and impairs colonic fluid and electrolyte absorption. Antibiotic-associated diarrhea is seen more frequently with the use of broad-spectrum antibiotics.[11] *C. difficile* is a toxin-producing organism that often causes diarrhea in the setting of antibiotic use, but is also being seen in increased frequency in the community without antibiotic exposure.[12] Toxins produced by *C. difficile* cause a pseudomembranous colitis (Figure 4–3) with bloody stools and abdominal pain. This illness occasionally can be fulminant, leading to an acute abdomen and

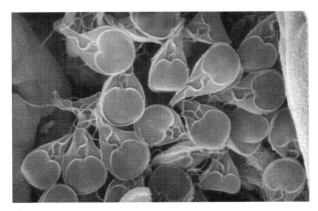

FIGURE 4–2 ■ Scanning electron micrograph of *Giardia intestinalis* on small bowel epithelial cells.

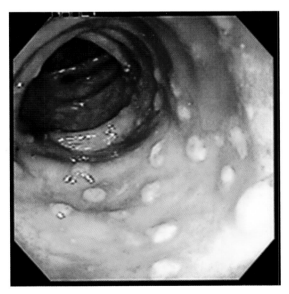

FIGURE 4–3 ■ Endoscopic view of pseudomembranous colitis secondary to *Clostridium difficile*. *Button-like pseudomembranes are present.*

Table 4–3.		
Differential Diagnosis of Chronic Diarrhea		
Infant	Toddler/Child	Adolescent
Acrodermatitis enteropathica	Enteric infection	Enteric infection
Enteric infection	Eosinophilic gastroenteritis	Eosinophilic gastroenteritis
Hirschsprung's disease	Hormone-secreting tumor	Inflammatory bowel disease
Hormone-secreting tumor (neuroblastoma)	Inflammatory bowel disease	Hormone/endocrine (hyperthyroidism, VIPoma, gastrinoma)
Intestinal lymphangiectasia	Small bowel bacterial overgrowth	Irritable bowel syndrome
Munchausen by proxy	Toddler's diarrhea	Laxative abuse
Pancreatic insufficiency (CF, Shwachman-Diamond)		Runner's diarrhea
Small bowel bacterial overgrowth		Small bowel bacterial overgrowth
Immune disorders		
Autoimmune enteropathy	Autoimmune enteropathy	Celiac disease
Primary immune deficiencies	Celiac disease	Secondary immune deficiencies (HIV, immunosuppression)
Secondary immune deficiencies (HIV, immunosuppression)	Primary immune deficiencies	
Congenital diarrheas	*Carbohydrate maldigestion*	*Carbohydrate maldigestion*
Microvillus inclusion disease	Lactose intolerance	Fructose intolerance
Tufting enteropathy	Sucrase–isomaltase deficiency	Lactose intolerance
Transport defects (congenital Cl or Na diarrhea, glucose–galactose malabsorption)		

toxic megacolon requiring colectomy. The presence of this organism and its toxins does not always lead to illness: 50–70% of neonates may exhibit asymptomatic colonization with *C. difficile*. Colonization rates decrease with age.[8]

Chronic Diarrheal Disorders

Neonates with failure to thrive and chronic diarrhea may have one of several, very rare *congenital disorders* of intestinal absorption (Table 4–3; Figure 4–4). These include congenital lactase deficiency, disorders of intestinal transport such as glucose–galactose malabsorption, congenital sodium diarrhea, congenital chloride diarrhea, and congenital enteropathies such as *microvillus inclusion disease* and *tufting enteropathy*. The diarrhea in these disorders is typically profuse and watery and may even be mistaken for urine.[13] A more common cause of chronic diarrhea with failure to thrive in infants is *cystic fibrosis* (see Chapter 32).

Infants with *intractable diarrhea of infancy* present with malnutrition and diarrhea that typically persists after an initial viral gastroenteritis. Decreased oral intake of nutrients impairs healing, leading to decreased absorptive capacity. Infants with this

condition have often been fed diluted formula or clear liquids for a prolonged period in response to the initial illness. Diarrhea improves with nutritional rehabilitation. Formulas that are lactose- and sucrose-free are needed because of carbohydrate malabsorption. Hydrolyzed or elemental formulas may also be considered. Sometimes parenteral nutrition is needed initially.[14]

Autoimmune enteropathy usually presents during the first year of life with symptoms of diarrhea and failure to thrive. It can be associated with immune deficiency disorders such as immune dysregulation, polyendocrinopathy, enteropathy, and X-linkage (IPEX). Small intestine biopsies are nearly identical to those of patients with celiac disease, with total villous atrophy and a lymphoplasmacytic infiltrate with intraepithelial lymphocytes. Serum antienterocyte antibodies can sometimes be detected. These patients have negative celiac serology and do not respond to a gluten-free diet.[13]

Preschool children are vulnerable to *toddler's diarrhea* (also called chronic non-specific diarrhea of childhood or functional diarrhea), a common cause of frequent, loose stools in this age group. It is defined as a functional disorder and criteria for diagnosis are

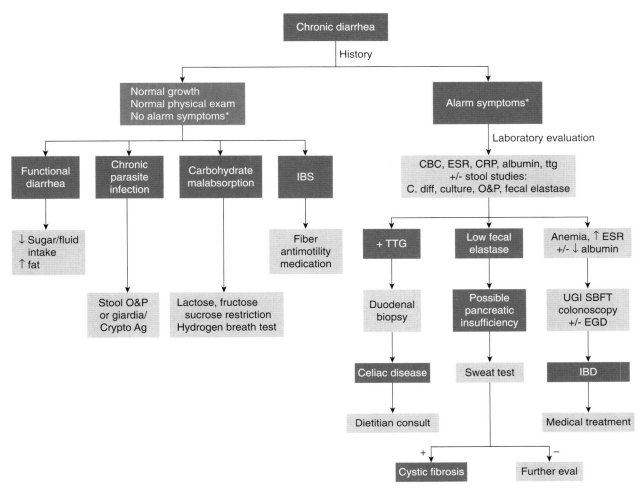

*Alarm symptoms: blood in stool, weight loss, poor growth, stooling or pain waking at night, pain away from umbilicus, mouth sores, joint pains/arthritis rashes, abdominal mass, perianal disease, unexplained fever

FIGURE 4–4 ■ Diagnostic algorithm for chronic diarrhea.

listed in Table 4–4.[15] These children have 3–10 loose to watery stools per day. Bowel movements may contain food particles or mucous and may run out the diaper. Despite the loose stools, they appear healthy and continue to grow well. A contributing factor in most, but not all, of these children is excessive intake of sweet beverages and juices or a diet low in fat with excessive carbohydrates.

Celiac disease should be considered in any child with diarrhea and weight loss, but particularly so in the preschool age group. Toddlers with a classic presentation of celiac disease experience frequent malodorous stools, a distended abdomen, thin extremities, and decreased activity or irritability. Children commonly present with more subtle symptoms as well. See Chapter 18 for further information.

Chronic parasite infections with *Giardia* or *Cryptosporidium* can also cause chronic diarrhea in the young child or those who are immunosuppressed.

School-age children with chronic diarrhea are more likely to have inflammatory bowel disease, celiac disease, lactose intolerance, and IBS.

Inflammatory bowel disease frequently presents in the peripubertal age group. The diarrhea may or may not contain gross blood, but frequently is occult blood

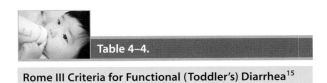

Table 4–4.

Rome III Criteria for Functional (Toddler's) Diarrhea[15]

Must include all of the following:
- Three or more large, unformed, painless stools per day
- Symptoms persisting for >4 weeks
- Onset of symptoms between 6 and 36 months of age
- Passage of stools occurs during waking hours
- No failure to thrive if caloric intake is adequate

positive. These patients may have any combination of weight loss, anemia, abdominal pain, and growth failure. See Chapter 16.

Lactose intolerance occurs when there is insufficient lactase available to hydrolyse lactose to its component simple sugars, glucose and galactose, leading to malabsorption and osmotic diarrhea. Lactase is located near the tips of the villi of the small intestine and, therefore, can result from intestinal injury (secondary lactose intolerance). *Primary lactose intolerance* has a genetic basis and occurs when there is decreased production of the enzyme. This can either be congenital (rare) or acquired as a normal aspect of maturation (*primary hypolactasia*).

Symptoms of lactose intolerance are abdominal cramping, bloating, gas, nausea, and diarrhea that occur within a short time of ingestion of lactose-containing foods or beverages. These symptoms are dose dependent, and many patients with lactose intolerance can still ingest small amounts of lactose without symptoms. The prevalence of primary hypolactasia increases with age and is more common in certain ethnic groups. It is estimated that about 70% of the world's population does not tolerate lactose as adults, and this should be considered a normal consequence of maturation. Persistence of lactase activity into adult life is uncommon in mammals, and in Europeans is thought to result from a mutation arising during the last Ice Age. The ability to digest unfermented animal milk in a cold climate favored survival and has persisted in their descendents. The prevalence of adult lactose intolerance is estimated to be 95–100% in Asians, and is also high in Native Americans, Africans, Ashkenazi Jews, and Hispanics. However, only 2–15% of Northern European adults are intolerant of dairy products. Ethnic groups with higher prevalence of lactose intolerance have earlier onset of symptoms that can occur before age 5 years. Patients in groups with lower prevalence usually present during adolescence or adulthood.[16]

Secondary lactose intolerance occurs in disorders causing damage to the villi, thus decreasing the density of lactase enzyme. The most common cause of secondary lactose intolerance is viral gastroenteritis. Secondary lactose intolerance may occur in infants and children with an acute viral gastroenteritis and may persist for about a week afterwards.[17] Symptoms resolve as the small intestine heals. Most children are still able to ingest lactose during and after these brief infections without significant symptoms. Any disease with injury to the villous such as celiac disease and Crohn's disease of the small intestine can cause secondary lactose intolerance. For patients with celiac disease, lactose tolerance resolves when adherent to the gluten-free diet. Crohn's patients may also find improvement with treatment.

Table 4–5.

Pediatric Rome III Diagnostic Criteria for Irritable Bowel Syndrome[19]

Must include all of the following:
- Abdominal discomfort or pain associated with two or more of the following at least 25% of the time:
  a) Improved with defecation
  b) Onset associated with a change in stool frequency
  c) Onset associated with a change in form of stool
- No evidence of an inflammatory, anatomic, metabolic, or neoplastic process that explains the patient's symptoms

Criteria must be fulfilled at least once per week for at least 2 months prior to diagnosis.

IBS is another common cause of chronic diarrhea, particularly in older children and adolescents. Patients with IBS present with chronic abdominal pain and changes in their bowel habits. It has been thought to be secondary to a dysregulation of the interaction between the enteric and central nervous systems that can lead to visceral hypersensitivity, pain, and altered gut motility. Visceral hypersensitivity may be triggered by infection, inflammation, changes in gut microbiota, intestinal trauma, food intolerances, and altered motility. There is likely a genetic component, with multiple family members often sharing the diagnosis. Psychosocial factors exacerbate symptoms for some patients.[18] IBS can be diagnosed if a patient fulfills the pediatric Rome III criteria (Table 4–5).[19] Patients with diarrhea-predominant IBS have loose to watery stools at least once per week with at least three stools in a day. Patients may complain of straining, urgency, or feeling of incomplete evacuation. Some patients may report passage of mucous. Bloating and abdominal distention may also be present. It is estimated that 10–15% of children have IBS.[18]

Table 4–6 lists symptoms, physical exam findings, and laboratory results in which to consider consultation with a pediatric gastroenterologist in the child with chronic diarrhea.

DIAGNOSIS

Acute Diarrhea

For the patient with acute symptoms, diagnosis is usually clinically based and laboratory studies are not required. Rotavirus can be diagnosed in the stool with antigen testing by ELISA. Bacterial infections can be identified via stool cultures. The bacterial pathogens identified by routine cultures vary among laboratories, and separate requests may need to be made to evaluate for some bacteria, especially *E. coli* O157:H7 and

Table 4–6.

Features in Patients with Chronic Diarrhea to Consider Pediatric Gastroenterology Consultation

History	Physical Exam Findings	Laboratory/Radiologic Findings
Weight loss	Weight loss	Anemia
Growth failure	Growth failure	Hemoccult positive stool
Blood in stool	Abdominal tenderness, mass or fullness	Hypoalbuminemia
Abdominal pain (especially if not centered near the umbilicus)	Perianal skin tags, fistulas, or fissures	Elevated inflammatory markers (ESR, CRP)
Delayed puberty	Digital clubbing	Positive celiac serology
Nighttime stooling	Delayed puberty	Abnormal fecal fat or fecal elastase
Abdominal pain waking patient at night	Joint swelling	Narrowing, dilation, or nodularity on a small bowel follow-through study
Unexplained fever	Erythema nodosum or pyoderma gangrenosum	Small bowel inflammation on abdominal CT
Joint pain or swelling	Edema	
Neonatal diarrhea with failure to thrive		

Y. enterocolitica. Giardia and *Cryptosporidium* can be diagnosed via stool antigen testing or ova and parasite exams. *C. difficile* is diagnosed based on toxin antigen assays. Testing for *C. difficile* in children under 1 year of age is not always reliable secondary to a high incidence of an asymptomatic carrier state. If pseudomembranous colitis is suspected in this age group, use of more than one diagnostic method (toxin assay, culture, or endoscopy with biopsy) is recommended.[20]

Chronic Diarrhea

Evaluation of the stool for diagnostic information is helpful in these patients. Ova and parasite examination may be done, and antigen testing for the more common North American culprits of *Giardia* and *Cryptosporidium* may be considered. A positive test (Clinitest) for stool-reducing sugars can point to carbohydrate malabsorption of glucose, fructose, or lactose. Fecal pH can be measured and, if low (<5.5) is suggestive of carbohydrate malabsorption. Stool osmolality and stool electrolytes to calculate the osmotic gap can help differentiate between osmotic and secretory diarrhea, as can a trial of fasting in the hospitalized patient (see Table 4–1). In addition, a high osmotic gap can be seen from osmotic laxatives such as lactulose. Low osmolality (<290 mOsm/kg) can be seen if stool is diluted after collection in cases of factitious diarrhea. The presence of white blood cells or positive occult blood in the stool is suggestive of an inflammatory diarrhea. Abnormal fecal fat studies (Sudan III stain or the technically difficult 72-hour stool collection) point to steatorrhea. Increased fecal alpha-1-antitrypsin is a marker of protein-losing enteropathy. Low fecal elastase is suggestive of pancreatic insufficiency.

A complete blood count may reveal anemia, which is common in inflammatory bowel disease or celiac disease. Elevated platelets, erythrocyte sedimentation rate, and C-reactive protein are suggestive of an inflammatory disorder. Low serum albumin is suggestive of a protein-losing enteropathy, which may be associated with inflammatory diarrhea. Serologic testing for celiac disease (antigliadin, endomysial, or tissue transglutaminase IgA antibodies) has high sensitivity and specificity (see Chapter 18). If malabsorptive or inflammatory disorders are suspected, evaluation of iron studies, folate, vitamin B_{12}, vitamins A, D, and E, calcium, and prothrombin time (marker of vitamin K deficiency) should be performed to evaluate the nutritional consequences of chronic diarrhea. To evaluate for immune deficiency, white blood cell differential, serum immunoglobulins, and HIV testing are initial tests to consider. Serum gastrin and VIP can be measured if hormone-secreting tumors are suspected.

Radiologic evaluation has a limited role in the evaluation of patients with chronic diarrhea. A barium upper gastrointestinal series with small bowel follow-through may show evidence of small bowel disease secondary to Crohn's disease. Typical findings include separation of bowel loops, nodularity, and strictures. Areas of stricturing with dilated proximal bowel may be sites of small bowel bacterial overgrowth, which can also be a cause of diarrhea. Abdominal computerized tomography can also show evidence of bowel wall thickening suggestive of inflammatory bowel disease.

Endoscopic evaluation is useful to evaluate for a number of causes of diarrhea. Duodenal biopsies showing villous atrophy with increased intraepithelial lymphocytes are considered the "gold standard" for the diagnosis of celiac disease. Upper endoscopy and colonoscopy with biopsies are used in the evaluation of patients suspected of having inflammatory bowel disease. Mucosal biopsies are also necessary for the diagnosis of autoimmune enteropathy and eosinophilic gastroenteritis. Electron microscopy of small bowel biopsies is needed for the diagnosis of tufting enteropathy and microvillus inclusion disease. Disaccharide enzyme quantification can be performed on flash-frozen duodenal biopsy specimens for the diagnosis of lactose intolerance or sucrase–isomaltase deficiency when breath hydrogen testing or dietary withdrawal is not sufficient.

For the patient with suspected lactose intolerance, a several-day trial of a lactose-free diet can be diagnostic. If desired, formal testing can be done using breath hydrogen analysis. In this test, the patient drinks 0.5–1 g/kg (maximum, 25 g) of lactose as a 10% solution, after first obtaining a baseline breath sample. Malabsorbed carbohydrates are fermented by colonic bacteria, producing hydrogen gas, which rapidly diffuses from the bowel into the bloodstream and then into the breath (Figure 4–5). To collect specimens, the patient exhales into special foil-lined bags at intervals of about every 30 minutes for 2–3 hours. The hydrogen in each specimen is then measured by gas chromatography. Lactose intolerance is diagnosed if the breath hydrogen concentration rises by at least 20 ppm over baseline.[17] Breath testing can also be used to diagnose sucrase–isomaltase deficiency, fructose malabsorption, and small bowel bacterial overgrowth.

TREATMENT

Acute Diarrhea

For patients with acute diarrhea, treatment is aimed at maintaining hydration. The degree of dehydration is best determined by percentage of weight loss; however, a recent pre-illness weight may not be available. Evaluation of heart rate, blood pressure, and possibly orthostatics as well as physical exam findings of dry mucous membranes, lack of tears, and abnormal skin turgor can give clues to the degree of dehydration (Table 4–7). Most patients are able to drink enough fluids to keep hydrated. Oral rehydration is preferred over parenteral hydration, especially when only mild dehydration is present, or when sophisticated medical care is not readily available.

For patients with mild to moderate dehydration, *oral rehydration therapy* is recommended. Oral rehydration solution, as recommended by the World Health Organization, is a glucose–electrolyte solution with 75 mEq/L of sodium and 75 mmol/L glucose and an osmolarity of 245 mOsm/L. Coupling of glucose and Na uptake in the small intestine improves the intestinal

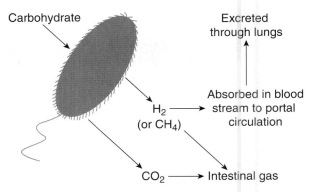

FIGURE 4–5 ■ Bacterial fermentation of carbohydrates: basis of breath hydrogen/methane test.

absorption of salt and water. In the United States, commercial rehydration solutions have less sodium and lower osmolarity, appropriate for treatment of non-cholera diarrhea. The fluid deficit can be calculated based on the estimated (or measured weight loss) degree of dehydration. For example, a 15-kg child who is 5% dehydrated requires 750 mL over 3–4 hours for replacement ($15,000\,g \times 0.05 = 750\,mL$). The oral rehydration solution should be given as 5 mL doses every 1–2 minutes. If the patient tolerates this well, the dose may be increased and given at longer intervals with a goal of about 30–80 mL/kg over 4 hours (Figure 4–6). Nasogastric tubes may also be used to hydrate patients who are unable to drink. Breastfed infants should be allowed to continue to nurse even through rehydration. Formula-fed infants should be fed their regular non-diluted formula once they are rehydrated. Children may eat a regular diet as tolerated once they are rehydrated, but should continue to receive oral rehydration solution to replace diarrheal losses.[21,22]

For patients who are unable to take fluids orally, have severe dehydration, or continue to have significant fluid losses, admission for IV or NG fluid therapy is often needed. These patients should be placed on contact isolation to prevent nosocomial spread of their infectious illness. A patient is considered severely dehydrated if there is decreased peripheral perfusion, altered mental status, >10% weight loss, or circulatory collapse. If severe dehydration is present, then IV hydration starting with a 20 mL/kg normal saline bolus is indicated, with frequent reassessment of vital signs, peripheral perfusion, urine output, and mental status. Repeat boluses may be required.[21,22]

Zinc has been studied in numerous trials as decreasing the severity and duration of acute infectious diarrhea. The mechanism is unknown.[23] WHO/UNICEF recommendation for zinc supplementation is 10–20 mg/day for 10–14 days for children and 10 mg/day for infants <6 months of age.[24]

Table 4–7.

Clinical Evaluation of Dehydration[21]

Symptoms	Mild Dehydration	Moderate Dehydration	Severe Dehydration
Weight loss	<3%	3–9%	>9%
Urine output	Normal to decreased	Decreased	Minimal
Pulse	Normal	Normal to increased	Increased (decreased in severe)
Blood pressure	Normal	May have orthostasis	Hypotensive
Respiratory rate	Normal	±Tachypnea, may have deep breathing	Tachypnea or deep breathing
Pulse quality	Normal	Normal to decreased	Weak, thready, or not palpable
Capillary refill	Normal	Slightly delayed (2–3 seconds)	Delayed (>3 seconds) or absent
Skin turgor	Instant recoil	Recoil <2 seconds	Recoil >2 seconds, tenting
Mental status	Alert	Normal, fatigued, or restless/irritable	Lethargic, apathetic, unconscious
Eyes	Normal	Slightly sunken	Deeply sunken
Mucous membranes	Normal or slightly dry	Dry	Parched
Extremities	Warm	Cool	Cold and mottled, may be cyanotic
Tears	Present	Decreased	Absent
Fontanelle (if open)	Normal	Mildly sunken	Sunken
Thirst	Drinks normally but may refuse	Thirsty and eager to drink	Drinks poorly, unable to drink

Probiotics have also been extensively studied for their potential to prevent and treat infectious diarrhea. *Lactobacillus* GG and *Saccharomyces boulardii* have been shown to decrease the duration of acute rotaviral diarrhea. The use of probiotics to prevent diarrhea acquired in daycare centers or nosocomially has less robust support in trials, but may be beneficial in preventing antibiotic-associated diarrhea.[25]

Antibiotic treatment is typically not recommended in most cases of bacterial infectious diarrhea. However, *Salmonella* should be treated in young infants and in patients who are immunocompromised to prevent sequelae such as sepsis and osteomyelitis. Antibiotics may also be used in other infections for patients who are more severely affected.[8] There is some evidence that antibiotic use may increase the risk of developing hemolytic uremic syndrome in patients with Shiga toxin-producing organisms and should be avoided if *E. coli* O157:H7 is suspected. Use of anti-motility and anti-diarrheal agents may also increase the risk for hemolytic uremic syndrome.[26]

Treatment with antibiotics is indicated for *C. difficile* colitis. First-line therapy for mild disease is metronidazole, dosed at 30 mg/kg/day divided four times a day for 10 days. This can be given orally or intravenously. Oral vancomycin should be considered as initial therapy for moderate to severe disease or if the child fails to respond to metronidazole at a dose of 40–50 mg/kg/day given orally for 7–10 days, divided into four daily doses. If disease is fulminant, intravenous metronidazole may be preferred because of poor delivery with ileus or toxic megacolon.[27] Newer non-absorbable antibiotics such as rifaximin and nitazoxanide are being studied.[28] A 2008 meta-analysis did not find sufficient evidence to support using probiotics as an adjunct treatment for *C. difficile* in adults.[29]

Giardia can be treated with metronidazole 15 mg/kg/day divided three times a day for 5 days, or nitazoxanide 100 mg twice daily for ages 1–3 years, 200 mg twice daily for ages 4–11 years, and 500 mg twice daily for greater than age 12 years for a total of 3 days. The same dose of nitazoxanide can be used for *Cryptosporidium*.[8]

Medication dosages are summarized in Table 4–8.

Chronic Diarrhea

Treatment for *toddler's diarrhea* starts with reassurance to the caregivers that this is a functional disorder and not infectious or inflammatory. Initial therapy involves limiting sweet beverage intake. Overall fluid intake may need

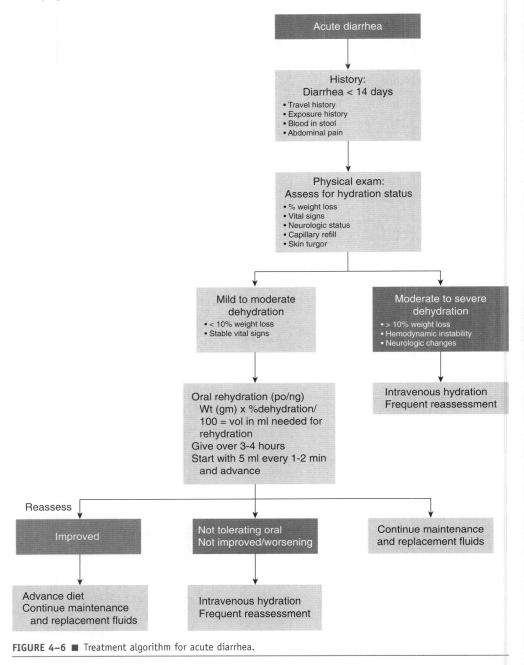

FIGURE 4–6 ■ Treatment algorithm for acute diarrhea.

to be limited in those children with excessive intake of water or milk. Increasing fat in the diet to 35–50% of their calories can help slow motility and reduce diarrhea.[30]

Lactose intolerance is treated by limiting lactose intake. Most patients with lactose intolerance are able to continue to eat small amounts of lactose-containing foods and drinks, but must be careful of the amount and type ingested. It is important to ensure that the patient continues to take adequate calcium and vitamin D. Lactase-treated milk and ice cream are available. Lactase enzyme supplements can be taken prior to dairy products, such as cheese, which cannot be

pretreated. Fortified milk alternatives such as soy or rice milk are lactose free and are good sources of calcium and vitamin D.[17] Yogurt is usually tolerated due to reduced lactose content and the presence of bacterial β-galactoside (lactase). Aged cheeses are often well tolerated secondary to decreased lactose content as compared to other cheeses.

Patients with diarrhea secondary to IBS may benefit from treatment with anti-motility agents, such as loperamide. These medications are best reserved for times that diarrhea is interfering with the child's ability to participate normally in their daily activities. Fiber

Table 4–8.

Medication Dosages

Medication	Dose
Zinc	10 mg/day for age <6 months
	10–20 mg/day for 10–14 days for age >6 months
Metronidazole (Flagyl) for *Clostridium difficile*— po/IV	30 mg/kg/day divided four times daily for 10–14 days
	Adult dose: 250–500 mg three to four times daily for 10–14 days
Vancomycin for *Clostridium difficile*	40–50 mg/kg/day divided four times daily for 7–10 days
	Adult dose: 125 mg/dose every 6 hours for 7–10 days
Metronidazole (Flagyl) for *Giardia* and *Cryptosporidium*	15 mg/kg/day divided three times daily for 5 days
	Adult dose: 250 mg three times daily for 5 days
Nitazoxanide (Alinia) for *Giardia* and *Cryptosporidium*	100 mg twice daily for age 1–3 years for 3 days
	200 mg twice daily for age 4–11 years for 3 days
	500 mg twice daily for age >12 years for 3 days
Lactase	Depends on manufacturer
Loperamide	1 mg three times daily for age 2–6 years (13–20 kg)
	2 mg two times daily for age 6–8 years (20–30 kg)
	2 mg three times daily for age 8–12 years (>30 kg)
	4 mg first dose, and then 2 mg/dose after each stool to maximum of 16 mg/day for age >12 years

supplementation may also decrease stool frequency and improve consistency in some patients with IBS. There are a few studies suggesting that the use of non-absorbable antibiotics (such as rifaximin) or probiotics may have some benefit in the treatment of IBS.[18]

SUMMARY

The differential diagnosis of diarrhea is broad, including functional and organic disorders. A complete clinical history and careful physical exam are important in helping to narrow down the potential causes. Laboratory evaluation including stool studies can provide further information about cause. Referral to a pediatric gastroenterologist should be considered for difficult or persistent cases, and whenever endoscopy is required for diagnosis.

REFERENCES

1. Sellin JH. The pathophysiology of diarrhea. *Clin Transplant.* 2001;15(suppl 4):2–10.
2. Guandalini S, Kahn SA. Acute diarrhea. In: Kleinman RE, Sanderson IR, Goulet O, et al., eds. *Walker's Pediatric Gastrointestinal Disease.* Hamilton: BC Decker, Inc.; 2008:253–258.
3. Viswanathan VK, Hodges K, Hecht G. Enteric infection meets intestinal function: how bacterial pathogens cause diarrhea. *Nat Rev Microbiol.* 2009;7:110–119.
4. Spiller R. Role of motility in chronic diarrhea. *Neurogastroenterol Motil.* 2006;18:1045–1055.
5. Rotavirus surveillance—worldwide. *MMWR.* 2001–2008;57(46):1255–1247.
6. Clark B, McKendrick M. A review of viral gastroenteritis. *Curr Opin Infect Dis.* 2004;17:461–469.
7. Vesikari T, Matson DO, Dennehy P, et al. Safety and efficacy of a pentavalent human-bovine (WC3) reassortant rotavirus vaccine. *N Engl J Med.* 2006;354:23–33.
8. Pickering LK, Baker CJ, Long SS, McMillan JA, eds. *Red Book: 2006 Report of the Committee on Infectious Diseases.* 27th ed. Elk Grove Village, IL: American Academy of Pediatrics; 2006.
9. Ina K, Kusugami K, Ohta M. Bacterial hemorrhagic enterocolitis. *J Gastroenterol.* 2003;38:111–120.
10. Huang DB, White AC. An updated review on *Cryptosporidium* and *Giardia. Gastroenterol Clin N Am.* 2006;35:291–314.
11. Coté GA, Buchman AL. Antibiotic-associated diarrhea. *Expert Opin Drug Saf.* 2006;5(3):361–372.
12. DuPont HL, Garey K, Caeiro JP, Jiang ZD. New advances in *Clostridium difficile* infection: changing epidemiology, diagnosis, treatment and control. *Curr Opin Infect Dis.* 2008;21:500–507.
13. Sherman PM, Mitchell DJ, Cutz E. Neonatal enteropathies: defining the causes of protracted diarrhea of infancy. *J Pediatr Gastroenterol Nutr.* 2004;38:16–26.
14. Keating JP. Chronic diarrhea. *Pediatr Rev.* 2005;26:5–13.
15. Hyman PE, Milla PJ, Benninga MA, Davidson GP, Fleischer DF, Taminiau J. Childhood functional gastrointestinal disorders: neonate/toddler. *Gastroenterology.* 2006;130:1519–1526.
16. Swagerty DL, Walling AD, Klein RM. Lactose intolerance. *Am Fam Physician.* 2002;65:1845–1850.
17. Heyman, MB. Lactose Intolerance in infants, children, and adolescents. *Pediatrics.* 2006;118;1279–1721.
18. McOmber MA, Shulman RJ. Pediatric functional gastrointestinal disorders. *Nutr Clin Pract.* 2008;23: 268–274.
19. Rasquin A, Di Lorenzo C, Forbes D, et al. Childhood functional gastrointestinal disorders: child/adolescent. *Gastroenterology.* 2006;130:1527–1537.
20. Bryant K, McDonald LC. *Clostridium difficile* infections in children. *Pediatr Infect Dis J.* 2009;28:145–146.
21. Armon K, Stephenson T, MacFaul R, Eccleston P, Werneke U, Baumer H. An evidence and consensus based guideline for acute diarrhea management. *Arch Dis Child.* 2001;85:132–142.
22. King CK, Glass R, Bresee JS, Duggan C. Managing acute gastroenteritis among children: oral rehydration,

maintenance, and nutritional therapy. *MMWR*. 2003; 52(RR–16) 1–16. Available at www.cdc.gov/mmwr/pdf/ RR/RR5216.pdf.

23. Lazzerini M, Ronfani L. Oral zinc for treating diarrhea in children. *Cochrane Database Syst Rev*. 2008;(3).

24. World Health Organization. *The Treatment of Diarrhea: A Manual for Physicians and Other Senior Health Workers*. 4th revision. Geneva: WHO Press; 2005:14. Available at http://whqlibdoc.who.int/publications/2005/9241 593180.pdf.

25. Allen SJ, Okoko B, Martinez E, Gregorio G, Dans LF. Probiotics for treating infectious diarrhea. *Cochrane Database Syst Rev*. 2003;(4).

26. Serna A, Boedeker EC. Pathogenesis and treatment of Shiga toxin-producing *Escherichia coli* infections. *Curr Opin Gastroenterol*. 2008;24:38–47.

27. Kelly CP, LaMont JT. *Clostridium difficile*—more difficult than ever. *N Engl J Med*. 2008;359:1932–1940.

28. Bartlett JG. New antimicrobial agents for patients with *Clostridium difficile* infections. *Curr Infect Dis Rep*. 2009;11:21–28.

29. Pillai A, Nelson RL. Probiotics for treatment of *Clostridium difficile*-associated colitis in adults. *Cochrane Database Syst Rev*. 2008;(1).

30. Kleinman RE. Chronic nonspecific diarrhea of childhood. *Nestle Nutr Workshop Ser Pediatr Program*. 2005; 56:73–84.

CHAPTER 5

Constipation

Uma Padhye Phatak and
Dinesh S. Pashankar

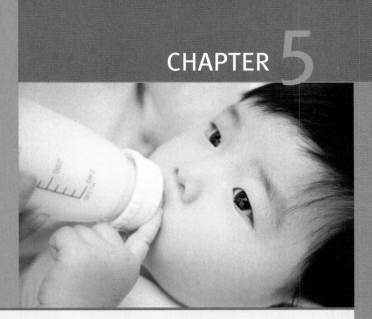

INTRODUCTION

Constipation is a common problem in childhood and is one of the most frequent reasons for a referral to pediatricians. It is termed functional or idiopathic in the absence of any organic etiology. Almost 95% of childhood constipation is functional in nature and only a small minority is due to an identifiable etiology. The diagnosis of functional constipation can usually be made with a detailed history and physical examination. Constipation can often be a chronic problem in children lasting for several months to years. Almost 50% of the patients presenting with constipation during childhood can remain constipated on long-term follow-up. Long-standing constipation and withholding often result into fecal incontinence. Constipation and incontinence can lead to low self-esteem and behavior problems, causing significant stress and anxiety to the patient and the parents. The therapeutic approach involves patient education, disimpaction, laxative therapy, and behavioral modification. The treatment typically lasts for months to years and relapses are common. A successful treatment outcome requires a team approach involving the patient, family, nurses, pediatricians, and the specialists. In this chapter, we will review the diagnostic evaluation and therapeutic approach to functional constipation.

DEFINITION

The term constipation is often defined differently by different parents. Constipation may mean infrequent bowel movements, hard stool consistency, large stool size, painful defecation, or voluntary withholding bowel movements. To most parents, constipation usually means infrequent bowel movements. It is important to remember that stool frequency varies in children with age.[1] Normally, the initial bowel movement is within the first 24 hours of birth. Delayed passage of stool should raise the suspicion for Hirschsprung's disease. Infants have approximately four stools per day during the first week of life. The frequency also differs between breast-fed and formula-fed infants. Some normal breast-fed infants can have only one stool per week. The stool frequency gradually changes to one to two stools per day by the age of 4 years. An adult defecation pattern is achieved after 4 years of age. The decrease in stool frequency is associated with an increase in stool size and prolonged gastrointestinal transit. The majority of children are toilet trained by 4 years of age. Girls tend to achieve toilet training slightly earlier than boys. *Encopresis* or *fecal incontinence* is defined as involuntary passage of stools after the developmental age of 4 years.

The North American Society for Pediatric Gastroenterology and Nutrition (NASPGHAN) defines constipation as a delay or difficulty in defecation, present for 2 or more weeks and sufficient to cause significant distress to the patient.[1]

The 2006 Rome III criteria for childhood functional gastrointestinal disorders describe the diagnostic criteria of functional constipation for neonate/toddler and for child/adolescent age groups as shown in Table 5–1.[2,3]

EPIDEMIOLOGY

Constipation is a common problem in children. The worldwide prevalence of childhood constipation in the general population ranges from 0.7% to 29.6%.[4] In a study done in Iowa, the prevalence was found to be as high as 23% in the pediatric primary care clinics. The

Table 5–1.

Diagnosis of Functional Constipation by Rome III criteria[2,3]

Older children/adolescents (>4 years of age)
Must include 2 months of two or more of the following occurring at least once per week:

- Two or fewer stools in the toilet per week
- At least one episode of fecal incontinence per week
- History of retentive posturing or excessive volitional stool retention
- History of painful or hard bowel movements
- Presence of a large fecal mass in the rectum
- History of large-diameter stools that may obstruct the toilet

Infants/toddlers (<4 years of age)
Must include 1 month of at least two of the following:

- Two or fewer defecations per week
- At least one episode per week of incontinence after the acquisition of toilet skills
- History of excessive stool retention
- History of painful or hard bowel movements
- Presence of a large fecal mass in the rectum
- History of large-diameter stools that may obstruct the toilet

Accompanying symptoms may include irritability, decreased appetite, and/or early satiety. The accompanying symptoms disappear immediately following passage of a large stool

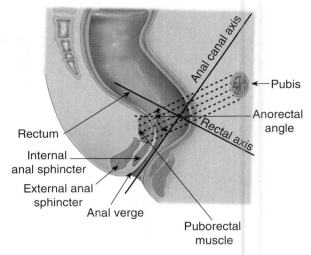

FIGURE 5–1 ■ Anatomy of the anorectal region.

prevalence of fecal incontinence was approximately 4.4% in these patients.[5] Constipation accounts for up to 25% of visits to pediatric gastroenterologists, and therefore causes a significant financial burden on the health care system. Children with constipation use more health care services amounting to a cost of an additional $3.9 billion/year as compared to children without constipation.[6]

The incidence of functional constipation appears to be rising over the last few decades. The reason for this increase is not well known, but may be due to changing patterns in toilet training, diminished dietary fiber intake, lack of exercise, or better access to health care services and improved diagnosis. Socioeconomic factors, such as lower income and family education, put children at risk for developing constipation. Another factor that appears to play a role in functional constipation is diet. A low-fiber diet and obesity are associated with an increased risk of functional constipation.[7]

PATHOGENESIS

It is important to explain the physiology of defecation and the pathogenesis of withholding and incontinence to parents. Figure 5–1 shows the anatomy of the anorectal region. The anorectal angle is formed by the internal and external anal sphincters with the puborectalis muscle. The angle is approximately 85–105° at rest. Normally, entry of stool into the rectum leads to relaxation of the internal anal sphincter. This is known as the rectoanal inhibitory reflex, and is an involuntary mechanism. The stool then passes into the anal canal, creating an urge to defecate which can be voluntarily suppressed until completed in a socially acceptable setting. Defecation begins with a voluntary increase in the intra-abdominal pressure and relaxation of the puborectalis and the levator ani muscles, straightening of the anorectal angle, allowing passage of the bowel movement through the voluntarily relaxed external anal sphincter.

Functional constipation is usually triggered by an experience of painful defecation. This pain leads to avoidance of defecation and voluntary stool-withholding behavior. Contraction of the pelvic muscles can prevent a bowel movement by pushing the stool proximally. The rectum can eventually accommodate this increasing stool mass. The colon absorbs fluid from the retained feces, causing dry and hard stools. Furthermore, these dry, hard stools may cause anal fissures or tears resulting in more pain during defecation. This vicious cycle continues to result in long-standing functional constipation. With time, the retained fecal mass leads to rectal distention and loss of the ability to voluntarily contract the external anal sphincter. Eventually, rectal distention also leads to decreased rectal sensation and therefore a decreased urge to defecate. Liquid stools from the proximal colon seep around this mass to cause fecal incontinence.

Constipation can begin at any time, although children are most vulnerable during certain developmental stages. Infants who are being weaned from breast milk to cereals and solids are at risk for developing constipation. Most commonly children who are being

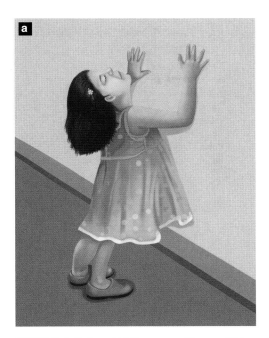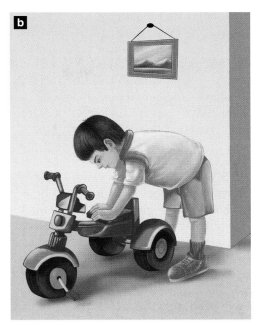

FIGURE 5–2 ■ (a and b) Common positions a child may take while struggling to retain bowel movement.

pressured into toilet training are likely to develop constipation. The American Academy of Pediatrics therefore strongly recommends that parents avoid forcing their child into toilet training.[8] Toilet training should be initiated only when the child shows interest. Older children may avoid bathrooms at school due to unhygienic conditions, lack of privacy, or even bullying, which puts them at risk for constipation.

CLINICAL PRESENTATION

A thorough history and examination are recommended in the evaluation of functional constipation. The first step is to find out what the family means when using the term constipation. The history should therefore include the frequency, size, and consistency of the stools. A common presenting symptom in children with functional constipation is abdominal pain. In one study, chronic constipation was found to be the most frequent cause of acute abdominal pain.[9] Toddlers may withhold stool and demonstrate typical posturing in the form of stiffening of the body and clenching of the buttocks. Children may assume a variety of positions and make bizarre movements while struggling to retain the bowel movement (Figure 5–2). The physician should determine the presence and frequency of fecal soiling. It is important to be aware that parents of children with fecal incontinence might seek medical attention for what they think is diarrhea. Table 5–2 shows common gastrointestinal symptoms and signs of functional constipation.

Children with constipation may also present with extraintestinal manifestations. Urinary tract symptoms may include frequency, enuresis, and infections. The prevalence of urinary incontinence is also higher in children with constipation.[5] When constipation causes fecal incontinence, depression and low self-esteem are common, and therefore obtaining a psychosocial and behavioral history is crucial. These children often have lower health-related quality of life scores due to lower emotional and social functioning.[10]

The history obtained should review the previous use of laxatives and the results of these treatments. The physician should inquire about intake of dairy products,

Table 5–2.

Symptoms and Signs of Functional Constipation

Symptoms
Infrequent bowel movements
Painful bowel movements
Hard stools
Abdominal pain
Fecal soiling
Blood in stools
Retentive posturing

Signs
Abdominal distention
Abdominal tenderness
Abdominal fecal mass
Anal fissure
Rectal fecal mass

such as cheese, which can predispose to constipation. The child should be asked whether he avoids using bathrooms at school. A family history of conditions such as celiac disease or thyroid disorders should raise the suspicion of organic causes of constipation. The physician should inquire about the family structure and dynamics as the family support is an important factor in the overall successful outcome of the patient.

Examination

A careful examination of all systems should be performed in a child who presents with constipation. Particular attention should be paid to the height and weight of the child. Poor growth may suggest the presence of organic conditions such as hypothyroidism or celiac disease. An abdominal exam should be performed to look for tenderness, distention, or mass. A rectal examination is recommended at the initial visit. It is helpful to explain the procedure to the child to decrease his anxiety. Rectal examination should be avoided in case of an uncooperative child, presence of neutropenia, or sexual abuse. A rectal examination might be difficult in certain circumstances such as with obese children. The perianal area should be first examined for presence of fecal soiling, anal fissures, position of the anus, and perianal sensation. Digital rectal examination can assess the presence, size, and consistency of stools in the rectum, the anal canal tone, and the size of the rectal vault. An empty rectal vault with explosive passage of stool on rectal exam is strongly suggestive of Hirschsprung's disease. The stool should be examined for presence of occult blood by guaiac testing. The lumbosacral spine should be examined for the presence of a sacral dimple or tuft of hair. An examination of the tone, strength, and

> ### Box 5–1. When to Refer to a Specialist
>
> ■ Constipation in age <3 months
> ■ Delayed passage of meconium
> ■ Empty rectal ampulla
> ■ Explosive passage of stool on rectal exam
> ■ Intermittent bloody diarrhea
> ■ Failure to thrive
> ■ Abnormal neurological signs and symptoms
> ■ Behavioral problems
> ■ Failure of conventional therapy

reflexes is also important to rule out any spinal cord lesions.

It is especially important to look for the presence of any symptoms or signs that might suggest an organic etiology. A referral to a specialist should be considered if the child has any of the 'red flag' clinical features shown in Box 5–1. In most cases, a referral should be made to a pediatric gastroenterologist when the conventional treatment fails or when there are features suggestive of Hirschsprung's disease. Sometimes a referral to a neurologist or a psychiatrist may be necessary if there are neurological or behavioral problems.

DIFFERENTIAL DIAGNOSIS

The diagnosis of functional constipation is usually straightforward. Almost 95% of childhood constipation is functional in nature. The remaining 5% can be attributed to wide variety of conditions, as shown in Table 5–3. Many of these etiologies are obvious by history and examination, and many have other specific symptoms besides constipation.

Table 5–3.

Organic Causes of Constipation

Anatomic malformations	Neuropathic conditions	Drugs
Imperforate anus	Meningomylocele	Opiates
Anteriorly displaced anus	Spinal cord tumor	Phenobarbital
Anal stenosis	Spinal cord trauma	Anticholinergics
Pelvic mass	Tethered cord	Sucralfate
	Cerebral palsy	Antacids
Systemic disorders		Antidepressants
Celiac disease	**Intestinal nerve or muscle**	Antihypertensives
Hypothyroidism	**disorders**	Chemotherapeutic agents
Hypercalcemia	Hirschsprung's disease	
Hypokalemia	Intestinal neuronal dysplasia	**Others**
Diabetes mellitus	Prune belly syndrome	Lead toxicity
Diabetes insipidus	Gastroschisis	Botulism
Cystic fibrosis		Vitamin D toxicity

Two other functional disorders should be considered in the differential diagnosis of functional constipation. *Infant dyschezia* presents as excessive crying and straining for at least 10 minutes that is followed by the passage of stool.[3] These babies do not have any underlying medical problems. This presentation is thought to be secondary to incoordination between abdominal muscle contraction and pelvic floor relaxation. These children outgrow this problem with age and do not require any therapy. The physician should provide reassurance to the parents.

Another condition is *non-retentive fecal incontinence,* which presents as intentional, socially inappropriate passage of stools at least once per month in children over 4 years of age.[2] These children do not have constipation, fecal retention, or any other medical problem. Laxatives are generally not recommended and therapy includes education and a toilet training program using behavior modification techniques.

DIAGNOSIS

Functional constipation can usually be diagnosed with a thorough history and physical examination using criteria as shown in Table 5–1.[2,3] Diagnostic tests are usually not required in most children with functional constipation. However, further testing is necessary when an organic etiology is suspected.

A plain abdominal X-ray is recommended in the practice guidelines by the NASPGHAN committee when there is doubt about the presence of constipation.[1] This may be obtained in case of an unreliable history or examination as in an obese child. An abdominal film is also useful when rectal examination is not performed due to the child's refusal, or when rectal examination might be traumatic, as in a history of sexual abuse. The abdominal X-ray is used to assess the amount and location of stools in the colon. Figure 5–3 shows an abdominal film showing significant fecal retention in the rectosigmoid colon and scattered stools in the entire colon. A plain X-ray of the lower spine might also be useful in children with fecal incontinence and urinary symptoms to look for spinal deformities.

Children who do not seem to respond to conventional treatment should have blood tests to look for organic etiologies such as hypercalcemia, hypothyroidism, and celiac disease prior to a referral to the specialist.[1] These tests should include serum calcium, thyroid function tests, and tissue transglutaminase with total serum IgA. A lead level should be obtained in children with anemia or pica.

Infants suspected of having Hirschsprung's disease should be referred to a pediatric gastroenterologist, and should have an evaluation consisting of a barium enema,

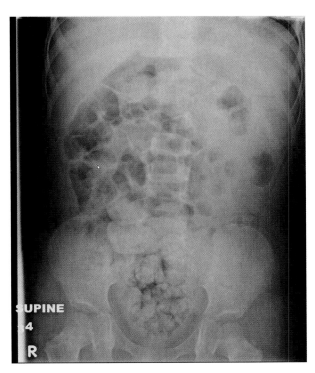

FIGURE 5–3 ■ Plain abdominal film showing fecal impaction.

rectal suction biopsy, or a full-thickness biopsy. Anorectal manometry may be useful in children with suspected Hirschsprung's disease or chronic intestinal pseudo-obstruction. Colonic transit time studies are usually used for research purposes and not in clinical settings.

TREATMENT

The goals of constipation treatment are to establish a regular defecation pattern, eliminate symptoms of pain, stop associated incontinence, and prevent relapses. The clinical practice guidelines by the NASPGHAN committee state that the management of constipation should involve a stepwise approach.[1] This approach consists of education, disimpaction, maintenance stool-softening therapy by diet and medications, behavioral modification, and regular follow-up. Figure 5–4 provides a simple algorithm of the therapeutic approach to a child with constipation.

Education

The physician should have a thorough discussion with the child and caregivers about the physiology of normal defecation. The pathogenesis of functional constipation and associated fecal incontinence should be emphasized. Drawings and diagrams may be used to better communicate with the family. Age-appropriate

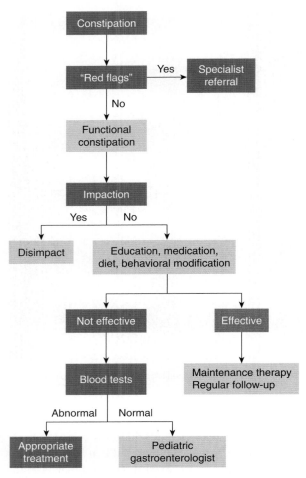

FIGURE 5–4 ■ Therapeutic approach to constipation.

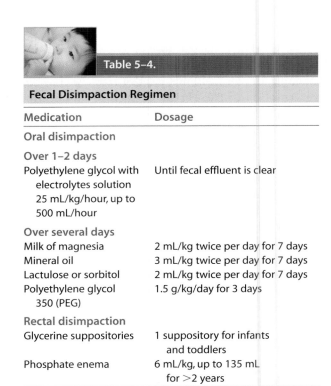

Table 5–4.	
Fecal Disimpaction Regimen	
Medication	Dosage
Oral disimpaction	
Over 1–2 days	
Polyethylene glycol with electrolytes solution 25 mL/kg/hour, up to 500 mL/hour	Until fecal effluent is clear
Over several days	
Milk of magnesia	2 mL/kg twice per day for 7 days
Mineral oil	3 mL/kg twice per day for 7 days
Lactulose or sorbitol	2 mL/kg twice per day for 7 days
Polyethylene glycol 350 (PEG)	1.5 g/kg/day for 3 days
Rectal disimpaction	
Glycerine suppositories	1 suppository for infants and toddlers
Phosphate enema	6 mL/kg, up to 135 mL for >2 years

terms should be used when explaining the problem to the child. It should be stressed that incontinence is an involuntary process due to fecal retention and that the child has no direct control over it. Improvement will result from adherence to the treatment regimen. Knowing this usually alleviates some of the conflict that typically exists between the child and his parents. The treatment plan should be discussed in detail. It is most important for the physician to maintain a positive and a supportive attitude. It should be stressed to the family that the problem is often chronic and relapses can occur, requiring long-term treatment for months to years. Ongoing education and constant support by the physician during regular follow-up visits are necessary to keep the patient and the family committed to their treatment plan.

Disimpaction

Fecal disimpaction can be achieved by the oral or rectal route. Disimpaction can be performed over a short duration (1–2 days) or a longer duration (1 week) as

shown in Table 5–4. The choice of therapy is primarily based on how quickly disimpaction needs to be achieved and on physician preference. Providing laxatives orally is non-invasive, but can take longer than other methods to achieve results. Enemas are invasive, unpleasant, and occasionally dangerous, but result in faster disimpaction.

Rapid disimpaction by the enteral route can be achieved by using a large volume of polyethylene glycol–electrolyte solution. The lavage is typically continued until the effluent is clear and may require up to 24 hours. This approach is effective, but few children are able to actually drink the solution, requiring hospitalization of the patient for nasogastric tube placement. Continuous lavage can also lead to nausea, vomiting, abdominal pain, and abdominal distention. Provision of intravenous fluids is required for prolonged disimpaction. Fortunately, polyethylene glycol 3350 without electrolytes (PEG) has been shown to be a palatable and effective oral therapy. A dose of 1.5 g/kg/day administered orally for 3 days has been found to be very effective for fecal disimpaction without causing significant side effects.[11] Other laxatives such as milk of magnesia, mineral oil, and lactulose have been used for disimpaction in doses higher than usual doses of maintenance therapy.

Although enemas and suppositories may lead to quicker disimpaction, these are unpleasant, and may aggravate the child's fear of defecation. Glycerine suppositories are convenient to use in infants and are safe and provide gentle stimulation and lubrication. Phosphate enemas are appropriate only for older children.

Table 5–5.

Commonly Used Laxatives in Children

Medication	Dosage	Proprietary Name
Osmotic laxatives		
Magnesium hydroxide	1–3 mL/kg/day	Milk of magnesia
Lactulose	1–3 mL/kg/day	Cephulac, Duphalac, Enulose
Polyethylene glycol 3350 (PEG)	0.8 g/kg/day (dilute 17 g/240 mL of liquid)	Glycolax, Miralax
Lubricant laxatives		
Mineral oil	1–3 mL/kg/day	Agoral Plain, Kondremul
Stimulant laxatives		
Senna	2.5–15 mL/day (short-term use only)	Ex-Lax, Senokot, Senna-gen
Bisacodyl	5–15 mg/day	Bisco-Lax, Dulcolax

Although these are usually well tolerated, they can rarely cause hyperphosphatemia and hypocalcemia, leading to convulsions, coma, and even death. The risk of these adverse effects is increased in younger children and hence phosphate enemas are not recommended for children less than 2 years of age. In older children, avoiding the use of consecutive enemas will minimize these risks.

Maintenance Therapy

Dietary intervention

Adequate intake of fluids and fiber is important in children with constipation. The recommended dietary intake of fiber in children older than 2 years of age is age plus 5 g/day. Addition of fiber such as glucomannan in a dose of 5 g/day to laxative therapy has been shown to be beneficial in children with constipation.[12] Cow's milk intolerance can lead to chronic constipation and elimination of cow's milk protein from diet has been shown to be effective in some children with intractable constipation. Children who have other associated conditions such as atopic disorders or perianal lesions are likely to show significant response to this form of dietary change.

Laxative Therapy

The goal of the therapy is for the child to have one to two soft bowel movements per day and to prevent relapse of constipation. There are many laxatives available for children. Laxatives can be divided into osmotic, lubricant, and stimulant types. Osmotic agents absorb water in the intestinal lumen and make stools soft. Lubricant laxatives facilitate the passage of stools through the colon. Stimulant laxatives induce colonic contractions and expel stools.

The list of commonly used laxatives and their doses is shown in Table 5–5.

In many children, the initial dose may need adjustment and parents should be taught to titrate the dose to achieve the aim of one to two soft, painless bowel movements per day. In children with chronic constipation, laxative therapy is required for months to years. Often parents will stop therapy prematurely after few months of improvement or because of concern about addiction to laxatives. Many of these children are likely to have relapses of constipation. Gradual weaning of laxatives can be tried in children who have been doing well for at least 6 months. An additional requirement is that they must have developed a reliable bowel habit, without reliance on reminders and with no evidence of reluctance to use the toilet.

Osmotic Laxatives

The most commonly used osmotic laxatives are magnesium hydroxide, lactulose, and PEG. These are generally safe, effective, and well tolerated when used over a long term.

Magnesium hydroxide (milk of magnesia)

Magnesium hydroxide is an osmotic laxative. It also acts by stimulating cholecystokinin release, increasing intestinal secretion and motility. This agent has been used successfully for both disimpaction and maintenance therapy.[13] Magnesium hydroxide is generally safe; however, it should be used with caution in patients with renal impairment and in infants. In these children, it can rarely cause hypermagnesemia. Magnesium hydroxide has a chalky taste, which many children find unpleasant, often resulting in poor compliance.

Lactulose

Lactulose is a synthetic non-digestible disaccharide containing galactose and fructose. Because it is not absorbed by the small bowel, it acts as an osmotic agent. It has been effectively used for long-term maintenance therapy in children.[1] Higher doses of lactulose for 3–7 days can be used for successful fecal disimpaction. Since lactulose is fermented by colonic bacteria to yield fatty acids, hydrogen, and carbon dioxide, children taking it may experience flatulence, bloating, nausea, and abdominal cramps. Some children may find this agent too sweet to take on a long-term basis. Because bacterial action can release free galactose, it should not be used in patients with galactosemia.

Polyethylene glycol 3350

PEG is a recent addition to the list of available laxatives. It is a non-toxic, highly soluble compound that is minimally absorbed in the gastrointestinal tract and, unlike lactulose, is not fermented by colonic bacteria. It is available as a virtually tasteless and odorless powder that can be dissolved in a variety of beverages. PEG therapy has been shown to improve stool frequency and soiling frequency in children with constipation and fecal incontinence.[14] The effective dose is around 0.8 g/kg/day although the range is quite wide (0.2–1.4 g/kg/day). Because PEG can be mixed in a beverage of the patient's choice and is virtually undetectable, long-term daily compliance is reported to be as high as 90% by parents. PEG is as effective as lactulose and milk of magnesia, but adherence to therapy is better.[13] It is generally well tolerated and has no major adverse effects.[15] Minor side effects include transient dose-dependent diarrhea (10%) and bloating (6%). PEG therapy has also been successfully and safely used in constipated children younger than 2 years of age.[16]

Lubricant Laxatives

Mineral oil

Mineral oil is derived from petroleum and acts as a lubricant laxative in children. This agent coats and lubricates stools, thereby reducing colonic absorption of fecal water and facilitating evacuation. It has been used as an effective long-term maintenance therapy for chronic constipation with incontinence and also for fecal disimpaction. Aspiration of mineral oil can cause severe lipoid pneumonia and it is contraindicated in infants and children with neurological impairment due to the possible risk of aspiration.[1] Mineral oil has an unpleasant texture, leading to compliance problems, and tends to leak from the anus, causing staining of clothing. For all of these reasons, it is less commonly used than the osmotic agents.

Stimulant Laxatives

Senna

Senna is a stimulant oral laxative from a group of drugs called anthraquinones. Long-term use of senna can cause adverse effects such as abdominal pain, melanosis coli, idiosyncratic hepatitis, and hypertrophic osteoarthropathy.[1] Senna can be used intermittently, but is not recommended for continuous long-term use in children.

Bisacodyl

Bisacodyl is a stimulant laxative and a polyphenolic derivative. It is available as a suppository for rectal use and as a tablet for oral use. Bisacodyl can be used as a short-term rescue therapy. It is not recommended for maintenance therapy as its chronic use can be associated with significant adverse effects such as abdominal pain, hypokalemia, renal mucosal abnormalities, and urolithiasis.

Newer Laxative

Lubiprostone

Lubiprostone is a novel selective chloride channel-2 activator that increases intestinal fluid secretion, and also increases gut motility. It has a very low systemic bioavailability. Lubiprostone has been effectively used for the treatment of chronic constipation and irritable bowel syndrome with constipation in adults.[17] It is usually well tolerated in a dose of 24 μg twice a day. The adverse effects are mild and include nausea and diarrhea. At present lubiprostone is approved by the FDA for use in adults only. Studies are currently underway to assess the role of lubiprostone in children.

Which Laxative to Use?

Because childhood constipation is usually a chronic problem, laxative therapy needs to be extended until the symptoms resolve completely. The choice of the medication depends on the child's preference, safety, cost, ease of administration, and the practitioner's experience. The actual choice of medication is not as important as the optimal dose and child's continuous compliance with the treatment regimen. It is also important to adjust the dose as required to achieve painless soft stools and avoiding diarrhea.

Osmotic and lubricant laxatives such as mineral oil, magnesium hydroxide, lactulose, and PEG are recommended for long-term use in children. PEG is available as a tasteless powder that can be mixed in any beverage. Its palatability and lack of significant adverse effects result in much greater acceptability by children and parents, compared to other laxatives. However, from a cost perspective, mineral oil and magnesium hydroxide are cheaper than PEG and lactulose. Stimulant laxatives, such as senna or bisacodyl, should only be used intermittently.

Behavioral Modification

Behavioral modification is a vital component of therapy, particularly for children with constipation and fecal incontinence. Physicians should stress the importance of regular toilet sitting for up to 5 minutes, three to four times a day after meals (when increased colonic motility provides assistance), to establish normal bowel habits. Toilet sitting should be done on a daily basis including weekends and holidays. The child should be encouraged to have a bowel movement at these sessions. Cooperation with toilet sitting and taking medications should be rewarded with praise and other age-appropriate positive reinforcers. Successful passage of stool on the toilet should result in additional positive reinforcement. A supportive attitude by the family is essential for a successful outcome, and therefore punishment (negative reinforcement) of lapses should be avoided. Children with constipation should also be allowed unrestricted toilet access at home and at school.

A combination of laxative therapy and behavioral modification has been found to be more effective than laxative therapy or behavioral modification alone for the treatment of children with incontinence.[18] Therefore, behavioral modification therapy is as important as laxative therapy for the optimal outcome in children with chronic constipation and incontinence.

PROGNOSIS

With a well-designed treatment plan, the majority of patients with functional constipation without incontinence will experience significant improvement. Relapses are common and children will often require chronic therapy for months to years. Constipation with fecal incontinence is a much more frustrating and chronic problem. Although the majority respond to treatment, approximately one-third of children can continue to have problems with constipation and incontinence beyond puberty.[19] Even with regular intensive treatment with laxatives and behavior modification, approximately only 50% of the children with constipation and incontinence will recover at 1 year. This stresses the chronic nature of this problem in children and the need for ongoing supportive management.

SUMMARY

Childhood constipation is one of the most common problems seen in pediatric practice. Organic causes of constipation are rare in children but should be ruled out by careful evaluation. Functional constipation with fecal incontinence is associated with significant physical morbidity and psychosocial stress in children. The chronic nature of the problem and frequent relapses make functional constipation a difficult and challenging problem. A physician should plan a systematic therapeutic approach involving patient education, appropriate use of laxatives, and behavior therapy for children with functional constipation. Long-term treatment is required in many children and patient compliance with medications and behavioral modification is essential for a successful outcome.

REFERENCES

1. Evaluation and treatment of constipation in infants and children: recommendations of the North American Society for Pediatric Gastroenterology, Hepatology, and Nutrition. *J Pediatr Gastroenterol Nutr.* 2006;43:e1–e13.
2. Rasquin A, Di Lorenzo C, Forbes D, et al. Childhood functional gastrointestinal disorders: child/adolescent. *Gastroenterology.* 2006;130:1527–1537.
3. Hyman PE, Milla PJ, Benninga MA, et al. Childhood functional gastrointestinal disorders: neonate/toddler. *Gastroenterology.* 2006;130:1519–1526.
4. Van den Berg MM, Benninga MA, Di Lorenzo C. Epidemiology of childhood constipation: a systematic review. *Am J Gastroenterol.* 2006;101:2401–2409.
5. Loening-Baucke V. Prevalence rates for constipation and faecel and urinary incontinence. *Arch Dis Child.* 2007;92: 486–489.
6. Liem O, Harman J, Benninga M, et al. Health utilization and cost impact of childhood constipation in the United States. *J Pediatr.* 2009;154:258–262.
7. Pashankar DS, Loening-Baucke V. Increased prevalence of obesity in children with functional constipation evaluated in an academic medical center. *Pediatrics.* 2005;116:e377–e380.
8. Toilet training methods, clinical interventions, and recommendations. American Academy of Pediatrics. *Pediatrics.* 1999;103:1359–1368.
9. Loening-Baucke V, Swidsinski A. Constipation as a cause of acute abdominal pain in children. *J Pediatr.* 2007;151: 666–669.
10. Bongers ME, van Dijk M, Benninga MA, et al. Health related quality of life in children with constipation associated fecal incontinence. *J Pediatr.* 2009;154:749–753.
11. Youssef NN, Peters JM, Henderson W, et al. Dose response of PEG 3350 for the treatment of childhood fecal impaction. *J Pediatr.* 2002;141:410–414.
12. Loening-Baucke V, Miele E, Staiano A. Fiber (glucomannan) is beneficial in the treatment of childhood constipation. *Pediatrics.* 2004;113:e258–e264.
13. Loening-Baucke V, Pashankar DS. A randomized, prospective, comparison study of polyethylene glycol without electrolytes and milk of magnesia for children with constipation and fecal incontinence. *Pediatrics.* 2006;118:528–535.

14. Pashankar DS, Bishop WP. Efficacy and optimal dose of daily polyethylene glycol 3350 for treatment of constipation and encopresis in children. *J Pediatr.* 2001;139:428–432.

15. Pashankar DS, Loening-Baucke V, Bishop W. Safety of polyethylene glycol 3350 for the treatment of chronic constipation in children. *Arch Pediatr Adolesc Med.* 2003;157:661–664.

16. Loening-Baucke V, Krishna R, Pashankar DS. Polyethylene glycol 3350 without electrolytes for the treatment of functional constipation in infants and toddlers. *J Pediatr Gastroenterol Nutr.* 2004;39:536–539.

17. Drossman DA, Chey WD, Johanson JF, et al. Clinical trial: lubiprostone in patients with constipation-associated irritable bowel syndrome-results of two randomized, placebo-controlled studies. *Aliment Pharmacol Ther.* 2009;29:329–341.

18. Brazzelli M, Griffiths P. Behavioral and cognitive interventions with or without other treatments for defaecation disorders in children. *Cochrane Database Syst Rev.* 2001;4:CD002240.

19. Van Ginkel R, Reitsma JB, Buller HA, et al. Childhood constipation: longitudinal follow-up beyond puberty. Gastroenterology 2003;125:357–363.

CHAPTER 6

Gastrointestinal Bleeding

Eyad Hanna

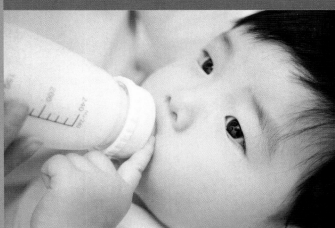

INTRODUCTION

Gastrointestinal (GI) bleeding can be occult (not readily visible) or overt. This chapter will focus on overt GI bleeding that is acute or subacute. Separate chapters (e.g., Chapters 13 and 16) will cover aspects of chronic or occult GI blood loss in more detail. The source of visible blood in stool or vomit may be from the upper GI (UGI) tract, lower GI (LGI) tract, extraintestinal (e.g., swallowed blood from a nosebleed), or an exogenous substance (e.g., red-colored foods). Regardless of the source, obvious blood from the GI tract tends to be a very distressing problem for patients and their families that quickly bring them to medical attention. GI bleeding can be serious and life threatening. Thankfully, serious GI bleeding is uncommon in the pediatric age group and the problem often resolves without specific intervention. The key to approaching a patient with GI bleeding is a rapid assessment of the severity of bleeding and hemodynamic status of the child. Given the nature of the content, this chapter will focus on differential diagnosis, diagnostic approach, and treatment based on clinical presentation: hematemesis or coffee ground emesis, hematochezia, and melena.

DEFINITIONS

UGI bleeding is defined as a source proximal to the ligament of Treitz (where the duodenum meets the jejunum). *LGI bleeding* is from a source distal to the ligament of Treitz (see Figure 6–1).

Hematemesis refers to vomiting bright red blood, usually indicating fairly brisk bleeding. *Coffee ground emesis* usually occurs with slower bleeding and coagulation of blood after exposure to gastric acid. *Melena* refers to stools that are jet black and tarry, and often have a distinctive foul odor. Melena occurs when intes-

tinal bacteria have time to oxidize heme to hematin, usually indicating a relatively slow bleed proximal to the cecum. *Hematochezia* refers to bright red or maroon blood in stools, usually from a colonic bleed but can occur with high-volume UGI bleeding with rapid transit time. Bleeding, if severe, can also become symptomatic (dizziness, syncope, pallor, tachycardia, and hypotension) before the passage of a bloody stool.

PATHOGENESIS

The pathogenesis of true GI bleeding varies greatly by etiology. A few broad categories of pathology underlie most causes of bleeding. Vascular anomalies (e.g., arteriovenous malformations or hemangiomas), collateral vessel formation (e.g., esophageal varices), or erosion of the intestinal mucosa (e.g., inflammation, ulceration, sloughing, and perforation) bring blood vessels in close proximity to the intestinal lumen and may make them prone to rupture. Acute or chronic vascular congestion, thrombosis, and/or ischemia may also lead to bleeding. Any illness (most often viral gastroenteritis) that causes persistent retching and vomiting can cause bleeding from mucosal tears in the lower esophagus and upper stomach (Mallory–Weiss tears) and/or broken capillaries in the gastric mucosa (emetogenic gastropathy).

KEY INITIAL STEPS IN THE EVALUATION OF GI BLEEDING

Determine the Severity of the Bleeding

Different diagnoses may be suggested by not only presenting signs and symptoms, but also patient age. Although the history is paramount, the initial history

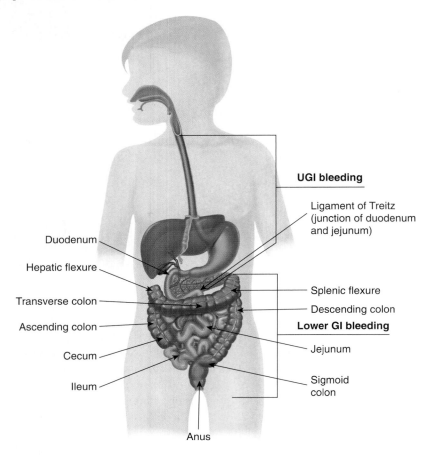

Duodenum

Hepatic flexure

Transverse colon

Ascending colon

Cecum

Ileum

UGI bleeding

Ligament of Treitz
(junction of duodenum
and jejunum)

Splenic flexure

Descending colon

Lower GI bleeding

Jejunum

Sigmoid
colon

Anus

FIGURE 6–1 ■ Position of ligament of Treitz. Bleeding above this point is considered upper GI and below is lower GI.

should be very brief followed by an assessment of vital signs and hemodynamic status. If it is obvious the child is ill or there is a large amount of bleeding, it is appropriate to initiate supportive management before completing the history and evaluation. Tachycardia is a sensitive indicator of blood loss but orthostasis tends to be more useful in assessment of hemodynamic status and response to therapy. Pulse and blood pressure should be obtained while supine. The patient then stands for at least 1 minute and measurements are repeated while standing. This must be done in a consistent manner (supporting staff may not do this correctly and specific instructions are a good idea). A pulse increase over 20 beats/minute *or* systolic blood pressure decrease of 10 mm Hg indicates intravascular volume depletion. Children have incredible reserve and although pulse may increase significantly, blood pressure may be stable in spite of severe blood loss. Dizziness, lethargy, pallor, diaphoresis, and nausea often accompany significant blood loss.

The unstable or actively bleeding patient should be resuscitated. Venous access is secured with two large-bore IV catheters or central venous access. Initial blood work should include type and cross to expedite transfusion if necessary. Key laboratory data include hemoglobin,

platelets, coagulation studies, and complete metabolic profile (see Table 6–1). The goal is to stabilize the patient for controlled evaluation. Transfer to the intensive care unit and/or a facility with surgical and endoscopic services is often warranted (see Box 6–1). Surgical consultation should be obtained early for patients who are hemodynamically unstable, especially if they have

Table 6–1.

Appropriate Considerations for Initial Evaluation of GI Bleeding

Guaiac testing: vomit, NG aspirate, stool

Apt–Downey Test (if suspect swallowed maternal blood): bright red vomit or stool

CBC with differential

PT/PTT

Complete metabolic profile: transaminases, albumin, electrolytes, BUN, creatinine

Blood type and crossmatch

Abdominal obstructive series (includes upright or decubitus films)

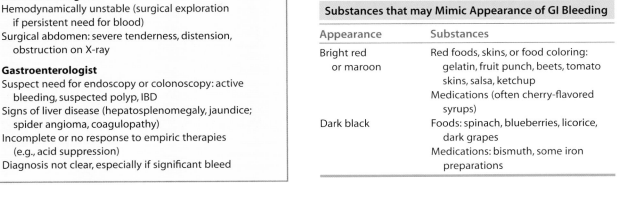

Table 6–2.	
Substances that may Mimic Appearance of GI Bleeding	
Appearance	Substances
Bright red or maroon	Red foods, skins, or food coloring: gelatin, fruit punch, beets, tomato skins, salsa, ketchup
	Medications (often cherry-flavored syrups)
Dark black	Foods: spinach, blueberries, licorice, dark grapes
	Medications: bismuth, some iron preparations

abdominal tenderness, distension, fever, or signs of obstruction on upright or decubitus abdominal films. Surgical exploration is indicated for signs of obstruction or ongoing blood loss (i.e., patient remains unstable requiring frequent blood transfusion, $\geq$85 mL/kg).[1,2]

For stable and/or asymptomatic patients, a thorough history is likely to be the most important part of the assessment. This should include a focused family history based on presentation (inflammatory bowel disease, atopic disease, polyposis or early colon cancer, bleeding disorders, and Hirschsprung's disease). For bloody diarrhea, recent antibiotic use and infectious exposures should be queried. Questions in plain English yield the most detailed information. Instead of asking about blood or bile in vomit, it is often more helpful to ask if they have seen anything that looks pink, red, bright yellow, bright green, or like coffee grounds. Similarly, for stool, ask about bright red, dark red (maroon), or tarry (jet) black color. Anxious patients or families often overestimate the amount of blood but a general approximation can be made. The severity of the bleeding is often reflected in the clinical presentation and hemodynamic status of the patient. In a clinically stable patient, minimal amounts of red blood or coffee grounds usually indicate slow bleeding (although large-volume bleeds can present with coffee ground vomit). Clots of blood or red blood mixed in the vomit may indicate higher volume bleeds. Melena may be slow or brisk bleeding depending on location and transit time. Large amounts of bright red blood in stool or pure blood usually are high-volume bleeds.

Determine if it is Blood

Exogenous substances may mimic blood. Identifying sources of confusion can appropriately redirect evaluation and management or avoid concern altogether (see Table 6–2). A commonly used antibiotic, cefdinir (Omnicef), may turn stool red causing concern. This is distinguished from *Clostridium difficile* colitis by the lack of ill appearance, fever, abdominal pain, and diarrhea.

Guaiac testing can usually determine if what we are seeing is blood or an exogenous substance. Guaiac is a natural resin that turns blue when oxidized after exposure to substances with peroxidase activity (e.g., heme) followed by hydrogen peroxide. The substance to be tested is placed on paper impregnated with guaiac followed by hydrogen peroxide after a few minutes. Gastroccult (Beckman Coulter, Inc., Fullerton, CA) is designed to detect heme in vomit with a low pH. Hemoccult (Beckman Coulter, Inc.) is used for stool. Hemoccult may produce false negatives if used to test vomit but a positive test should be reliable if Gastroccult is not immediately available. These tests are inexpensive and reliable for the most part. False positives no longer occur with iron preparations. However, since the reaction is based on peroxidase activity, rare false positives may occur with certain foods (e.g., red meats, turnips, horseradish, artichokes, mushrooms, radishes, broccoli, bean sprouts, cauliflower, melons, and grapes). Newer immunochemical or heme–porphyrin tests can detect human blood more specifically but are not in wide use due to higher cost, slower turnaround, and possible false positives due to high sensitivity.[2,3]

Determine if Blood Originated from the GI Tract

Extraintestinal sources of blood can include spit or swallowed blood (nasopharyngeal, oropharyngeal, and hemoptysis) and blood that only appears to come from the rectum (anal fissure, excoriated skin, and vaginal or urinary tract bleeding). The history is key in determining the origin of the blood. Clues to nasopharyngeal origin include frequent nosebleeds, recent surgery (e.g., tonsillectomy or adenoidectomy), dental work, facial trauma, or traumatic nasogastric tube placement. Infants with denuded skin from diaper dermatitis may have intermittent bleeding. Vaginal bleeding may be normal in the first week of life and is sometimes mistaken for LGI bleeding. Similarly, onset of menstruation in adolescents may be confused with hematochezia.

Determine if it is the Child's Blood

Infants may swallow maternal blood during birth or breastfeeding. Physiologic reflux (normal infant spitting) is common, so this is often spit up. It may also manifest as hematochezia or melena. For breastfeeding infants, the mother should be asked if she has had any breast tenderness, sores, or bleeding (blood on the bra or seen in the baby's mouth before spitting up are useful clues). Significant anxiety can be avoided by distinguishing fetal from maternal blood early by this history or diagnostic testing.

The Apt–Downey Test can be used to detect maternal hemoglobin in vomit or stool containing bright red blood. This is based on the fact that fetal hemoglobin is resistant to alkali denaturation. The bloody vomit or stool is mixed with 1–5 mL of water and centrifuged yielding a pink hemolysate; 1 mL of 1% NaOH is then added and the solution's color is observed after a few minutes. Fetal hemoglobin is alkali resistant and the solution remains pink. Maternal hemoglobin A is denatured and the solution turns yellow to dark brown indicating that further evaluation in a well-appearing infant is unnecessary. The test requires grossly visible bright red blood. Melena or coffee grounds contain already denatured blood and may falsely indicate maternal hemoglobin. The infant's blood (especially for older breastfeeding infants) can be tested as a control to exclude the presence of significant hemoglobin A in which case the test would not be helpful.

CLINICAL PRESENTATION

Upper GI Bleeding

Table 6–3 lists common diagnoses and typical characteristics of presentation for both UGI and LGI bleeding. Most patients with overt UGI bleeding present with

Table 6–3.

Typical Presentations of Common Diagnoses

Diagnosis	Severity/Character of Bleeding	Character of Vomit and/or Stool	Appearance/Status of Patient
Swallowed blood	Mild to moderate, red vomit, red or black stool	Effortless reflux Normal stools	Healthy
Mallory–Weiss tear	Mild, red or coffee ground vomit	Frequent, forceful vomiting	Relatively well, typical of viral illness
Acid peptic disease	Usually mild, red or coffee ground vomit Severe if ulcer with arterial bleeding	Intermittent, sometimes forceful	Healthy, epigastric pain, heartburn Signs of hypotension if severe
Esophageal varices	Moderate to severe, red vomit or black stool	Vomit may be forceful Normal stools initially followed by melena	Pain sometimes precedes vomiting
Anal fissure	Mild, red streaks	Hard stool	Healthy, anal pain
Juvenile polyp	Mild to moderate, red, coats outside of stool Rarely severe	Normal	Healthy Signs of hypotension if severe
Colitis*	Mild to moderate, red mixed in with stools	Loose, frequent, urgent stools with mucus	Crampy, diffuse pain worse with stools
Meckel's diverticulum	Severe, maroon, red or black stools	Painless stools	Healthy, often signs of hypotension
Intussusception (ischemia#)	Moderate, red, black or currant jelly stool	Normal consistency, "currant jelly" appearance Vomiting may occur	Often toxic. Severe, episodic pain
Henoch–Schoenlein purpura	Mild to moderate, red or black stool	Normal stools	Abdominal pain often severe; can precede rash
Hirschsprung's enterocolitis	Mild to moderate, maroon, red or black stool	Loose stools often with forceful vomiting	Toxic: abdominal pain, distension, fever

*Colitis includes: allergic, infectious, and inflammatory bowel disease.
#Ischemia with gut injury can also include: volvulus, incarcerated hernia, and thrombosis.

Table 6–4.

Etiology of Hematemesis or Coffee Ground Emesis by Age and Presentation

Age	Ill Appearing	Well Appearing	
		High Rate	Low Rate
Newborn (up to a couple of months)	Hemorrhagic gastritis Volvulus		Swallowed maternal blood Vitamin K deficiency Mallory–Weiss tear (e.g., pyloric stenosis) Vascular anomaly
Infants (<2 years)	Hemorrhagic gastritis Esophageal varices Volvulus or bowel obstruction	Esophageal varices Intestinal duplication	Acid peptic disease Mallory–Weiss tear Swallowed blood (e.g., epistaxis) Food protein allergy
Child to adolescent	Esophageal varices Caustic ingestion Hemorrhagic gastritis Bowel obstruction Crohn's disease	Esophageal varices	Mallory–Weiss tear Acid peptic disease Chemical gastritis Ingestion (caustic or foreign body) Swallowed blood Vasculitis (e.g., HSP) Crohn's disease

Swallowed blood may include: maternal blood, epistaxis, recent surgery (tonsillectomy, adenoidectomy, and dental work), and hemoptysis. Acid peptic disease includes: erosive reflux esophagitis, gastritis (including H. pylori), and gastric or duodenal ulcer. Hemorrhagic gastritis has the following risk factors: ICU admission, burns, trauma, mechanical ventilation, and multi-organ failure. Chemical gastritis has the following risk factors: NSAID use, alcohol, and bile reflux.

hematemesis or coffee ground emesis. This can include bleeding from the intestinal tract and rarely from the biliary system (hemobilia) or pancreatic ductal system (hemosuccus pancreaticus). Occasionally, UGI bleeding will present as melena without vomiting. If there is massive UGI bleeding and/or rapid intestinal transit (e.g., infants, short bowel), hematochezia may be seen. Finally, a severe bleed may present with hypovolemic shock before hematemesis or the passage of a bloody stool. Depending on the etiology and severity of bleeding, children may appear completely asymptomatic or quite ill.

Lower GI Bleeding

Overt LGI bleeding can present as hematochezia or melena depending on etiology and severity. The amount and character of blood loss (bright red, black, or currant jelly) is important in suggesting specific diagnoses and possible need for urgent intervention. Stool frequency and consistency (normal, large and hard, or loose) should be investigated. Streaks of red blood coating hard or normal stool suggest a distal source (e.g., anal fissure and polyp). Presence of abdominal or anal pain can also be helpful. Non-bloody vomiting may occur with certain etiologies (e.g., bowel obstruction and inflammatory bowel disease). As with UGI bleeding, LGI bleeding can present with signs of severe blood loss before passage of a bloody stool.

DIFFERENTIAL DIAGNOSIS BASED ON PRESENTATION

Memorizing the differential diagnosis for UGI and LGI bleeding is less useful than a thoughtful approach based on the clinical presentation. Tables 6–4 and 6–5 provide a guide for hematemesis and hematochezia, respectively. It should be remembered that some diagnoses can have variable presentations and occur in different age groups. Tables 6–6 and 6–7 list rare causes separately. Variables besides presentation may include the age of the patient, the type and character of bleeding, and the clinical status of the child. The key initial steps described above should be undertaken no matter the presentation.

APPROACH TO DIAGNOSIS AND MANAGEMENT

See Tables 6–8 and 6–9.

Hematemesis or Coffee Ground Emesis

Hematemesis or coffee ground emesis indicates an UGI bleed. An algorithm for approaching the child with UGI bleeding is shown in Figure 6–2. In the hemodynamically stable child, a controlled approach in the outpatient

Table 6–5.

Hematochezia or Melena by Age and Presentation (Always Consider UGI Sources)

Age	Ill Appearing	Well Appearing	
		High Rate	Low Rate
All age groups	Infectious colitis		Anal fissure
			Infectious colitis
Newborn (up to a couple of months)	Necrotizing enterocolitis		Swallowed maternal blood
	Hirschsprung's enterocolitis		Benign rectal bleeding (lymphoid hyperplasia)
	Volvulus		Allergic colitis
Infants (<2 years)	Intussusception	Meckel's diverticulum	Allergic colitis
	Meckel's diverticulum		Lymphonodular hyperplasia (LNH)
	Volvulus or bowel obstruction		Swallowed blood (e.g., epistaxis)
	Hirschsprung's enterocolitis		
Preschool (2–5 years)	Meckel's diverticulum	Meckel's diverticulum	Juvenile polyp
	Bowel obstruction	Juvenile polyp with autoamputation	Swallowed blood
			Vasculitis (e.g., HSP)
	Inflammatory bowel disease	Ulcerative colitis	Inflammatory bowel disease
			LNH
Child to adolescent	Inflammatory bowel disease	Ulcerative colitis	Juvenile polyp
	Bowel obstruction	Juvenile polyp with autoamputation	Swallowed blood
		Meckel's diverticulum	Vasculitis (e.g., HSP)
			Inflammatory bowel disease
			LNH

Inflammatory bowel disease refers to either Crohn's disease or ulcerative colitis. HSP = Henoch–Schoenlein purpura; LNH = lymphonodular hyperplasia.

Table 6–6.

Rare Causes of UGI Bleeding

Radiation gastritis or esophagitis
Vascular abnormalities: hemangioma, hemangioendothelioma, arteriovenous malformations, Dieulafoy lesion, aortoesophageal fistula
Hemobilia (biliary bleeding) or hemosuccus pancreaticus (pancreatic bleeding)
Tumors: teratoma, leiomyosarcoma
Graft versus host disease (GVHD): common with bone marrow transplant
Munchausen syndrome by proxy: intentional poisoning, factitious bleeding

Table 6–7.

Rare Causes of Hematochezia or Melena

See rare causes of UGI bleeding in Table 6–6
Perianal group A beta-hemolytic streptococcus
Hemorrhoids: internal or external
Vascular abnormalities: hereditary hemorrhagic telangiectasia, Turner syndrome (telangiectasias), angiodysplasia, Dieulafoy lesion, blue rubber bleb nevus syndrome
Polyposis syndromes: familial adenomatous polyposis, Peutz–Jeghers syndrome, Gardner syndrome, Turcot syndrome
Clotting disorders: hemophilia, von Wilebrand's disease
Vasculitis: lupus erythematosus, Churg-Strauss syndrome, polyarteritis nodosa
Related to prior surgery: diversion colitis, perianastamotic ulcer
Cancer related: colorectal carcinoma, GVHD, neutropenic colitis (typhlitis)
Solitary rectal ulcer syndrome
Abuse with traumatic anal fissures
Intestinal duplication

setting may be appropriate. If the bleeding is significant by history or the patient is hemodynamically unstable, an NG saline lavage can determine if there is still active bleeding. (*Note*: Room temperature saline should be used as iced saline lavage is no longer considered useful or safe.)

For unstable patients, attention should be focused on supportive care (see the section "Key Initial Steps in the Evaluation of GI Bleeding"). Transfer to an intensive care setting and/or a tertiary care center with surgical and

endoscopic services should be initiated early. Surgical exploration is indicated for signs of obstruction or ongoing blood loss uncontrolled by medical therapy. Causes of severe UGI bleeding most often include: esophageal

Table 6–8.

Physical Exam Findings Suggestive of Specific Diagnoses

Portion of Exam	Findings	Suggested Diagnoses
Vital signs	Impaired linear growth or weight gain; weight loss	Crohn's disease; Hirschsprung's disease; Turner syndrome
	Fever	Infectious colitis, IBD
Abdomen	Hepatosplenomegaly, ascites, caput medusa	Portal hypertension
Rectal exam	Midline anal fissures or tags; dilated rectal vault	Constipation
	Anal fissures or tags without constipation. Fissures not in midline. Abscess, fistula	Crohn's disease; chronic granulomatous disease
	Rectal mass on a stalk	Polyp
	Circumscribed erythema	Perianal group A streptococcus
Miscellaneous	Jaundice, spider angioma, palmar erythema	Cirrhotic liver disease
	Pigmented oral or buccal lesions	Peutz–Jeghers syndrome
	Fingernail clubbing	Cirrhotic liver disease, IBD
	Arthritis	IBD, HSP
	Palpable purpura	HSP

Table 6–9.

Laboratory Findings Suggestive of Specific Diagnoses

Laboratory Test	Findings	Suggested Diagnoses
CBC	Microcytic anemia, elevated platelets	IBD
	Elevated WBC, no anemia	Infectious colitis
	Low platelets, leucopenia	Portal hypertension
ESR, CRP	Elevated ESR or CRP	IBD, infectious colitis
Metabolic profile	Elevated transaminases, bilirubin	Liver disease
	Low albumin	Liver disease, Crohn's disease
Stool studies	Culture, C. difficile toxin	Infectious colitis
Urinalysis	Positive for blood	HSP

varices due to portal hypertension, hemorrhagic gastritis in the ICU setting (e.g., trauma, burns, and mechanical ventilation), and ischemic bowel injury (malrotation with volvulus, bowel obstruction, and intussusception).

Selected conditions leading to UGI bleeding

Acid peptic disease Acid peptic disease is one of the more common causes of UGI bleeding in older children (>6–12 months) or those in a critical care setting. However, it is important to remember that this is a common problem that does not usually present with overt GI bleeding, but rather with more typical symptoms (regurgitation, heartburn, acid brash, epigastric pain, and poor feeding). Reflux esophagitis or gastritis is rare in infants <6 months old in spite of the fact that over half of all infants have frequent spitting (physiologic reflux of infancy). This is probably due to frequent milk intake buffering gastric acid. However, it can occur, especially in older infants who eat less frequently with less milk intake. They are usually fussy and may have a decline in oral intake. Other conditions may contribute (e.g., eosinophilic esophagitis or food allergy).

Helicobacter pylori may cause gastritis but not usually ulcers as it may in adults. Gastritis may also be caused by frequent NSAID use, often for another chronic problem (e.g., headaches, juvenile rheumatoid arthritis, and cystic fibrosis). If an NSAID is prescribed as a daily medication for some of these problems, there are data that concurrent use of a proton pump inhibitor (PPI) reduces the incidence of gastritis or ulceration.

Mallory–Weiss tear Retching from any cause (e.g., viral gastroenteritis, pyloric stenosis, or anatomic

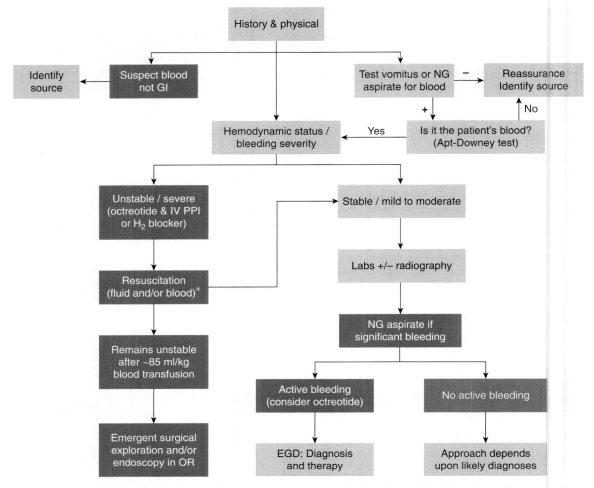

FIGURE 6–2 ■ Approach to hematemesis, coffee ground emesis, or rectal bleeding with positive NG aspirate. (*) The unstable or actively bleeding patient should be resuscitated (IV access, fluid, and/or blood) while obtaining key laboratory and radiographic data if possible. The goal is to stabilize for controlled evaluation and possible transfer to the ICU and/or a facility with surgical and endoscopic services. Endoscopy is technically challenging with active bleeding but can be therapeutic (e.g., esophageal varices).

obstruction) can lead to mucosal tears and bleeding. Coffee ground emesis in an infant under 4 months of age should prompt one to investigate for a history of progressively worsening retching during or after feeding (pyloric stenosis).

Esophageal varices Large-volume, bright red UGI bleeding is most commonly caused by esophageal variceal bleeding and may present as hematemesis or melena. Interruption or slowing of portal venous flow (portal hypertension, portal venous thrombosis, etc.) leads to shunting of blood to the systemic circulation (Figure 6–3). Flow is reversed through the left gastric vein into gastric and esophageal venous plexuses that then drain into the azygous vein. The engorged submucosal esophageal veins are most prominent near the gastroesophageal junction and lower esophagus.

Although variceal bleeds frequently resolve spontaneously, rebleeding is a common problem without prophylactic therapy. The history should investigate risk

factors for liver disease (neonatal history, family history, infectious exposure, blood transfusions, and jaundice) and portal vein thrombosis (omphalitis, sepsis, and umbilical catheter). The examination should focus on findings consistent with portal hypertension and liver disease: hepatosplenomegaly, ascites, caput medusa, jaundice, and spider angiomata.

Ingestions Foreign body ingestion can cause bleeding if there is a sharp edge. A foreign body in the esophagus for over 24 hours may cause erosion and bleeding. A chronic foreign body in the stomach may cause an ulcer. Caustic ingestions may also cause UGI or LGI bleeding. This is usually a late occurrence for accidental ingestions (usually a small amount) after stricture formation. However, intentional ingestions (larger amounts with more significant injury) may present as bloody vomiting.[4] Similarly, overdose with certain medications (e.g., iron) can cause ulceration and bleeding.

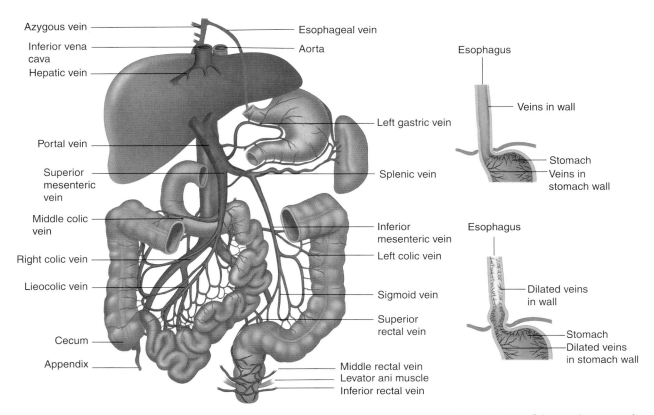

FIGURE 6–3 ■ Portal hypertension and development of esophageal varices. The portal vein is formed by the junction of the superior mesenteric and splenic veins. The left gastric vein inserts into the portal vein. Impeded flow in the portal vein may lead to systemic shunting (e.g., to azygous vein via left gastric vein to gastric and esophageal veins) and development of esophageal varices. These develop distally and propagate upwards. Less commonly seen are caput medusa (abdominal wall veins) and hemorrhoids.

Malrotation with intermittent midgut volvulus Crying or screaming in infants before vomiting blood and/or bile is worrisome for obstruction, especially malrotation with volvulus (twisting of midgut that usually obstructs the superior mesenteric artery and blood flow to almost the entire small bowel). This is a surgical emergency as it can lead to necrosis of the entire small bowel and part of the colon. Patients will appear ill, often with distension, diminished bowel sounds, tachycardia, and poor perfusion. The highest risk for volvulus is in the first few months of life but can occur at any age. Diagnosis is often confirmed at surgery if the child is not stable for radiographic studies.[5]

Hemorrhagic gastritis In critically ill patients, shock (e.g., sepsis or heart failure) can commonly lead to ischemic injury causing gastritis or stomach ulcers. However, significant UGI bleeding is uncommon (<2%) even in this setting.[6] Major risk factors include mechanical ventilation, burns, trauma, and multi-organ failure.

Coagulopathy Although coagulopathy alone does not usually cause GI bleeding, hemorrhagic disease of the newborn (vitamin K deficiency) or other bleeding disorders (e.g., von Willebrand's disease) can present this way. Fat malabsorption (e.g., cystic fibrosis or other pancreatic insufficiency, and cholestasis) leading to vitamin K deficiency in infancy is rare.

Food protein allergy Food allergies can occasionally present with gastritis and hematemesis although blood-streaked stools are much more common.[7]

Other causes Crohn's disease can involve any part of the intestinal tract with ulcerations causing GI bleeding. Upper tract involvement is not common in children. This will usually be accompanied by other signs and symptoms such as growth impairment, abdominal pain, iron deficiency anemia, and hypoalbuminemia. Other causes of overt UGI bleeding in children are rare: Henoch–Schoenlein purpura, vascular anomalies (e.g., Dieulafoy lesion and aortoesophageal fistula), hemosuccus pancreaticus, and gastric polyps or tumors. Hemangiomas are common skin lesions but rarely symptomatic when present in the gut. Skin lesions are usually obvious when intestinal hemangiomas are present and can be a clue. As with skin lesions, gut hemangiomas often fade with time. Intestinal duplications are a rare cause of UGI bleeding if there is gastric mucosa present.

Hematochezia or Melena

Blood in stools can be from either an UGI or LGI source. The character of bleeding provides vital clues (see Table 6–5). Bloody diarrhea is usually due to infectious or inflammatory colitis. Large amounts of maroon stools are most often due to a Meckel's diverticulum or other source of brisk bleeding in the small bowel. Currant jelly stools are typical of ischemic injury, most often seen with intussusception or volvulus in infants. Dark black stools are unlikely to originate distal to the cecum and may represent UGI bleeding up to 15% of the time. An approach to the child with hematochezia or melena is shown in Figure 6–4. As with UGI bleeding, outpatient evaluation may be appropriate in the hemodynamically stable child with mild bleeding. With melena or significant hematochezia, NG lavage can identify an UGI source (most sources not identified this way can be diagnosed by upper endoscopy). As with UGI bleeding, stabilizing the patient is the primary goal while initiating evaluation and management.

Again, for unstable patients, supportive care should be initiated and specialist consultation considered (see the section "Key Initial Steps in the Evaluation of GI Bleeding"). Surgical consultation is reasonable in unstable patients. Surgical exploration is indicated with signs of obstruction or ongoing blood loss not responsive to medical management. Causes of severe LGI bleeding most often include: Meckel's diverticulum, Hirschsprung's enterocolitis, and ischemic bowel injury (malrotation with volvulus, bowel obstruction, and intussusception).

Age of presentation is very important when considering causes of LGI bleeding. There can be significant overlap with certain problems seen in different age groups: traumatic anal fissure (usually due to constipation), infectious colitis, Meckel's diverticulum, Henoch–Schoenlein purpura, malrotation with volvulus, allergic colitis, intussusception, and lymphoid nodular hyperplasia. As discussed above, UGI bleeds can present with hematochezia or melena which may be demonstrable by nasogastric lavage or upper endoscopy. The characteristics of the bleed-

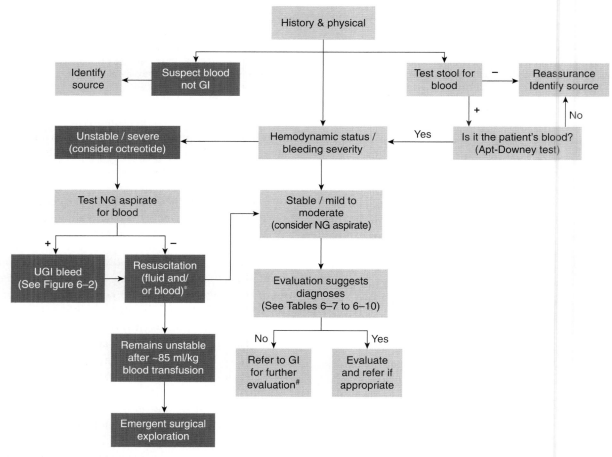

FIGURE 6–4 ■ Approach to hematochezia or melena. (#) Any patient with health-threatening bleeding (hemodynamically significant or large volume) should be referred to a gastroenterologist if an obvious source is not immediately found and treated. Mild, isolated bleeding without an obvious cause after limited evaluation (stool studies and radiographic studies) should also be referred. (*) The unstable or actively bleeding patient should be resuscitated (IV access, fluid, and/or blood) while obtaining key laboratory and radiographic data if possible. The goal is to stabilize for controlled evaluation and possible transfer to the ICU and/or a facility with surgical and endoscopic services.

ing, clinical presentation, and history often yield a diagnosis with the aid of minimal, directed diagnostic studies.

Certain conditions are seen almost exclusively in newborns and infants: necrotizing enterocolitis, Hirschsprung's enterocolitis, hemorrhagic disease of the newborn, allergic colitis, and idiopathic intussusception. In contrast, certain problems are rarely, if ever, encountered during infancy: inflammatory bowel disease and juvenile polyps.

Selected conditions leading to LGI bleeding

Specific conditions may cause both hematemesis and hematochezia: volvulus, allergy, IBD, HSP, vascular anomalies (e.g., Dieulafoy lesion), hemosuccus pancreaticus, hemobilia, tumors, hemangiomas, and intestinal duplications.

Allergic colitis and benign rectal bleeding

Infants with streaks of blood and mucus in stools have usually been considered to have allergic colitis if stool cultures are negative. They are empirically switched to non-cow's milk-based formulas, often with resolution of bleeding. However, we have come to recognize many of these infants have a benign problem usually associated with lymphoid hyperplasia of the rectum often unrelated to allergy.[8] This resolves with time and is not dangerous. Clues to a diagnosis of allergic colitis include eczema, frequent diarrhea, and poor weight gain. Even then, if there is improvement with diet change (for mother or infant), a rechallenge to confirm the diagnosis is useful as formula changes usually mean increased expense for the family. In addition, many mothers stop breastfeeding or lose weight when restricting their diet. If allergy is not causative, bleeding may continue intermittently for a couple of months leading the mother to agonize about what mistakes she is making in her diet.

Hirschsprung's disease

Hirschsprung's enterocolitis may present with abdominal distension, fever, vomiting, and loose stools which may become bloody. This diagnosis needs to be evaluated in any infant who did not have spontaneous passage of stool in the first 24–48 hours of life (most normal infants will pass stool in the first 36 hours of life). However, up to 25% of patients with Hirschsprung's disease will pass stool in the first 48 hours, so this cannot be used to exclude the diagnosis.[9] Typically, infants will have infrequent, explosive passage of liquid stools from birth. They rarely pass large or hard stools.

Anal fissures

Anal fissures are usually in the midline, caused by traumatic passage of a large, hard stool. This is exquisitely painful and one should expect to hear a history consistent with painful passage of hard stools. The blood is expected to be on the outside of the stool. Fissures that are not in the midline should prompt an evaluation for Crohn's disease or traumatic injury (e.g., abuse).

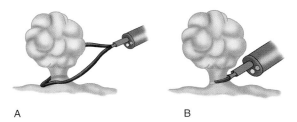

FIGURE 6-5 ■ Colonoscopic snare polypectomy. Juvenile polyps almost always occur as a round mass (as large as a couple of centimeters) on a narrow stalk or pedicle. (A) The snare is introduced through the scope and maneuvered over the polyp. (B) The snare tightens around the stalk and thermal energy is delivered as it is transected to promote coagulation and minimize bleeding risk. The polyp is retrieved for histologic confirmation of diagnosis. Risks are low but include perforation and bleeding which may occur up to a couple of weeks after polypectomy.

Juvenile polyps A juvenile polyp is a non-malignant, hamartomatous overgrowth of tissue that is highly vascular and intermittently bleeds. As they increase in size, they become rounded masses on a stalk. These most frequently occur in school-aged children with painless, intermittent bleeding that is not significant. Sometimes, if the child or parent reports a polyp prolapsing with bowel movements, it can be felt on rectal exam (small, mobile mass on a stalk). They are almost always distal and solitary (three or less) unless associated with a polyposis syndrome. They may bleed significantly if they slough spontaneously and are usually removed at colonoscopy (see Figure 6–5).[10]

Meckel's diverticulum Meckel's diverticulum is the most common congenital GI abnormality occurring in ~2% of the population.[11] It is the remnant of the omphalomesenteric duct (connecting the yolk sac and intestine during embryogenesis) located in the distal ileum (see Figure 6–6). About 50% contain ectopic gastric tissue which can cause ulceration and bleeding of the adjacent, normal intestinal mucosa. Luckily, a minority of these become symptomatic. The rule of 2's is commonly used to recall typical features of a Meckel's diverticulum: present in *2%* of the population, located within *2* ft (60–100 cm) of ileocecal valve, usually *2* in. (3–5 cm) long, and most (well over 50%) present before age *2* years.

Infectious colitis Invasive pathogens have the potential to cause GI bleeding. These will mostly be bacteria (*E. coli* O157:H7, *Salmonella*, *Shigella*, *Campylobacter*, and *Yersinia*). See Chapter 4 which covers diarrheal diseases in detail. Viral infections (i.e., rotavirus and Norwalk virus) rarely cause overt blood loss in the stool. However, CMV can cause ulcerations and GI bleeding in immunocompromised patients.

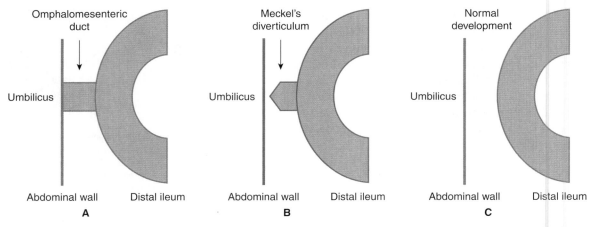

FIGURE 6–6 ■ Meckel's diverticulum. (A) Omphalomesenteric duct during normal development. (B) Abnormal, incomplete obliteration of the duct. (C) Normal condition.

Necrotizing enterocolitis Loss of mucosal barrier allows bacterial invasion into the intestinal wall. Although most risk factors are associated with prematurity (low birth weight, sepsis, and hypoxia), necrotizing enterocolitis also occurs in term infants. It is imperative to rule out this diagnosis in any newborn with rectal bleeding. There are frequently systemic signs and symptoms of illness (hypothermia, apnea, tachy- or bradycardia, bilious vomit, distension, and poor feeding). Abdominal films may show air in the bowel wall (pneumatosis intestinalis) and dilated loops of bowel. Colonoscopy is contraindicated as there is a high risk of progression and perforation.

Intussusception Most cases of intussusception occur before 1 year of age (65%). Most are ileocolic and idiopathic or associated with lymphoid hyperplasia of the ileum (often after a viral illness). Only 20% of cases occur after 2 years of age but these more often have an identifiable cause. An intestinal mass can act as a lead point (e.g., polyp, Meckel's diverticulum, and HSP). Certain diseases are associated with recurrent episodes of intussusception (e.g., celiac disease, cystic fibrosis, and Ehlers–Danlos syndrome). Diagnosis may be suspected with episodic pain, vomiting, and currant jelly stools. An abdominal mass may be felt. Ultrasonography, in the right hands, has near 100% sensitivity and specificity. Air or contrast enema may provide diagnosis and be therapeutic in up to 80% of cases. A pediatric surgeon should be immediately available as there is risk of perforation.[12]

DIAGNOSTIC TESTS OF INTEREST

Radiography

Plain radiography is appropriate in most cases of significant GI bleeding. It may identify some foreign bodies, obstructive processes, and perforation, and give clues to other diagnoses. Contrast studies are not appropriate first-line investigations as they may delay evaluation by other means (endoscopy, colonoscopy, and nuclear medicine scans) and lead to complications (perforation if done in setting of obstruction).

Ultrasonography

Ultrasound is very helpful if certain diagnoses are suspected: intussusception (almost 100% sensitive and specific), portal hypertension (hepatosplenomegaly and portal vein flow), and vascular anomalies or duplication cysts.

Endoscopy and Colonoscopy

Endoscopy is the best method to evaluate UGI bleeding and will yield a diagnosis in most cases.[13] Therapeutic techniques have advanced greatly allowing hemostasis via coagulation (e.g., heater probe or argon plasma coagulation), injection (e.g., epinephrine or sclerosing agents), and mechanical occlusion (e.g., variceal banding, hemostatic clips, and detachable loops).[14] Many of these techniques may be also used during colonoscopy.[10] Endoscopy is rarely urgent in pediatrics and has high risk in the hemodynamically unstable patient making medical management important prior to endoscopic therapy. Colonoscopy can also be diagnostic (e.g., IBD) and therapeutic (e.g., polypectomy and hemostasis of vascular lesions). Contraindications include: suspected obstruction, ischemia perforation, or peritonitis; pneumatosis intestinalis; and intussusception. Push enteroscopy or double balloon enteroscopy allows examination of almost the entire small bowel but has limitations in children. Wireless capsule endoscopy has emerged as a useful tool for evaluation of the small bowel, especially if no source is found on upper endoscopy and colonoscopy.[15] Laparotomy or laparoscopy-assisted endoscopy is reserved for cases in which other modalities have not yielded a diagnosis.

Nuclear Medicine Scans

The radionuclide technetium 99m pertechnetate is taken up by ectopic gastric mucosa in a Meckel's diverticulum in up to 90% of symptomatic patients (sensitivity may be improved with administration of a histamine$_2$ antagonist). A negative scan should not be a deciding factor against exploratory surgery in a toddler or even older child with classic symptoms and health-threatening bleeding.[16] Red blood cells can be tagged with the radionuclide and reinjected into the blood stream. Rough localization of the bleeding site can be made using a gamma camera, which shows extravasation into the intestine at the site of bleeding. The rate of bleeding must be significant to allow visualization; often, the bleeding has often stopped or slowed by the time the study is performed.

Angiography

A bleeding rate of 0.5 mL/min is required to identify a bleeding site. It may also diagnose vascular abnormalities and can be therapeutic by embolization of the feeding vessel. This is reserved for cases in which most other modalities have not yielded a diagnosis.

TREATMENT

The major points regarding supportive treatment were previously discussed (e.g., stabilizing patient with fluid and/or blood resuscitation). The roles of surgery and interventional radiologic techniques have also been discussed.

Medical Therapy for Minor Upper GI Bleeding

Table 6–10 lists some common medications and doses used to control peptic injury in GI bleeding (there are little data in children to guide dosing). Conservative, empirical treatment is reasonable for minimal UGI bleeding with normal initial evaluation. If there is a history of reflux symptoms (regurgitation, acid brash, heartburn, and epigastric pain) or suspected Mallory–Weiss tear, then a trial of acid suppression is reasonable. PPIs tend to be cleared faster by children, so they tend to need higher doses than adults per body weight. These medications are most effective when taken on an empty stomach and eating 30 minutes later. Liquid preparations are unpalatable but there are alternatives. Soluble tablets may be dissolved in water. Capsules may be opened and sprinkled on applesauce or yogurt. Significant improvement is not usually seen for at least a week (a couple of days to suppress acid production and a few days for mucosal healing to begin). If there is no improvement of symptoms within a couple of weeks or more bleeding is seen, then endoscopy is indicated.

Alternatively, for suspected mucosal disruption (ulcer and pill esophagitis), sucralfate can be used. This is a cytoprotective agent that binds to injured tissue creating a protective barrier and promoting tissue healing. The dose is 40–80 mg/kg/day in four divided doses (up to 1 g four times a day). It is best given as a liquid, especially for esophageal injury and may result in rapid improvement in symptoms (chest pain and dysphagia). The tablet dissolves easily in water but children may not find this palatable. The liquid formulation is accepted by most. It should be given about 1 hour before meals since binding to injured tissue is enhanced in an acidic environment. It is for this reason that concurrent therapy with a PPI is not recommended. Sucralfate is typically given for a couple of weeks with transition to a PPI that can be given once a day. Side effects are minimal. It may reduce bioavailability of other drugs and there is potential for aluminum toxicity in patients with renal insufficiency. Long-term use can affect absorption of fat-soluble vitamins.

 Table 6–10.

Oral Medications for Minimal GI Bleeding

Medication	Class	Dose*
Omeprazole	PPI	1–1.5 mg/kg/day (maximum 40 mg) divided once or twice daily
Lansoprazole	PPI	1–1.5 mg/kg/day (maximum 60 mg) divided once or twice daily
Ranitidine	H$_2$ blocker	2–4 mg/kg/day (maximum 300 mg) divided twice daily
Famotidine	H$_2$ blocker	0.5–1 mg/kg/day (maximum 40 mg) divided twice daily
Sucralfate	Cytoprotection	40–80 mg/kg/day (maximum 4 g) divided four times daily
		Liquid preparation preferable for esophageal lesions

PPI = proton pump inhibitor; H$_2$ blocker = histamine$_2$ antagonist.
* Note: PPI dosing is not based on stringent data. Some practitioners may use higher doses in select cases based on experience and available data.

Table 6–11.		
Intravenous Medications for Active GI Bleeding		
Medications	Class	Dose*
Pantoprazole	PPI	0.5–1 mg/kg/day (maximum 40 mg) divided once or twice daily
Lansoprazole	PPI	1–1.5 mg/kg/day (maximum 30 mg) divided once or twice daily
Ranitidine	H₂ blocker	Bolus: 2–4 mg/kg/day (maximum 200 mg) divided q 6–8 hours
		Continuous: 1 mg/kg bolus, and then 2–4 mg/kg/day (maximum 200 mg/day)
Octreotide*	Vasoactive	1 mcg/kg bolus (maximum 50 mcg), and then 1 mcg/kg/hour
		Titrate by 1 mcg/kg/hour q8 hours as needed (maximum 5 mcg/kg/hour)

PPI = proton pump inhibitor; H_2 blocker = histamine$_2$ antagonist.
Note: PPI dosing is not based on stringent data. Some practitioners may use higher doses in select cases based on experience and available data.
*Octreotide dosing is based on limited data. Monitor for hyperglycemia.

Medical Therapy for Active GI Bleeding

Table 6–11 lists some common medications and doses used in active GI bleeding. Octreotide is the most useful vasoconstrictive medication for patients with active, hemodynamically significant bleeding. It reduces splanchnic blood flow and has minimal side effects (hyperglycemia). It is usually given initially as a 1 mcg/kg bolus (maximum 50 mcg) followed immediately by 1 mcg/kg/min continuous infusion. The infusion may be increased every 8 hours if necessary by 1 mcg/kg/min to a maximum of 4–5 mcg/kg/min[17]. If successful, this will stop active bleeding and allow stabilization for further evaluation and therapy. Two intravenous PPIs are available for patients who cannot take oral medication.

Endoscopic Therapy for Active GI Bleeding

Gastric lavage before endoscopy may clear blood and clots that otherwise make endoscopic therapy challenging. Erythromycin given IV may also enhance gastric emptying clearing blood from the stomach. If possible, endoscopy should be performed shortly after bleeding stops to maximize diagnostic yield.

Endoscopic therapies continue to evolve.[14] Most available data are in adults with a growing body of experience in pediatrics. Injection of epinephrine (1:10,000) into the tissue surrounding a non-variceal bleeding lesion may slow or stop bleeding but it is not thrombogenic. Contact probes (heater probes or bipolar probes) allow direct pressure to be applied to a bleeding vessel. This collapses the vessel and the delivery of thermal energy fuses the walls of the vessel together. Current data suggest improved outcomes if injection is followed by thermal coagulation (need for surgical intervention

with combination therapy is <10% in adults). Due to risk of perforation, less thermal energy is utilized for lesions in the thin-walled colon than the stomach.

Endoscopic clip placement achieves hemostasis by grasping and compressing tissue surrounding a bleeding vessel. Mechanical ligation (loops and bands) works similarly. Again, most experience is with adults but this is being used more in pediatrics as it is a straightforward technique with high success and low complication rate. Other hemostatic therapies are used less commonly in children (argon plasma coagulation, fibrin glue injection, and laser photocoagulation).

Management of Variceal Bleeding

Esophageal variceal bleeding that does not resolve spontaneously is frequently controlled with octreotide and/or endoscopic therapy. Slowing or stopping the bleeding with octreotide while stabilizing the patient often makes endoscopic visualization and treatment much easier. If these measures are not successful, temporary control of bleeding may be achieved by balloon tamponade devices.[3] This is infrequently required but may be life saving for the unstable patient. This is a delicate procedure performed in the ICU setting with sedation and control of the airway. As brisk bleeding makes endoscopy technically challenging, this maneuver can make endoscopic therapy more successful if the bleeding can be slowed or stopped. The balloon tamponade device is removed before endoscopy.

Treatment for bleeding varices includes sclerotherapy and band ligation. Both focus on obliterating esophageal varices at their most distal aspect near the lower esophageal sphincter (see Figure 6–3). Sclerotherapy has been used for decades and has a high success rate. An injection needle is introduced through the endoscope and small volumes of sclerosing agents are injected into the varix leading to obliteration of the vessel and, hopefully, the smaller feeding vessels. Complications are more common than with banding (ulcers, strictures, and perforation).

The concept of variceal banding is a simple one adapted from a proven treatment for hemorrhoids. The banding device is placed on the endoscope. Suction is applied to pull the varix into the device. An elastic band is released compressing the varix leading to obliteration. Up to six bands can be placed in one session. Adult studies suggest banding is just as effective as sclerotherapy with less complications (no such comparative data exist in children). The major limitation is the size of the device which does not allow it to be introduced in smaller children and infants.

Rebleeding of varices is frequent (up to 50%). However, sclerotherapy or banding can be repeated on an elective basis to eradicate varices and prevent rebleeding (multiple sessions may be required). Prophylaxis of rebleeding may include non-selective beta blockers to reduce portal pressures. They are effective in adult studies but may significantly limit exercise tolerance. Surgery to decompress the portal system or liver transplantation may be helpful in selected patients.

SUMMARY

GI bleeding in children is rarely life threatening but can be severe. The keys to approaching these patients are rapid assessment of severity and stabilization. In the majority of cases, this will allow a controlled evaluation yielding a diagnosis and/or consultation with a specialist.

REFERENCES

1. Gilger M, Whitfield K. Upper gastrointestinal bleeding. In: Kleinman E, Walker WA, eds. *Walker's Pediatric Gastrointestinal Disease: Physiology, Diagnosis, Management.* Hamilton, Ont./Lewiston, NY: BC Decker; 2008:1285.
2. Turck D, Michaud L. Lower gastrointestinal bleeding. In: Kleinman E, Walker WA, eds. *Walker's Pediatric Gastrointestinal Disease: Physiology, Diagnosis, Management.* Hamilton, Ont./Lewiston, NY: BC Decker; 2008:1309.
3. Boyle JT. Gastrointestinal bleeding in infants and children. *Pediatr Rev.* 2008;29:39–52.
4. Mas E, Olives JP. Toxic and traumatic injury of the esophagus. In: Kleinman E, Walker WA, eds. *Walker's Pediatric Gastrointestinal Disease: Physiology, Diagnosis, Management.* Hamilton, Ont./Lewiston, NY: BC Decker; 2008:105.
5. Applegate KE. Evidence-based diagnosis of malrotation and volvulus. *Pediatr Radiol.* 2009;39(suppl 2): S161–S163.
6. Deerojanawon J, Peongsujarit D, Vivatvakin B, Prapphal N. Incidence and risk factors of upper gastrointestinal bleeding in mechanically ventilated children. *Pediatr Crit Care Med.* 2009;10(1):91–95.
7. Maloney J, Nowak-Wegrzyn A. Educational clinical case series for pediatric allergy and immunology: allergic proctocolitis, food protein-induced enterocolitis syndrome and allergic eosinophilic gastroenteritis with protein-losing gastroenteropathy as manifestations of non-IgE-mediated cow's milk allergy. *Pediatr Allergy Immunol.* 2007;18(4):360–367.
8. Arvola T, Ruuska T, Keranen J, et al. Rectal bleeding in infancy: clinical, allergological, and microbiological examination. *Pediatrics.* 2006;117(4):e760–e768.
9. Lewis NA, Levitt MA, Zallen GS, et al. Diagnosing Hirschsprung's disease: increasing the odds of a positive rectal biopsy result. *J Pediatr Surg.* 2003;38(3):412–416.
10. Walker TM. Ileocolonoscopy and enteroscopy. In: Kleinman E, Walker WA, eds. *Walker's Pediatric Gastrointestinal Disease: Physiology, Diagnosis, Management.* Hamilton, Ont./Lewiston, NY: BC Decker; 2008:1291.
11. Thurley PD, Halliday KE, Somers JM. Radiological features of Meckel's diverticulum and its complications. *Clin Radiol.* 2009;64(2):109–118.
12. Waseem M, Rosenberg HK. Intussusception. *Pediatr Emerg Care.* 2008;24(11):793–800.
13. Schappi M, Mougenot JF, Belli D. Upper gastrointestinal endoscopy. In: Kleinman E, Walker WA, eds. *Walker's Pediatric Gastrointestinal Disease: Physiology, Diagnosis, Management.* Hamilton, Ont./Lewiston, NY: BC Decker; 2008:1265.
14. Kay MH, Wyllie R. Therapeutic endoscopy for nonvariceal gastrointestinal bleeding. *J Pediatr Gastroenterol Nutr.* 2007;45(2):157–171.
15. Melmed GY, Lo SK. Capsule endoscopy: practical applications. *Clin Gastroenterol Hepatol.* 2005;3(5): 411–422.
16. Kiratli PO, Aksoy T, Bozkurt MF, Orhan D. Detection of ectopic gastric mucosa using 99mTc pertechnetate: review of the literature. *Ann Nucl Med.* 2009;23(2):97–105.
17. Siafakas C, Fox VL, Nurko S. Use of octreotide for the treatment of severe gastrointestinal bleeding in children. *JPGN.* 1998;26(3):356–359.

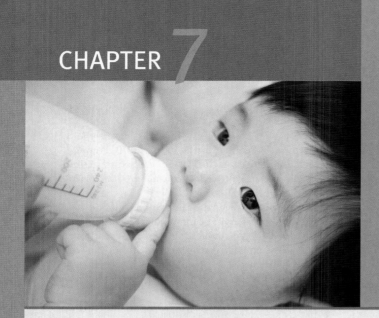

CHAPTER 7

Jaundice and Neonatal Cholestasis

Riad M. Rahhal

DEFINITIONS AND EPIDEMIOLOGY

Jaundice comes from the French word "jaune," meaning yellow. Jaundice refers to the yellow staining of the sclera, mucous membranes, and skin by bilirubin. It is not a disease by itself but rather a manifestation that accompanies different diseases. Jaundice is caused by elevated serum bilirubin levels with subsequent tissue deposition. In infants, it is usually apparent with bilirubin levels above 4–5 mg/dL (68–86 mmol/L). In older children, jaundice can be noted at levels above 2–3 mg/dL (34–51 mmol/L). The color of the sclera and skin varies depending on the serum bilirubin level. Jaundice involves the head first and progresses caudally with higher levels.

Total serum bilirubin is the sum of the unconjugated (or indirect) and conjugated (or direct) bilirubin fractions. The terms direct and conjugated hyperbilirubinemia are often used interchangeably, but this is not always accurate. Direct bilirubin is measured in the laboratory using a diazo dye-binding assay, and, depending on the method used, can include both conjugated bilirubin and delta bilirubin. Delta bilirubin is formed by covalent bond formation between serum conjugated bilirubin and albumin. Clearance of delta bilirubin can therefore be prolonged, reflecting the half-life of albumin, and may lag behind other signs of clinical improvement.

Cholestasis is defined as diminished bile formation or flow, and is manifested by conjugated hyperbilirubinemia. The guidelines of the North American Society for Pediatric Gastroenterology, Hepatology and Nutrition (NASPGHAN)[1] define an abnormal conjugated bilirubin level as:

- a conjugated bilirubin >1.0 mg/dL, if the total bilirubin is <5 mg/dL, or
- a conjugated bilirubin level >20% of the total bilirubin, if the total bilirubin is >5 mg/dL.

Neonatal jaundice is common, observed in the first week of life in about 50% of term infants and 80% of preterm infants. This is usually harmless, often related to physiological jaundice or breastfeeding, and is characterized by unconjugated hyperbilirubinemia. Rarely, however, severe unconjugated hyperbilirubinemia can lead to bilirubin encephalopathy or kernicterus.[2] On the contrary, cholestasis (or conjugated hyperbilirubinemia) is much less commonly seen but often results from conditions with serious hepatobiliary dysfunction. Cholestatic jaundice affects approximately 1 in every 2500 infants.[3] The challenge for physicians is to identify infants with cholestasis who will need additional evaluation and treatment. Early detection of cholestatic jaundice and accurate diagnosis of its etiology are vital for successful treatment and a favorable prognosis.

PATHOGENESIS

Bilirubin is the end product of heme moiety metabolism from hemoglobin and other heme-containing proteins (Figure 7–1). After unconjugated bilirubin is formed, it is transported with albumin in blood to the liver. Inside hepatocytes, unconjugated bilirubin is conjugated with glucuronic acid by uridine diphosphate glucuronosyltransferase (UGT) to increase water solubility. Conjugated bilirubin, along with cholesterol, bile acids, and phospholipids, is transported through the bile canalicular system to the gallbladder and later into the small intestine. Conjugated bilirubin cannot be reabsorbed by enterocytes and is degraded by the intestinal flora into colorless urobilinogen, which is excreted with feces. Urobilinogen is oxidized to urobilin and stercobilin, which are responsible for the brown color of stools. A portion of conjugated bilirubin is deconjugated by beta-glucuronidase and is reabsorbed into the

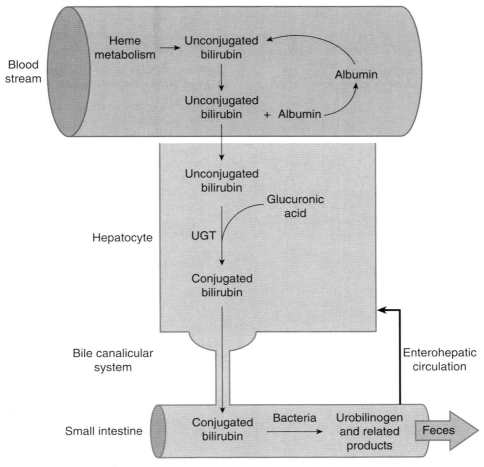

FIGURE 7–1 ■ Bilirubin metabolism: following transport from the blood stream into the hepatocytes, unconjugated bilirubin is converted by the action of uridine diphosphate glucuronosyltransferase (UGT) to mono- and diglucuronide that are excreted into the small intestine.

portal circulation and liver, a normal process called the enterohepatic bilirubin circulation. In the liver, this can be conjugated again and excreted into the bile.[4]

Any disease process that leads to increased bilirubin production and/or limits bilirubin excretion can potentially manifest by visible jaundice from underlying hyperbilirubinemia. Depending on the etiology and pathogenesis, this can lead to unconjugated or conjugated hyperbilirubinemia.

Hyperbilirubinemia in healthy, full-term infants is often attributed to physiological immaturity of bilirubin metabolism, leading to elevated unconjugated bilirubin levels. In actuality, neonatal jaundice is often due to a combination of one or more of the following (Table 7–1):

- increased bilirubin production;
- decreased bilirubin clearance;
- increased enterohepatic circulation.

Increased bilirubin production is seen with hemolytic disease processes such as ABO incompatibility, inherited membrane defects or enzyme abnormalities of red blood cells, hyperviscosity (polycythemia)

syndrome, or resorption of a large hematoma. Decreased bilirubin conjugation is seen in Crigler–Najjar syndrome and Gilbert's syndrome that are due to the absence or reduction of UGT activity, leading to unconjugated hyperbilirubinemia.[5] Delayed intestinal transit can enhance the enterohepatic circulation of unconjugated bilirubin contributing to unconjugated hyperbilirubinemia. This can be seen in breast milk jaundice, inadequate breastfeeding, and impaired intestinal motility or intestinal obstruction. In neonates, the inadequately developed anaerobic intestinal flora may also enhance the enterohepatic circulation as less bilirubin is converted to urobilinogen for excretion.[6]

Cholestasis, or conjugated hyperbilirubinemia, results from diminished bile flow or excretion. In infants, the etiologies vary and can be divided into two main categories: obstructive/structural and hepatocellular (Table 7–2). The category of obstructive/structural cholestasis includes biliary atresia and choledochal cysts. The etiology of *biliary atresia* is unknown, but several mechanisms (infectious, genetic, and immunologic) have been proposed to explain the inflammatory process

Table 7–1.

Differential Diagnosis of Unconjugated Hyperbilirubinemia in Neonates and Infants

- Increased bilirubin production
  - Intravascular hemolysis
    - Infection
    - ABO blood group incompatibility
    - Drug-induced hemolysis
    - Hemoglobinopathies: sickle cell disease
    - Red blood cell membrane defects: spherocytosis, elliptocytosis/ovalocytosis
    - Hemoglobin synthesis disorders: thalassemia
    - Red blood cell enzyme deficiencies: G6PD deficiency, pyruvate kinase deficiency
    - Hyperviscosity (polycythemia) syndrome
  - Extravascular hemolysis
    - Hematoma
- Decreased bilirubin clearance
  - Crigler–Najjar syndrome (types I and II)
  - Gilbert's syndrome
  - Drug induced
  - Cardiac failure
- Increased enterohepatic circulation
  - Breast milk jaundice
  - Inadequate breastfeeding
  - Impaired intestinal motility

Table 7–2.

Differential Diagnosis of Conjugated Hyperbilirubinemia in Neonates and Infants

- Obstructive or structural causes
  - Biliary atresia
  - Choledochal cyst
  - Alagille syndrome
  - Non-syndromic duct paucity
  - Choledocholithiasis
  - Spontaneous biliary perforation
  - External compression
    - Tumor
  - Neonatal sclerosing cholangitis
- Hepatocellular causes
  - Idiopathic neonatal hepatitis
  - Infections
    - Viral: CMV, toxoplasmosis, rubella, parvovirus B19, herpes simplex, syphilis, human herpesvirus-6, Enteroviruses, hepatitis B, hepatitis C, HIV
    - Bacterial: sepsis, urinary tract infection
  - Metabolic/genetic disorders
    - Disorders of carbohydrate metabolism: galactosemia, hereditary fructose intolerance, glycogen storage disease
    - Disorders of amino acid metabolism: type I tyrosinemia
    - Disorders of lipid metabolism: Niemann–Pick disease, Wolman syndrome
    - Peroxisomal disorders: Zellweger syndrome
    - Alpha 1-antitrypsin deficiency
    - Cystic fibrosis
    - Progressive familial intrahepatic cholestasis
    - Disorders of bile acid synthesis
    - Dubin–Johnson syndrome, Rotor syndrome
  - Endocrine disorders
    - Hypothyroidism
    - Panhypopituitarism
  - Toxic
    - TPN-associated cholestasis
    - Drug induced

that leads to bile duct obliteration.[7] Biliary atresia is described in more detail in Chapter 23. *Choledochal cysts* are rare congenital anomalies of the bile ducts characterized by cystic dilatation of the biliary tree.[8] Conditions that lead to hepatocellular cholestasis are numerous and include idiopathic neonatal hepatitis, infections, metabolic, genetic, and endocrine disorders.

CLINICAL PRESENTATION

History

The parents or caregivers should be asked about the onset, duration, and progression of jaundice. Jaundice is considered to be pathologic if it is detected before 24 hours of age or persists beyond 14 days of age. Dark urine color and light or acholic stools are often present with conjugated hyperbilirubinemia and can indicate a serious underlying hepatobiliary disorder. Inspection of a stool sample by the physician may be more accurate rather than solely relying on the parents' description. However, in some countries parents are given stool color cards as a screening method for obstructive cholestasis. Parents can compare their child's stool color with examples on the card, and contact their physician, if stools exhibit too light a color. This has led to earlier detection and referral, timely intervention, and better outcome for patients with biliary atresia.[9]

The physician should inquire about the infant's feeding pattern, type and amount of milk intake, and the presence of vomiting and irritability. Jaundice should not be attributed to dehydration in an infant who seems to be taking adequate amount of milk (>100 mL/kg/day), so further workup may be needed. Feeding intolerance and irritability can be seen with infections and metabolic disorders. The appearance of a thriving but jaundiced infant beyond 2 weeks of age should not delay evaluation, as a serious condition such as biliary atresia may be present in early life without other obvious signs and symptoms.

The maternal and perinatal history should be reviewed, looking for signs of maternal illness during pregnancy or delivery (fever, skin rashes, and respiratory symptoms), traumatic delivery, and birth asphyxia. The neonate's size relative to gestational age is important; small-for-gestational-age neonates may have polycythemia, and large-for-gestational-age neonates have an increased incidence of birth trauma that can be accompanied by hematomas. Pertinent family history should be obtained, including that for jaundice, liver diseases, anemia, hemolysis, metabolic disorders, or splenectomy.

Physical Examination

Different etiologies of hyperbilirubinemia can be accompanied by a variety of clinical manifestations. The physical evaluation should focus on confirming the presence of jaundice and looking for risk factors and for associated signs that can help delineate the cause. Evidence of complications such as portal hypertension, coagulopathy, thrombocytopenia, and failure to thrive should be sought.

Jaundice may be the only manifestation of hyperbilirubinemia. It should be assessed with adequate ambient light. Blanching the skin by applying finger pressure over a bony part can help detect jaundice. The extent of body jaundice can provide a rough estimate of bilirubin level. This, however, may not be accurate, especially in infants with dark skin color. Carotenemia, or pseudojaundice, can occur with excessive ingestion of foods rich in beta-carotene (such as squash and carrots). This is common in older infants and toddlers, and is manifested by a yellow-orange skin color without scleral icterus or hyperbilirubinemia. Infants whose jaundice is caused by ongoing hemolysis may also appear pale and lethargic.

The presence of skin rashes can suggest infection, especially those that are perinatally acquired. Clinical manifestations of congenital cytomegalovirus (CMV) can include a petechial rash, jaundice, hepatosplenomegaly, and central nervous system involvement with microcephaly, seizures, and cerebral calcifications. Infants born with congenital toxoplasmosis may have a maculopapular rash, jaundice, fever, hepatosplenomegaly, microcephaly, and seizures. Congenital rubella can present with purpuric skin lesions, growth retardation, and hepatosplenomegaly. Blueberry muffin lesions, described as maculopapular reddish-blue- or magenta-colored lesions related to persistent dermal erythropoiesis, have been reported in neonates with CMV, rubella, and parvovirus. The presence of vesicular skin lesions should raise suspicion for a herpes virus infection.[10]

Cataracts can be associated with metabolic disorders and congenital infections. Metabolic disorders associated with cataracts and liver diseases include galactosemia and peroxisomal disorders (Zellweger syndrome). Infectious causes include toxoplasmosis, rubella, CMV, herpes, and syphilis.

Liver size and consistency should be assessed. Hepatomegaly can be present with disorders leading to liver damage and with storage diseases. A firm or hard liver can suggest advanced liver disease with cirrhosis. The presence of edema, ascites, coagulopathy, or encephalopathy may also suggest advanced liver disease. Splenomegaly is seen with infections (such as CMV), hematological disorders (such as hereditary elliptocytosis), and storage disorders (such as cholesteryl ester storage disease and glycogen storage diseases).

In certain conditions, if the underlying process is not treated, progression to liver failure can occur, leading to ascites, hypoglycemia, coagulation abnormalities, and encephalopathy. Encephalopathy may not be easily diagnosed in a young infant but should be suspected with poor feeding, irritability, and reversal of day/night sleep patterns.

DIFFERENTIAL DIAGNOSIS

The differential diagnosis for jaundice is age-specific. This chapter will mostly address conditions associated with jaundice in neonates and infants. Etiologies of jaundice from unconjugated and conjugated hyperbilirubinemia in this population are summarized in Tables 7–1 and 7–2. Causes of cholestatic jaundice occurring in older children and adolescents are briefly summarized in Table 7–3.

Causes of Unconjugated Hyperbilirubinemia

Increased bilirubin production

Increased bilirubin production can result from increased breakdown of hemoglobin and other heme-containing proteins. Ongoing hemolysis, both intravascular and extravascular, can contribute to unconjugated hyperbilirubinemia. Intravascular hemolysis can occur in the setting of infection, autoimmune and drug-induced hemolysis, hemoglobinopathies (such as sickle cell disease), red blood cell membrane defects (such as elliptocytosis and spherocytosis), hemoglobin synthesis disorders (such as thalassemia), and red blood cell enzyme deficiencies of the glycolysis pathway (such as glucose-6-phosphate dehydrogenase deficiency or G6PD). Extravascular hemolysis is often related to hematomas (such as a cephalhematoma following traumatic delivery).

Decreased bilirubin clearance

Certain drugs, including sulfonamides, can displace bilirubin from albumin. Other drugs, such as rifampicin

Table 7–3.

Differential Diagnosis of Cholestatic Jaundice in Older Children and Adolescents

- Obstructive or structural causes
  - Choledocholithiasis
  - Biliary sludge
  - Choledochal cyst
  - Alagille syndrome
  - External compression
    - Tumor
  - Parasitic infestations
    - Ascaris
- Hepatocellular causes
  - Infections
    - Viral: CMV, hepatitis B, hepatitis C, HIV
    - Bacterial: sepsis
  - Metabolic
    - Alpha 1-antitrypsin deficiency
    - Cystic fibrosis
    - Wilson disease
  - Toxic
    - Drug induced
    - Herbal supplements
    - TPN-associated cholestasis
  - Autoimmune
    - Autoimmune hepatitis
    - Primary sclerosing cholangitis
  - Other
    - Budd Chiari syndrome

and probenecid, can impair hepatic bilirubin uptake, promoting hyperbilirubinemia. Conditions reducing hepatic blood flow, such as cardiac failure, can also result in decreased bilirubin uptake by hepatocytes. Few inherited conditions such as Crigler–Najjar syndrome are known to impair bilirubin conjugation. Crigler–Najjar syndrome types I and II are autosomal recessive disorders characterized by deficiency in UGT, the enzyme responsible for bilirubin conjugation (Figure 7–1). These disorders result in severe and chronic unconjugated hyperbilirubinemia with onset in the first few days of life for type I, and later for type II. Typically these patients have otherwise normal liver tests and normal liver histology. Unconjugated bilirubin levels range between 20 and 25 mg/dL in type I, which is associated absence of UGT enzyme activity. In type II, UGT activity is significantly reduced (<10% of normal) with unconjugated bilirubin levels rarely exceeding 20 mg/dL.[5] Kernicterus and death can occur within months in untreated patients, especially with type I Crigler–Najjar syndrome. When the diagnosis is suspected, treatment with phototherapy should be started until the evaluation is completed; exchange transfusion is required for dangerously high levels of bilirubin. The diagnosis is

often made on clinical grounds in the face of unremitting unconjugated hyperbilirubinemia that is dependent on phototherapy. It can be confirmed by mutation analysis on genomic DNA. A phenobarbital challenge will help differentiate type I from type II, as infants with type II will have at least a 30% decrease in serum bilirubin levels while on phenobarbital, which induces the partially deficient UGT activity. Phenobarbital is not effective in type I patients as UGT activity is absent. Other ways to differentiate between types I and II include the determination of residual bilirubin glucuronidating activity in a liver biopsy or analysis of bile composition; however, these are invasive and rarely used.[11] Most patients with type I Crigler–Najjar syndrome eventually require liver transplantation as phototherapy becomes less effective over time.[12,13] It is hoped that gene therapy or an alternative, such as hepatocyte transplantation, may someday prove useful.

Increased enterohepatic circulation

Increased enterohepatic circulation can lead to reabsorption of bilirubin and elevated serum levels. This occurs in the setting of inadequate fluid and/or caloric intake, including suboptimal breastfeeding, typically in the first few days after birth. Another common cause for increased enterohepatic circulation is breast milk jaundice. This usually occurs after the third day of life and peaks by 2 weeks (to a level of 15–25 mg/dL) and is followed by a slow but gradual resolution. The mechanism of breast milk jaundice is still a matter of debate. Suggested theories include inhibition of hepatic bilirubin conjugation (by a maternal metabolite) or increased intestinal hydrolysis of conjugated bilirubin (by maternal beta-glucuronidase in breast milk). In the majority of breast-fed infants, breast milk jaundice remains a harmless and physiological phenomenon. Intervention is needed when high bilirubin levels are reached or in the presence of other contributing factors.

Causes of Conjugated Hyperbilirubinemia

Obstructive/structural

Biliary atresia (Chapter 23) is the leading cause of extrahepatic obstructive jaundice in newborns. It is a progressive obliterative inflammatory process involving the bile ducts, resulting in obstruction of bile flow leading to cholestasis, hepatic fibrosis, and eventually cirrhosis. Patients with biliary atresia often seem well nourished and present with jaundice and acholic stools. Over time, fat malabsorption, fat-soluble vitamin deficiencies, poor growth, hepatosplenomegaly, and other signs of liver dysfunction become apparent. If untreated, the outcome is uniformly fatal. A portoenterostomy (known as the Kasai procedure) is the treatment of choice for biliary atresia with favorable outcome if performed early. This can restore bile flow and, if successful, may have a 10-year survival of 90% with a native liver. It is therefore essential to establish the diagnosis of biliary atresia early and refer such patients for surgical intervention before the first 8 weeks of age. Those who do not undergo or fail a portoenterostomy procedure will develop fibrosis progressing to end-stage cirrhosis and death, unless liver transplantation is performed.[7]

Choledochal cysts (Chapter 23) are congenital cystic lesions involving the bile ducts that can result in impairment of bile flow. Different types of choledochal cysts have been described based on the anatomy. Type 1, accounting for 80–90% of lesions, involves the entire or segments of the common hepatic and common bile ducts. Infants typically present with jaundice and acholic stools. A palpable right upper quadrant mass can sometimes be appreciated. Treatment is surgical.[8]

Alagille syndrome is an autosomal dominant disorder characterized by paucity of interlobular bile ducts. Affected patients can have peculiar facies with a broad nasal bridge, triangular facies, and deep set eyes. Associated features include cardiac anomalies (mostly with peripheral pulmonic hypoplasia or stenosis), posterior embryotoxon (prominent Schwalbe line) on ophthalmologic exam, and butterfly vertebrae. Less frequent characteristics include growth retardation, mental retardation, developmental delay, and renal and pancreatic insufficiency. Alagille syndrome is associated with mutations of the Jagged-1 gene on chromosome 20p. These mutations arise de novo in >50% of the cases.[14]

Other rare structural abnormalities that can affect bile flow leading to conjugated hyperbilirubinemia include choledocholithiasis, external compression by another organ or mass, and spontaneous biliary perforation.

Hepatocellular

Idiopathic neonatal hepatitis is a term used to describe a clinical syndrome manifested by prolonged neonatal cholestasis without a clear etiology. The subset of infants diagnosed with idiopathic neonatal hepatitis has been decreasing with discovery of more specific disorders leading to cholestasis. The onset of cholestasis in idiopathic neonatal hepatitis may be later compared to biliary atresia and acholic stools are less commonly reported. Cholestasis may still be severe requiring supportive care but prognosis is generally good.[10]

Neonatal infections can result in cholestasis, and should be promptly identified and treated whenever possible. Infections can be bacterial, viral, and even parasitic in origin. Sepsis and extrahepatic bacterial infections, including urinary tract infections, can be insidious. Evaluation for common congenitally acquired pathogens should include toxoplasmosis, rubella, CMV, herpes simplex, and syphilis, depending on the exam findings and risk factors. Other possible infections include parvovirus 19, human herpes virus 6, HIV, varicella, hepatitis B and C, adenovirus, and coxsackie viruses.

Alpha 1-antitrypsin deficiency (Chapter 26) is the most common inherited liver disease that presents with neonatal cholestasis. It is an autosomal recessive disorder that has been implicated in 5–15% of cases of neonatal cholestasis. Liver disease results from accumulation of the mutant protein within the endoplasmic reticulum of hepatocytes. In addition to cholestasis, other manifestations may include elevated aminotransferase levels, hepatomegaly, and other signs of progressive liver dysfunction. Lung involvement from alpha 1-antitrypsin deficiency occurs later in life.[15]

Cystic fibrosis (Chapter 32) can occasionally present with cholestasis. Obstruction of bile ducts with inspissated secretions is thought to play a major role in the pathogenesis. A history of meconium ileus or the presence of hepatomegaly, steatorrhea, or poor growth should raise concern for cystic fibrosis.

Galactosemia (Chapter 28) is an autosomal recessive disorder of carbohydrate metabolism arising from abnormalities in galactose metabolism. The classic form results from deficiency of the enzyme galactose-1-phosphate uridyl transferase, leading to accumulation of metabolites that can be toxic to the liver and other organs. Progressive cholestasis and liver dysfunction are often noted during the first 1–2 weeks of life. Other signs include feeding intolerance, hypoglycemia, diarrhea, and poor weight gain. Hemolysis may be present further contributing to hyperbilirubinemia. If untreated, galactosemia often leads to progressive liver disease, cataracts, and severe mental retardation. It is associated with sepsis due to *Escherichia coli* infection. When suspected, exclusion of lactose-containing milk (both human milk and cow's milk-based formulas) is needed.[16] Patients presenting in early infancy with liver dysfunction should also be evaluated for type I tyrosinemia, a disorder of amino acid metabolism. This disorder can be devastating leading to liver failure, renal dysfunction, neurologic crises, rickets, poor growth, and death. A characteristic "boiled cabbage" odor has sometimes been described.

Congenital hypothyroidism can contribute to hyperbilirubinemia through decreased bilirubin excretion. Clinical presentation may include prolonged jaundice, lethargy, poor feeding, hypotonia, constipation, and enlarged fontanelles. If untreated, adverse long-term developmental consequences are likely to occur. Hypopituitarism can also present with cholestasis. Other associated features of hypopituitarism may include hypoglycemia, poor weight gain, and temperature instability.[17]

Defects in transporters in the bile canalicular membrane of hepatocytes have been described as causes of cholestasis. These are categorized under progressive familial intrahepatic cholestasis (PFIC) and can lead to severe liver dysfunction and cirrhosis. Unlike PFIC I and II, children with PFIC III have elevated gamma-glutamyl transferase (GGT) levels. Bile acids play a major role in bile flow and intestinal digestion of fat and fat-soluble vitamins. Several specific defects in bile acid metabolism have been identified. Other disorders include Dubin–Johnson syndrome, an autosomal recessive disorder, that is associated with defective hepatic secretion of conjugated bilirubin through the canalicular membrane and marked liver pigmentation (usually later in childhood).[10] Rotor syndrome, another autosomal recessive disorder, is characterized by decreased intracellular bilirubin storage with modest impairment of bilirubin excretion. In both disorders, affected children are usually asymptomatic except for jaundice.

Infants maintained on parenteral nutrition frequently develop cholestasis (TPN-associated cholestasis) as well as steatosis and cholelithiasis. This can progress to hepatic fibrosis, cirrhosis, development of portal hypertension, and liver failure. Factors contributing to TPN-associated cholestasis include prematurity, low birth weight, lack of enteral feeding, sepsis, intestinal bacterial translocation, and duration of parenteral nutrition.[18]

DIAGNOSIS

Depending on the clinical scenario, evaluation of a jaundiced child may include blood tests, urine tests, imaging studies, and histological assessment. A summary of possible tests is provided in Table 7–4.

Blood and Urine Testing

Physiological jaundice with unconjugated hyperbilirubinemia remains the most common cause of neonatal jaundice. The presence of certain risk factors should raise concern for the development of severe hyperbilirubinemia. These include jaundice observed in the first 24 hours of age, blood group incompatibility, or other known hemolytic disease, previous sibling requiring phototherapy, cephalhematoma, significant bruising, East Asian race, and a bilirubin level plotting in the high-risk zone on published age-specific normograms.[19]

Initial blood testing should include measurement of direct and total bilirubin levels to determine

Table 7–4.

Evaluation of a Jaundiced Child

Workup for unconjugated hyperbilirubinemia

- CBC with differential
- Blood smear
- Reticulocyte count
- Heptoglobin level
- Blood group testing
- Coomb's test
- Newborn screen
- Infectious workup
    - Blood culture
    - Urinalysis, urine culture

Workup for conjugated hyperbilirubinemia

- GGT, Alk phos, ALT, AST
- Albumin and prothrombin time
- Glucose level
- Serum bile acid analysis
- Newborn screen
- TSH and free T4 levels
- Urine-reducing substances, erythrocyte galactose-1-phosphate uridyl transferase analysis
- Plasma amino acid profile
- Urinary succinylacetone and/or urine organic acid analysis
- Alpha 1-antitrypsin level and phenotype

what type of hyperbilirubinemia is present. With unconjugated hyperbilirubinemia, assessment for hemolysis is needed, including a complete blood count, blood smear, reticulocyte count, and possibly a haptoglobin level. Blood group testing and a direct antiglobulin test (Coomb's test) should be performed, if not already obtained with cord blood. Checking a G6PD level (for G6PD deficiency) is recommended in patients not responding to phototherapy or with appropriate ethnic or family history. Infection can contribute to hemolysis and should be considered in the workup (white blood cell count and differential, blood and urine cultures).

With conjugated hyperbilirubinemia, further workup is always warranted. An algorithm for evaluating a cholestatic infant is provided in Figure 7–2. Assessment of liver injury should include GGT, alkaline phosphatase (AP), alanine aminotransferase (ALT), and aspartate aminotransferase (AST). Conditions mainly affecting the biliary tree, such as biliary atresia, are often accompanied by proportionately higher GGT and AP elevations compared to the hepatocellular enzymes, ALT, and AST. Albumin and prothrombin time should be checked to assess liver synthetic function. Hypoglycemia can be a sign of liver dysfunction but is also a prominent feature of metabolic disorders (galactosemia and

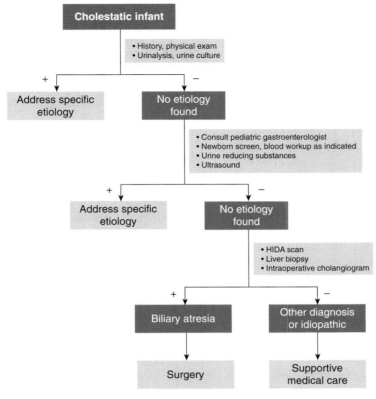

FIGURE 7–2 ■ Suggested algorithm for evaluating a cholestatic infant.

hereditary fructose intolerance). Serum levels of primary bile acids are usually elevated with biliary obstruction and generally normal or low in infants with disorders of bile acid synthesis. Fast atom bombardment mass spectroscopy may be needed to detect specific bile acid intermediates when a primary bile acid synthetic disorder is suspected.

The newborn screen results should be checked promptly for hypothyroidism, galactosemia, and tyrosinemia. Certain newborn screen programs include only thyroid-stimulating hormone (TSH) and not thyroxine (free T4) that can miss central hypothyroidism. If any suspicion exits, testing for hypothyroidism should include TSH and free T4 levels. In cases of suspected galactosemia, testing for urine-reducing substance is usually positive, but this is not a specific finding. Definitive diagnosis of galactosemia is based on a quantitative erythrocyte galactose-1-phosphate uridyl transferase analysis.[16] Because this assesses enzyme activity in red blood cells, false negatives can result with recent blood transfusions. In *tyrosinemia*, the plasma amino acid profile reveals elevated tyrosine, phenylalanine, and methionine levels. However, an increased tyrosine level on newborn screen or plasma amino acid profile is not specific for tyrosinemia, but rather a general reflection of liver disease. Confirmatory testing for tyrosinemia includes increased urinary succinylacetone excretion,

which is often included in urine organic acid analysis, but may need to be ordered separately. Further confirmation can be determined by documenting decreased fumarylacetoacetate hydrolase activity in red blood cells or fibroblasts.[20]

The diagnosis of alpha 1-antitrypsin deficiency is suggested by a low-level serum alpha 1-antitrypsin level. Serum level alone is not sufficient, as it is an acute phase reactant and may rise above the deficient range in some subjects. An abnormal alpha 1-antitrypsin phenotype (PiZZ), as determined by electrophoresis, confirms the diagnosis of alpha 1-antitrypsin deficiency.[15] Infants with cystic fibrosis often have elevated blood levels of immunoreactive trypsin on newborn screening. Sweat chloride iontophoresis is the standard for diagnosis. If adequate quantities of sweat cannot be collected, mutation analysis can be performed.

Infectious workup should include a urinalysis and urine culture sent to look for bacterial infections. Evaluation for specific viral infections can be guided by the maternal and perinatal history. In the infant, serologic IgM testing should be sought as IgG is often of maternal origin. CMV infection can also be assessed by a urine CMV culture.[10] Polymerase chain reaction testing for certain infectious agents can be useful. When indicated blood bacterial culture and cerebral spinal fluid analysis and culture may be obtained.

Radiologic Testing

Radiologic evaluation is needed in the setting of conjugated hyperbilirubinemia to assess the biliary anatomy. Ultrasonography is the first test of choice as it does not involve radiation exposure. Accuracy depends on operator experience, and is better performed in a pediatric center. It should include determination of the liver size and echotexture, and assessment of the intrahepatic and extrahepatic biliary systems. Normally, the common bile duct measures <1 mm in neonates and <2 mm in infants. Ultrasonography can help exclude anatomical anomalies, mainly choledochal cysts and biliary stones or extrinsic compression by masses or other organs. Most, but not all, patients with biliary atresia will not have a gallbladder visible on ultrasonography. A triangular echogenic structure (also known as the triangular cord sign) is sometimes visualized in the porta hepatis, and is attributed to fibrous tissue seen with biliary atresia. The finding of polysplenia or situs inversus should raise concern for the embryonic form of biliary atresia.[21]

Hepatobiliary imaging using technetium-labeled diisopropyl iminodiacetic acid nuclear tracer can be useful in the evaluation of cholestasis. Intestinal excretion of the tracer confirms patency of the biliary system and rules out biliary atresia. Serial images should be taken for up to 24 hours or until intestinal excretion is visualized. The test sensitivity is high and improved by pretreatment with phenobarbital, given at a dose of 5 mg/kg/day for at least 5 days prior to imaging.[22] However, the test specificity remains low, as hepatocellular dysfunction in a jaundiced patient often prevents tracer excretion even without an anatomical obstruction.

An intraoperative, or less often percutaneous, cholangiogram can be performed to assess the morphology and patency of the biliary tree. This is often helpful if the diagnosis of biliary atresia remains unclear.

Histological Assessment

Percutaneous liver biopsy can be extremely valuable in the evaluation of neonatal cholestasis. The main histological features of biliary atresia are bile plugging, bile duct proliferation, portal edema, and fibrosis. Biliary atresia is thought to be an evolving inflammatory process, so biopsies performed early in the disease course, especially before 2 weeks of age, may not be diagnostic. Giant cell transformation and lobular disarray are often seen in idiopathic neonatal hepatitis but can also be seen with other causes of neonatal cholestasis, including biliary atresia. In Alagille syndrome, reduced number of small bile ducts can be appreciated on liver biopsy, although this may not be apparent in newborns. Liver histology can also help in assessment of metabolic or genetic disorders including alpha 1-antitrypsin deficiency and some types of storage diseases. When a storage disease is suspected, a small part of the specimen should be sent for transmission electron microscopy. If the liver biopsy findings suggest an obstructive etiology, an intraoperative cholangiogram is helpful to further assess the biliary tree.[23]

TREATMENT

Medical interventions in cases of unconjugated hyperbilirubinemia aim at supporting the infant, addressing reversible causes of hyperbilirubinemia, and avoiding complications. Such complications may include the development of severe anemia, and deposition of unconjugated bilirubin in the central nervous system, leading to bilirubin-induced neurologic dysfunction, kernicterus, and death. The standard treatment of unconjugated hyperbilirubinemia is phototherapy that induces photoisomerization of unconjugated bilirubin to a water-soluble form that is excreted into bile. Bilirubin hour-specific monograms are available to guide clinicians to the need for phototherapy and exchange transfusions.[19] Exchange transfusions may be required with ongoing hemolysis, when phototherapy fails to maintain low enough bilirubin levels to avoid kernicterus. Fluid and calorie intake should be optimized if dehydration is present. Concerns for underlying infection should be addressed and drugs contributing to the hyperbilirubinemia should be withdrawn. Surgical treatment is very rare and restricted to certain cases of intestinal obstruction and liver transplantation for Crigler–Najjar syndrome.

Treatment approaches for cholestatic infants include general supportive care and specific interventions related to the underlying etiology. Nutritional support should be optimized and weight should be monitored closely. Administration of medium-chain triglyceride (MCT)-containing formulas or supplements added to breast milk can increase fat absorption and help maintain good growth and development. In contrast to long-chain triglycerides, intestinal MCT absorption is not dependent on bile acid secretion, which is compromised in cholestasis. Prolonged use of exclusive MCT formulas may place patients at risk of developing essential fatty acid deficiency.

Increasing the caloric density of infant formula can also increase daily caloric intake. Supplementation with nasogastric tube feedings may sometimes be needed to reach needed intake goals. Weaning of parenteral nutrition while advancing enteral feedings can significantly help resolve cholestasis that is TPN induced, in addition to reducing the risk of catheter-related infections that contributes to liver disease. Fat-soluble vitamin supplementation and serial level assessments are essential to avoid vitamin deficiencies. Table 7–5 summarizes the signs and treatment of fat-soluble

Table 7–5.

Fat-soluble Vitamin Supplementation

Vitamin	Signs of Vitamin Deficiency	Oral Replacement Dose	Signs of Vitamin Toxicity
A	Night blindness, Bitot's spots, keratomalacia, follicular hyperkeratosis	5000–25,000 IU/day*	Hepatotoxicity, headache, erythematous or peeling skin, pseudotumor cerebri
D	Myalgia, osteomalacia, rickets, tetany	Cholecalciferol: 2500–5000 IU/day 25-OH cholecalciferol: 2–5 mcg/kg/day	Hypercalcemia, hypercalciuria, nephrocalcinosis
E	Hemolytic anemia, neurologic deficits (ophthalmoplegia, loss of DTRs, vibration and position senses, ataxia)	α-Tocopherol: 15–25 IU/kg/day	Fatigue, nausea, diarrhea, bleeding
K	Bleeding, easy bruising	Phytonadione: 2.5–5 mg twice weekly up to 5 mg/day	Phytonadione is non-toxic

DTRs = deep tendon reflexes.
*mcg retinol equivalent (0.3 mcg retinol = 1 unit vitamin A).

vitamin deficiencies and signs of vitamin toxicity that may occur with overdosing.[23,24]

Pruritis associated with cholestasis can be severe, affecting the child's quality of life by interference with sleep and social interaction. This is usually addressed medically, but when medical approaches fail surgical interventions can be considered. A conservative approach includes the use of topical soothing creams. Histamine blockers are often ineffective in controlling pruritis. More effective antipruritics include ursodeoxycholic acid and cholestyramine that are relatively safe and inexpensive. Others include rifampin, phenobarbital, and naltrexone (Table 7–6).[25] Surgical interventions can be effective in controlling pruritis and include partial external biliary diversion and ileal exclusion. The external biliary diversion involves creating a conduit between the gallbladder and skin to allow for bile drainage.[26] Ileal exclusion involves creating an ileo-colonic anastomosis that bypasses the distal ileum interrupting the enterohepatic circulation.[27] Liver transplantation has also been used to treat severe intractable pruritis associated with liver disease.[28]

In infants with suspected or confirmed galactosemia, galactose-containing feedings and medications should be stopped immediately. Such infants should be placed on a soy formula or other lactose-free formula.[16] Treatment of tyrosinemia includes dietary restriction or elimination of foods rich with phenylalanine and tyrosine along with nitisinone or NTBC, 2-(2-nitro-4-fluoromethylbenzoyl)-1,3-cyclohexanedione, which blocks an enzyme proximal in the catabolic pathway of tyrosine. Liver transplantation can be effective. An experienced nutritionist working with a geneticist should manage the nutrition of infants with metabolic disorders requiring special diets.[20] Hypothyroidism and hypopituitarism should be treated promptly with appropriate hormonal supplementation to avoid adverse non-reversible consequences. Such infants are best followed by a pediatric endocrinologist.

Table 7–6.

Medications Used for Treatment of Pruritis Associated with Liver Disease

Medication	Dose	Potential Side Effects
Ursodeoxycholic acid	15–20 mg/kg/day, in two divided doses	Diarrhea
Cholestyramine	240 mg/kg/day, in three divided doses	Constipation, electrolyte abnormalities, fat malabsorption, intestinal obstruction
Rifampin	10 mg/kg/day (maximum 600 mg/day), in two divided doses	Hypersensitivity reactions, thrombocytopenia, orange-red fluid color, hepatotoxicity, drug interactions
Phenobarbital	5–10 mg/kg/day	Sedation, behavioral side effects, respiratory depression

If a diagnosis of biliary atresia is confirmed, a portoenterostomy is the only therapeutic intervention, besides liver transplantation. This aims at restoring biliary drainage through a Roux-en-Y anastomosis to the hepatic hilum. The main factor for success is the infant's age at the time of surgery. Best results are achieved with surgical intervention before 60 days of age and poor results are encountered with surgery beyond 90 days of age. Otherwise liver transplantation is the only available treatment option for biliary atresia.[7]. Other etiologies leading to severe liver dysfunction may also benefit from liver transplantation. Treatment of choledochal cysts is also surgical. Excision is performed, often with reconstruction of a Roux-en-Y anastomosis for biliary drainage, depending on the type of the choledochal cyst.

Infants should have serial developmental assessments. Physical therapy can be introduced to help improve motor skills if needed. Immunizations should be kept up to date, and include vaccination for hepatitis A and B. Accelerated immunization programs are sometimes implemented, especially for live virus vaccines if liver transplantation is anticipated in the future. Assessment and management of complications of advancing liver disease and portal hypertension are needed by an experienced pediatric gastroenterologist.

CONCLUSIONS

Jaundice is the consequence of hyperbilirubinemia. Physicians should be able to distinguish between unconjugated and conjugated hyperbilirubinemia based on published guidelines. Rapid diagnosis, appropriate referral, and intervention are keys to good patient outcome.

REFERENCES

1. Moyer V, Freese DK, Whitington PF, et al. North American Society for Pediatric Gastroenterology, Hepatology and Nutrition. Guideline for the evaluation of cholestatic jaundice in infants: recommendations of the North American Society for Pediatric Gastroenterology, Hepatology and Nutrition. *J Pediatr Gastroenterol Nutr.* 2004;39(2): 115–128.
2. Palmer C, Mujsce DJ. Common neonatal illnesses. In: Hoekelman RA, ed. *Primary Pediatric Care.* St. Louis: Mosby; 2001:587–599.
3. Dick MC, Mowat AP. Hepatitis syndrome in infancy—an epidemiological survey with 10 year follow up. *Arch Dis Child.* 1985;60(6):512–516.
4. Watson RL. Hyperbilirubinemia. *Crit Care Nurs Clin North Am.* 2009;21(1):97–120.
5. Nowicki MJ, Poley JR. The hereditary hyperbilirubinaemias. *Baillieres Clin Gastroenterol.* 1998;12(2):355–367.
6. Tiribelli C, Ostrow JD. Intestinal flora and bilirubin. *J Hepatol.* 2005;42(2):170–172.
7. Bassett MD, Murray KF. Biliary atresia: recent progress. *J Clin Gastroenterol.* 2008;42(6):720–729.
8. Miyano T, Yamataka A. Choledochal cysts. *Curr Opin Pediatr.* 1997;9(3):283–288.
9. Hsiao CH, Chang MH, Chen HL, et al. Taiwan Infant Stool Color Card Study Group. Universal screening for biliary atresia using an infant stool color card in Taiwan. *Hepatology.* 2008;47(4):1233–1240.
10. Roberts EA. Neonatal hepatitis syndrome. *Semin Neonatol.* 2003;8(5):357–374.
11. Bosma PJ. Inherited disorders of bilirubin metabolism. *J Hepatol.* 2003;38(1):107–117.
12. Van der Veere CN, Sinaasappel M, McDonagh AF, et al. Current therapy for Crigler–Najjar syndrome type 1: report of a world registry. *Hepatology.* 1996; 24:311–315.
13. Yohannan MD, Terry HJ, Littlewood JM. Long term phototherapy in Crigler–Najjar syndrome. *Arch Dis Child.* 1983;58:460–462.
14. Piccoli DA, Spinner NB. Alagille syndrome and the Jagged1 gene. *Semin Liver Dis.* 2001;21(4):525–534.
15. Fairbanks KD, Tavill AS. Liver disease in alpha 1-antitrypsin deficiency: a review. *Am J Gastroenterol.* 2008;103(8):2136–2141.
16. Bosch AM. Classical galactosaemia revisited. *J Inherit Metab Dis.* 2006;29(4):516–525.
17. Choo-Kang LR, Sun CC, Counts DR. Cholestasis and hypoglycemia: manifestations of congenital anterior hypopituitarism. *J Clin Endocrinol Metab.* 1996;81(8):2786–2789.
18. Btaiche IF, Khalidi N. Parenteral nutrition-associated liver complications in children. *Pharmacotherapy.* 2002;22(2):188–211.
19. American Academy of Pediatrics Subcommittee on Hyperbilirubinemia. Management of hyperbilirubinemia in the newborn infant 35 or more weeks of gestation. *Pediatrics.* 2004;114(1):297–316.
20. Scott CR. The genetic tyrosinemias. *Am J Med Genet C Semin Med Genet.* 2006;142C(2):121–126.
21. Gubernick JA, Rosenberg HK, Ilaslan H, Kessler A. US approach to jaundice in infants and children. *Radiographics.* 2000;20(1):173–195.
22. Majd M, Reba RC, Altman RP. Effect of phenobarbital on 99mTc-IDA scintigraphy in the evaluation of neonatal jaundice. *Semin Nucl Med.* 1981;11(3):194–204.
23. Balistreri WF. Neonatal cholestasis. *J Pediatr.* 1985;106(2):171–184.
24. Novy MA, Schwarz KB. Nutritional considerations and management of the child with liver disease. *Nutrition.* 1997;13(3):177–184.
25. Cies JJ, Giamalis JN. Treatment of cholestatic pruritus in children. *Am J Health Syst Pharm.* 2007;64(11):1157–1162.
26. Ekinci S, Karnak I, Gürakan F, et al. Partial external biliary diversion for the treatment of intractable pruritus in children with progressive familial intrahepatic cholestasis: report of two cases. *Surg Today.* 2008;38(8):726–730.
27. Modi BP, Suh MY, Jonas MM, Lillehei C, Kim HB. Ileal exclusion for refractory symptomatic cholestasis in Alagille syndrome. *J Pediatr Surg.* 2007;42(5):800–805.
28. Engelmann G, Schmidt J, Oh J, et al. Indications for pediatric liver transplantation. Data from the Heidelberg pediatric liver transplantation program. *Nephrol Dial Transplant.* 2007;22(suppl 8):viii23–viii28.

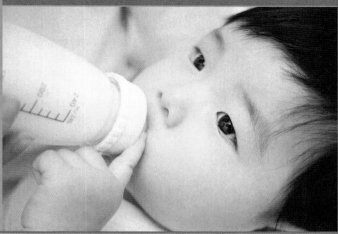

CHAPTER 8

Nutrition

Robert D. Baker and Susan S. Baker

NUTRITION IN HEALTH

According to the American Academy of Pediatrics, the goal of pediatrics is "to attain optimal physical, mental, and social health and well-being for all infants, children, adolescents, and young adults." It is self-evident that maintaining good nutrition is a prerequisite to attaining this goal. Appropriate nutrition supplies the "building blocks" for healthy physical growth. Optimal mental health and mental capacity rely on adequate nutrition, from conception to old age. D.J.P. Barker theorized that fetal nutrition is associated with a number of chronic conditions of later life. The Barker hypothesis, in its expanded form, proposes that infant nutrition, as well as fetal nutrition, has long-term health effects reaching into adulthood and old age. Some of the parameters that may be affected by nutrition in infancy include cardiovascular health, blood pressure, bone mineralization, low-density lipoprotein cholesterol, split proinsulin, and cognitive development. While these observations are tantalizing, they are observational. A causal relationship has not been established. The Barker hypothesis continues to be debated, but to the extent that it proves true, early nutrition gains tremendous importance.

Much of the early work on establishing nutritional requirements focused on preventing diseases and deficiencies. It was assumed that if a child were given adequate amounts and varieties of foods, good nutrition would automatically follow. The present obesity epidemic that has affected all age groups in our society has proven this assumption incorrect. It has become clear that we need to monitor the nutritional health of our youth and encourage good nutrition for all. In order to accomplish this, we must know the nutritional requirements for optimal growth and to avoid future nutrition-related complications, not merely to avoid deficiency states.

NUTRITIONAL NEEDS AND REQUIREMENTS

Recommended Dietary Allowances (RDAs) were first established in 1941 and first published in 1943. The RDAs were based on scientific evidence and intended to serve as goals for good nutrition. Over the years the RDAs have changed according to the needs of the country. When first devised, the country was struggling with war-time shortages and the RDAs were used to guide priorities and to avoid widespread deficiencies in *groups of people.* Over time, the emphasis changed to goals for individuals. The eighth edition of the RDAs published in 1974 included the following definition of RDA: "the levels of essential nutrients that, on the basis of scientific knowledge, are judged by the Food and Nutrition Board to be adequate to meet the known nutrient needs of *practically all healthy persons.*" The exception to the "practically all healthy persons" rule is the RDA for energy. Since it would not be reasonable to recommend the high end of the distribution curve for energy, in this case the RDA was set at approximately the average. Planning for the present *Dietary Reference Intakes* (DRIs), that have superseded the RDAs, began in 1993 with the realization that RDAs need to be "continuously" updated rather than periodically reviewed and updated and that values beyond RDAs were necessary. Among other things, Upper Limits (UL) needed to be established. The DRIs are now the accepted reference standard for most nutrient requirements for all age groups. There is now a standing committee of the

Table 8–1.

Dietary Reference Intakes

Term	Definition
Estimated Average Requirement (EAR)	The average daily intake level of a nutrient that, based on scientific evidence, is estimated to meet the requirements of half the healthy individuals of a particular gender and in a particular age group
Recommended Dietary Allowance (RDA)	The average daily nutrient intake level that meets the nutrient requirement of nearly all healthy individuals of a particular gender and in a particular age group. Usually the RDA is the EAR plus two standard deviations
Adequate Intake (AI)	The recommended average intake level based on experimental or observed approximations or estimates of apparently adequate nutrient intakes by groups of individuals assumed to be healthy. AI is used when there is insufficient scientific knowledge to establish an EAR and therefore no RDA can be calculated
Tolerable Upper Intake Level (UL)	The highest average daily intake level of a nutrient that is likely to pose no risk of adverse health outcome to almost all individuals of a particular gender and in a particular age group
Acceptable Macronutrient Distribution Range (AMDR)	Range of macronutrient intakes for a particular energy source that is associated with reduced risk of chronic disease while providing adequate intakes of essential nutrients

Institute of Medicine (IOM) that sets DRIs as directed by the Food and Nutrition Board (FNB). The IOM has published these references in a series of eight volumes that cover more than 40 nutrient substances.[1] These books can be purchased or are available free online at www.USDA.gov. Table 8–1 lists and defines the reference values included in the DRIs. As with earlier versions, the DRIs list energy requirements (Table 8–2) at

Table 8–2.

Dietary Reference Intakes

Nutrient	Age	RDA	AI	UL
Carbohydrate (g/day): total digestible; acceptable macronutrient distribution range: 45–65	0–6 months	130	60	Sugars ≤25% of calories
	7–12 months	130	95	
	1–3 years	130		
	4–8 years	130		
	9–13 years			
	14–18 years			
Total fiber (g/day)	0–6 months	ND	19	
	7–12 months	ND	25	
	1–3 years		31 (m), 26 (f)*	
	4–8 years		38 (m), 26 (f)	
	9–13 years			
	14–18 years			
Total fat (g/day)	0–6 months	30–40	31	
	7–12 months	25–35	30	
	13 years			
	4–8 years			
	9–13 years			
	14–18 years			
n-6 PUFAs (g/day) (linoleic acid)	0–6 months	ND	4.4	
	7–12 months	ND	4.6	
	1–3 years		7	
	4–8 years		10	
	9–13 years		12 (m), 10 (f)	
	14–18 years		16 (m), 11 (f)	

Table 8–2. (Continued)

Dietary Reference Intakes

Nutrient	Age	RDA	AI	UL
n-3 PUFAs (g/day) (α-linolenic acid)	0–6 months	ND	0.5	
	7–12 months	ND	0.5	
	1–3 years		0.7	
	4–8 years		0.9	
	9–13 years		1.2 (m), 1.0 (f)	
	14–18 years		1.6 (m), 1.1 (f)	
Saturated and *trans* fatty acids, and cholesterol	0–6 months	ND		
	7–12 months	ND		
	1–3 years	ND		
	4–8 years	ND		
	9–13 years	ND		
	14–18 years	ND		
Protein (g/day)	0–6 months	ND	1.52 (g/kg/day)	
	7–12 months	11		
	1–3 years	13		
	4–8 years	19		
	9–13 years	34		
	14–18 years	52 (m), 46 (f)		
Biotin (mcg/day)	0–6 months		5	
	7–12 months		6	
	1–3 years		8	
	4–8 years		12	
	9–13 years		20	
	14–18 years		25	
Choline (mg/day)	0–6 months		125	ND
	7–12 months		150	ND
	1–3 years		200	1000
	4–8 years		250	1000
	9–13 years		375	2000
	14–18 years			3000
Folate (mcg/day)	0–6 months	150	65	ND
	7–12 months	200	80	ND
	1–3 years	300		300
	4–8 years	400		400
	9–13 years			600
	14–18 years			800
Niacin (mg/day)	0–6 months	6	2	ND
	7–12 months	8	4	ND
	1–3 years	12		10
	4–8 years	16 (m), 14 (f)		15
	9–13 years			20
	14–18 years			30
Pantothenic acid (mg/day)	0–6 months		1.7	
	7–12 months		1.8	
	1–3 years		2	
	4–8 years		3	
	9–13 years		4	
	14–18 years		5	
Riboflavin (mg/day) (vitamin B$_2$)	0–6 months	0.5	0.3	
	7–12 months	0.6	0.4	
	1–3 years	0.9		
	4–8 years	1.3 (m), 1.0 (f)		
	9–13 years			
	14–18 years			

(continued)

Table 8–2. (Continued)

Dietary Reference Intakes

Nutrient	Age	RDA	AI	UL
Thiamin (mg/day) (vitamin B₁)	0–6 months	0.5	0.2	
	7–12 months	0.6	0.3	
	1–3 years	0.9		
	4–8 years	1.2 (m), 1.0 (f)		
	9–13 years			
	14–18 years			
Vitamin A (mcg/day)	0–6 months	300	400	600
(Retinol Activity Equivalent)	7–12 months	400	500	600
	1–3 years	600		600
	4–8 years	900 (m), 700 (f)		900
	9–13 years			1700
	14–18 years			2800
Vitamin B₆ (mg/day) (pyridoxine)	0–6 months	0.5	0.1	ND
	7–12 months	0.6	0.3	ND
	1–3 years	1.0		30
	4–8 years	1.3 (m), 1.2 (f)		40
	9–13 years			60
	14–18 years			80
Vitamin B₁₂ (mcg/day) (cobalamin)	0–6 months	0.9	0.4	
	7–12 months	1.2	0.5	
	1–3 years	1.8		
	4–8 years	2.4		
	9–13 years			
	14–18 years			
Vitamin C (mg/day) (ascorbic acid)	0–6 months	15	40	ND
	7–12 months	25	50	ND
	1–3 years	45		400
	4–8 years	75 (m), 65 (f)		650
	9–13 years			1200
	14–18 years			1800
Vitamin E (mg/day) (α-tocopherol)	0–6 months	6	4	ND
	7–12 months	7	5	ND
	1–3 years	11		200
	4–8 years	15		300
	9–13 years			600
	14–18 years			800
Vitamin D (mcg/day) (calciferol)	0–6 months		5	25
(1 mcg calciferol = 40 IU vitamin D)	7–12 months		5	25
	1–3 years		5	50
	4–8 years		5	50
	9–13 years		5	50
	14–18 years		5	50
Arsenic	0–6 months	ND	ND	
	7–12 months	ND	ND	
	1–3 years	ND	ND	
	4–8 years	ND	ND	
	9–13 years	ND	ND	
	14–18 years	ND	ND	
Boron (mg/day)	0–6 months	ND	ND	ND
	7–12 months	ND	ND	ND
	1–3 years	ND	ND	3
	4–8 years	ND	ND	6
	9–13 years	ND	ND	11
	14–18 years	ND	ND	17

Table 8–2. (Continued)

Dietary Reference Intakes

Nutrient	Age	RDA	AI	UL
Calcium (mg/day)	0–6 months		210	ND
	7–12 months		270	ND
	1–3 years		500	2500
	4–8 years		800	2500
	9–13 years		1300	2500
	14–18 years		1300	2500
Chromium (mcg/day)	0–6 months		0.2	
	7–12 months		5.5	
	1–3 years		11	
	4–8 years		15	
	9–13 years		25 (m), 21 (f)	
	14–18 years		35 (m), 24 (f)	
Copper (mcg/day)	0–6 months	340	200	ND
	7–12 months	440	220	ND
	1–3 years	700		1000
	4–8 years	890		3000
	9–13 years			5000
	14–18 years			8000
Fluoride (mg/day)	0–6 months		0.01	0.7
	7–12 months		0.5	0.9
	1–3 years		0.7	1.3
	4–8 years		1	2.2
	9–13 years		2	10
	14–18 years		2	10
Iodine (mcg/day)	0–6 months	90	110	ND
	7–12 months	90	130	ND
	1–3 years	120		200
	4–8 years	150		300
	9–13 years			600
	14–18 years			900
Iron (mg/day)	0–6 months	11	0.27	40
	7–12 months	7		40
	1–3 years	10		40
	4–8 years	8		40
	9–13 years	11 (m), 15 (f)		40
	14–18 years			45
Magnesium (mg/day)	0–6 months	80	30	ND
	7–12 months	130	75	ND
	1–3 years	240		65†
	4–8 years	410 (m), 360 (f)		110†
	9–13 years			350†
	14–18 years			350†
Manganese (mg/day)	0–6 months		0.003	ND
	7–12 months		0.6	ND
	1–3 years		1.2	2
	4–8 years		1.5	3
	9–13 years		1.9 (m), 1.6 (f)	6
	14–18 years		2.2 (m), 1.6 (f)	9
Molybdenum (mcg/day)	0–6 months	17	2	ND
	7–12 months	22	3	ND
	1–3 years	34		300
	4–8 years	43		600
	9–13 years			1100
	14–18 years			1700

(continued)

Table 8–2. (Continued)

Dietary Reference Intakes

Nutrient	Age	RDA	AI	UL
Nickel (mg/day)	0–6 months	ND	ND	ND
	7–12 months	ND	ND	ND
	1–3 years	ND	ND	0.2
	4–8 years	ND		0.3
	9–13 years	ND		0.6
	14–18 years	ND		1.0
Phosphorus (mg/day)	0–6 months	460	100	ND
	7–12 months	500	275	ND
	1–3 years	1250		3000
	4–8 years	1250		3000
	9–13 years			4000
	14–18 years			4000
Selenium (mcg/day)	0–6 months	20	15	45
	7–12 months	30	20	60
	1–3 years	40		90
	4–8 years	55		150
	9–13 years			280
	14–18 years			400
Silicon	0–6 months	ND	ND	
	7–12 months	ND	ND	
	1–3 years	ND	ND	
	4–8 years	ND	ND	
	9–13 years	ND	ND	
	14–18 years	ND	ND	
Vanadium (mg/day)	0–6 months	ND	ND	ND
	7–12 months	ND	ND	ND
	1–3 years	ND	ND	ND
	4–8 years	ND	ND	ND
	9–13 years	ND	ND	ND
	14–18 years	ND	ND	ND
Zinc (mg/day)	0–6 months	3	2	4
	7–12 months	3		5
	1–3 years	5		7
	4–8 years	8		12
	9–13 years	11 (m), 9 (f)		23
	14–18 years			34

*(m) = male; (f) = female.
†Supplemental.

approximately the average, rather than two standard deviations above the average. The DRIs take into consideration both gender and age in establishing requirements. This discussion will adhere to the age groups used in the DRIs. They are: 0–6 months, 7–12 months, 1–3 years, 4–8 years, 9–13 years, and 14–18 years. Table 8–2 lists the DRIs for a number of nutrients. Table 8–3 shows how to calculate energy requirements and Table 8–4 lists approximate energy requirements from infancy to adolescence.

Infant Requirements (0–6 and 7–12 months)

In establishing values for infants, the IOM relied heavily on clinical trials including dose–response, balance, depletion/repletion, prospective observational, case–control studies, and clinical observations in humans. Greater emphasis was placed on studies that measured actual dietary and supplement intake than those that depended on self-reported food and

Table 8–3.

Calculated Energy Requirements from Infancy to Adolescence

Category	Calculation of Estimated Energy Requirements (EER)
0–3 months	(89 × weight [kg] − 100) + 175 kcal
4–6 months	(89 × weight [kg] − 100) + 56 kcal
6–12 months	(89 × weight [kg] − 100) + 22 kcal
13–35 months	(89 × weight [kg] − 100) + 20 kcal
Boys, 3–8 years	88.5 − (61.9 × age [years] + PA* × (26.7 × weight [kg] + 903 × height [m])) + 20 kcal
Girls, 3–8 years	135.3 − (30.8 × age [years] + PA* × (10.0 × weight [kg] + 934 × height [m])) + 20 kcal
Boys, 9–18 years	88.5 − (61.9 × age [years] + PA* × (26.7 × weight [kg] + 903 × height [m])) + 25 kcal
Girls, 9–18 years	135.3 − (30.8 × age [years] + PA* × (10.0 × weight [kg] + 934 × height [m])) + 25 kcal

PA* = physical activity: sedentary = 1.00; low activity = 1.16; active = 1.31; very active = 1.56.

supplement intake. All studies were published in peer-reviewed journals. For some nutrients, the available data did not provide a basis for proposing different requirements for various life stages or genders, most notably infants less than 6 months of age. For infants 0–6 months, only Adequate Intakes (AI) (Table 8–1) exist. For infants, the AI is based on the reported intake of human milk (780 mL/day) determined by test weighing of full-term infants and by the reported average human

Table 8–4.

Estimated Energy Requirements in Infants to Adolescents

Category	Estimated Energy Requirements (EER; kcal/kg/day)
0–3 months	102–110
4–6 months	82–84
6–12 months	78–82
13–35 months	81–83
Boys, 3–8 years	60–85
Girls, 3–8 years	60–85
Boys, 9–18 years	36–47
Girls, 9–18 years	34–40

EER calculated using median weight and median height for age from CDC growth charts.

milk concentration of a specified nutrient after 1 month of lactation. While this is an intuitively logical approach, it provides information only for breastfed infants. Human milk is a matrix of interacting factors and each factor may be more or less biologically available in this matrix compared to the biological availability of the factor when not in the human milk matrix. This means that there are no reference values applicable to non-breastfed infants (Tables 8–2 and 8–3). The AIs, based solely on estimates of nutrients in human milk, may result in frank deficiency for some nutrients if those nutrients are fed to non-breastfed infants at the level of AI. Further, this approach assumes that the mother has no nutrient deficiency, that all events surrounding the birth were optimal (cord clamping, etc.), and that the mother's milk has at least the average amount of nutrients. If any of these assumptions are not correct and the infant is not supplemented, nutrient deficiency can occur. Nevertheless, the DRIs are the best estimates of infant nutrition needs available.

Toddler Requirements (1–3 years)

There is no widely accepted definition of "toddler." The term is taken from the wide-based gait seen in children who are just learning to walk. While it is generally agreed that "toddlerhood" begins at 12 months of age, the upper boundary of this age bracket is poorly defined. In this discussion, it will be assumed that toddlerhood ends at 36 months. Thus, a child less than 12 months is an infant and after 36 months a toddler becomes a "preschooler." Growth and therefore nutritional requirements peak during the first year of life. Growth rate during the second 12 months of life continues to be high. The second year of life is one of transition from an infant diet to a modified adult diet. There is a paucity of studies and guidelines on toddlers' nutrition, although there are a number of studies that describe what toddlers eat. These have included studies documenting a change in eating patterns of toddlers over time, and there have been reports on the psychological and behavioral aspects of toddler nutrition. There are, however, few studies to determine actual nutritional requirements for children of this age group. There are also few published guidelines, but those that are available often use data extrapolated from other age groups.

School Age Requirements (4–8 years)

This age group is characterized by very much slower rate of growth than in the infant and toddler age groups. Children at this age are typically in a formal education system and are often making some nutritional choices independently. School age children are often viewed as "picky eaters." This may be merely a perception as, because of their slower growth rate, the rate of increase in the consumption slackens.

Pre-teen Requirements (9–13 years)

The genders in this age group grow at different rates, as many girls will have completed their growth spurt by age 13 years, while many boys have not entered this rapid growth phase. This means that requirements for boys and girls may be substantially different. Because there is a wide range of normal progression of puberty and because nutritional requirements, in part, depend on pubertal status, making fixed recommendations in this age group is difficult.

Teenager Requirements (14–18 years)

Nutritional requirements vary by gender in this age category as well. During teenage years, nutritional requirements can vary with requirements for growth and with physical activity. Teenagers have a keen sense of their body image. This can result in either healthy eating habits or unhealthy ones. Nutritional syndromes such as anorexia and obesity become very important.

Nutritional Assessment

The four elements of nutritional assessment are: (1) history, including social history and medications, (2) physical examination and anthropometrics, (3) laboratory tests, and (4) observation including general behavior, feeding behavior, and familial interactions.

History

A nutritional history focuses on the potential reasons for undernutrition or for overnutrition. Causes of undernutrition at any age fall into the same categories: decreased intake, increased losses, malabsorption, increased requirements, and decreased synthetic function, such as might accompany inborn errors of metabolism. Similarly, causes of overnutrition at all ages are increased intake and decreased energy expenditure. Recent literature has highlighted genetic predisposition to obesity and overweight. These genetic differences have existed for many generations and therefore do not explain the recent "epidemic of obesity." Another recent finding is that obese individuals have an identifiably different microbiome. Their GI flora are said to consist of "obesogenic bacteria." There remains a debate as to which come first, diets predisposing to weight gain, the weight gain itself, or the altered bacterial flora.

Physical Examination

For the most part, physical findings other than changes in growth parameters are late findings in malnutrition. Physical evidence of single-nutrient deficiencies are not commonly encountered in the developed world. These are listed in Table 8–5.

Anthropometrics

Anthropometry is the measurement of the physical dimensions of the human body at different ages. In children it is one of the best indicators of nutritional status and overall health. Accurate measurements of weight, length, head circumference, and skin fold thickness are an important part of a nutritional evaluation. When these measurements are available over time, showing trends, they become even more informative. The correct equipment is essential as is proper training of personnel performing these measurements. When accurate methods and appropriate comparison data are used, anthropometry is reliable, non-invasive, and inexpensive. Derivatives of these basic measures such as weight for height and body mass index (BMI) give an indication of altered patterns of growth.

Length/height

Children less than 2 years of age are measured recumbent, while those over 2 years are measured standing. For accuracy in both age groups, a stadiometer is necessary.

Weight

This is a simple and reproducible measurement that reflects both short-term and chronic nutritional status. When serial measurements are taken, care should be given to assure consistent values. The child should be measured on the same scale and at the same time of day. Preferably the child should be naked or, at least, with same amount of clothes.

Skin fold thickness

This is a measure of body fat. While it is inexpensive to perform, it is difficult to assure accuracy. Skin fold thickness is measured with calipers that require frequent calibration. Training of personnel and consistency of technique is crucial. Because of these difficulties, many centers have given up performing skin fold thickness measurements.

Weight for height

Weight for height is used as a measure of adiposity in children under 1 year of age, where BMI percentile data are not available.

Table 8–5.

Physical Findings in Nutrient Deficiencies

Area	Signs Associated with Malnutrition	Possible Nutrient Deficiency
General	Growth failure, lethargy	Calories, protein, zinc
Hair	Dull and dry, thin and sparse, color changes (flag sign), easily plucked	Protein, calories
Face	Depigmentation, dark skin over cheeks and under eyes, lumpiness or flaking of skin of the nose and mouth, swollen face, nasolabial seborrhea	Calories, protein, riboflavin, niacin
Eyes	Redness of membranes, Bitot's spots, angular palpebritis, corneal xerosis, keratomalacia, scar on cornea, eye membranes pale and dry	Vitamin A, anemia (iron, folate, vitamin B_{12})
Lips	Redness and swelling of the mouth or lips, chelosis, angular stomatitis	Niacin, riboflavin, vitamin B_6
Tongue	Swollen, scarlet, raw, magenta (purplish), smooth, swollen sores, hyperemic papillae, hypertrophic papillae, atrophic papillae	Riboflavin, niacin
Teeth	Missing, erupting abnormally, gray spots, black spots, caries	Fluoride
Gums	Spongy, bleeding, recession	Vitamin C
Neck	Swollen, enlarged thyroid, enlarged parotid	Iodine, protein
Skin	Xerosis, follicular hyperkeratosis, flaky, ecchymosis, swollen pigmentation of exposed areas (pellagrous dermatosis), dyspigmentation (light or dark), petechiae, decreased subcutaneous fat	Proteins, calories, zinc, niacin, riboflavin, vitamin A, vitamin B_6, essential fatty acids
Nails	Koilonychia, brittle, ridged	Iron, protein
Musculoskeletal system	Muscle wasting, craniotabes, frontal and parietal bossing, epiphysial enlargement, beading of ribs, prolonged open anterior fontanel, knock-knees or bowlegs, bleeding into muscle, unable to walk	Calories, proteins, vitamin D, vitamin C
Cardiovascular system	Tachycardia, enlarged heart, abnormal rhythm, elevated blood pressure	Potassium, selenium, phosphorus, thiamine
Gastrointestinal system	Enlarged liver	Calories, protein
Nervous system	Irritable, confused, paresthesia, loss of position and vibratory sense, weakness, tenderness of muscles, decrease and loss of reflexes, tetany	Protein, thiamine, vitamin B_{12}, vitamin E, calcium, magnesium

BMI percentile

The ratio of the weight (kg) to the height (m) squared is the BMI. In adults the BMI should be relatively constant over time; this is not true for children. Therefore, there are age-adjusted charts of BMI percentiles or of BMI z-scores. BMI is a surrogate measure of adiposity.

Growth Charts

It is important to understand the difference between the terms "growth reference" and "growth standard." Until recently all growth charts have been "references," that is, they describe the growth patterns of infants and children. The widely used Centers for Disease Control (CDC) growth charts are examples of "reference" curves (http://www.cdc.gov/nchs/about/major/nhanes/growthcharts/clinical_charts.htm). The CDC charts are an amalgamation of data obtained from many observational studies of infant and childhood growth. The World Health Organization (WHO) has completed an ambitious project in which it created growth curves depicting how infants should grow (growth standards) rather than how they actually grow. To do this, infant–mother pairs were selected to be followed from several sites around the world. The infants had to be full-term, breastfed, and of middle to upper socioeconomic status. The last requirement was imposed so that obtaining adequate food would not be a factor in successful breastfeeding. These infants were followed and measured repeatedly until they were 1 year of age. The resulting curves show that the WHO babies were heavier than the CDC babies for the first several months, but in the second half of the first year the trend reversed. Likewise, the WHO infants grew faster for several months, but by a year of age the linear difference had disappeared. Interestingly, despite ethnic, cultural, and geographic differences, the WHO babies exhibited very similar growth.[2]

Table 8–6.				
Proteins Used for Nutritional Assessment				
Protein	Half-life	Reference Range (mg/dL)	Advantages	Disadvantages
Albumin	20 days	2.8–5.8	Easy to obtain, inexpensive	Long half-life, affected by non-nutritional factors
Transferrin	8–9 days	130–280	Easy to obtain, inexpensive	Affected by iron status, imprecise normal values
Prealbumin (transthyretin)	2–3 days	2–42	Short half-life, easy to obtain	Affected by renal and liver disease
Retinol-binding protein	12–25 hours	0–60	Short half-life, easy to obtain	Affected by renal and liver disease, expensive
Fibronectin	4–24 hours	220–400	Short half-life	Expensive, difficult to measure
Insulin-like growth factor I (IGF-1)	2–6 hours	0.1–0.4	Short half-life	Expensive, not easily obtained

Laboratory Tests

In theory laboratory tests should be able to confirm nutritional deficiencies that are suspected by history or physical exam (Table 8–6). Because nutritional deficiencies usually manifest in blood or body tissues before physical findings are present, laboratory tests should be able to identify sub-clinical malnutrition. In reality, interpretation of laboratory tests is difficult. Levels can be affected by many biological and technical factors that may make interpretation difficult. In these situations, measuring the response to a therapeutic trial of a suspected nutrient deficiency may be the best method of assessment. In terms of the laboratory assessment of nutrition, tests can be divided into: (1) tests that measure the levels (body, blood, serum, or plasma) of nutrients, (2) tests that measure biochemical or physiologic changes that result from nutrient deficiencies, and (3) tests that measure compositional changes that result from nutrient deficiencies.

Observation of Feeding Behavior

Much can be learned by merely observing a child and parent during a meal. The reason for malnutrition in a child may become obvious by watching a single meal. There are child-specific factors, such as inability to maintain proper position for successful feeding. There are parent-specific factors such as not allowing a child time to consume sufficient food. And there are child–parent interactions that may interfere with proper nutrition such as power struggles over eating. The interplay of these factors varies with the age of the child, the social context, and cultural norms, to name a few. Because of the complexity, we have found that it is beneficial for an expert in child–parent feeding interactions to take the lead in this evaluation. In our institution it is the speech therapist who has this expertise. In other institutions it might be a child psychologist or a physical therapist.

NUTRITION SUPPORT

Definition

Nutrition support (NS) is the assistance provided to an individual to assure that adequate nutrition is supplied to promote health, prevent deficiencies, treat deficiencies, and rehabilitate malnourished individuals. NS can be delivered by eating, through a tube (nasogastric, nasojejunal, gastric, gastrojejunal, or jejunal), or through a central or peripheral vein.

Pathogenesis and Clinical Presentation

NS is indicated when nutritional needs cannot be met by eating a healthy diet. Nutritional needs depend on the individual's nutritional state. The nutritional state may vary because of decreased intake, increased requirements, altered absorption, or increased losses. Table 8–7 outlines some of the conditions that can lead to the need for NS. Immediate NS is indicated for infants born prematurely or of low birth weight, in any child with weight loss of more than 10% of usual body weight, decrease in two growth channels within 1–4 weeks, no weight gain for 3 or more months, or serum albumin less than 2.8 g/dL. When these findings are present, it is important to enlist the aid of a dietitian and a physician trained in NS. They can assist with patient assessment, decisions about type and administration of NS, monitoring, avoiding complications, and assuring growth is optimal. NS includes providing dietary advice, oral supplements, and

Table 8–7.

Examples of Indications for Nutrition Support

- Decreased intake
  - Congenital or acquired abnormalities of the face, mouth, throat, esophagus, or stomach
  - Congenital or acquired oral-motor dysfunction
  - Prematurity (<34 weeks)
  - Low birth weight
  - Anorexia associated with chronic disease
  - Psychosocial disorders
    - a) Anorexia nervosa
    - b) Non-organic failure to thrive
- Increased metabolic requirements
  - Burns
  - Sepsis
  - Trauma
  - Congenital heart disease
  - Bronchopulmonary dysplasia
  - Inflammatory states
- Altered absorption or metabolism
  - Short bowel syndrome
  - Liver disease
  - Congenital or acquired small bowel mucosal abnormalities
  - Glycogen storage disease (types I and III)
  - Gastrointestinal dysmotility
  - Pancreatic insufficiency
  - Amino or organic acidopathies
  - Cystic fibrosis
- Increased losses
  - Diarrhea
  - Vomiting
  - Burns
  - Fistula
  - Abscess
  - Chylous thorax/ascites
  - Congenital skin lesions
  - Protein-losing enteropathy
  - Lymphangectasia

enteral (tube feeds) and parenteral feedings. This discussion focuses on enteral and parenteral support.

Treatment

Figure 8–1 offers a decision tree for the most appropriate type of NS. In general, NS that is the most physiologic and has the least possible serious complications is the treatment of choice. Table 8–8 outlines fundamentals of NS.

Dietary Supplements

Dietary supplements are defined by the Dietary Supplement Health and Education Act of 1994[3] as a product

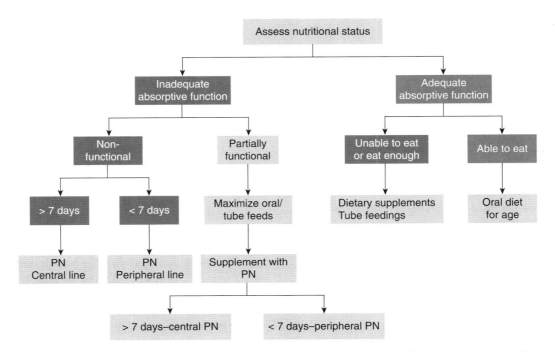

FIGURE 8–1 ■ Algorithm for initiating nutrition support. PN = parenteral nutrition. Baker RD, Baker SS, Davis AM: *Pediatric Parenteral Nutrition*. New York, Chapman and Hall, 1997. With kind permission of Springer Science and Business Media.

Table 8–8.

Fundamentals of Nutrition Support

- ■ **Assess patient**
  - ■ Anthropomorphics
  - ■ Biochemistry
  - ■ Determine if malnourished
  - ■ Determine level of stress
  - ■ Determine expected level of gastrointestinal function
  - ■ Consider anticipated changes in above (planned surgery, chemotherapy, etc.)
- ■ **Set goals**
  - ■ Provide for basal metabolism
  - ■ Rehabilitate malnourished states
  - ■ Correct mineral/electrolyte imbalance
    - a) Initiate catch-up growth
    - b) Support growth
    - c) Support through a metabolic stress (surgery, chemotherapy, sepsis, etc.)
    - d) Account for nutrient needs of disease processes (cystic fibrosis, inflammatory bowel disease, etc.)
  - ■ Maintain gastrointestinal mucosal structure and function
- ■ **Design written therapeutic plan**
  - ■ Which nutrients and how much
    - a) Fluids
    - b) Electrolytes
    - c) Minerals
    - d) Protein
    - e) Carbohydrate
    - f) Lipids
    - g) Trace elements
    - h) Vitamins
  - ■ How administered
    - a) By mouth, tube, or intravenous
    - b) Continuously or cycled
    - c) Rate of delivery of solution
    - d) Rate of advancement
    - e) Decide on tools to evaluate and monitor patient
- ■ **Monitor**
  - ■ Daily review flow sheets
  - ■ Record fluid from every source (all intravenous lines, medications, tube or oral intake)
  - ■ Record amount of solution administered at rate administered
  - ■ Record fluid composition
  - ■ Calculate percent of nutrients from therapeutic plan actually delivered
  - ■ Record adverse reactions
- ■ **Reassess**
  - ■ Repeat initial assessment
  - ■ Reevaluate goals in light of nutritional therapy and changes in metabolic/disease state
  - ■ Reaffirm goals and therapeutic plan
  - ■ Modify plan

Baker RD, Baker SS, Davis AM: Pediatric Parenteral Nutrition. New York, Chapman and Hall, 1997. With kind permission of Springer Science and Business Media.

other than tobacco that is intended to supplement the diet. For children who are not growing adequately, or have a disease that is associated with increased nutrient requirements, sometimes supplementing the diet with nutritionally dense foods is all that is needed to initiate nutritional rehabilitation. These children can be identified by poor or inadequate nutrient intake. Intake can be confirmed with a 24-hour dietary recall or a 3-day food record with a fecal fat collection. If these assessments show inadequate intake for the child's needs and no fat malabsorption, food sources of nutrients can be used as an initial step in NS. For infants formula can be concentrated to 24, 27, or 30 kcal/oz. This assures that the child receives all the nutrients necessary for growth in a small volume and the ratio of nutrients is the same as in the original formula. It is not advisable to concentrate beyond 30 kcal/oz in the first year of life as inadequate free water may be supplied and acidosis and growth failure ensue.

For older children, foods or flavored nutritionally complete beverages may be the easiest and most acceptable way to increase nutrient intake. A complete beverage is one that contains all the required nutrients for growth and development if at least 1 L or more is consumed in 24 hours. Complete beverages are available as soy- or milk-based products. If modular dietary components, such as proteins or a carbohydrate–fat powder, are deemed absolutely essential, then a dietitian must calculate the ratios of the macro- and micronutrient components of the final diet to be sure a nutritional imbalance will not occur. Table 8–9 lists some nutrient dense foods that are often palatable for children.

ENTERAL NUTRITION

Enteral nutrition[4] is the delivery of nutrition directly into the stomach or small bowel. Enteral feeds can be used for infants, children, or adolescents who have a functional gastrointestinal tract and cannot or will not sustain AI to permit normal growth or if total feeding time is greater than 4–6 hours a day. Enteral feeds can also be used to supplement oral feedings to overcome increased requirements or malabsorption. Enteral feedings require the placement of a feeding device into the gastrointestinal tract. Jejunal tubes are more difficult to place and keep in position than gastric tubes, but offer protection from severe gastroesophageal reflux and are useful in certain other conditions, such as gastroparesis (poor gastric emptying) and in mechanically ventilated patients. Table 8–10 lists possible tube placements and some of their advantages and disadvantages.

When long-term NS is necessary, a feeding schedule that best fits the family's lifestyle is an important factor in achieving compliance. Slow continuous feedings are associated with better tolerance and absorption than bolus feedings, and are required when transpyloric

Table 8–9.

Examples of Palatable Foods to Enhance Nutrient Intake

Nutrient	Nutritional Attribute
Whole milk	Calories, protein, fat, vitamins, minerals
Meats	Proteins, iron, zinc, minerals
Eggs	Protein, calories, minerals, vitamins
Mayonnaise	Calories, minerals, vitamins
Full-fat yogurt, cottage cheeses, or sour cream	Calories, protein, fat, vitamins, minerals
Unsaturated oils	Calories
Butter	Calories
Peanut butter	Calories, protein, minerals
Avocado	Calories
Full-fat cheeses	Calories, proteins, vitamins, minerals
Instant breakfast powders	Calories, proteins, vitamins, minerals
Milk-based complete, balanced nutritional drinks	Complete diet
Soy-based complete, balanced nutritional drinks	Complete diet

tubes are used. Feedings can be administered as a continuous drip either over a 24-hour period or on a nocturnal schedule. Table 8–11 lists some schedule choices and advantages and disadvantages of each.

Hundreds of formulas are available, and deciding on the best one can seem overwhelming. In general, the age and underlying disease determine the choice of formula. Some factors that should be considered are

nutritional requirements, fluid requirements, age, activity level, presence of a chronic disease, gastrointestinal function, route of delivery, food intolerance, allergy, and family lifestyle/schedule. Formulas are usually designed for age groups: premature infants, term infants, children aged 1–6 years, and children older than 6 years.

Special formulas are available for prematurely born infants and have higher calories, and protein, vitamin, and mineral concentrations than the usual infant formula. These formulas are recommended until the premature infant reaches a weight of 2–2.5 kg and has normal serum alkaline phosphatase and albumin levels. Premature infant formulas should not be used to increase the caloric intake in full-term infants because the calcium and phosphorus content is too high for them. Breast milk is not adequate as a sole nutrient source for prematurely born infants. It must be supplemented with calories, protein, vitamins, and minerals, especially zinc, calcium, and phosphorus. This can be accomplished using human milk fortifiers.

Term infants with normal gastrointestinal function can be fed breast milk or infant formula during the first year of life for infants less than 4–6 months only.[5] However, if the condition of the infant precludes the introduction of solid foods at 4–6 months of age, then human milk becomes inadequate as a sole source of nutrition and a complete formula must be added to the diet. If breast milk is used for continuous enteral feeds, care must be taken to adjust for nutrient losses caused by separation of the fat that adheres to tubing. Table 8–12 outlines formulas types and some indications for each. Formulas can be further modified by adding modular components such as fat, carbohydrates, and proteins. If modification of formulas is indicated, it is best to have a dietitian review the final content of the prescription to be sure all nutrients are provided in appropriate concentrations and ratios to each other.

Table 8–10.

Types of Feeding Tubes

Type of Appliance	Advantages	Disadvantages
Nasogastric (NG)	Position easily, temporary, easily changed, family/patient can be taught	Appliance on face, can be associated with oral feeding problems
Gastrostomy tube (G-tube, PEG)	No appliance on face, minimally invasive placement procedure, tube can be used immediately after placement	Minimal skin care, tube can dislodge, skin infections
Nasojejunal tube (NJ)	Easily positioned and removed, temporary	Appliance on face, usually requires radiation or endoscopy to place/confirm position, tube can clog easily
Jejunal tube (J-tube, PEJ)	Easily placed in procedure similar to PEG, no appliance on face, easily removed	Skin care, dislodgement, skin infections
Gastric–jejunal tube (G–J tube)	Uses gastrostomy to position a tube into the jejunum	Tube must be positioned radiographically or endoscopically, clogs easily

Table 8–11.

Formula Schedules

Feeding Schedule	Advantages	Disadvantages
Continuous feedings over 24 hours	Maximal nutrient absorption and physiologic tolerance, recommended for jejunal feeds	Little mobility, no cycling of hormones, requires pump, bag, and tubes, child is tied to feeding equipment
Nocturnal continuous	Excellent nutrient absorption, free during day to eat with family, etc., does not interfere with normal hunger–satiety cycles	Sleep can be disrupted for family and patient, requires pump, bag, and tubes, child is tied to feeding equipment at night, may wake to void
Bolus feeds	Convenient, mimics normal feeding, does not require pump, maximal mobility	Increased risk of aspiration, poor tolerance of volume, may not be recommended if reflux, vomiting, or delayed gastric emptying, normal social interactions are lost, decreases interest in food

For children aged 1–6 years, formula choices are limited. The most desirable formula contains 1.0 Kcal/mL, and has more iron, zinc, calcium, phosphorus, and vitamin D than formulas prepared for older children and adults. For children older than 6 years, adult formulas are acceptable.

Formulas can also be grouped according to protein, carbohydrate, or fat content. With respect to protein, there are several types of formulas: cows' milk, soy, partially or extensively hydrolyzed casein (a cows' milk protein), and formula composed of single amino acids. Formulas contain one or more different carbohydrates: lactose, sucrose, hydrolyzed cornstarch, glucose polymers, fiber, tapioca, and maltodextrins. Fat sources can include medium-chain triglycerides, soybean oil, safflower oil, sunflower oil, canola oil, structured lipids, lecithin, corn oil, and coconut oil.

Complications of enteral feedings include mechanical, gastrointestinal, metabolic, and biochemical. Mechanical complications include tube dislodgement or inappropriate tube positioning, pump failure, and tube occlusions.

Gastrointestinal complications include vomiting, diarrhea, aspiration of gastric contents, and constipation. Vomiting can occur because of poor motility, rapid or excessive administration of feedings, hypoproteinemia, central nervous system problems, or metabolic abnormalities. The development of diarrhea requires careful assessment. Infection, osmotic load from medications, and errors in formula dilution or in the rate of delivery can cause diarrhea. Constipation may occur in children on long-term feeding. Causes include increased transit time, decreased physical activity, poor abdominal muscle tone, and lack of dietary fiber.

Metabolic complications occur infrequently with enteral feedings because the formulas are complete foods and the gastrointestinal tract and liver provide a buffer between the formula and the circulation. However, over- and underhydration, over- and underfeeding, and, in specific situations, single-nutrient deficiencies can occur. For example, iron deficiency can develop when chronic blood loss occurs and additional iron is not supplied. With careful monitoring, these are usually easily correctable.

Drug–nutrient interactions can occur with enteral feeds and the outcomes of these interactions can be desirable, benign, or unwanted. Major adverse outcomes are occlusion of tubes, acute reactions, and drug-induced nutritional deficiencies. Risk factors include administration of drugs via the feeding tube, high osmolality of the formulations, the use of drugs or feeding products that produce histamine release, prolonged use of antibiotics, and use of drugs that are vitamin antagonists or are likely to deplete nutrients via the renal tract. Treatment requires recognition and discontinuation of the regimen that caused the reaction. Prevention requires careful monitoring of nutritional status and blood levels of drugs and nutrients as changes in regimens are instituted.

PARENTERAL NUTRITION

Parenteral nutrition (PN) is a highly specialized therapy for which the indications are limited and serious complications can result in morbidity and mortality. Therefore, unless one routinely provides this type of nutrition therapy, it is best to consult with a NS team if PN is necessary.

PN is indicated if the gastrointestinal tract cannot be used, or cannot fully support the pediatric patient.[6,7] Before initiating PN, a careful assessment of the enteral route for NS should be made and the enteral route used whenever possible (Figure 8–1). The largest group for

Table 8–12.

Pediatric Enteral Formulas

Clinical Condition	Formula Description	Comments
Premature infant (<1800 g)	Premature formula—12% protein, contains MCT oil, carbohydrate, lactose/glucose polymers, calcium, and phosphorus	Breast milk must be mixed with a breast milk fortifier since human milk is inadequate in calories, protein, vitamins, and minerals for preterm infants. Soy formulas are not indicated for premature infants
Term infant		
Primary (very rare) or secondary lactose intolerance	60:40 whey:casein or casein formula	The food of choice is breast milk as the sole food for the first 4–6 months and the sole beverage until 1 year of age. Infants must be supplemented with vitamin D and fluoride, if indicated. Human milk is low in iron and zinc and supplementation may be needed. First solid food should be meat to prevent deficiency
Casein sensitivity, vegetarian family	Lactose-free cow milk	Formulas are complete foods and supplementation is not necessary
Organ dysfunction (e.g., renal, cardiac)	Soy protein formula	
Steatorrhea associated with bile acid deficiency, ileal resection, or lymphatic anomalies	Low electrolyte/renal solute load	
Cow's milk protein and soy protein sensitivity, abnormal nutrient absorption, digestion, and transport, intractable diarrhea or protein–calorie malnutrition	Infant formula with MCT	
	Hypoallergenic, hydrolyzed casein, or chemically defined protein (elemental), lactose and sucrose free	
1–6 years old		
Oral supplement	Acceptable taste, different flavors	For many disabled children the calorie content of formulas is high relative to requirements. There is no low-calorie formula that is complete in all other nutrients. Careful monitoring and adjusting of nutrients is necessary to prevent obesity
Tube feeding	Complete nutrition in 1100 mL, 1.0 Kcal/mL caloric density, gluten free, lactose free, isotonic	
Protein sensitivity/compromised GI/pancreatic function	Elemental or chemically defined	
Over 6 years		
Normal GI function	Hypercaloric (1.0–2.0 Kcal/mL) formula	
Abnormal bowel movement	Added fiber	
Pulmonary/diabetes	High fat	
High stress, trauma, sepsis, burns	Hypercaloric, high protein	
Lactose intolerance	Lactose-free formula	
Compromised GI/pancreatic function, protein allergy	Elemental formula	
Organ failure (renal or liver), pre-dialysis	Low protein, essential amino acids, low or no electrolytes, consider formula with increased branched chain amino acids	

whom PN is indicated is premature infants. The gastrointestinal tract development of these infants may not be sufficient to allow for full enteral nutrition. PN is generally not necessary for children with cancer or pancreatitis, as preparation for surgery, or for rehabilitating malnourished children. However, PN is indicated if hypoproteinemia is present and sufficient enteral nutrition to meet all requirements is not tolerated. Gastrointestinal tract dysfunction, whether caused by anatomic abnormalities, absorptive inadequacies, or motility disorders, can be an indication for PN. For children with short bowel that have not adapted sufficiently to maintain nutrition, consideration should be given to a small bowel transplant, because the likelihood of developing cholestasis and eventual liver failure is high.

PN can be administrated through a peripheral or a central vein. If PN is required for less than 7 days and the child is not malnourished, peripheral support can be used. If the child is malnourished, or it is anticipated that PN will be required longer than 7 days, the PN must be administered into a central vein because adequate nutrients to rehabilitate a malnourished child or support growth cannot be sustainably delivered through a peripheral vein. Unless it is anticipated that PN will be needed for more than 3–5 days, little benefit derives from its use. Protein sparing can be accomplished in both malnourished and fully nourished individuals with the administration of a 10% dextrose solution. The administration of 10% dextrose may offer protein sparing while a determination of the necessity for PN is made. Caution, however, must be exercised because use of a protein-deficient diet for longer than 5–7 days in well-nourished children or 3–5 days in malnourished children can lead to the development of kwashiorkor, further impairing the rehabilitation of malnourished children.

PN solutions are necessarily nutritionally complete, containing water, calories, protein, electrolytes, minerals, vitamins, and trace elements. In general, PN solutions should be used only to consistently deliver estimated requirements. When changes in solution content are required over a short period of time, such as to correct an electrolyte imbalance, a separate solution designed to correct the problem can be run concurrently with the pre-mixed solution, rather than discarding and remixing an expensive preparation.

Estimation of fluid requirements can be made on a volume/weight, volume/surface area, or volume/calorie basis (Table 8–13). Table 8–14 lists recommended daily parenteral requirements for electrolytes.

Glucose is the only clinically available carbohydrate source for PN in children. Table 8–15 lists guidelines for glucose delivery in PN. To prevent hyperosmolality and hyperinsulinemia, glucose infusions are initiated in a stepwise manner. Similarly, when cycling, discontinuing, or interrupting PN solutions, a stepwise decrease in car-

Table 8–13.

Fluid Requirements

Method	Body Weight (kg)	Amount/Day
Volume/weight	0–10	100 mL/kg
	10–20	1000 + 50 mL/kg for weight >10 kg
	>20 kg	1500 + 20 mL/kg for weight >20 kg
Volume/surface area	0–70	1500–1700 mL/m²
Volume/ kilocalorie	0–70	100 mL/100 kcal metabolized

Baker RD, Baker SS, Davis AM: Pediatric Parenteral Nutrition. New York, Chapman and Hall, 1997. With kind permission of Springer Science and Business Media.

bohydrate is necessary to prevent hypoglycemia. Glucose intolerance develops in critically ill patients and careful monitoring of urine and serum glucose is necessary.

Intravenous lipids are a necessary calorie source and prevent and treat essential fatty acid (EFA) deficiency. To prevent EFA deficiency, 2–4% of non-protein calories (0.5–1.0 g/kg/day) must be provided. In balanced PN solutions, 30–40% (3–4 g/kg/day), but not more than 60%, of non-protein calories is provided as lipid. Intravenous lipids currently available are an emulsion of soy bean oil and egg phospholipids. In a few anecdotal studies in children, a new lipid composed of fish oils shows promise in preventing PN-induced cholestasis, but is not readily available in the United States. Lipid should be infused over 24 hours. Lipid solutions are available as 10% or 20% emulsions and in general should be provided as 20%. The 20% emulsion has a slightly higher ratio of phospholipid to triglyceride. This may increase lipoprotein lipase activity, so serum triglycerides and

Table 8–14.

Intravenous Requirements for Electrolytes and Minerals

Nutrient	Daily Requirement
Sodium	2–4 mEq/kg
Potassium	2–3 mEq/kg
Chloride	2–3 mEq/kg
Calcium	0.5–2.5 mEq/kg
Phosphorus	1–2 mM/kg
Magnesium	0.25–0.5 mEq/kg

Table 8–15.

Complications of Carbohydrates in PN

Complication	Usual Cause	Prevention or Treatment
Cholestasis	Infant fed exclusively by PN	Enteral feedings
CO_2 retention	High glucose infusion rate in patient with respiratory failure	Decrease glucose infusion rate
Hepatosteatosis	All calories provided as glucose	Provide 30% of calories as lipid
Hyperglycemia	High glucose infusion rate, stress, burns, sepsis, incorrect glucose concentration	Decrease glucose infusion rate, add insulin, improve quality control in pharmacy
Hypoglycemia	Abrupt discontinuation of PN or decrease in child <3 years of age	Taper PN
Phlebitis	High osmolarity of peripherally infused solutions	Keep concentration of glucose 12.5% or less for peripheral infusions
Refeeding syndrome	Rapid refeeding of a malnourished patient	Refeed slowly. Monitor serum P, Ca, K, Mg

other lipids are lower with the 20% emulsion. There are no contraindications to infusion of lipids. In patients with significant metabolic stress such as sepsis or multiorgan failure, intolerance to higher doses may occur.

Proteins are administered as amino acids, and are necessary for maintenance and synthesis of structural proteins, as well as for enzymes, peptide hormones, immunoglobulins, neurotransmitters, transport proteins, and other proteins important in metabolism. The protein requirement of parenterally fed infants and children is dependent on energy intake, amino acid profile and availability of vitamin and mineral cofactors, age, clinical conditions, and medications. If energy intakes are low, protein will not be effectively retained. Parenteral protein requirements are 3.0–3.5 g/kg/day for prematurely born infants, 2.5 g/kg/day for full-term infants, 1.5–2.0 g/kg/day for children 2–13 years, and 1.0–1.5 g/kg/day for adolescents. There are many types of parenteral amino acid solutions. In general, pediatric amino acid solutions have a higher ratio of essential amino acids to total amino acids and contain tyrosine, cystine/cysteine, and glutamine, which are not usually found in adult protein solutions but are essential for preterm infants. In addition, pediatric amino acid solutions yield more normal serum amino acid profiles than adult PN solutions, as defined by amino acid profiles in human milk-fed infants or in cord blood. The addition of cysteine allows for better solubility of calcium and phosphorus by lowering the pH. A non-protein calorie to nitrogen ratio of 150–250:1 is optimal. Under certain conditions such as sepsis or burns, the ratio may be optimal at 100:1. Protein status is followed with serum prealbumin, albumin, and blood urea nitrogen.

Several pre-mixed solutions of essential trace elements and vitamins designed for children are available and must be added to PN. For children who are totally

dependent on PN, iron and carnitine must also be added. Some medications are compatible with PN. The dietitian and pharmacist members of the NS team can help with decisions about which products to choose.

Complications of PN include infections, mechanical problems with lines, and metabolic abnormalities. Some of the complications, such as air embolus, lipid thrombus, catheter perforation of the heart, etc., can be life threatening. Hence, it is important for a NS team including physicians, dietitians, and pharmacists trained and experienced in NS to oversee the patient receiving PN.

The goal of NS is to replete malnourished children, sustain children through a metabolic stress (burns, trauma, and surgery), provide the extra nutrition demanded by a chronic disease (liver, inflammatory bowel disease, cystic fibrosis, and cancer), and ensure normal growth. The best outcome measure is sustained normal growth.

NUTRITION NEEDS IN DISEASE

Malabsorption and Nutrition

Malabsorption is defined by the inadequate digestion or absorption of nutrients. It occurs if there is dysfunction of one or more of the three main organs (liver, pancreas, or small bowel) that are necessary for normal digestion of foods and absorption of nutrients into the bloodstream. Malabsorption can be limited to a single nutrient, or can involve several or all nutrients. For children, fat malabsorption is a serious situation, since inadequate uptake of calories, vitamins, and minerals has severe consequences for growth and development. In general, careful attention must be paid to supplying adequate nutrients, especially energy and protein for growth, monitoring vitamin and mineral status, and protecting bone health and cognitive development.

The principles of NS, as outlined in Table 8–8, apply to all infants and children with malabsorption. Additional monitoring (dual energy X-ray absorptiometry (DEXA)) and supplementation of specific nutrients, such as fat-soluble vitamins and minerals, are necessary (see Table 8–16).

Nutrition in Liver Disease

Clinical presentation

The liver has two main functions—synthesis and degradation or detoxification of a variety of substances. Hence, liver disease has a profound effect on nutritional status and can alter nutritional requirements. Liver disease can be caused by infections, anatomic abnormalities, inborn errors, and autoimmune disorders, and can

Table 8–16.

Vitamins and Minerals in Malabsorption Disease*

Nutrient	How to Monitor	Desired Level	Estimated Amount to Supplement	How to Supplement
Vitamin A[†]	Retinol:retinol-binding protein molar ratio	≥0.8	1000 IU/kg/day up to 25,000 IU	Aqueous vitamin A
Vitamin D[†,‡]	Serum 25 (OH) vitamin D	>30 ng/mL	Weight <20 kg, 400–800 IU/day	Liquid for infants
			Weight ≥20 kg, 800–1000 IU/day	Capsules and pills for older children and adults
Vitamin E[†]	Vitamin E:total lipid (sum of triglyceride, cholesterol, and phospholipids) ratio	Adults and adolescents: ≥0.8 total tocopherol/g total lipids	20–25 IU/kg/day	D-α-Tocopheryl polyethylene glycol–1000 succinate
		Children <12 years: ≥0.6 total tocopherol/g total lipid		
Vitamin K[†]	Prothrombin time	12–15 seconds	2.5–5 mg/day three times per week	Phytonadione 5 mg pills
	International normalized ratio (INR)	0.8–1.2		
	Proteins induced by vitamin K absence (PIVKA)	<2 ng/mL		
Calcium[‡]	Serum level	9.0–11.0 mg/dL up to 24 months	Infant/child 20 mg/kg/day[§]	Calcium salts
		8.8–10.8 mg/dL for >2 years	Adult 500–1000 mg/day[§]	
Phosphorus[‡]	Serum level	4.5–6.7 mg/dL up to 24 months	30–90 mg/kg/day	Phosphorus salts
		4.5–5.5 mg/dL for 24 months to 12 years		
		2.7–4.5 mg/dL for >12 years		
Magnesium	Serum level	1.3–2.0 mEq/L	65–130 mg/kg/dose to maximum of 2 g for adults in four divided doses	Magnesium salts
Zinc	Serum level	70–120 mcg/dL	0.5–1 mg/kg/day to a maximum of 50 mg in three divided doses[§]	Zinc salts
Iron	Soluble transferring receptor	9.6–29.6 nmol/L	6 mg/kg/day[§]	0.85–2.00 mg/L

Frequent, careful monitoring with dose adjustments as necessary is absolutely essential.
†*Or use ADEK vitamin preparation where each soft gel capsule contains 9000 IU vitamin A, 400 IU vitamin D, 150 IU vitamin E, and 10 mg vitamin K; and 1 mL contains 3170 IU vitamin A, 400 IU vitamin D, 40 IU vitamin E, and 100 mcg vitamin K.*
‡*Or use Posture-D® that contains 600 mg calcium as tricalcium phosphate, 125 IU vitamin D, and 266 mg phosphorus as tricalcium phosphate.*
§*Elemental.*

be acute or chronic. Acute liver disease such as viral hepatitis does not require special nutritional interventions, as the disease is generally short lived and does not confer a lasting disability. Metabolic liver diseases, such as galactosemia, tyrosinemia, and glycogen storage diseases, require lifelong adherence to a strict diet that has been developed specifically to prevent toxicity and support normal growth and development. Sometimes liver transplantation is required. Please see Chapter 28 for an in-depth discussion of these diseases.

Cholestatic liver diseases present a complicated nutritional challenge.[8] *Cholestasis* is defined as reduced bile flow into the small bowel. Because bile acids are reduced or even absent, emulsification of fats is impaired, leading to malabsorption of dietary lipids and causing inadequate calorie and fat-soluble vitamin absorption. In addition, most children with chronic liver disease experience anorexia, leading to decreased dietary intake. In liver disease, anorexia is further aggravated by ascites that can cause nausea, vomiting, and early satiety, and the unpalatability of diets necessarily rich in medium-chain triglycerides and low in sodium. In addition, chronic disease itself, especially one that is associated with an increased risk of infections, increases nutritional requirements. Medications such as cholestyramine, neomycin, and lactulose can cause decreased nutrient absorption or osmotic diarrhea that further potentiates the malabsorption of nutrients. Nutritional management for these children begins as outlined in Table 8–8, with special attention to aspects of liver disease that make some of the assessment tools unreliable. For example, in children with ascites, weight is not a reliable estimate of nutritional status and, because the synthetic function of the liver is compromised, serum proteins do not provide an accurate assessment of visceral protein status.

Treatment

In general, the following recommendations should be followed. *Energy* should be supplied at about 130–150% of the RDA, based on ideal dry weight, and should contain at least 50% of fat as medium-chain triglycerides. Medium-chain triglycerides are absorbed directly into the portal vein and do not require bile acid emulsification for absorption, as do long-chain triglycerides. Even so, at least 10% of total energy must be supplied as long-chain fatty aids to prevent EFA deficiency. In fact, total lipids should not be restricted because reducing fat intake adversely affects overall caloric intake and hastens the development of malnutrition. To achieve the necessary increase in energy intake, infant formulas must be concentrated. This can be accomplished by dissolving the formula powder in less water and/or adding modular nutrition components. In either case, a dietitian is an absolutely necessary part of the care team to

assure that the formulas are correctly constructed. The amount and type of protein that should be supplied for liver disease has been controversial, especially in end-stage liver disease. Enough protein must be provided to prevent tissue catabolism. The breakdown of lean body mass in protein-undernourished liver patients contributes to blood ammonia levels and reduces their capacity to metabolize ammonia. Infants require at least 3 g/kg/day and can tolerate up to 4 g/kg/day without encephalopathy. For older children and adolescents, receiving the RDA for protein will maintain nitrogen balance, and does not adversely affect the underlying liver disease. Protein is best offered as whole foods, because these are more palatable than dietary supplements. The use of branched chain amino acids is controversial and mostly limited to end-stage disease.

Vitamin and mineral nutrition is vitally important in children with liver disease (Table 8–16). Deficiency of the fat-soluble vitamins (A, D, E, and K) is commonly found in cholestatic liver disease, and can have a significant negative impact on health. These vitamins must be monitored on a routine basis, every 3 months, and adjustments in supplementation made accordingly. Mineral supplementation, especially with calcium, zinc, and iron, is frequently required.

Pancreas and Nutrition

Clinical presentation

The pancreas has endocrine and exocrine functions and dysfunction of either can have severe nutritional consequences. The following discussion focuses on exocrine function. Exocrine pancreatic dysfunctions most commonly occurs in cystic fibrosis, Shwachman–Diamond Syndrome, and after long-standing pancreatic disease that causes destruction of the parenchyma (see Chapter 32). Exocrine pancreatic insufficiency is a cause of malabsorption that can be partially overcome in infants by mother's milk because it contains lipase, and, to a lesser degree, by salivary and brush border amylases and lingual lipase in older children.

Protein digestion begins in the stomach by acid hydrolysis and continues by brush border proteolytic enzymes. Similarly, starch digestion can be initiated by salivary amylase and continued by brush border oligosaccharidoses. Protein and starch digestion are maintained even when virtually all pancreatic function is ineffective. However, fat malabsorption is most important in pancreatic insufficiency and is associated with abdominal pain, steatorrhea, flatulence, diarrhea, and deficits in energy and the fat-soluble vitamins A, D, E, and K. Malabsorption causes growth failure and specific nutrient deficiencies in children.

Delivery of free fatty acids into the proximal small bowel stimulates the release of cholecystokinin and this in turn stimulates pancreatic secretion. The pancreas has a high reserve capacity. In healthy individuals, 10–20 times more enzymes are secreted than are required and, in fact, only 5–10% of normal prandial enzyme output is sufficient for normal digestion. Clinically significant malabsorption is usually not detectable until 90–95% of the secreting parenchyma is destroyed. Treatment of malabsorption requires delivery of sufficient enzyme activity into the duodenal lumen simultaneously with a meal.

The most accurate estimate of pancreatic function is the secretin–pancreozymin stimulation test.[9] This test requires duodenal intubation and collection of fluid before and after intravenous hormonal stimulation of the pancreas. It is invasive, expensive, and time consuming. Most commonly a 72-hour fecal fat collection and food diary from which the coefficient of fat absorption can be calculated is used. This test does not discriminate among hepatobiliary, mucosal, or pancreatic causes for fat malabsorption, intake must be carefully recorded, and many people find the stool collection onerous. Table 8–17 outlines how to conduct a 72-hour fecal fat collection for clinical purposes. Serum immunoreactive trypsinogen accurately discriminates pancreatic insufficiency in patients over 8 years of age. Stool chymotrypsin analysis requires that pancreatic enzyme supplements be discontinued for at least 5 days before the stool collection. Assessment of fecal elastase, an ELISA for the human protein, provides an excellent, non-invasive estimate of pancreatic exocrine function that can be obtained without stopping enzyme supplementation and can be used for infants as young as 2 weeks of age.

Table 8–17.

Seventy-two-hour Fecal Fat Collection and Calculation of Coefficient of Fat Absorption*

- Forty-eight hours prior to the beginning of stool collection, subject is started on a high-fat diet (>2 g/kg/day and minimum of 50 g/day fat)
- All stools are collected into a single container for a full 72 hours. Stool container is kept refrigerated during collection
- During the collection, all food and fluid intake is recorded. A record of all bowel movements is kept. Intake record is analyzed for total dietary fat intake
- Collected stool is homogenized and analyzed for fat by the method of Van de Kamer. Medium-chain triglyceride will not be measured by this method
- Coefficient of fat absorption (CFA) is calculated as follows: CFA = (Dietary fat − Stool fat)/Dietary fat

This protocol is intended for clinical use. For research proposes this protocol is not adequate.

Treatment

After identification of pancreatic insufficiency, the most important therapy is enzyme replacement even though the clinically available enzyme replacement products are not ideal from either a manufacturing or a pharmacological viewpoint, while carefully monitoring nutritional status including growth, minerals, and vitamins (Table 8–16). There are two methods to estimate the amount of pancreatic enzyme to be prescribed, a weight-based and a dietary fat-based method. The weight-based method can be used at any age. The starting dose for children less than 4 years of age is 1000 lipase units/kg body weight per meal and for children older than 4 years of age is 500 lipase units/kg body weight per meal. Smaller doses are offered with fat-containing snacks eaten between meals. Dosing is increased based on symptoms of pancreatic insufficiency to a maximum of 2500 lipase units/kg body weight per meal to avoid fibrosing colonopathy. The fat-based method is useful for infants who take a known amount of formula or for patients who receive tube feedings. The dose starts at approximately 2000 lipase units/120 mL of formula or per breastfeeding (about 1600 lipase units/g of fat ingested per day).

The estimate of 130% of RDA calories for patients with cystic fibrosis is a simplification of their requirements. Recent studies show that increased energy expenditure correlates with increased severity of disease and with decrease in pancreatic function. However, a wide range of energy expenditures are reported, from normal to 150% of RDA depending on the individual and the circumstances of that individual. Therefore, each patient with CF needs an individually tailored regimen, based on their genetic defect, past medical history, and the degree of lung involvement.

EFA deficiency is well described in cystic fibrosis and has been associated with symptoms including scaly dermatitis, alopecia, thrombocytopenia, a hemolytic anemia, and growth failure because long-chain polyunsaturated fatty acids of the omega-3 and the omega-6 series cannot be synthesized by humans and must be supplied by the diet. Presently, EFA deficiency is defined by a triene:tetraene ratio (eicosatrienoic acid:arachadonic acid) of greater than 0.4. However, serum linoleic acid (omega-6), expressed as a molar percent of total serum phospholipid fatty acids, is a more clinically relevant biomarker of EFA deficiency than triene:tetraene ratio. Linoleic acid concentration above 21 mol% was associated with better growth, body composition, and FEV_1. Fatty acids of the omega-3 series are found as components of cell membranes and exhibit profound anti-inflammatory effects. Fish oil is a rich source of the metabolically active, omega-3 fatty acid, docosahexaenoic acid (DHA), and has been found to be efficacious in a number of conditions that include chronic inflammatory states such as rheumatoid arthritis and inflammatory bowel disease. A recent Cochrane Database Review concluded that omega-3 supplements in patients with CF were beneficial with few adverse effects.

Since aggressive NS is associated with improved outcomes in cystic fibrosis, children who are not maintaining normal growth are candidates for nutritional support using dietary supplements and enteral feedings. There are very few instances when PN would be useful for children with cystic fibrosis.

Small Bowel and Nutrition

Clinical presentation and treatment

The intestine serves two opposed and important functions, that of absorption and a barrier. The intestine digests molecules, polypeptides, and carbohydrates and transports nutrients across the mucosa and into the systemic circulation, blood, or lymph. There are several causes of intestinal malfunction including a shortened bowel, disordered motility, abnormal mucosa because of inflammation, allergy, infection, and medications, or congenital abnormalities. Some diseases of the intestine cause such dysfunction that the enteral route of nutrient delivery is not and will never be adequate to support health. In most instances it is important to identify the cause of the intestinal dysfunction as the disease process will drive the therapy. For example, in short bowel, congenital abnormalities (lymphangectasia, microvillar inclusion disease, etc.) and motility disorders preference should be given to transplantation since long-term reliance on PN eventually results in liver failure. For food allergy or food intolerance, such as celiac disease, the food can simply be avoided and for inflammatory states, such as occur with Crohn's disease, reducing inflammation positively affects nutritional status. Sometimes it is unclear if the small bowel will be able to adapt, for example, in short bowel, and in these instances, careful prescription of enteral feedings and meticulous overall nutritional management may lead to weaning from dependence on PN over a year or longer. This is a slow and difficult process that requires the intimate management by gastroenterologists and nutritionists.

REFERENCES

1. Institute of Medicine, Food and Nutrition Board. *Dietary Reference Intakes*. Washington, DC: National Academy Press; 2000.
2. de Onis M, Onyango AW. The Centers for Disease Control and Prevention 2000 growth charts and the growth of breastfed infants. *Acta Paediatr*. 2003;92(4):413–419.
3. http://www.health.gov/dietsupp/execsum.htm.
4. Bankhead R, Boullata J, Brantley S, et al. Enteral nutrition practice recommendations. *JPEN*. 2009;67:122–167.
5. Kleinman R, ed. *Pediatric Nutrition Handbook*. Elk Grove Village, IL: American Academy of Pediatrics; 2008:113–121.
6. ASPEN Board of Directors and the Clinical Guidelines Task Force. Guidelines for the use of parenteral and enteral nutrition in adult and pediatric patients. *JPEN*. 2002;26(suppl):1SA–138A.
7. Mehta NM, Compher C. A.S.P.E.N. clinical guidelines: nutrition support of the critically ill child. *JPEN*. 2009;33:260–276.
8. Wieman RA, Balistreri WF. Nutrition support in children with liver disease. In: Baker SS, Baker RD, Davis AM, eds. *Pediatric Nutrition Support*. Sudbury, MA: Jones and Bartlett Publishers; 2007:459–476.
9. Baker SS. Delayed release pancrelipase for the treatment of pancreatic exocrine insufficiency associated with cystic fibrosis. *J Ther Risk Manage*. 2008:4(5) 1079–1084 (http://www.dovepress.com/articles.php?article_id=2428&l=KaoMHpGIqeNL7xnWoAh70K4F1852).

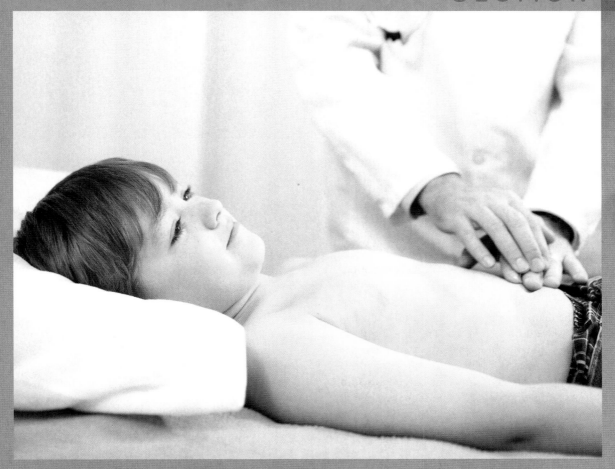

Diagnostic Techniques in Gastroenterology

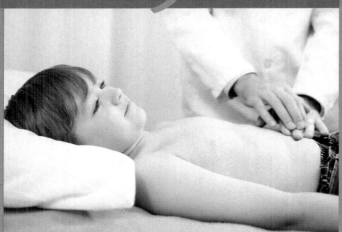

CHAPTER 9

Imaging in Pediatric Gastroenterology

Yutaka Sato and Achint K. Singh

IMAGING TECHNIQUES

Introduction

Imaging provides significant contribution in evaluation, diagnosis, and follow-ups of pediatric gastrointestinal (GI) problems. Children truly are not merely small adults, and the many unique imaging features of pediatric problems should be recognized. The imaging techniques used to evaluate the pediatric patients with GI symptoms are significantly different from those applied to adults. Radiologists and clinicians should work in concert to select the most appropriate modality, as well as optimal timing of the examination to maximize the benefits and minimize the risks and costs. When imaging modalities requiring radiation are selected, the "as low as reasonably achievable" (*ALARA*) principle should always be observed to minimize the radiation exposure.[1]

Radiographs

The technique of using X-rays to evaluate disease is over a century old, having been demonstrated first by Professor Wilhelm Conrad Roentgen in 1895, using a cathode ray tube and photographic emulsion. Despite its antiquity, radiography continues to be used as the first-line imaging technique to evaluate various abdominal conditions, providing important clues directing subsequent workups. Modern X-ray equipment is vastly different from those used during the first decades of development, and uses sensitive digital imaging techniques to minimize exposure to ionizing radiation.

The X-ray machine can be positioned above a supine patient (vertical beam), or can be directed horizontally. Radiographs using a horizontal beam technique are essential to detect a small amount of free air (*pneumoperitoneum*). This can be most easily accomplished in many patients by obtaining erect frontal films. Patient who cannot stand up may have either decubitus frontal or supine cross-table lateral views. Free air can be detected at the highest part of the peritoneal cavity, under the diaphragm on an erect frontal projection, along the non-dependent flank on a decubitus frontal projection (Figure 9–1), or along the anterior abdominal wall on cross-table lateral projection. Larger amounts of free air can even be diagnosed on routine supine frontal views (using a vertical beam) by outlining intestinal walls sandwiched between the intraluminal and extraluminal air ("double wall" or Rigler sign). Other structures that can be seen in this situation include the falciform ligament of the liver and occasionally the umbilical arterial ligaments. In the neonate, a large amount of free air can dissect into the scrotal cavity on one or both sides through an incompletely closed processus vaginalis.[2,3]

The radiological hallmark of *necrotizing enterocolitis* is multiple air bubbles in the intestinal wall (*pneumatosis intestinalis*) (Figure 9–2). It can be seen as bubbly lucency along the intestine or curvilinear/ring-like lucency.[4] The intramural gas eventually finds the way to the portal veins via the mesenteric veins (Figure 9–3). When the findings are equivocal, consider sonographic observation of the liver. Air bubbles carried by the mesenteric veins circulating into portal veins can be demonstrated even before visualization of portal venous gas on radiographs. Once the diagnosis of necrotizing enterocolitis is established and treatment has initiated, sequential follow-up abdominal radiographs, usually a single right-side-up decubitus frontal view every 12 hours, are obtained to detect perforation. Free

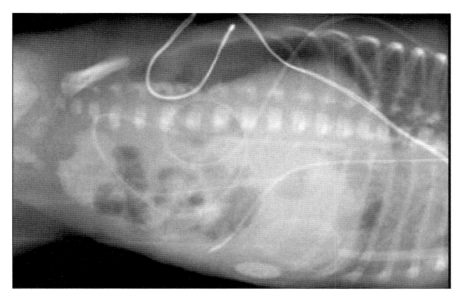

FIGURE 9–1 ■ Ileal perforation. A left-side down decubitus frontal view shows free air along the right flank.

air can be seen in the non-dependent peritoneal cavity along the right lateral flank against the soft tissue window provided by the liver.

Congenital upper GI obstruction, such as duodenal and proximal jejunal atresia, is often detected by in utero ultrasound (US) demonstrating dilated, fluid-filled intestinal loops with associated polyhydramnios.

In distal ileal atresia (Figure 9–4), postnatal radiographs show progressively dilating intestinal loops. Distinction from colonic obstruction or from *Hirschsprung's disease* (see Figure 19–6) requires a contrast enema, because in neonates, differentiation between dilated small intestine and colon is often impossible.[3] In acquired mechanical obstruction, radiographs show progressive intestinal distention with multiple air–fluid levels, with the absence of distal gas. One should be cautious that, in case of strangulated,

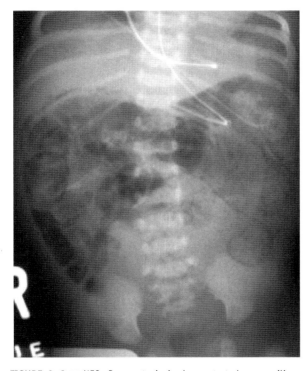

FIGURE 9–2 ■ NEC. Pneumatosis is demonstrated as curvilinear lucencies at the edge of the intestine.

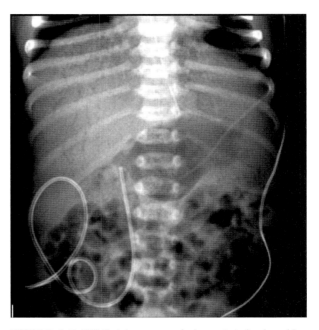

FIGURE 9–3 ■ NEC. Portal venous gas is demonstrated as branching air density in the right lobe of the liver.

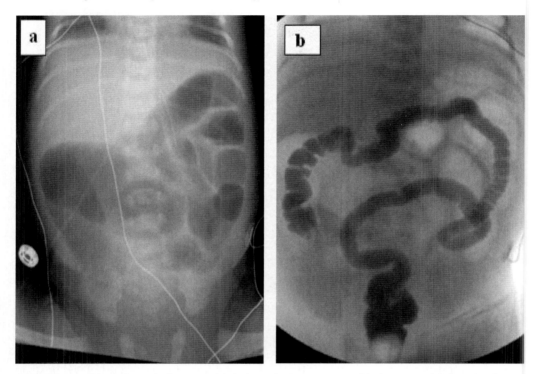

FIGURE 9–4 ■ "Distal obstruction" pattern. (a) Ileal atresia. Contrast enema (b) shows unused "microcolon."

vascular-compromised mechanical obstruction, dilated segments of affected intestine contain large amounts of fluid without significant gas (fluid-filled loops). When this condition is suspected, sonography can be used for verification.

In acute abdominal conditions, one should look for *calcified lesions*, including appendicoliths, gallstones, renal/ureteric stones, and calcification/ossification of pelvic masses. A typical appendicolith is seen in the right lower quadrant as a round, laminated calcification. A diagnosis of acute appendicitis can be made in these patients, when they present with appropriate clinical and laboratory findings. Many patients with incidentally found appendicolith and without symptoms of appendicitis undergo elective appendectomy because of high prevalence of rupture once appendicitis occurs. Torsion of the ovary containing dermoid or teratoma should be suspected when formed teeth or small skeletal structures are seen in the pelvis in a female with acute lower abdominal pain. Sonography can confirm the diagnosis. When gallstone and renal/ureteric stones are suspected, sonography can verify the diagnosis.

Upper Gastrointestinal Series

Preparation for a barium upper GI series for children is minimal, withholding feeding for 2–6 hours, depending on the age[3] (Table 9–1). Digital low-dose pulsed fluoroscopy with "last screen capture," small field size, and gonadal shielding minimize the radiation exposure. Barium is the contrast material of choice because of its superior contrast, mucosal coating, and biological inertness. When perforation is suspected, low-osmolar non-ionic water-soluble contrast is used. High-osmolar contrast material such as Gastrografin (osmolarity of 1900 mmol/L, which is approximately six times the normal serum osmolarity) should not be used because of its potential to cause a significant fluid shift, resulting in hypovolemia, or if aspirated, severe pulmonary irritation.

Table 9–1.

Preparation for GI Procedures

1. Upper GI series, small bowel follow-through
   - ■ Newborn to 6 months: NPO 2–3 hours
   - ■ 6 months to 3 years: NPO 3–4 hours
   - ■ Over 3 years: NPO 6 hours
2. Barium enema: no preparation
3. Ultrasound
   - ■ Abdomen: NPO 4 hours (infants: NPO 1–2 hours)
   - ■ Pelvis: 24–32 oz of fluid, 2 hours before the exam
4. CT: NPO 4 hours except for oral contrast
5. MRI: NPO 4 hours

Modified from Ref. (3).

Small Bowel Follow-through

Small bowel follow-through is performed by having the patient ingest additional barium after routine upper GI evaluation, and watching its progress as motility carries it through the entire small bowel. The most common indication is suspicion of Crohn's disease. Other indications include evaluation of polyps, malabsorption, protein-losing enteropathy, and intestinal dysmotility.

Sequential overhead radiographs are taken every 30–60 minutes, supplemented by fluoroscopic observation and spot radiographs when abnormalities are suspected. Occasionally, continuous infusion of barium into the small bowel through a nasoduodenal or nasojejunal tube (enteroclysis and small bowel enema) is performed to evaluate subtle obstructive lesions, such as multiple strictures and adhesions, which are difficult to be elucidated otherwise. Enteroclysis is particularly helpful when surgical intervention is contemplated in patients with incomplete small bowel obstruction.

Contrast Enema

Barium provides excellent contrast and it is most commonly used unless there is a contraindication, such as the possibility of perforation. Because of its poor contrast density and high osmolarity, *hyperosmolar water-soluble contrast* material such as Gastrografin (sodium/meglumine diatrizoate) has only limited use in the pediatric age group.

Lower osmolarity, *non-ionic water-soluble contrast* agents (such as Isovue/iopamidol) are commonly used instead of barium when there is concern of perforation. Water-soluble, low-osmolar contrast should also be used to evaluate a segment that has limited function, such as colon downstream from a colostomy, or a region with diminished motility. In these situations, barium may become inspissated. When neonatal distal intestinal obstruction is suspected, a barium enema should be performed to differentiate colonic from distal ileal obstruction.[3] Hirschsprung's disease is characterized by a small rectum and dilated proximal colon above the aganglionic segment (see Figure 19–6), while distal ileal obstruction such as ileal atresia and meconium ileus would show unused small colon (microcolon) (Figure 9–4).

The traditional use of contrast enema for the evaluation of polyposis syndromes and colonic inflammatory bowel disease including Crohn's disease and ulcerative colitis has been in major part replaced by endoscopic evaluation, including capsule endoscopy of the small intestine (see Chapter 10).

Sectional Imaging

US is a highly useful sectional imaging modality in evaluation of pediatric GI disorders. In some cases, US provides diagnostic findings, and in others it can provide information useful in formulating the differential diagnosis. US can be performed at the bedside and, in contrast to computerized tomography (CT), is free of ionizing radiation. It does require an expert operator, capable of directing the US probe at the desired structures, recognizing abnormalities, and recording the selective images. This often limits the full utility of US in many smaller facilities. Nevertheless, US should be considered as the first study when sectional imaging is required in pediatric patients.

CT provides exquisite anatomical information without the factor of operator dependence that is problematic in US studies. However, we should recognize that CT is the largest source of ionizing radiation in diagnostic imaging. Genetic effects and risk of carcinogenesis due to ionizing radiation is proportional to the dose, without any threshold effect. Further, the radiation risk for children is much greater than that of adults because of higher tissue radiosensitivity, a longer lifetime in which to manifest radiation-induced injury, and the cumulative effects of repeated examinations. The typical radiation dose from an abdominal CT study is approximately 500 times that of a single chest radiograph, and is equal to about 2 years of background radiation exposure. Thus, clinicians must be cautious about ordering CT studies. When CT is performed, appropriate pediatric technical parameters should be used, rather than using adult techniques for children.

Magnetic resonance imaging (MRI) is another imaging modality that, like US, does not use ionizing radiation. It is increasingly used in place of CT with recent advancement of faster data acquisition techniques and widespread availability. The basic principle of MRI is the interaction between applied magnetic field and hydrogen atoms in water in the body. T1 weighted and T2 weighted are two commonly used sequences. T1-weighted images best demonstrate anatomy, while T2-weighted images best demonstrate pathology. On T1-weighted images water appears dark; this is the reason for low T1 signal of most pathologies such as infection, infarction, or tumors. Only few tissues can produce high signal on T1-weighted images, for example, fat, methemoglobin, and cyst with proteinaceous contents. On T2-weighted images water appears bright; hence, most pathologies appear bright on this sequence as they have increased water content. Hemosiderin appears low signal on T2-weighted images. Air, calcification, fast-flowing blood, and cortical bone do not produce any signal on T1/T2-weighted images and appear black. Contrast material is required to increase the contrast between normal tissue and pathology. Gadolinium (Gd) is the most commonly used MRI contrast media that increased the signal intensity of water molecules on T1-weighted images. Gd is mainly used when tumors and infection are suspected. Chemical shift imaging (in-phase and opposed-phase image) is another technique mainly used for liver and adrenal imaging. On in-phase images, the signal from both water and fat protons contributes to tissue signal intensity. On opposed-phase images, signal from fat protons cancels that of water protons. In other words, signal of fat drops out on opposed-phase images. This technique is used to detect focal or diffuse fatty liver infiltration, fat-containing liver tumors, and adrenal adenomas. Because MR image acquisition is much slower than CT, requiring the patient to remain perfectly still for the best images, and because the machines tend to be noisy and can frighten young children, sedation or anesthesia is commonly required for young children undergoing MRI.

Nuclear Medicine

In the workup of lower GI bleeding the "Meckel's scan" using 99mTc-pertechnetate is often used. 99mTc-pertechnetate is taken up by gastric mucosa and, because about one-half of the Meckel's diverticulum also contains gastric mucosa, it can be demonstrated (Figure 9–5). When performed non-emergently, pretreatment of the patient with an H2 blocker can improve the sensitivity of this test. Intestinal duplications containing gastric mucosa can also be detected.

Acute GI bleeding can be evaluated using *99m technetium-labeled red blood cells* (the patient's own red blood cells are labeled in vitro and re-infused) or *99m Tc-sulfur colloid*, consisting of tiny particles that extravasate at the bleeding site, may be used.

In neonates and young infants with suspected biliary atresia, a *hepatobiliary scan* using 99mTc–imino-diacetic acid (IDA) is often useful to suggest the diagnosis of biliary atresia (Figure 9–6) or neonatal hepatitis. The same technique is also used for verification of choledochal cyst, diagnosis of acalculous cholecystitis, and assessment of hepatoenterostomy (Kasai procedure).

IMAGING FEATURES OF PEDIATRIC GASTROINTESTINAL DISORDERS

Acute Abdominal Emergencies

Vomiting of infancy is a common indication for upper GI examination. In this context, the main questions to be answered are: (1) Is there gastric outlet obstruction? (2) Is the ligament of Treitz normally located? Prototypic entities under consideration are *hypertrophic pyloric stenosis* and *midgut volvulus.*

Midgut malrotation is suspected when the ligament of Treitz is abnormally placed. The *ligament of Treitz* is the point where the retroperitoneal duodenum reenters the peritoneal cavity and forms the proximal retroperitoneal attachment of the mesenteric root. On upper GI, the ligament of Treitz should be on the left side of the vertebral column and at or above the level of the duodenal bulb (Figure 9–7).[3] If the location of the ligament of Treitz is abnormal, the study should be continued to visualize the rest of the small intestine to the ileocecal junction, the distal end of the mesenteric root.[1] Elective surgery is indicated in infants with repeated vomiting and imaging evidence of malrotation.

Midgut volvulus is true acute abdominal emergency resulting from strangulation of mesenteric vessels requiring urgent surgery. It occurs among patients with intestinal malrotation. The midgut is twisted around the narrow mesenteric root, which contains its vascular pedicle, namely the superior mesenteric artery and vein. When torsion of the mesenteric vascular pedicle occurs,

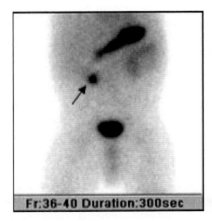 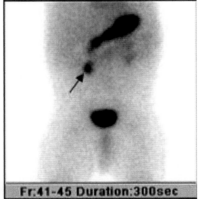 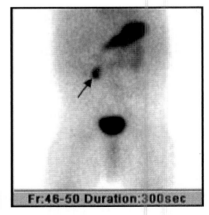

Fr:36-40 Duration:300sec   Fr:41-45 Duration:300sec   Fr:46-50 Duration:300sec

FIGURE 9–5 ■ Positive "Meckel's scan" using 99mTc-pertechnetate. Ectopic gastric mucosa in the Meckel's diverticulum (arrow).

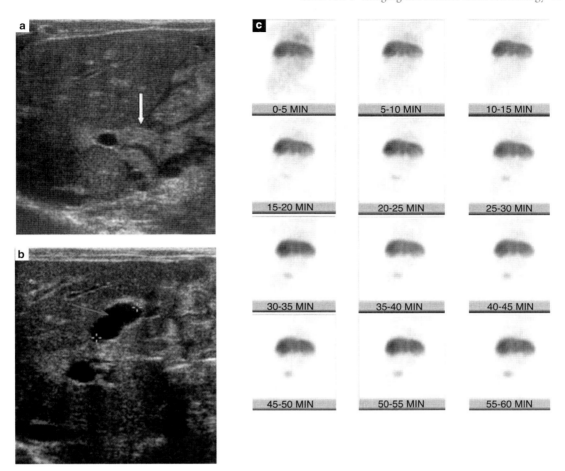

FIGURE 9–6 ■ Biliary atresia. US of the hepatic hilus (a and b) shows triangular hyperechogenicity (white arrow) correlating an area of fibrosis and vestigial gallbladder (black arrow). Biliary scan (c) using 99mTc HIDA shows rapid hepatic tracer uptake but failure of excretion into the intestinal tract.

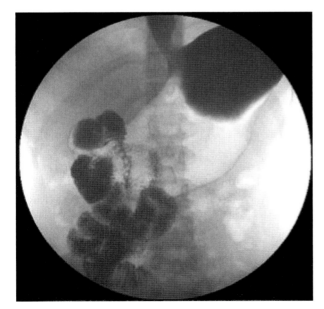

FIGURE 9–7 ■ Malrotation. A supine view from upper GI shows no fixation of the ligament of Treitz and the proximal jejunum is in the right upper quadrant.

the superior mesenteric vein is compressed and collapsed, while more elastic superior mesenteric artery continues to allow the inflow of blood into the volvulated segment, which becomes markedly congested. Once the congestion becomes severe enough, the tissue pressure of the volvulated intestine eventually surpasses the blood pressure and results in necrosis of the entire midgut. This "strangulation sequence" may complete merely in a few hours. Thus, neonates and infants with bilious vomiting should be evaluated immediately and the possibility of midgut volvulus should be ruled in or ruled out. The upper GI series is the appropriate diagnostic procedure and, when positive, the distal duodenal obstruction can be demonstrated, with the volvulated segment as a spiral column (*cork-screw appearance*).[2]

Hypertrophic pyloric stenosis

US is the modality of choice when congenital hypertrophic pyloric stenosis is suspected. The stomach should be filled at the time of examination; if it is empty, then

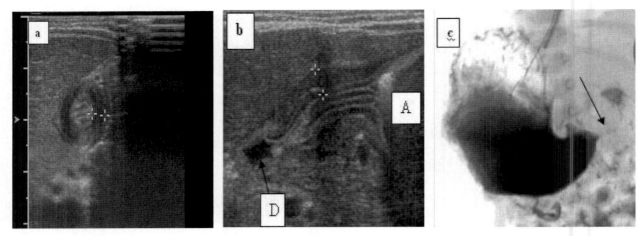

FIGURE 9–8 ■ Idiopathic hypertrophic pyloric stenosis. A short-axis and a long-axis pyloric US (a and b) show thickened hypoechoic muscular layer with the elongated pylorus (A: gastric antrum; D: duodenal bulb). A prone view from upper GI (c) demonstrates elongated narrow pyloric channel (arrows) and characteristic deformity of the gastric antrum.

5% dextrose solution can be given orally prior to the study. Typical signs include pyloric muscle thickness >4 mm, pyloric channel length >17 mm, protrusion of pyloric mucosa in the fluid-filled antrum (*antral nipple sign*), and gastric hyperperistaltis with failure of passage of gastric contents through the pylorus (Figure 9–8). The numeric value for the lower limit of muscle thickness is variable in the literature, ranging between 3.0 and 4.5 mm. According to some of the authors, actual numeric value is less important than the overall morphology of the canal and the real-time observations.[5] When US is not available or results are equivocal, an upper GI study can be helpful. This is able to demonstrate the presence of increased gastric peristalsis, a narrow, elongated pyloric channel, and characteristic compression deformity at the distal gastric antrum and at the base of the duodenal bulb caused by the enlarged pyloric muscle.

Acute appendicitis

Both US and CT are adequate for evaluation of appendicitis and imaging strategy should be conformed considering resources available at the individual institution. US has a sensitivity of 80% with a specificity of 94%.[6] A graded compression technique is used where compression is applied during scanning utilizing the basic principle that normal appendix is easily compressible while inflamed appendix cannot be compressed. Compression also displaces the bowel gas and thus helps in visualizing the appendix. Typical diagnostic findings are a dilated, non-compressible, non-peristaltic appendix with a diameter of >6 mm. Additional findings sometimes seen are the presence of an appendicolith, increased vascularity, and periappendiceal fluid. Some of the limitations of US are: (1) *retrocecal appendix*, which is difficult to find on US

due to overlying gas in the cecum, (2) patients with *high body mass index*, and (3) *perforated appendix* in which the typical findings may be absent due to decompression and disintegration of the appendix. CT with intravenous contrast is more sensitive (97%) than US for appendicitis and is helpful in those cases where US is difficult to perform or equivocal. Positive CT findings are an enlarged appendix with a diameter of >6 mm, presence of an appendicolith, adjacent fat stranding, and prominent enhancement of its wall. The full extent of perforated appendicitis, and abscess formation can be better visualized on CT (see Chapter 21, Figure 21-16).

Intussusception

US is the diagnostic modality of choice when intussusception is suspected. The typical findings are intraabdominal mass with concentric rings of high and low echogenicity known as "target sign" on transverse plane and "pseudokidney sign" on the longitudinal plane (Figure 9–9). The presence of trapped fluid in intussusception correlates significantly with ischemia and irreducibility.[7] Lead points causing secondary intussusceptions, such as Meckel's diverticulum, polyps, duplication cysts, or lymphoma, can also be visualized on US. Once the diagnosis is established, fluoroscopically guided hydrostatic or pneumatic reduction is indicated (Figure 9–10). CT and MRI are not utilized in the workup of intussusception. When the diagnosis is confirmed on US, then fluoroscopic-guided reduction should be done. Pneumatic reduction is preferred over hydrostatic reduction as it is safer, faster, and cleaner. During reduction, air pressure should not exceed 120 mm Hg. Successful reduction rate is around 80% using the pneumatic technique, while the perforation rate <1%.

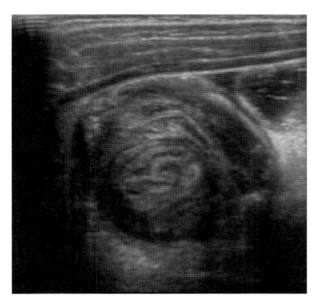

FIGURE 9–9 ■ Intussusception: transverse US image shows target sign (concentric rings of hyperechogenicity and hypoechogenicity).

Meconium ileus

When congenital bowel obstruction due to cystic fibrosis is suspected, use of a moderately hyperosmolar water-soluble contrast enema, such as a half-strength Gastrografin, can not only demonstrate the abnormality, but can also hydrate and dislodge impacted tenacious meconium in the dilated distal ileum. This is successful in about one-third of cases, avoiding surgery.

Hirschsprung's disease evaluation requires a barium enema. In this case, no cleansing enema should be given prior to the study, as the dilation of the rectum caused by this intervention could mask the characteristic findings. In an unprepped barium enema, Hirschsprung's is suggested when the maximum diameter of the rectum is less than that of the proximal sigmoid (rectosigmoid ratio <1). The aganglionic segment may show tonic contraction ("saw-toothing") (see Figure 19–6).

Acute pancreatitis

US is less sensitive than CT for the evaluation of pancreatitis. The most common finding is focal or diffuse enlargement of the gland with a dilated pancreatic duct. Other findings are peripancreatic fluid collection and decreased pancreatic echogenicity. CT is the investigation of choice for the evaluation of pancreatitis. Typical findings are pancreatic enlargement with heterogenous appearance (normal pancreas appears homogenous on CT), peripancreatic fat stranding, and dilatation of the pancreatic duct (Figure 9–11a). Other findings may include extrapancreatic or intrapancreatic fluid collections. Complications of pancreatitis can also be visualized on CT. *Pancreatic pseudocysts* are seen as walled-off fluid collections, most commonly in the lesser sac (Figure 9–11b).

Acute cholecystitis

US is the modality of choice for the diagnosis of both calculous and acalculous cholecystitis. Typical findings include the *sonographic Murphy's sign* (point tenderness at the gallbladder fossa during examination), gallbladder wall thickening, and edema. Intramural edema appears as a band of hypoechogenicity in the wall. Gallbladder wall thickening can be seen in other conditions

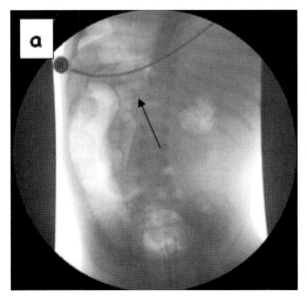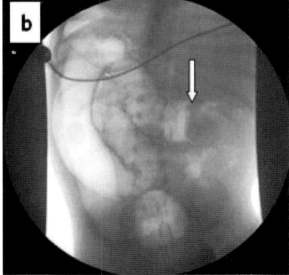

FIGURE 9–10 ■ Pneumatic reduction of intussusception (prone views). Image "a" shows soft tissue density (black arrow) in the region of splenic flexure. Image "b" shows subsequent migration of soft tissue density (white arrow) that is now lying in the region of hepatic flexure.

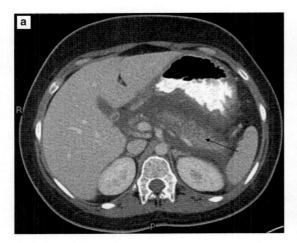
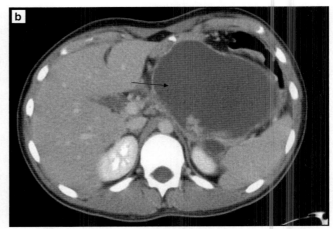

FIGURE 9–11 ■ (a) Acute pancreatitis: axial CT image shows enlarged heterogenous pancreas (arrow) with peripancreatic fluid. (b) Pseudocyst: axial CT image shows fluid collection (arrow) in the lesser sac behind the stomach in a patient with history of acute pancreatitis.

including hepatitis, ascites, and heart failure but intramural edema is not seen and wall thickening in these conditions is typically homogenous.

Cholelithiasis

US is the primary modality for evaluation of gallstones. They are typically echogenic, mobile, and produce a prominent acoustic shadow (Figure 9–12).Choledocholithiasis is usually due to migration of stones from the gallbladder to the common bile duct. US can demonstrate stones in the common bile duct but sometimes it is difficult due to interposing gas in duodenum. US can also demonstrate biliary ductal dilatation secondary to choledocholithiasis. The internal diameter of the common bile duct should not be >2 mm in infants or 4 mm in children older than 1 year.[8] Biliary sludge on US appears echogenic without acoustic shadowing.

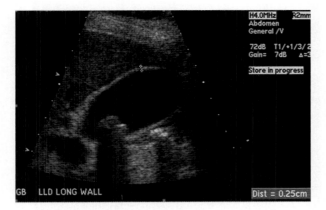

FIGURE 9–12 ■ Cholelithiasis: longitudinal US image shows distended gallbladder with calculi with prominent shadowing. Wall thickness is normal (<3 mm).

Congenital Malformations

Choledochal cyst

The US appearance varies depending on the type of choledochal cyst. A type 1 cyst (fusiform enlargement of the bile duct) appears as an anechoic fluid collection separated from the gallbladder and communicating with the CBD without vascular flow on Doppler. A type 2 cyst (an outpouching of the bile duct) appears as an eccentric cyst with narrow communication with the common bile duct. Diagnosis is confirmed by radionuclide biliary scan.

Biliary atresia

A triangular-shaped echogenic density (*triangular cord sign*),[9] representing a fibrous remnant of the biliary tract, can be seen on US adjacent to the portal vein bifurcation. The gallbladder is usually absent or rudimentary in size. Indeed, the finding of a normal gallbladder in case of persistent jaundice in newborn is suggestive of neonatal hepatitis rather than biliary atresia.[10] Diagnosis is further consolidated by radionuclide scan (*see above*).

Pancreas divisum

US is usually not used for the evaluation of pancreas divisum. On CT, dorsal duct can be seen in the anterior part of head and draining into the minor papilla, which is located anterior to the common bile duct. Ventral duct located posteriorly can be visualized and its caliber must be less than that of dorsal duct (*dominant dorsal duct sign*).[11] Ventral duct drains into the duodenum with the common bile duct. MRCP is a highly sensitive and specific study for pancreas divisum.

Annular pancreas

The diagnosis is best made on CT or MRI, which show a thick circumferential band of pancreatic tissue around the duodenum. T1-weighted fat-suppressed image is a particularly useful sequence on which pancreas appears as high signal intensity in contrast to the lower signal intensity of duodenum.

Enteric duplication cyst

The most common location of duplication cyst is in the region of the terminal ileum followed by duodenum and stomach. On US, it appears as an anechoic fluid-filled mass with typical double wall sign with inner echogenic layer representing mucosa–submucosa and outer hypoechoic layer representing muscular layer.

Infections

Liver abscess

Pyogenic abscesses are variable in appearance, but typically are ill defined, may be solitary or multiple, and are hypoechoic. Internal debris is usually present. Air–fluid levels, if present, should raise concern for a GI connection. Doppler examination reveals an avascular center with increased vascularity in the wall. *Amebic abscesses* are solitary, tend to lie near the capsule, and on US are well-defined hypoechoic collections with low-level internal echoes and distal acoustic enhancement. In early stages, amebic abscess may appear solid and hyperechoic, but devoid of any central blood flow. On CT, differentiation between pyogenic and amebic abscess is difficult, as both appear as hypodense lesions with peripheral enhancement (Figure 9–13). *Echinococcal disease* has certain characteristic features on US. These include an anechoic cyst with a collapsed membrane within it (water lily sign), multiple echogenic foci falling to the dependent part of the cyst on repositioning the patient (snowstorm sign),[12] septated or multicystic appearance due to daughter cyst formation, and calcification of the cyst wall. On CT, it is usually seen as a

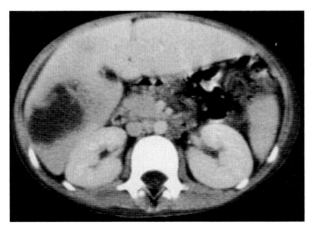

FIGURE 9–13 ■ Pyogenic abscesses: axial CT image shows well-defined hypodense lesion in the right lobe with peripheral enhancement.

multiloculated, hypodense lesion with peripheral enhancement. Daughter cysts can also be seen. *Cat-scratch disease* involves the liver in 5–10% of cases and reveals multiple small hypoechoic, circular homogenous lesions.

Hepatitis

Imaging is usually not essential in the diagnosis when clinical suspicion is very high, but it can be useful to differentiate between obstructive and non-obstructive causes of jaundice. In mild hepatitis, imaging is usually normal. On US, findings in severe hepatitis include hepatomegaly, decreased echogenicity of the liver parenchyma, and increased echogenicity of portal vein branches, giving a "starry sky" pattern. Other associated findings are gallbladder wall thickening, periportal lymphadenopathy, and ascites. CT findings are hepatomegaly, periportal edema, and gallbladder wall thickening.

Tumors

Hepatoblastoma

US appearance is non-specific. This tumor is a well-defined intrahepatic mass. It is usually hyperechoic with small internal calcifications. Increased vascularity is usually present on Doppler. An intravascular tumor thrombus can sometimes be seen in hepatic veins or portal veins as an echogenic density. On CT, the tumor is usually hypodense on non-contrast scan, with heterogenous enhancement on contrast administration. Calcification is seen in 50% of cases. Metastasis may be present at the time of diagnosis, with lungs being the most common site. On MRI, it is usually hypointense on T1-weighted images and hyperintense on T2-weighted images. Calcification, hemorrhage, and fibrosis also influence the signal intensity. Vascular invasion, if present, can be easily seen on CT or MRI.[13]

Hepatocellular carcinoma

US findings are usually similar to those of hepatoblastoma, but calcifications are less common. On Doppler, these lesions are vascular with pulsatile flow. Imaging findings on CT/MRI are usually similar to hepatoblastoma. Fibrolamellar carcinoma (FLC) usually appears as a well-defined lobulated mass with heterogenous echotexture and a typical hyperechoic central scar. On CT, it is hypodense with heterogenous enhancement.

The central scar, if present, does not enhance. On MRI, HCC is hypointense on T1, and hyperintense on T2 with enhancement. The central scar of FLC is hypointense on T1 and T2 images; this feature allows the differentiation between FLC and fibronodular hyperplasia (FNH). Another differentiating feature is that the central scar of FLC usually does not show delayed enhancement, as it typically does in FNH.

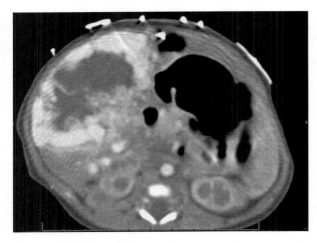

FIGURE 9–14 ■ Infantile hemangioma of liver: axial CT image (early phase) shows hypodense lesion with peripheral nodular enhancement of its wall. Hepatic veins were also enlarged in this case (not shown).

Infantile hemangioma

Infantile hemangioma is the most common benign hepatic tumor in children. It usually presents before 6 months of age. On US, it is of variable echogenicity with high intratumoral vascularity. Multiple feeding arteries can be seen. On CT and MRI, the signal pattern corresponds to the blood vessels. The pattern of contrast enhancement is typical, with early peripheral nodular enhancement and delayed centripetal filling. Other findings are enlarged feeding arteries and draining veins, and a small aorta distal to the origin of the celiac artery. The latter finding is caused by the shunting of a large part of the cardiac output to the tumor (Figure 9–14).

Hepatic metastases

The most common causes of metastases to the liver in children are Wilms tumor, neuroblastoma, lymphoma, and leukemia. On US most metastases are multiple, hypoechoic, and well defined without any vascularity. Neuroblastoma and lymphoma metastases can present as diffuse infiltration with distortion of hepatic architecture with hepatomegaly. On CT, most hepatic metastases are hypoattenuating with peripheral enhancement.

Pancreatic tumors

Pancreaticoblastoma is typically large at the time of presentation. On US it is hypoechoic and heterogenous with solid and cystic components. On CT, it is usually hypodense and multiloculated with enhancing septations. Calcifications can be seen. MRI features are variable.

Solid–cystic papillary tumor of the pancreas is usually solid with cystic components with hemorrhagic

areas. Calcification is common. Hemorrhage leads to a heterogenous appearance on US and CT. The vascular enhancement pattern is variable. On MRI, it can appear hyperintense on T1 images and heterogenous on T2 images due to hemorrhage.

Islet cell tumors

Insulinomas are the most common islet tumors in children. They are usually small at the time of presentation. On US, they are typically small, well-defined, hypoechoic lesions. Large tumors can have central necrosis. On CT, they are typically homogenous and hypervascular in the arterial phase. Larger lesions have peripheral-enhancing solid components with central non-enhancing necrotic areas. On MRI, they are hypointense on T1 and highly hyperintense on T2 with early phase enhancement.

Inflammatory Bowel Disease

In *Crohn's disease*, US can delineate bowel wall thickening, lymphadenopathy, and abscess formation. The major limitation of US is bowel gas that obscures underlying areas. In addition, bowel evaluation on US is highly operator dependent. Hence, CT is almost always recommended for cross-sectional bowel imaging. A target appearance is seen on intravenous contrast-enhanced CT, caused by enhancement of the inflamed, vascular mucosa and muscularis propria, separated by hypodense, edematous submucosa. Fibrofatty proliferation in the mesentery appears as increased attenuation and streaking of mesenteric fat. Mesenteric vessels show increased vascularity and dilatation (comb sign) (see Chapter 16, Figure 16–10). Complications of Crohn's disease such as abscess, fistulae, perforation, or bowel obstruction can be easily evaluated by CT. Upper GI series with small bowel follow-through is the standard technique for evaluation of the extent of small bowel involvement in this disorder. Typical findings include nodularity and narrowing of involved segments, with separation (effacement) from adjoining loops of bowel due to bowel wall thickening (see Figures 16–8 and 16–9).

Ulcerative colitis extends upward from the anus to involve part or the entire colon. Radiographically, it appears as wall thickening without skip lesions. Unlike ulcerative colitis, Crohn's disease tends to involve the colon asymmetrically with skip lesions. In contrast to ulcerative colitis, the right colon is most commonly involved and the rectum is usually spared. Mean colonic wall thickness is typically greater in Crohn's disease than ulcerative colitis. Abscess and fistula formation are more common in Crohn's disease than in ulcerative colitis.

REFERENCES

1. Bloom DA, Slovis TL. Congenital anomalies of the gastrointestinal tract. In: Slovis TL, ed. *Caffey's Pediatric Diagnostic Imaging.* 11th ed. Philadelphia, PA: Mosby Elsevier; 2008:188–246.

2. Buonomo C, Taylor GA, Share JC, Kirks DR. Gastrointestinal tract. In: Kirks DR, Griscom NT, eds. *Practical Pediatric Imaging: Diagnostic Radiology of Infants and Children.* 3rd ed. Philadelphia, PA: Lippincott-Raven; 1998:821–995.

3. Epelman M, Daneman A, Navarro OM, et al. Necrotizing enterocolitis: review of state-of-the-art imaging findings with pathologic correlation. *Radiographics.* 2007;27: 285–305.

4. Hernanz-Schulman M. Infantile hypertrophic pyloric stenosis. *Radiology.* 2003 227:319–331.

5. Kaiser S, Frenckner B, Jorulf HK. Suspected appendicitis in children: US and CT—a prospective randomized study. *Radiology.* 2002;223:633–638.

6. Del-Pozo G, Albillos JC, Tejedor D, et al. Intussusception in children: current concepts in diagnosis and enema reduction. *Radiographics.* 1999;19:299–319.

7. Siegel MJ. Liver. In: Siegel MJ, ed. *Pediatric Body Sonography.* 3rd ed. Philadelphia, PA: Lippincott William and Wilkins; 2002:213–273.

8. Choi SO, Park WH, Lee HJ, Woo SK. "Triangular cord": a sonographic finding applicable in the diagnosis of biliary atresia. *J Pediatr Surg.* 1996;31:363–366.

9. Ranson M, Hiew C, Babyn PS. Pediatric biliary imaging. In: Stringer DA, Babyn PS, eds. *Pediatric Gastrointestinal Imaging and Intervention.* 2nd ed. Hamilton, Ont.: B.C. Decker Inc.; 2000:551–598.

10. Soto JA, Lucey BC, Stuhlfaut JW. Pancreas divisum: depiction with multi-detector row CT. *Radiology.* 2005;235: 503–508.

11. Martin GS, Chiesa JC. Falling snowflakes, an ultrasound sign of hydatid sand. *J Ultrasound Med.* 1984;3:257–260.

12. Moore CW, Lowe LH. Hepatic tumors and tumor-like conditions. In: Slovis TL, ed. *Caffey's Pediatric Diagnostic Imaging.* 11th ed. Philadelphia, PA: Mosby Elsevier; 2008:1929–1945.

13. Slovis TL, ed. ALARA conference proceedings. The ALARA concept in pediatric CT intelligent dose reduction. *Pediatr Radiol.* 2002;32:217–317.

CHAPTER 10

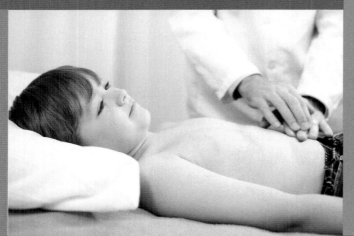

Endoscopy

Michael A. Manfredi and
Jenifer R. Lightdale

INTRODUCTION

Gastrointestinal endoscopy involves examining the inside of the gastrointestinal tract using a lighted flexible or rigid instrument called an endoscope. An endoscope is generally introduced into the body through the mouth or anus. As a medical procedure, endoscopy has been performed since the early nineteenth century, and originally involved the use of alcohol or turpentine lamps as light sources for rigid instruments.[1] The birth of modern endoscopy can be dated to the 1960s with the development of flexible fiberoptic instruments. These allowed visualization of areas beyond the reach of rigid instruments and greatly improved patient comfort. The development of fiberoptic illumination further improved endoscopic safety by removing thermal and electrical complications from the procedure. Flexible fiberoptic endoscopes were further modified in the 1980s by replacing fiberoptic image bundles with a charge-coupled device (CCD) video camera, which provided greater image detail and display on a video screen. CCD chip size has become smaller over time, further allowing the size of endoscopes to become smaller.

In the 1970s, the diameter of endoscopes became small enough to allow investigation of children.[2] Prior to the use of endoscopy, gastrointestinal diseases were diagnosed mostly by fluoroscopic contrast studies. Over the past four decades, gastrointestinal endoscopy has been shown to be safe and effective in diagnosis and treatment of children. In the 1980s, endoscopes were designed specifically for use in children, thereby cementing the importance of endoscopy in the field of pediatric gastroenterology.

Today, the diagnosis of gastrointestinal diseases in children can be made more accurately and quickly as a result of direct visualization of tissue and targeted tissue biopsies. In addition, therapeutic endoscopy has allowed for safe, minimally invasive treatments that were once only performed by open surgical techniques with longer recovery periods. As a result of endoscopy, the field of pediatric gastroenterology has grown tremendously. The contributions of endoscopy to pediatric gastroenterology will continue to grow as technology continues to progress.

In this chapter, we review the fundamentals of pediatric endoscopy. In particular, we describe the endoscopy unit as a clinical resource for children with gastrointestinal disease, as well as necessary steps that must be followed by both clinicians and families in preparation for endoscopic procedures. We also provide descriptions of different diagnostic and therapeutic procedures, as well as indications for their performance, and discuss post-endoscopy care.

THE ENDOSCOPY UNIT

Generally speaking, a pediatric endoscopy unit is comprised of a reception and waiting area, preprocedure preparation facilities, procedure rooms, and a recovery suite.[3] The waiting area allows patients to check in and families to gather while their child is having a procedure. This area should be a fun and inviting place where young children will feel comfortable. Most units have an initial preparation area where the patient will undress and informed consent is obtained. The next area of the unit is the procedure area (see Figure 10–1). This is often composed of multiple rooms where multiple providers can be performing endoscopic procedures simultaneously. After their procedure, patients will be taken to a recovery area where they are closely monitored. An endoscopy unit also must have facilities for endoscope and equipment storage,

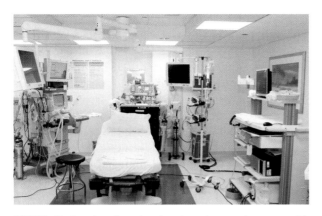

FIGURE 10–1 ■ A well-equipped endoscopic procedure room with multiple monitors, procedure cart, and general anesthesia equipment.

as well as an area for scope cleaning and disinfecting. Endoscopy units may be exclusively for pediatrics or a shared unit, where both adult and pediatric endoscopies are performed. Pediatric endoscopy may also be performed in operating rooms; this procedure location may be preferable for patients with high anesthesia risk. In acute medical situations, procedures may also be performed in intensive care settings.

The endoscopy procedure room should also be child-friendly. Equipment consists of an endoscopy station with a video processor and endoscope light source (see Figure 10–2), an air, water, and suction pump, and at least one video monitor, although two monitors, preferably on boom towers, are preferable. The procedure room should have an examining table as well as anesthesia capabilities, ideally allowing for anesthetic gas administration. In addition, an electrosurgical generator should be present for therapeutic procedures, such as polypectomy or hemostasis. Although not mandatory, it is helpful if at least one procedure room also has fluoroscopic capabilities with either a fixed fluoroscopy table or a fluoroscopic C-arm unit.

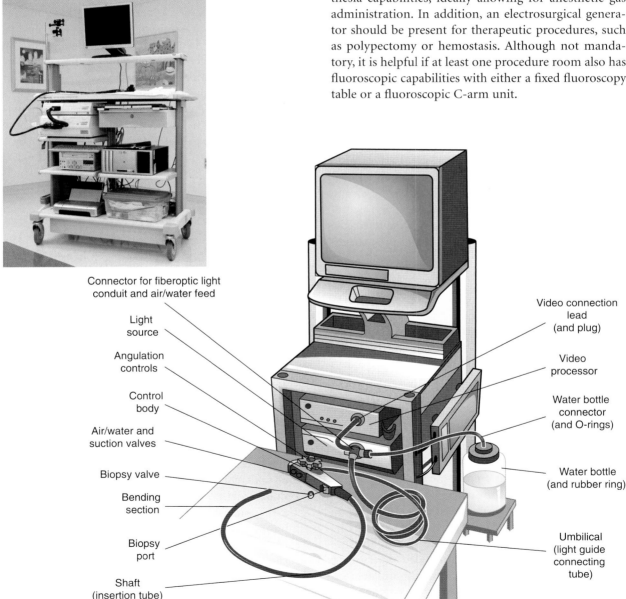

FIGURE 10–2 ■ Endoscopic equipment cart.

PREPARING CHILDREN FOR ENDOSCOPY

Preparing children and their families for an endoscopic procedure ideally begins well ahead of the procedure day.[3] Both electively and urgently scheduled procedures should involve a careful explanation by the patient's primary gastroenterologist about indications that warrant its performance, as well as basic information about endoscopy itself. The gastroenterologist should also communicate with the child's primary care provider. Gastrointestinal endoscopy, as a concept, can be introduced to patients by describing the endoscope as a camera that allows the inspection of the lining of the gastrointestinal tract, thereby providing a unique means of imaging this part of the body. It is also appropriate for physicians to discuss early on in the planning process that small biopsies from multiple sites in the inspected intestinal tract will likely be obtained.

Once the procedure has been scheduled, the patient's family will be contacted by the procedural unit staff. Initial contact by unit staff often occurs via telephone for electively scheduled procedures, and serves to allow the endoscopy unit personnel to: (1) determine individual needs of the patients, (2) obtain a medical history, and (3) review prior procedural experiences. The preprocedure telephone call is also important for expanding upon anticipatory guidance for children and their families regarding the day of the procedure, including what monitoring equipment will be applied, the need for intravenous line placement, and the patient's sedation plan.

PREPARING FOR COLONOSCOPY

Children undergoing colonoscopy will require complete cleansing of stool from the colon before the day of the procedure. Cleansing of the colon can take up to 3 days and involve a number of different preparation regimens. Most regimens use a combination of osmotic laxatives, such as magnesium citrate or polyethylene glycol (PEG), and stimulants, such as biscodyl tablets, to aid in the efficiency of purging. Rectal irrigation with saline or phosphosoda enemas may be used on the morning of the procedure to further prepare the bowel. In general, the goal of any colonoscopy prep is to have watery output on the day of the procedure that is clear with no sediment apparent in the toilet bowl or diaper.

Preprocedure information with specific instructions for bowel cleansing may be provided in person, or over the telephone, and is increasingly available on institutional websites. This information is often also reiterated in an information packet that is mailed to the patient's home. Generally speaking, bowel cleansing involves asking children to follow a clear diet for at least 1–2 days prior to the procedure, and to take specific doses of laxatives at defined intervals in advance of the procedure. A clear diet consists of broth, clear fruit juices (without pulp or sediment), popsicles, and flavored gelatin desserts (without added fruit). In general, it is best if children can avoid eating red-colored liquids, popsicles, and gelatin, as these tend to transiently stain the mucosa red and make it difficult for the endoscopist to identify true erythema or hemorrhage.

Ensuring safety of preparation regimens is paramount. All bowel cleansing approaches carry some risk of electrolyte imbalance and dehydration, and must be employed carefully in ill patients. If patients are significantly ill, unstable, at significant risk for dehydration, or at risk for hypoglycemia, it may be appropriate to perform bowel preparation in the hospital, where intravenous fluids can be administered simultaneously. Inability of patients to tolerate the bowel preparation, because of an inability either to comply with the instructions or to tolerate the preparation, may also be identified as indications for admission for bowel cleansing. Nevertheless, most children are able to prepare for ambulatory colonoscopy at home, as regimens have become increasingly more palatable and well tolerated in recent years.

Sedation

A careful plan for sedation is also fundamental to preparing for pediatric gastrointestinal endoscopy.[4] The primary goals of sedation regimens for pediatric endoscopic procedures are to ensure a patient's safety, comfort, and cooperation continuously throughout the procedure. Secondary and often desirable goals of sedation are to provide periprocedural amnesia, maximize procedural efficiency, minimize recovery times, and maintain cost-effectiveness.

The two primary types of sedation available for children undergoing gastrointestinal procedures are general anesthesia and intravenous sedation. Both are considered safe and effective, especially when patient's physical status, age, and cognitive development are taken into account. Institutions may vary in which sedative regimens are standard for otherwise healthy children undergoing endoscopy. In many institutions, intravenous sedation may be administered by either an anesthesiologist or the endoscopists themselves. Most intravenous sedation combines a fast-acting anxiolytic, such as the benzodiazepine, midazolam, with a narcotic, such as fentanyl. Alternatively, some institutions prefer to use ketamine, a dissociative hallucinogenic that is fairly effective at rendering children quiet and still. Anesthesiologists may choose to work with fast-acting inhalational anesthetics, such as sevoflurane, or use a total intravenous propofol sedation regimen, often in combination with midazolam. Propofol is a fast-acting sedative hypnotic that can be used to induce a full spectrum of sedation depths, from light sedation to general anesthesia. In children undergoing gastrointestinal procedures, propofol is generally administered as a constant infusion (by a pump), which allows for careful drug titration.

To aid in guiding which patients should receive anesthesiologist-administered sedation, the American Society of Anesthesiologists (ASA) has designed a patient classification system that ranges from Status 1 (healthy patient) to Status 5 (moribund patient) (Table 10–1). Children who are Status 1 and 2 and thus either healthy or known to have a systemic illness (i.e., asthma) that is under good control can be considered good candidates for endoscopist-administered sedation. All ASA Status 3 patients with severe or unstable systemic diseases should be evaluated carefully, on an individual basis, for either sedation or general anesthesia. Many of these are safe for sedation in the endoscopy suite, and may not require the operating room. Status 4 and 5 patients with either a severe systemic disease that is a threat to their life

or who are moribund should receive general anesthesia, generally in an operating room setting.

One increasing practice trend among pediatric endoscopists is the employment of anesthesia support to perform endoscopy in children outside of the main operating room, often in a dedicated outpatient endoscopy suite, using propofol. This approach is again used in children who would be classified as ASA I or II, and are stable and otherwise healthy. Very small infants, very ill children, and those with significant co-morbidities, including cardiac or respiratory diagnoses, are best served with general anesthesia in the operating room.

Prophylactic Use of Antibiotics Prior to Endoscopy

All children with congenital heart disease should receive cardiac clearance prior to undergoing gastrointestinal procedures, as well as guidance as to whether or not they require prophylactic antibiotics to prevent subacute bacterial endocarditis (SBE). In recent years, the American Heart Association (AHA) has altered their recommendations. They no longer recommend antibiotic prophylaxis in patients undergoing gastrointestinal procedures for the sole purpose of preventing infective endocarditis.[5] This departure of the AHA from previous guidelines refers to the fact that no data exist demonstrating a link either between endoscopy and endocarditis or between antibiotic prophylaxis and the prevention of endocarditis. Nevertheless, a cardiologist may recommend that some children with cardiac disease receive a dose of amoxicillin or other antibiotic prior to the procedure.

UPPER GASTROINTESTINAL ENDOSCOPY

Upper gastrointestinal endoscopy allows for the direct inspection of the esophagus, stomach, duodenal bulb, and the second and third portions of the duodenum.[6] Upper gastrointestinal endoscopy is therefore otherwise known as esophagogastroduodenoscopy (EGD). An EGD is the most common procedure performed in pediatric gastroenterology, and can be performed in children of all ages, including premature neonates.

Instruments

Endoscopes are commercially available by Olympus, Pentax, and Fujinon and in general are similar in design, with only subtle differences. Today's modern gastroscopes have four-way directional tip control that ranges from 180° to 210° in the up direction and 90° to 120° in the down direction with 100–120° deflection in both the left and right directions (see Figure 10–3). This tip mobility allows

Table 10–1.

American Society of Anesthesiologists (ASA) Patient Classification Scheme

ASA Class	Description
I	The patient is normal and healthy
II	The patient has mild systemic disease that does not limit their activities (e.g., controlled diabetes or controlled seizure disorder without systemic sequellae)
III	The patient has moderate or severe systemic disease, which does limit their activities (e.g., diabetes or asthma with systemic sequellae)
IV	The patient has severe systemic disease that is a constant potential threat to life (e.g., severe cyanotic heart disease, end-stage renal failure)
V	The patient is morbid and is at substantial risk of death within 24 hours, especially if procedure is not performed
E	Emergency status: in addition to indicating underlying ASA status (1–5), any patient undergoing an emergency procedure is indicated by the suffix "E." For example, a fundamentally healthy patient undergoing an emergency procedure is classified as 1-E. If the patient is undergoing an elective procedure, the "E" designation is not used

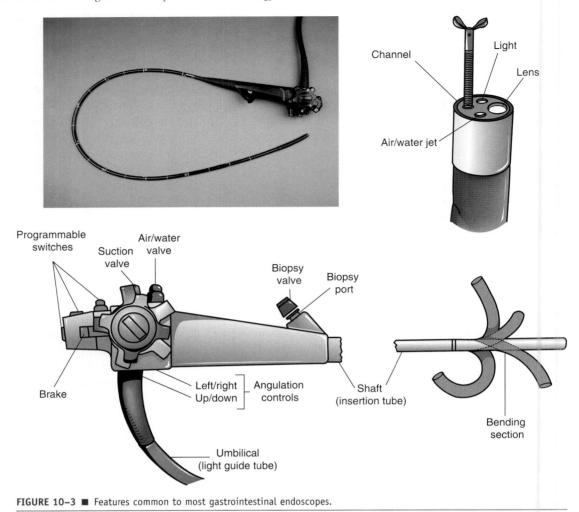

FIGURE 10–3 ■ Features common to most gastrointestinal endoscopes.

a complete inspection of the upper GI tract. The endoscope diameter size can vary from 6 to 9.8 mm in diameter. The 9.8-mm scope can provide high-definition quality images; both have a fiberoptic light source, an instrument/suction channel that ranges in size from 2 to 2.8 mm in diameter, and an air/water nozzle. Larger diameter endoscopes geared for therapeutics are also available, and have a diameter from 11 to 13 mm. Larger instruments also have larger instrument/suction channels, as well as separate suction and instrument channels. Therapeutic endoscopes are the ideal scopes to use for gastrointestinal bleeding. However, their large size makes them difficult to use in young children.

Indications for Upper Endoscopy

Indications for upper endoscopy can be divided by diagnostic and therapeutic purposes (Table 10–2). It is important to note that, in many cases, diagnostic endoscopy is indicated only after medical therapy has failed, or if symptoms relapse after discontinuation of medical therapy.

Contraindications for Upper Endoscopy

There are relatively few contraindications to upper endoscopy. In children, the size of the patient is rarely a contraindication. The only absolute contraindication for endoscopy is when bowel perforation is suspected. Most other conditions that might give an endoscopist pause before starting a procedure represent relative contraindications, and should be weighed in terms of whether the benefits of performing a procedure outweigh its risks. Coagulopathy is only a relative contraindication for diagnostic endoscopy, although extra care is certainly required and biopsies would be contraindicated until the coagulopathy is corrected.

Neutropenia is another relative contraindication. Cardiopulmonary issues may also preclude the performance of endoscopy, with the exception of gastrointestinal hemorrhage since endoscopy may be used to address the problem. Even in these situations, initial

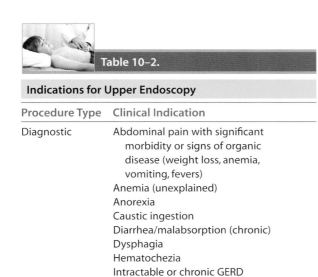

Table 10–2.

Indications for Upper Endoscopy

Procedure Type	Clinical Indication
Diagnostic	Abdominal pain with significant morbidity or signs of organic disease (weight loss, anemia, vomiting, fevers)
	Anemia (unexplained)
	Anorexia
	Caustic ingestion
	Diarrhea/malabsorption (chronic)
	Dysphagia
	Hematochezia
	Intractable or chronic GERD (including surveillance for Barrett's esophagus)
	Odynophagia
	Vomiting/hematemesis
	Weight loss/failure to thrive
Therapeutic	Dilation of esophageal and upper GI strictures
	Esophageal variceal eradication
	Foreign body removal
	Upper GI bleeding control

resuscitation steps with crystalloid and blood products should be attempted first.

Upper Endoscopy Examination Basics

Patient positioning

The preferred position of the patient is on the left side, especially for sedation cases. The supine position is an alternative position, and is especially safe in intubated patients.

Oropharynx

The preferred method of inserting the endoscope is under direct visualization. Generally speaking, the palate, epiglottis, and arytenoid cartilages should all be visualized prior to entry into the esophagus. In the non-intubated patient, it should also be possible to visualize the vocal cords (see Figure 10–4).

Esophagus

The esophagus starts at the cricopharyngeus muscle at the level of C5–C6. The normal-appearing esophagus has a mucosa that is white to pinkish in color and is slightly transparent, so that the underlying blood vessel pattern is evident. The lower esophageal sphincter marks the gastroesophageal junction, and is

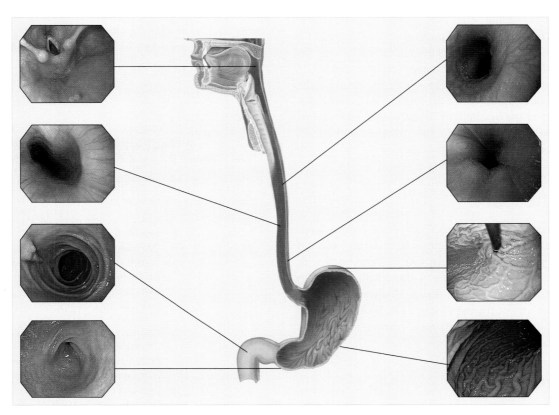

FIGURE 10–4 ■ Visual landmarks in upper endoscopy (esophagogastroduodenoscopy, EGD).

located at or below the diaphragmatic hiatus. The squamocolumnar junction marks this area, with a characteristic color change from the white color of the squamous epithelium to the salmon-colored columnar epithelium of the stomach. This transition area is commonly called the "Z line" due to the serrated appearance of this area when the esophagus is partially distended.

Stomach

The stomach is divided in three areas: the fundus, corpus, and antrum. The mucosa of the stomach is salmon in color and typically is not transparent, rendering poor visualization of blood vessels. The corpus is usually seen on entering the stomach, and has folds called rugae, which start in the upper corpus and course to the antrum. The folds should flatten out on insufflation of the stomach. The fundus is dome-shaped and is located above the corpus. The fundus is best seen with the tip of the scope angulated back upon itself, a position called retroflexion. The antrum is distal to the corpus and is free of gastric folds. The antrum leads to the ring-like pylorus.

Duodenum

The duodenum is divided into four sections. On passing through the pylorus, the duodenal bulb, or first part of the duodenum, is entered and duodenal villi can first be visualized. The second portion of the duodenum contains the major duodenal papilla also known as ampulla of Vater. The third portion of the duodenum is just past the papilla, and is characterized by circular folds with villi. These first three sections curve in a "C"-loop, forming a concavity in which the head of the pancreas lies. The fourth portion of the duodenum is narrowed at the ligament of Treitz. Most upper endoscopies will be advanced to the third portion of the duodenum.

COLONOSCOPY

Colonoscopy allows inspection of the entire large intestine and the terminal ileum.[7] In children 3 years of age and younger, colonoscopy can be performed with an upper endoscope, which is of smaller diameter than current pediatric colonoscopes. Preference for the small diameter of the upper scope needs to be weighed against its relative stiffness compared to the colonoscope.

Instruments

Colonoscopes, like gastroscopes, are commercially available by Olympus, Pentax, and Fujinon. Like gastroscopes, colonoscopes have four-way directional tip control. In comparison, colonoscopes offer more range in all four directions with 180° in the up and down directions and 160° deflection in both the left and right directions. The enhanced tip mobility of colonoscopes allows passage throughout the colon and ileum.

Colonoscope diameter size can vary from 11.6 to 13.2 mm. The modern colonoscope is capable of producing high-definition quality images. These scopes have a fiberoptic light source, an instrument/suction channel that ranges in size from 3.2 to 4.2 mm in diameter, and an air/water nozzle. Colonoscopes also have an auxiliary water jet that enables stool, mucus, and debris in the colon to be washed away at a touch of a button on the scope, or on a footswitch unit when an optional flushing pump is connected. The Olympus colonoscopes also have a variable stiffness dial that increases the stiffness of the insertion tube and can be helpful in difficult looping colon.

Indications for Colonoscopy

The indications for colonoscopy are listed in Table 10–3, by diagnostic and therapeutic purposes. The main indication of performing colonoscopy in children is to look for evidence of colitis and ileitis, as well as intestinal polyps. Symptoms associated with these conditions, such as rectal bleeding and chronic diarrhea, warrant colonoscopy. Polypectomy and hemostasis represent standard therapeutic techniques that can be performed by endoscopists in the lower colon.

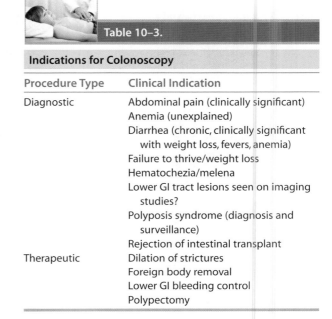

Table 10–3.

Indications for Colonoscopy	
Procedure Type	**Clinical Indication**
Diagnostic	Abdominal pain (clinically significant)
	Anemia (unexplained)
	Diarrhea (chronic, clinically significant with weight loss, fevers, anemia)
	Failure to thrive/weight loss
	Hematochezia/melena
	Lower GI tract lesions seen on imaging studies?
	Polyposis syndrome (diagnosis and surveillance)
	Rejection of intestinal transplant
Therapeutic	Dilation of strictures
	Foreign body removal
	Lower GI bleeding control
	Polypectomy

Contraindications for Colonoscopy

As with upper endoscopy, there are relatively few contraindications to colonoscopy. The only absolute contraindication is again suspected intestinal perforation. Relative contraindications include severe fulminant colitis, which may place a patient at high risk for perforation. Coagulopathy, neutropenia, and cardiopulmonary issues may increase anesthetic risks and outweigh the benefits of the procedure. As always, the endoscopist must weigh the risks and benefits of the procedure when performing colonoscopy.

Colonoscopy Examination Basics

Patient positioning

The preferred position of the patient is on their left lateral side (Figure 10–4). Nevertheless, it is common to reposition patients during procedures to successfully complete colonoscopy.

Inspection and digital rectal examination

A colonoscopic examination actually begins by inspecting the perianal area, with careful attention to hemorrhoids, fissures, skin tags, and fistulae. A digital rectal exam is performed to assess the anus and anal canal and to detect polyps, mass lesions, and strictures close to the anal verge that could be missed on insertion of the colonoscope. Performance of a rectal exam also helps establish the orientation of the colonoscope tip insertion.

Anal canal

The dentate line marks the separation of the anal canal and rectum. This area is characterized by a mixture of squamous and columnar epithelium. The squamous epithelium can become thickened, forming finger-like anal papilla. This area is best viewed with retroflexion of the colonoscope in the rectum.

Colon

The colon is a tubular structure that is approximately 60 cm in length in the newborn and reaches up to 150 cm in adults. The colon is characterized by three separate strap-like thick longitudinal bands called the teniae coli. The contractions of the teniae give the colon outpocketings known as haustra. In the middle of the haustra, the wall is thrown into crescentic folds, the plicae semilunares, which project into the lumen of the colon.

The colon is divided into anatomic segments (rectum, sigmoid, descending, transverse, ascending, and cecum). The rectum has three prominent semilunar folds called the valves of Houston. The sigmoid colon has an "S" shape and a round lumen, due to strong muscle contractions. The descending colon has a circular to oval shape that leads to the classic triangular folds seen in the transverse colon. The ascending colon is noted for its thick triangular folds and large caliber lumen. The cecum is marked by the star-like formation that is formed by the convergence of the three teniae coli. The appendiceal orifice and ileocecal valve are other landmarks of the cecum.

The mesentery fixates the cecum, ascending, and descending colon to the posterior abdominal wall, making those colonic segments retroperitoneal (Figure 10–5a). The sigmoid and transverse colon are intraperitoneal, and have a mobile mesenteric attachment. The rectum is primarily retroperitoneal.

The combination of having fixated and freely moving portions of the colon allows for loop formation during colonoscopy that can make endoscope advancement difficult and even impossible if the loop is not reduced (Figure 10–5b). Excessive looping of the

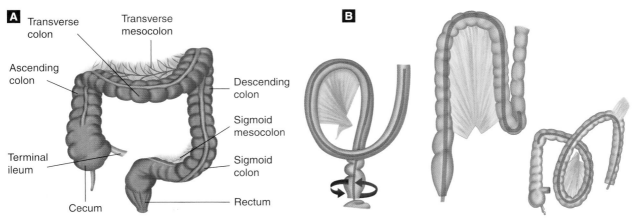

FIGURE 10–5 ■ (a) Normal colon prior to endoscope insertion; (b) 3 types of loops encountered during colonoscopy (L to R) alpha loop, N loop, reverse alpha loop.

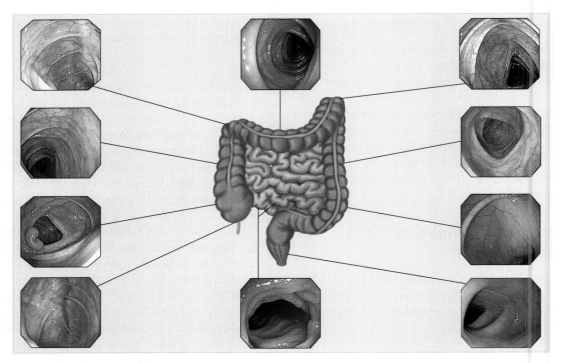

FIGURE 10–6 ■ Visual landmarks in colonoscopy.

colonoscope poses an increased risk of perforation of the bowel. Loop formation during colonoscopy will give the sensation of pain to a patient who is not completely anesthetized, and may help indicate to the endoscopist that loop reduction is necessary. Of course, a majority of pediatric colonoscopy is performed under general anesthesia or deep propofol sedation, and patients may not be able to communicate pain with loop formation. This adds an additional challenge to the pediatric endoscopist. Experienced endoscopists can recognize loop formation by feeling resistance to endoscope advancement, experiencing paradoxical loss of progress as the endoscope is pushed forward, and requiring excessive endoscope length to arrive at a particular segment.

The mucosa of the colon is smooth and shiny due to its reflective nature (Figure 10–6). The color of the mucosa can vary from a pale pink to yellow, depending on the amount of serosal fat. The vascular pattern of the colon is easily seen in healthy mucosa. At the splenic and hepatic flexures, the bluish hue of spleen and liver can be seen.

Ileum

The ileum enters the cecum from the side at the ileocecal valve, which is usually a prominent yellowish polyp-like structure. Villi in the terminal ileum lend it a granular appearance. In many children, lymphatic follicles are prominently visible as small polypoid structures. Unlike in the colon, the blood vessel pattern in the terminal ileum is less easily seen and the folds are less pronounced.

DIAGNOSTIC TECHNIQUES IN UPPER ENDOSCOPY AND COLONOSCOPY

A mainstay of diagnostic endoscopy in children consists of obtaining mucosal biopsies. Patients will feel no discomfort during or after taking biopsies. Biopsy forceps vary in size and ability to obtain multiple biopsies. The sizes of biopsies vary by forceps size, but in general are 0.5–2 mm in length (see Figure 10–7a). The risks of biopsy are bleeding and perforation; fortunately both are extremely rare.

If *Candida* or other fungal agents are suspected, cytology brushes are commonly used to culture them. Suction traps can also be temporarily connected to the suction line, and allow for sampling of bile, intestinal, and gastric secretions for microbiology, chemistry, or cytology.

POST-PROCEDURE CARE

Recovery from standard pediatric upper endoscopy and colonoscopy is usually uneventful. The child will be drowsy for a variable period of time, depending on the anesthetic. Once they are awake, patients are given clear liquids in the recovery area. Patients can resume their regular diet when they return home. After the procedure, they should plan to refrain from activities that may be dangerous when not fully alert, such as bike

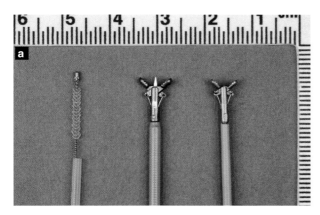

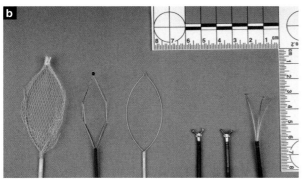

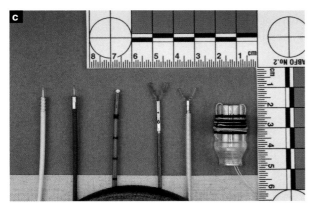

FIGURE 10–7 ■ (a) Sampling instruments, including a brush for cytology and biopsy forceps; (b) Snares and forceps for polypectomy/foreign body retrieval; (c) Needles, coagulator, clips, and band ligator for control of hemorrhage.

riding, rollerblading, swimming, and driving. In general, patients can resume all normal activities the day after the procedure. The most common complaint from an upper endoscopy is a minor sore throat, and from a colonoscopy is a bloated feeling from trapped gas. Both of these can be minimized by gentle technique and by avoiding excess insufflation of air during the procedure. Children are encouraged to walk to help pass the gas. If the patient develops fever, severe abdominal pain, persistent vomiting, or bleeding, they should be evaluated by a physician.

THERAPEUTICS PROCEDURE IN ENDOSCOPY

Foreign Body

Foreign body removal is a common endoscopic therapy in children. Esophageal foreign bodies require urgent attention because of risk of perforation. There are three areas of normal physiologic esophageal narrowing where a foreign body can get lodged. The first and most common location is the proximal esophagus at the level of the thoracic inlet (Figure 10–8). The second location is the mid-esophagus at the level of aortic arch, and the third location is the distal esophagus, slightly proximal to the gastroesophageal junction. Foreign bodies that pass through the esophagus will usually pass unimpeded. Other locations where objects can become lodged more distally are the pylorus, the distal duodenum, and the ileocecal valve.

It is generally recommended that foreign body removal be done under general endotracheal anesthesia to protect the airway from aspiration. Common exceptions to this are coins, which are easily removed without risk of airway compromise. Emergent foreign body removal would include any symptomatic esophageal foreign body as well as asymptomatic esophageal button battery due to the high risk of esophageal tissue necrosis and risk of fistula formation. Asymptomatic esophageal foreign bodies and gastric button batteries should be removed within 24 hours.

Gastric foreign bodies that should be removed include large objects (with a diameter 20 mm or greater and or a length greater than or equal to 30 mm), sharp objects that are at risk of causing bleeding or perforation, and battery ingestion. In most other instances, a conservative approach of observation for up to a month can be taken to see if the object passes before attempting endoscopic removal.

There are a variety of instruments to remove foreign bodies. These include retrieval nets, rat tooth and alligator forceps, polyp snares, wire baskets, and graspers (Figure 10–7b). All attempts should be made to try to find a similar object to the one ingested in order to find the ideal instrument to remove it.

Percutaneous Endoscopic Gastrostomy (PEG)

The PEG tube procedure was developed by Ponsky and Gauderer in the 1980s. This procedure is associated with faster recovery time and less pain than open gastrostomy tube placement. PEG placement is indicated for pediatric patients who are unable to ingest adequate calories or medications. Many of these children

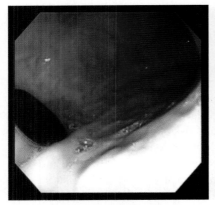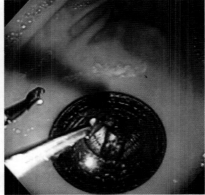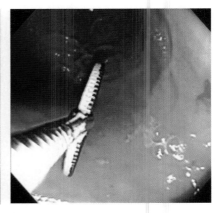

FIGURE 10–8 ■ Retrieval of a foreign object (United States 25-cent coin) from the stomach using endoscopic forceps.

have neurologic impairment. PEGs may also be indicated in patients who aspirate liquids, or who have higher metabolic needs that cannot be met orally, due to cystic fibrosis, congenital heart disease, and other conditions.

Technique

PEG placement requires two physicians, one performing the endoscopy and the other acting as a surgical assistant (Figure 10–9). The first advances the endoscope into the stomach and a site is identified by transillumination of the skin by the endoscope light. The assistant indents the chosen spot with a finger, which is observed internally with the endoscope. The finger may be moved anywhere in the transilluminated region until an ideal location within the stomach is decided upon. Once the spot is identified and the area has been surgically cleansed and draped, an angiocatheter is inserted through the skin into the stomach, and a looped guidewire is inserted through the catheter. The guidewire is grasped using a snare or forceps, and is pulled out through the mouth as the endoscope is withdrawn. The gastrostomy tube is

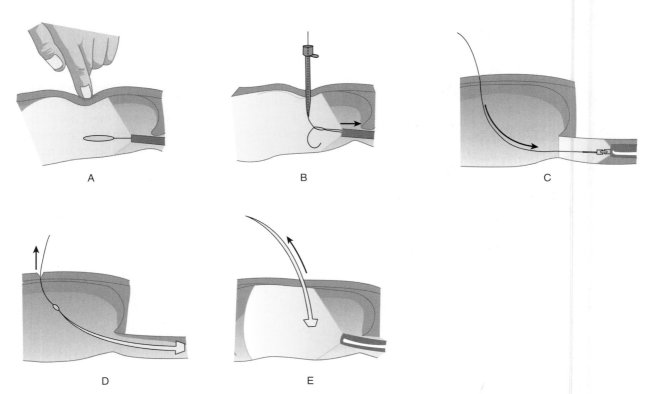

FIGURE 10–9 ■ Technique of percutaneous endoscopic gastrostomy (PEG). (A–C): An over-needle is placed into stomach under endoscopic visualization, wire placed through catheter is grasped and pulled out through mouth. (D–E) Gastrostomy tube is tied to wire and pulled back into the stomach and out through the needle tract.

attached to the wire at the mouth, and is then pulled down through the esophagus and out through the abdominal wall by the assistant. An inner disk or "bumper" prevents the tube from being accidentally pulled out, and a similar bolster is placed at the skin to prevent inner migration of the tube.

Contraindications

Absolute contraindications to PEG placement include inability to achieve successful transillumination of the stomach or to visualize the finger indentation, presumably for anatomic reasons, such as the presence of an overlying liver or colon. Relative contraindications that may preclude a PEG are ascites, peritoneal dialysis catheter, prior abdominal surgery, hepatomegaly, splenomegaly, scoliosis, ventriculoperitoneal shunt, situs inversus, and gastric varices.

Complications

Since the placement of the gastrostomy tube is somewhat blind, complications can occur early or late. A rare late complication is the development of gastrocolocutaneous fistula due to placement of the PEG tube through the colon and stomach. Other complications include tube migration into the abdominal wall (buried bumper), intrahepatic placement, peritonitis, hemorrhage, necrotizing fasciitis, pneumoperitoneum, leakage around the G-tube, and wound infection.

Stricture Dilation

Esophageal stricture is the most common indication for endoscopic dilation in children. The causes of esophageal strictures in children are usually benign: narrow anastomoses after surgical repair of esophageal atresia, peptic injury, eosinophilic esophagitis, congenital lesions, Schatzki's rings, and caustic injury. Strictures can also be found in the proximal or distal small bowel and colon related to Crohn's disease and previous surgical anastomoses. Dilation is also indicated for achalasia.

Endoscopic dilation can be performed by through the scope (TTS) balloon dilation or by Savary–Gillard dilators. There are a variety of available TTS balloon dilators available in either single or multiple diameters. The balloon is inflated with gastrograffin or water under pressure to a preset maximum diameter. TTS balloon dilation gives the benefit of direct visualization of the balloon passage through the stricture. Savary dilators are hollow, flexible polymer cylinders of various sizes with a tapered tip. The Savary dilator is advanced over a guidewire that has been placed endoscopically through the stricture and the procedure is usually done under fluoroscopic guidance. The most serious complication of esophageal dilation is perforation. The perforation rate for esophageal strictures after dilation has been reported to be 0.1–0.4%.

Management of GI Bleeding

Significant gastrointestinal bleeding in children is a rare event, but can be life threatening. Endoscopy within the first 24 hours can reduce morbidity and mortality from gastrointestinal hemorrhage. Prior to endoscopy, the patient should be stabilized with aggressive fluid resuscitation using crystalloid or colloid solutions and transfusion as required. Different approaches to gastrointestinal bleeding can be categorized as injection techniques, thermal coagulation, and mechanical therapies. All three modalities may be incorporated in an individual case if necessary.

Injection therapy

Injection therapy is a common treatment used to achieve hemostasis. Various chemical agents can be injected depending on the indication, and each has recommended aliquot volumes to administer and maximum doses (Table 10–4). All sclerosing agents are administered via endoscopic needles (Figure 10–7c). Epinephrine in a 1:10,000 dilution is the most commonly used agent.

Table 10–4.

Indications and Doses of Common Sclerosing Agents for Therapeutic Endoscopy

Solution	Indications	Volumes Per Injection, Maximum Total Dose
Epinephrine (1:10,000 concentration)	Bleeding ulcer	0.5–2 mL aliquots injected around bleeding site. Maximum total dose of 10 mL
Ethanol (98%)	Varices	0.1–0.2 mL aliquots surrounding bleeding site. Maximum total dose 0.6–1.2 mL
Sodium morrhuate (5%)	Varices	0.5–1.0 mL aliquots, watching for effect. Maximum total dose 5–10 cm³mL per session
Sodium tetradecyl sulfate (1–3%)	Varices	0.5–1.0 mL aliquots, watching for effect. Maximum total dose 3–5 cm³mL per session

It has three major modes of action: local vasoconstriction, platelet aggregation, and mechanical tamponade. Epinephrine is not tissue-destructive, so relatively large volumes can be administered.

Sclerosing agents such as sodium tetradecyl sulfate and sodium morrhuate induce tissue destruction by causing local inflammation, thrombus formation, and scarring. These agents and others can be injected directly into varices for the treatment of variceal hemorrhage. Complications of sclerotherapy include stricture formation, tissue ulceration, bleeding, perforation, infection, and fistula formation. This mode of treatment has been replaced largely by band ligation, but is still useful in infants and small children in whom the band ligator is too large to pass through the oropharynx.

Thermal coagulation

Thermal coagulation can be divided into contact and non-contact devices. Examples of contact devices are bipolar coagulation probes and heater probes (Figure 10–7c). Heater probes provide a constant temperature of 250°C and deliver a set programmed amount of energy. Bipolar probes transmit current between two electrodes in the probe, limiting the depth of tissue injury compared to monopolar probes, which are less commonly used. The goal of contact therapy (coaptive coagulation) is to provide steady heat to coagulate the local tissue and the bleeding vessel. This treatment is useful in bleeding ulcers and vascular lesions. Complications of coaptive coagulation include increased bleeding and deep tissue injury, including perforation. Argon plasma coagulation (APC) is a newer non-contact thermal modality that has the benefit of covering larger areas with less risk of deep tissue injury.

Mechanical therapy

Mechanical clips are devices that apply mechanical tamponade to a lesion. They are effective in closing mucosal defects as well as applying mechanical compression to a visible bleeding vessel. There are several types of clips commercially available and range in opening size from 9 to 11 mm. Some clips can open and close multiple times, while others are rotatable to facilitate accurate placement (Figure 10–7c). Clip placement may be difficult depending on the location of the lesion. All clips are designed to slough off in a few days to weeks.

Band ligation

Band ligation is a hemostatic approach used for varices (Figure 10–10). A band ligator consists of a cylindrical cap, preloaded with multiple elastic bands, which is placed over the tip of the endoscope. The varix is sucked into the cap and a band is released onto the tissue. Band ligation has replaced sclerotherapy in most instances since it causes less ulceration and stricturing, but may be difficult to perform in small children.

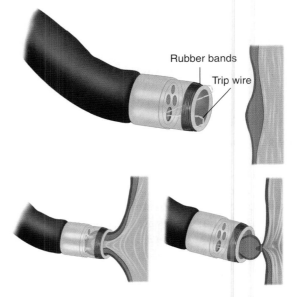

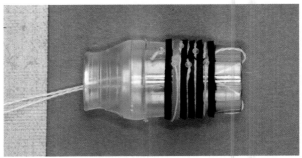

FIGURE 10–10 ■ Band ligation of esophageal varices-technique and close-up view of device.

Polypectomy

Polypectomy is one of the most common procedures performed in endoscopy. The technique of polyp removal depends on the shape and size of the polyp. The most common polyps encountered in pediatrics are pedunculated polyps, which have stalks of varying size. Polyps 2 mm or less can be removed with forceps. Most polyps are removed with a snare. The snare can have monopolar cautery current applied to it ("hot snare"), or can be used without current ("cold snare"). As a rule, polyps 2–5 mm can be removed with a cold snare. Polyps greater than 5 mm are best removed with a hot snare. When applying cautery to a polyp, it is best to use pure coagulation current, rather than cutting or blended current, from an electrosurgical generator to minimize bleeding.

Once resected, small polyps can be suctioned through the channel and captured in a suction trap. Large polyps need to be removed with a net or other grasping device. Sessile polyps generally require submucosal injection of saline to lift the polyp from the colon wall. These polyps are rarely encountered in pediatrics.

Complications of polypectomy include bleeding, bowel perforation, and post-polypectomy syndrome, which occurs if cautery causes full thickness burns to the colon, resulting in peritoneal symptoms.

ADVANCED PROCEDURES

Endoscopic Retrograde Cholangiopancreatography (ERCP)

ERCP involves the passage of a side-viewing endoscope into the second portion of the duodenum and cannulation of the major duodenal papilla.[8] After cannulation of the papilla, radiopaque contrast is injected under fluoroscopy to visualize the biliary tree and the pancreatic duct (Figure 10–11a). Biliary indications for ERCP include choledocholithiasis, evaluation of primary sclerosing cholangitis, choledochal cyst, biliary strictures, bile plug syndrome, intra- or extrahepatic ductal dilation, and bile leak after liver transplantation or cholecystectomy. ERCP can also be used to diagnose biliary atresia. Pancreatic indications for ERCP include persistent acute pancreatitis, recurrent episodes of acute pancreatitis, chronic pancreatitis, pancreatic divisum, annular pancreas, and pancreatic trauma. In addition to diagnostic capabilities, ERCP has therapeutic capabilities such as biliary or pancreatic sphincterotomy, stone removal, stricture dilation, and stent placement. Complications of ERCP include pancreatitis, bleeding, perforation, and cholangitis.

Endoscopic Ultrasound

Endoscopic ultrasound (EUS) utilizes an ultrasound transducer attached to the endoscope and can be used to obtain high-resolution images of the GI tract layers, submucosal lesions, liver, bile ducts, and pancreas, as well as extraluminal masses and lymph nodes in the mediastinum and peritoneal cavity. A miniprobe has been developed that can be passed through conventional endoscopes and has increased the potential for this procedure in children. EUS is particularly useful for assessment of submucosal lesions, and its indications include cancer staging, pancreatic and biliary disease, and anorectal malformations. Needle aspiration of cystic lesions can be accomplished via EUS, and chronic pancreatitis and autoimmune pancreatitis can be diagnosed (Figure 10–11b). Since the incidence of esophageal, gastric, biliary, and pancreatic cancer is low in children, pediatric EUS is typically performed with the help of adult gastroenterologists.

Small Bowel Imaging

The small bowel distal to the duodenum was once thought to be an unreachable area for an endoscope. However, the recent development of double and single balloon enteroscopy now allows exploration of the small bowel. Balloon enteroscopy involves sequentially inflating and deflating the balloon or balloons, which allows the endoscope to be advanced using a device called an overtube. The enteroscope can be advanced by pulling or pleating the small bowel, like an accordion, onto the instrument. Indications for enteroscopy are both therapeutic and diagnostic. Hemostasis for small bowel bleeding, small bowel polypectomy, and balloon dilation are possible therapies that can be performed with this procedure. Complications of enteroscopy include bleeding, perforation, and pancreatitis.

Wireless video capsule endoscopy has emerged in the last 5 years as a non-invasive technology that can also provide diagnostic imaging of the small intestine.[9]

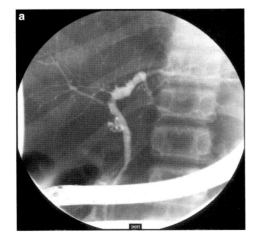
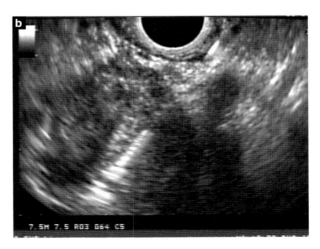

FIGURE 10–11 ■ (a) ERCP in patient with primary sclerosing cholangitis; (b) endoscopic ultrasound.

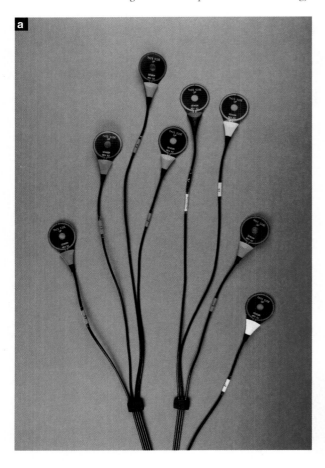

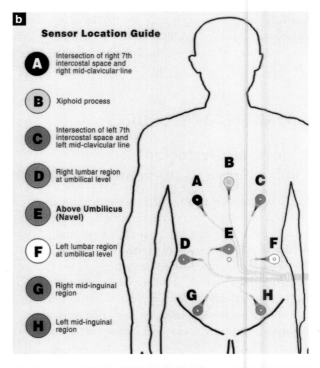

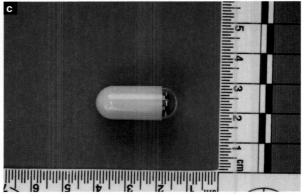

FIGURE 10–12 ■ Wireless capsule endoscopy (a) Antenna array (b) antenna placement diagram (c) closeup view of capsule endoscope, with clear optical dome and LED lights on the right side.

Small bowel capsules are commercially available from Given Imaging (PillCam SB) and Olympus (EndoCapsule). Both capsules take two video images per second, which are transmitted wirelessly to a recorder, which can acquire up to 55,000 images over approximately 8 hours. The patient wears an eight-lead sensor array that picks up the signal and also provides information about capsule location within the abdomen. The array is connected to a recording device, which is worn on a belt (Figure 10–12a). The video capsules from both companies currently measure 11 × 26 mm (Figure 10–12b).

Preparation for capsule endoscopy is variable, and at our institution involves a regular diet until noon on the day before the procedure. Non-red clear liquids can be taken up to 3 hours prior to the procedure. A mild bowel prep consisting of 17 g of PEG-3350 in the afternoon and again at bedtime is administered in order to minimize the amount of dark bile and secretions. Capsules are swallowed with water. A clear liquid diet can be resumed after 2 hours; food and medication can be ingested 4 hours after the video capsule is swallowed.

Indications for capsule endoscopy include looking for an obscure source of gastrointestinal bleeding, suspected Crohn's disease, celiac disease, and polyps in patients with hereditary polyposis syndromes. Capsule endoscopy is FDA approved for children 10 years of age and older; however, capsule studies have been done in patients as young as 2.5 years, with one case report of successful capsule in an 18 month old. Young patients who cannot swallow the capsule can have it placed endoscopically using a delivery device. The main risk associated with capsule endoscopy is capsule retention, which is clinically significant in less than 1% of patients.

REFERENCES

1. Hirschowitz BI, Modlin IM. History of endoscopy: the American perspective. In: Classen M, Tytgat GNJ, Lightdale CJ, eds. *Gastroenterological Endoscopy*. Stuttgart, Germany: Thieme; 2002:2–16.

2. Gilger MA. Gastroenterologic endoscopy in children: past, present, and future. *Curr Opin Pediatr*. 2001;13:429–434.

3. Heard L. Taking care of the little things: preparation of the pediatric endoscopy patient. *Gastroenterol Nurs*. 2008;31:108–112.

4. Fredette ME, Lightdale JR. Endoscopic sedation in pediatric practice. *Gastrointest Endosc Clin N Am*. 2008;18:739–751.

5. Wilson W, Taubert KA, Gewitz M, et al. Prevention of infective endocarditis: guidelines from the American Heart Association: a guideline from the American Heart Association Rheumatic Fever, Endocarditis, and Kawasaki Disease Committee, Council on Cardiovascular Disease in the Young, and the Council on Clinical Cardiology, Council on Cardiovascular Surgery and Anesthesia, and the Quality of Care and Outcomes Research Interdisciplinary Working Group. *Circulation*. 2007;116:1736–1754.

6. Cotton PB, Williams CB. Upper endoscopy: diagnostic techniques. In: Cotton PB, Williams CB, eds. *Practical Gastrointestinal Endoscopy: The Fundamentals*. Singapore: Markono Print Media Pte Ltd; 2008:37–58.

7. Gershman G, Ament M. Pediatric colonoscopy. In: Gershman G, Ament M, eds. *Practical Pediatric Gastrointestinal Endoscopy*. Malden, MA: Blackwell Publishing Inc.; 2007:132–168.

8. Fox V. Pediatric endoscopy. In: Classen M, Tytgat G, Lightdale CJ, eds. *Gastroenterological Endoscopy*. New York: Thieme; 2002:720–748.

9. Lee KK, Anderson MA, Baron TH, et al. Modifications in endoscopic practice for pediatric patients. *Gastrointest Endosc*. 2008;67:1–9.

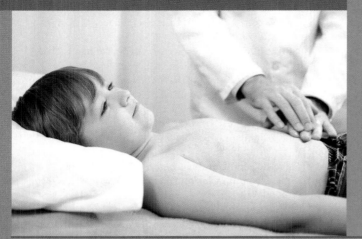

CHAPTER 11

Esophageal pH and Impedance Monitoring

Rachel Rosen, Eric Chiou, and Samuel Nurko

INTRODUCTION

Gastroesophageal reflux (GER), defined as the passage of gastric contents into the esophagus, occurs on a daily basis as a normal process in infants, children, and adults. Most episodes of physiologic reflux are transient, asymptomatic, and reach only the distal esophagus. Gastroesophageal reflux disease (GERD) is distinguished by reflux into the esophagus resulting in well-defined symptoms or medical problems (see Chapter 12). When children present with atypical complaints or extraesophageal symptoms, testing may be necessary to document the presence or absence of pathologic reflux, or the association between reflux events and specific symptoms.[1]

While endoscopy can be helpful in documenting acid damage to the esophageal mucosa in the form of erosions or ulcers, the majority of patients with symptoms of GERD do not have endoscopic or pathologic evidence of esophagitis.[2] Tests designed to detect the presence of GER have been developed.

The first test utilized was esophageal pH monitoring, in which an electrode designed to detect changes in pH is used to assess the frequency and duration of acidic reflux present in the distal esophagus. Over the years the advantages, disadvantages, and limitations of traditional, catheter-based esophageal pH monitoring have become better defined, with a subsequent evolution of newer diagnostic techniques. Wireless methods to detect acidic contents in the esophagus have now become available (Bravo capsule). Additionally, we have seen the development of the technical possibility of measuring both acidic and non-acidic reflux with multichannel intraluminal impedance (MII). In the present chapter we will review the current techniques that are being used for the dynamic detection of reflux episodes.

CATHETER-BASED ESOPHAGEAL pH MONITORING

Esophageal pH monitoring, which quantifies the frequency and duration of acidic reflux episodes, can be used to confirm abnormal esophageal acid exposure and/or correlate symptoms with acidic reflux episodes. Testing may be especially helpful in patients who present with atypical symptoms, patients with persistent symptoms despite pharmacologic treatment, or patients without evidence of mucosal damage on endoscopy. Other diagnostic approaches, such as barium contrast upper GI series or nuclear scintigraphy, have had variable sensitivity and specificity when compared to esophageal pH monitoring.[1] Unacceptably high false-positive and false-negative rates seen with these radiographic tests have made esophageal pH monitoring preferable over barium contrast and scintigraphy studies for the diagnosis of reflux.

Equipment

Over the years, the methodology of esophageal pH monitoring in children has become relatively standardized as evidenced by the publication of professional practice guidelines.[1,3] In addition to a catheter-based pH sensor, a portable data logger that records intraesophageal pH as well as events during the study such as symptoms, meals, position changes, and activity is required. As technology has improved and as electronic devices have become smaller, pH monitoring is now conducted on an ambulatory basis, even for pediatric patients.

Electrode Placement

The catheter-based pH electrode is placed through the nose into the distal esophagus.[3] There are several types of pH electrodes available, including glass and antimony-based electrodes. Proper placement of the pH electrode relative to the lower esophageal sphincter (LES) is very important for accurate data. The closer the electrode is to the esophagogastric junction, the greater the acid exposure that is recorded. Similarly, as pH electrodes are placed at higher and higher locations in the esophagus above the LES, there is a linear decrease in acid exposure time, which ultimately decreases the sensitivity of the test. In adult studies, the pH electrode is typically inserted through the nose and positioned 5 cm above the superior margin of the LES.[2] Ideally, localization of the LES is best achieved with stationary esophageal manometry prior to placement of the catheter. Because of the two required nasal intubations, this additional procedure is difficult in children, however, so manometry has not become standard procedure before pH-probe placement in children. As a result, there are other methods for localization of the pH electrode in children, including calculation of the esophageal length according to Strobel's formula[4] and fluoroscopy. If using Strobel's formula [length from nares to LES (cm) = 5 + 0.252(height)], the tip should be placed at 87% of the distance between the nares and the LES (the rationale being that 5 cm is 13% of the standard adult esophageal length). Because of concerns about the accuracy of applying Strobel's formula to children over 1 m in height, the Working Group of the European Society of Pediatric Gastroenterology and Nutrition recommended use of an X-ray or fluoroscopy to confirm placement of the pH electrode so that the sensor or tip lies over the third vertebral body above the diaphragm throughout the respiratory cycle.[3] In general, in the absence of manometry, radiographic verification of catheter placement is necessary and adjustments can be made to the catheter location accordingly.

Recording Conditions

From a clinical standpoint, in order to best study GER, recording conditions should follow the patient's normal daily routine as much as possible in terms of activity and diet. On the other hand, the monitoring protocol should be somewhat standardized to reduce variability and the effect of confounding factors, especially if the study is also being conducted for research purposes.

The optimal duration of monitoring should be at least 18 hours, including a day and a night period.[3] Depending on the aim of the study, H_2-blockers and proton-pump inhibitors should be stopped at least 3 or 7 days prior to the study, respectively.[2] Performing a pH monitoring study while "on-medications" may be indicated if the investigator desires to evaluate the efficacy of acid-blocking medications in patients who have persistent symptoms despite maximal medical therapy.

Depending on the clinical question in mind, prokinetics may also be stopped at least 48 hours before pH monitoring,[5] although they do not interfere with reflux detection.

Instructions for feeding during the study should again represent a balance between maintaining a degree of standardization and recreating normal circumstances with minimal restrictions. Although a strict standardized diet is generally not necessary, acidic drinks and foods should be minimized and documented in the diary. Investigators may consider excluding meal times from analysis, since it is difficult to distinguish episodes of GER from pH changes secondary to swallowing acidic foods during periods of eating, one of the major limitations of pH monitoring. The study period should include at least three discrete meals with minimal snacking in between meals. Given the buffering effect of formula or food, an interval of 3–4 hours in between meals is recommended. Very hot and cold beverages should be avoided, since extreme fluctuations in temperature can affect the sensitivity of the pH electrode. Chewing gum or hard candy should also be avoided because these activities increase saliva production and therefore induce additional swallowing and peristalsis that can affect the detection of GER. Documentation of patient position and activity (e.g., sleeping) during the study should also be recorded since the effect of body position on different patterns of GER has been well-reported in infants, children, and adults.[1]

Definitions and Criteria

Once a pH monitoring study is completed, data are downloaded from the data logger and analyzed with validated software on a computer. A pH of 4 is generally accepted as the optimum cutoff in both children and adults. This pH threshold was based on early observational studies that showed that perfusion of acid into the esophagus, resulting in a drop in intraesophageal pH below 4, corresponded with symptoms of heartburn.[6] In adults, using a cutoff of pH 4 also provided the best discrimination in terms of sensitivity and specificity between subjects with proven reflux disease and asymptomatic controls, when compared to other threshold values.[1,2] The identification of a reflux episode typically starts when the pH drops below the cutoff limit, lasts for at least 5 seconds, and ends when the pH returns to the cutoff limit.[7] Several parameters based on this pH cutoff have been studied, including the total number of reflux episodes, number of reflux episodes lasting >5 minutes, duration of the longest reflux episode, and the reflux index, which is the percentage of time of the entire duration of the investigation during which the pH <4. Complex scoring systems, such as the ones proposed by Johnson and DeMeester for adults[8] and by Jolley et al.

for children,[9] incorporate several of these parameters. The reflux index, however, is generally considered the single most important variable in clinical practice for both adults and children.[1,2]

Normal Ranges

Once reflux episodes have been identified in a pH monitoring study, often the next step is to determine where on the continuum between physiologic reflux and pathologic GERD a particular patient should be placed. Normative data are therefore needed to guide interpretation of pH monitoring results. Although published pediatric data are rather limited, few would debate the occurrence of asymptomatic episodes of reflux in normal infants and children. In a study of 509 infants 1–11 months old, the upper limit of normal for the number of acidic reflux episodes was 73 episodes daily, and the upper limit of normal for the reflux index pH <4 was 11.7%.[10] Normative values for older children are relatively scarce, limited by the difficulty in obtaining data from truly healthy and asymptomatic volunteers. In some cases, "normals" were obtained from children hospitalized for GER evaluations who turned out to be asymptomatic during the time of pH monitoring[11] or were found to have other causes for their gastrointestinal symptoms.[12] As a result, caution should be used when comparing results. Overall, these studies suggest that physiologic acidic reflux is a common occurrence in infants during the first year of life, with decreased acid exposure found in older children and adults (Table 11–1). Based on the available data, the North American Society for Pediatric Gastroenterology, Hepatology and Nutrition (NASPGHAN) developed the following recommendations in the assessment

of normal versus abnormal pH monitoring studies in infants and children: an upper limit of normal of the reflux index up to 12% in the first year of life and up to 6% thereafter.[1]

Diagnostic Accuracy

Although endoscopy and histology remain the gold standard for diagnosis of esophagitis, in the absence of erosive or biopsy-proven esophagitis, there is no gold standard for the definition of GERD, since not all patients with GERD will have esophagitis. In comparing adults with endoscopic esophagitis with normal volunteers, esophageal pH monitoring was found to have 77–93% sensitivity and 85–97% specificity.[1,2] In children, estimated sensitivity of pH monitoring to predict esophagitis has been similar to adults, ranging from 83% to 100%.[1]

For the subset of symptomatic patients without evidence of esophagitis, diagnosis using reflux monitoring is arguably even more crucial in distinguishing between reflux disease and functional heartburn. However, when acid exposure times were compared between normal adult controls and patients with GERD symptoms but negative endoscopic findings, pH testing was able to discriminate between the two groups, but with considerable overlap in the percentage of time that the pH <4; the sensitivity was decreased to only 61–64%, and specificity was 85–91%.[2] The clinical utility of pH monitoring in children with non-erosive reflux disease has not been well studied. Although esophagitis is clearly associated with abnormal acid exposure in children, the severity of esophagitis or symptoms has not been found to correlate with the severity of reflux as measured by pH monitoring.[1,2]

 Table 11–1.

Esophageal pH Data from Asymptomatic Infants, Children, and Adults (Mean Upper Limit of Normal = Mean + 2SD)

Reference	n	Mean Age (range)	No. of Reflux Episodes/24 Hours	Reflux Index (% Time pH < 4)
Infants				
Vandenplas et al.[10]	509	2 months (0–11 months)	73	11.7
Children				
Boix-Ochoa et al.[11]	20	19 months (2 months to 3 years)	27	5.1
Sondheimer[65]	6	61 months (1–24 months)	22	2.7
Euler and Byrne[66]	22	15 months (1–108 months)	14	3.1
Cucchiara et al.[12]	63	24 months (2 months to 12 years)	28	3.4
Adults				
Vitale et al.[67]	50	25 years		7.2
Richter et al.[68]	110	38 years		5.8

Reproducibility

In pediatrics, results from studies looking at the intrasubject reproducibility of esophageal pH results are variable. Vandenplas et al. studied 30 infants and children over two consecutive 24-hour periods; the Pearson correlation coefficients for the reflux index and number of reflux episodes between day 1 and day 2 were 0.95 and 0.98, respectively.[13] In contrast, the Spearman correlation coefficient for the reflux index reported by Mahajan et al. was only 0.62 between day 1 and day 2, and for the number of reflux episodes it was 0.71.[14] In yet another study that consisted of two consecutive 24-hour pH monitoring studies, 9 out of 30 children had discordant (normal versus abnormal) results between the 2 recording days, yielding an overall reproducibility of 70%.[15] Similar studies in adults have reported slightly higher degrees reproducibility ranging from 77% to 89%.[2] Overall, there appears to be some degree of day-to-day variability among patients; whether these differences are clinically significant is debatable. Esophageal pH monitoring results in isolation of clinical history should certainly be interpreted with caution, and consideration should be given for repeat testing when the clinical picture is unclear.

Symptom Correlation

For patients with typical symptoms of reflux, such as heartburn or regurgitation, clear findings of erosive disease on endoscopy, or histologic evidence of esophagitis, the diagnosis of GERD can usually be made without further diagnostic testing. Care should be taken in those patients that may have eosinophilic esophagitis. On the other hand, for patients with non-specific symptoms such as irritability and crying in infants, or extraesophageal symptoms of cough or wheezing, pH monitoring studies may be indicated to assess the relationship of symptoms with reflux episodes. There is currently no consensus on the time window that should be used to link a recorded symptom with a preceding or simultaneous reflux event. Based on analysis of time windows of various durations, most investigators recommend looking for symptom correlation during a 2-minute window beginning 2 minutes before onset of symptoms, although both longer and shorter intervals of between 30 seconds and 5 minutes have been proposed.[2]

Several statistical methods have also been proposed over the years to better quantify the association of symptoms and reflux episodes; there are no conclusive data, however, proving one index to be superior to the others. The symptom index (SI) is defined as the percentage of symptom episodes that are related to reflux[16]:

$$\frac{\text{Number of reflux-related symptom episodes}}{\text{Total number of sympton episodes}} \times 100$$

In adults, a SI score of scores $\geq 50\%$ suggests a relationship between symptom and reflux.[2,16] One drawback of using this method is that it does not take into account the total number of reflux episodes. For example, if a subject was found to have an abnormally elevated number of reflux episodes but only one or two symptoms that happened to coincide with an episode of reflux by chance, the relationship between symptoms and reflux may be overestimated by the SI.

The symptom sensitivity index (SSI), which was subsequently developed, is the percentage of reflux episodes that are associated with symptoms[2,16]:

$$\frac{\text{Number of symptom-associated reflux episodes}}{\text{Total number of reflux episodes}} \times 100$$

An arbitrary cutoff of 10% or higher is commonly used to indicate a significant association between symptoms and reflux episodes. One disadvantage is that the SSI is more likely to be positive when the number of symptom episodes is high.

Most recently, the symptom association probability (SAP) was developed; this method statistically compares pH data temporally related to symptoms with pH data obtained during symptom-free periods and expresses the likelihood that the patient's symptoms are related to reflux.[2] Each 24-hour study is divided into consecutive 2-minute periods; these periods and the 2-minute periods preceding the onset of symptoms are then evaluated for the occurrence of reflux. Fisher's exact test is then applied to calculate the probability (p) that reflux and symptom episodes are unrelated. SAP is calculated as $(1 - p) \times 100\%$. By statistical convention, SAP $\geq 95\%$ is considered positive.

Both SAP and SSI were recently shown to be significantly related to symptomatic response to high-dose omeprazole, albeit with a significant number of discordant cases. Diaz et al. also showed that SAP is an independent predictor of the success of antireflux surgery.[17] Although patients with a positive relationship between symptoms and reflux have been shown to more likely respond to medical and surgical therapy, further prospective validation studies are needed. Ultimately, these indices can be helpful in evaluating the relationship between symptoms and reflux, but they do not directly take into account other factors that also influence the perception of symptoms, such as inherent esophageal mucosal sensitivity, duration of acid exposure, and proximal extent of reflux.[2]

The evaluation of the association between reflux and aerodigestive disorders has been challenging. Traditional 24-hour esophageal pH monitoring with a probe placed in the distal esophagus has not been shown to be sensitive for supraesophageal symptoms.[18] Dual-probe pH monitoring adds a second pH electrode for measurement of pH changes in the proximal esophagus. There are several limitations, however, with dual-probe pH monitoring. At the present time, there is no consensus on the best location for proximal probe placement. Various studies report probe placement below the upper esophageal sphincter (UES), at or above the UES, or even above the esophagus in direct contact with the pharynx. There is also no agreement on the definition of a proximal reflux event; conventionally, it has been defined as a drop in pH below 4, based on the pH threshold for distal esophageal reflux. Recent data, however, have suggested that non-acidic or weakly acidic reflux with pH between 4 and 7 may also play a clinically significant role in aerodigestive disease,[16,19] and there have been proposals to revise the pH criteria for proximal reflux. These various issues have ultimately made the establishment of normative values for proximal reflux elusive. Studies employing dual-probe pH monitoring in children and adults have had mixed results in terms of sensitivity and specificity for extraesophageal manifestations of reflux as well as intrasubject reproducibility.[18] Newer diagnostic modalities, such as oropharyngeal or nasopharyngeal pH monitoring, and the non-invasive measurement of exhaled breath condensates for the detection of aspiration of gastric contents are currently under investigation. At the current time, however, the clinical advantage of dual-probe pH monitoring in children is not yet clearly proven; more research is needed before these new methodologies can become part of the routine evaluation of children with extraesophageal manifestations of reflux.

Limitations of Catheter-based pH Monitoring

Nasally passed pH catheters can be uncomfortable and cumbersome for the patient. In some cases, patients may restrict their daily routines and activity levels during the performance of the test, leading to the potential for "false-negative" outcomes.[2,20] To avoid this possibility and to increase patient's compliance, wireless methods for measuring intraesophageal pH have been developed, as discussed below.

There are also patients with intractable symptoms who remain refractory despite aggressive medical therapy or have normal results on traditional esophageal pH monitoring studies. These patients have been shown to ultimately benefit from fundoplication,[16] suggesting that pH monitoring may be missing some important information, most notably non-acidic reflux. The advent of multichannel intraluminal impedance with pH (MII-pH) technology has allowed for the detection of non-acidic reflux and will also be discussed later.

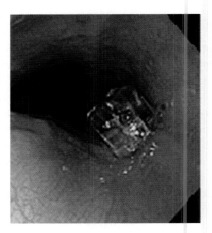

FIGURE 11–1 ■ Bravo capsule shown attached to the esophageal mucosa.

WIRELESS pH MONITORING

The Bravo pH system (Medtronic, Shoreview, MN) consists of an antimony pH electrode contained within a small capsule that transmits pH data wirelessly to a portable receiver using radio telemetry. In adults, the capsule is securely attached to the mucosal wall of the distal esophagus 6 cm above the squamocolumnar junction, with placement confirmation by endoscopy. This location was selected based on the understanding that the proximal border of the high-pressure zone, representing the LES, is 1–1.5 cm above the squamocolumnar junction (Figure 11–1). Since the capsule remains securely pinned to the esophageal mucosa for at least 48 hours, there is less chance for displacement of the pH sensor than with a transnasal catheter with changes in body position, swallowing, or vomiting. The Bravo system also allows for prolonged monitoring over a 48-hour period, and is expelled from the body into the stool after 3–5 days. Compared to catheter-based technique, the Bravo system has been shown to have less effect on daily routines, diet, and activity levels.[2,21]

The wireless pH capsule currently samples data at 6-second intervals (0.17 Hz), which is slower than the 4-second intervals (0.25 Hz) used by the catheter-based equipment.[2,21] The 95th percentile for distal esophageal acid exposure in normal adults using the wireless pH system was 5.3%, a value higher than values reported in several (although not all) catheter-based system studies.[2,21] The higher acid exposure threshold reported in healthy controls using the wireless pH system may be the consequence of less restriction in daily activities. No similar information is available for control children.

In published studies of children older than 4 years old, distal esophageal pH monitoring with the Bravo capsule has been found to be well tolerated, with no significant complications other than mild chest discomfort.[20,22–25] Case reports have mentioned the possibility of applying the Bravo capsule even in smaller children. The capsule has been significantly better tolerated than a transnasal catheter in terms of appetite, activity, and satisfaction.[20] There is currently no consensus on proper location for placement of the capsule in children, with one group confirming position by fluoroscopy similar to ESPGHAN recommendations for pH catheters, for example,[25] and another group using Strobel's formula to estimate 87% of the length of the esophagus between incisors and the LES.[20]

In terms of reproducibility and accuracy, relatively few studies have been performed in children. Only one study to date has compared the Bravo capsule side-by-side with a simultaneous transnasal pH catheter in children. Croffie et al. found no significant difference in the reflux index obtained by the two devices on day 1; on day 2, however, the median reflux index recorded by the Bravo capsule was significantly higher compared to day 1 of both the capsule and catheter.[20] The clinical significance of this is unclear, with only one patient having discordant (abnormal versus normal) results between the 2 days of recording. Gunnarsdottir et al. also studied the use of 48-hour monitoring with a wireless capsule in children and found no statistically significant difference in the fraction of time with pH <4 between the first 24 hours and the entire 48-hour recording.[23] In contrast, in our own series of 145 Bravo studies in children, there were significantly higher values on day 1 versus day 2 for the number of long reflux episodes, duration of longest episode, and fraction of time with pH <4 in the upright position.[22] Figure 11–2 shows a representative tracing in a normal patient, while Figure 11–3 shows the results in a patient with pathologic acidic reflux.

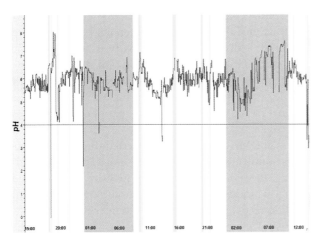

FIGURE 11–2 ■ Representative tracing from a normal 48-hour Bravo study. The y-axis shows the pH measurements, and the x-axis represents time. Areas shaded in green represent periods of sleep or supine position.

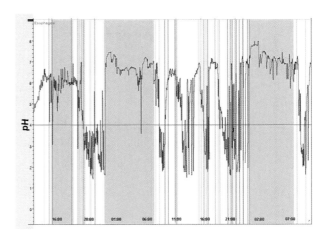

FIGURE 11–3 ■ Representative Bravo tracing showing pathologic reflux. The y-axis shows the pH measurements, and the x-axis represents time. As can be seen, there are multiple pH drops to <4. There is evidence of pathologic reflux in both days.

Day-to-day variability between the first and second 24-hour periods could be due to the effect of anesthesia or to differences in lifestyle and dietary intake.[22,23] It is not yet clear if these differences are clinically significant. Likewise, there is no consensus on how 48-hour data should be interpreted in children, whether the average of 2 days or only the 24-hour period with the greatest acid exposure (worst day analysis) should be used. In adults, studies have shown a slight increase in the sensitivity with a small decrease in the specificity of pH testing when utilizing the worst day data compared with either the initial 24-hour or overall 48-hour data.[2,21,26]

There are still some limitations of the wireless system. Given the size of the capsule it is not recommended for use in small and young children, so caution needs to be exercised if considering placement in a child <4 years of age. In general, the placement requires endoscopy, although it can be placed without endoscopy via the oral route. The risk of perforation needs to be considered, and although there have been no pediatric reports of perforation, there was a single case report in the adult literature.[27] Early detachment of the capsule, with subsequent recording of intragastric pH, is also possible and could lead to misinterpretation of the acid exposure time (Figure 11–4). This occurred in 9 out of 85 subjects prior to 36 hours in one adult series.[2,21]

Overall, the Bravo system appears to be a reasonable alternative for older children to conventional 24-hour catheter-based pH monitoring given the potential advantages in terms of patient tolerance and compliance. In addition, the advantage of performing an extended 48-hour study to help minimize the effects of day-to-day variability should be weighed against the

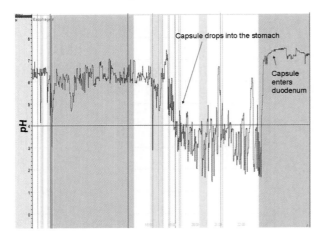

FIGURE 11-4 ■ Early detachment of a Bravo capsule. It can be seen when the capsule detached from the esophagus and fell into the stomach, and eventually migrated into the small intestine. The y-axis shows the pH measurements, and the x-axis represents time.

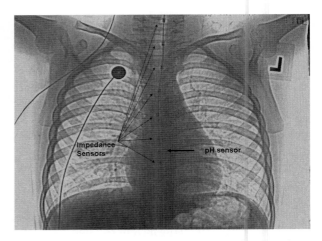

FIGURE 11-5 ■ Chest X-ray showing placement of an impedance catheter. The longitudinal array of the impedance sensor can be observed. The catheter is positioned such that pH electrode is at the third vertebral body above the diaphragmatic angle.

unknown effects of anesthesia, which is typically required for endoscopy and capsule placement.

MULTICHANNEL INTRALUMINAL IMPEDANCE

Despite the widespread use of pH monitoring, there are other limitations to pH-probe testing that are not be addressed by either catheter-based or wireless pH monitoring systems. First, the pH sensor is not able to differentiate swallowed contents from refluxed contents, which limits its utility. As a result, it fails to detect the majority of postprandial reflux events that have a pH >4 secondary to the buffering effects of swallowed saliva and food. In patients who are continuously tube-fed into the stomach and therefore have a pH >4 for the majority of the recording time, this is a particular problem. Second, for patients who depend on acid-suppression medication for symptom control, routine discontinuation of medications prior to pH testing is often difficult. Finally, for measurement of proximal reflux in the context of extraesophageal symptoms, dual-channel pH probes with a proximal pH sensor are unreliable because of frequent discordance between the two sensors such that there are drops in pH reported by the proximal sensor with no associated distal drops.

MII-pH overcomes many limitations of the pH probe because it is able to measure all refluxed material, whether acidic, weakly acidic, or non-acidic. This is a particular advantage in the pediatric population where the majority of reflux occurs in the postprandial period when reflux is likely to be non-acidic.[28-30] Impedance sensors measure changes in resistance to electrical current in either direction across the catheter (Figure 11-5). The electrical impedance value that is measured between each pair of adjacent sensors is inversely proportional to the ionic concentrations of esophageal contents. Air has the highest impedance measurements while liquids have relatively lower values; it is possible therefore to also differentiate between liquid (Figures 11-6 and 11-7) and gas reflux (Figure 11-8).

In most catheters there are seven impedance sensors placed in series that generate six impedance waves, one for each pair of adjacent sensors (Figure 11-5). This array is capable of differentiating antegrade versus retrograde transit of esophageal contents (Figures 11-6 and 11-7). Sensors are distributed throughout the esophagus at different spacing depending on the size of the catheter that is used (2–4-cm spacing on adult catheter, 2-cm spacing on the pediatric catheter, and 1-cm spacing on infant catheter). The presence of sensors throughout the esophagus also allows for the determination of the proximal extent of the reflux (Figure 11-6). Given that impedance by itself cannot differentiate between acid and non-acid material, a distal pH sensor has been added on the catheter. This allows the clinician to determine whether the flow across the catheter is acidic, weakly acidic, or non-acidic, depending on the pH value (Figures 11-6 and 11-7). This technique is known as MII-pH.

The MII-pH catheter is inserted through the nose in the same fashion as traditional esophageal pH monitoring. Placement relative to the LES can be confirmed using manometry, fluoroscopy, or chest X-ray. As with traditional pH monitoring in children, the MII-pH catheter is placed so that the distal pH sensor rather than the impedance sensors is at the third vertebral body above the diaphragmatic angle.[3] The pH sensor, on chest X-ray, has the appearance of a horizontal line, which differentiates it from the impedance sensors (Figure 11-5). The

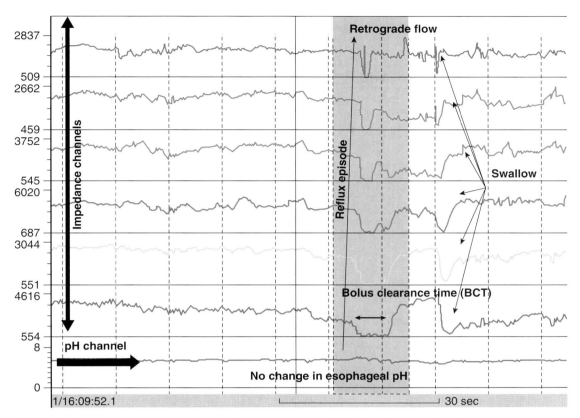

FIGURE 11–6 ■ A representative impedance tracing showing a non-acidic liquid reflux event. The six upper channels are the impedance measurements (in ohms), and the lower ones the ph tracing (in pH units). The ↑ arrow shows this was an episode with retrograde esophageal flow of liquid, that reaches the upper most pair of sensors (full column). The pH remains above 4 at all times. Therefore, this represents a full-column, non-acidic liquid reflux episode. The figure also shows a clearing swallow, characterized by the antegrade progression of the impedance drops.

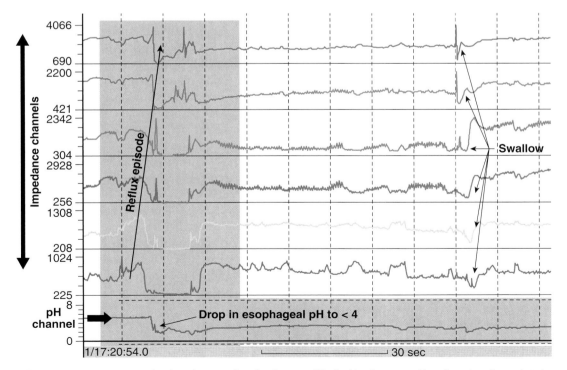

FIGURE 11–7 ■ A representative impedance tracing showing an acidic liquid reflux event. The pH tracing shows that the pH drops below 4 at the same time as the impedance detected episode, indicating this is an acidic reflux event.

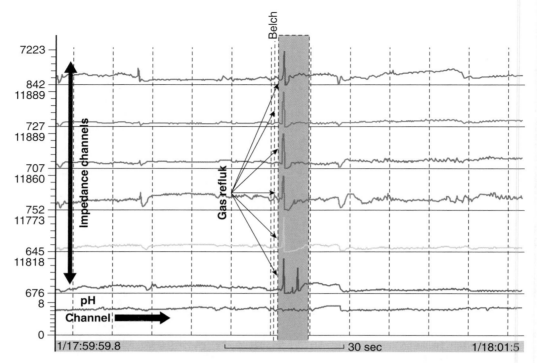

FIGURE 11–8 ■ Impedance tracing that shows a gas reflux event, shown as a simultaneous increase in ohms to >8000 in at least two channels. There is also evidence of liquid reflux, so this represents a mixed reflux episode (gas and liquid).

catheter is secured to the patient's face with tape and remains in place for 24 hours. Unlike with pH data, there have not been studies to show the optimal length for MII-pH recording, so currently standards for pH monitoring have been adopted. As with traditional pH monitoring, there are symptom buttons, recumbent/upright buttons, and meal buttons in the impedance recorder.

Because MII-pH detects both acidic and non-acidic reflux, it is possible and often ideal to study patients while taking acid-suppression medications in order to assess therapeutic efficacy. Adult studies have shown that acid-suppression therapy with proton-pump inhibitors does not decrease the total number of reflux events but rather converts them from acid to non-acid events.[31] Because the total number of events is unchanged, it is still possible to see correlations with symptoms and both acid and non-acid events, though some literature suggests that symptom correlation may be higher if studies are performed while off acid-suppression therapy.[32]

Definitions

The advantage of MII-pH is that it allows clinicians to determine the type of reflux (acidic, non-acidic, and weakly acidic reflux), as well as the composition of reflux. By convention, the majority of reflux is liquid. A liquid episode is defined as a drop in impedance to 50% of the baseline value or below, with a subsequent recovery back

to 50% of the baseline value (Figures 11–6 and 11–7). This drop in impedance needs to be visualized in at least the distal two channels to be considered reflux. Gas reflux is defined as simultaneous increases in impedance to >8000 Ω in two or more channels (Figure 11–8). Mixed reflux has components of both liquid and gas (Figure 11–8). Reflux detected by impedance is further classified into acidic, non-acidic, and weakly acidic reflux. Acidic reflux is reflux detected by the impedance sensors that also has a simultaneous drop in pH to <4 (Figure 11–7). There is some inconsistency in the literature over the definitions of non-acidic reflux. Some papers define non-acidic reflux as any reflux event with a pH >4 (Figure 11–6), whereas others divide non-acidic reflux into two groups, weakly acidic reflux (pH 4–7) and alkaline reflux (pH > 7). By using a combined MII and pH catheter, there are mainly three types of episodes that can be detected: (a) acidic reflux events detected by both the impedance and the pH sensor, (b) non-acidic reflux events, which are detected only by the impedance probe, and (c) pH-only events, which are detected only by the pH sensor, without any impedance changes.

Sensitivity

Early studies of MII-pH were combined with fluoroscopy to insure that MII-pH accurately detected when a liquid bolus was in the esophagus. Imam et al. found that the correlation between impedance and bolus transit by radiographic imaging is excellent in 97% of swallows and Peter et al. found that impedance sensors were able to detect volumes as little as 0.1 cm³ in the esophagus.[33]

Studies have suggested that MII-pH has a sensitivity equal to or greater than that of a standard pH probe.[34,35] Hila et al. found that MII-pH detected 1133 acidic reflux episodes, whereas pH analysis alone in the same patients detected 2307 acid episodes; 81% of the episodes that were not detected by MII-pH occurred in the setting of swallows, whereas 19% were true pH drops with no associated MII-pH changes. The pH probe alone did significantly worse than MII-pH in detecting weakly acidic and non-acidic reflux events. The pH probe had a sensitivity of 28% for detecting non-acidic or weakly acidic reflux demonstrated by MII-pH; conversely, 83% of weakly acidic events detected by pH probe were not detected by MII-pH.[36] Aanen et al. also looked at the sensitivity of the pH probe to detect reflux as compared to MII-pH. They found that the sensitivity of a 0.5 pH drop had a sensitivity of 76% in detecting reflux. The sensitivity dropped to 53% when a 1.5 pH drop was used to define a reflux episode compared to the gold standard MII-pH.[37]

In our own studies, we found that the sensitivity of MII-pH in pediatric patients who were not taking acid-suppression therapy was 76 ± 13% compared to the pH probe whose sensitivity was 80 ± 18%. When patients taking acid suppression were studied, the sensitivity of the pH probe dropped to 47 ± 36%, whereas the sensitivity of MII-pH in treated patients was 80 ± 21%.[34] Additionally, Wenzl et al. found that, in untreated infants, the sensitivity of MII-pH to detect acidic reflux events was 54% compared to the pH probe.[38] Failure of MII-pH to report reflux events detected by pH probe was primarily due to episodes where there was a persistent drop in pH <4 even after the bolus had been cleared by impedance or because the pH was hovering around 4 with multiple drops to <4.

Reproducibility

Aanen et al. studied the reliability of MII-pH to detect reflux and the reliability of MII-pH to detect reflux-associated symptoms. The authors conducted two 24-hour MII-pH studies (separated by a minimum of 1 week) on 21 adults. The authors found that the number of acidic, weakly acidic, and total events was extremely constant between the 2 days with a Kendall's W-value of 0.9, 0.9, and 0.92 (where a value of 1 indicates perfect concordance). Additionally, the reproducibility of symptom indices using the SAP, SI, and SSI was 0.9, 0.73, and 0.86, respectively.[39] In another study of 27 adults that underwent repeated studies, Zerbib et al. showed good

reproducibility for the number, acidity, and air–liquid composition of reflux events (Kendall's W-values = 0.72–0.85).[40] No similar information is available in children.

Interpretation

The interpretation of impedance tracings is time-consuming and, in most research laboratories, is still done by hand even though there is commercially available analysis software. Recently, commercial software has been developed to make the analysis of the tracing automatic. Roman et al. studied the reproducibility of the automated software to detect reflux events compared to a manual scoring of the events. Detection of esophageal acid exposure and acidic reflux events was similar with both analyses. Agreement between visual and automated analysis was good (Kendall's coefficient W > 0.750, p < 0.01) for all parameters. They also analyzed symptom detection, and concluded that despite good agreement with manual analysis, automatic analysis overestimated the number of non-acidic reflux events. Manual analysis remains the gold standard to detect an association between symptoms and non-acidic reflux events.[41] The recent possibility of displaying impedance events in contour plots may (Figure 11–9) enhance the recognition of reflux episodes, improve the ease of measurement, and reduce analysis time.[7] At this point, the use of software is an auxiliary tool for interpretation of impedance. Manual analysis is still the gold standard, and caution should be exercised before relying only on software interpretation. The software performs particularly poorly if there is esophagitis present or if there is a motility disorder such as achalasia or esophageal atresia all of which lower impedance baselines. This

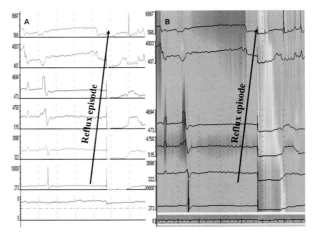

FIGURE 11–9 ■ (Panel A) Standard view of a non-acidic reflux episode. (Panel B) Contour plot of the same reflux episode where the colors represent the percent impedance change from baseline: yellow and orange colors represent a larger percentage drop and blue and purple represent smaller drops.

low-impedance baseline result is significant underestimation of the amount of reflux present.

Normal Values

One of the current limitations to MII-pH monitoring is the lack of normal values to differentiate physiologic from pathologic reflux. Adult normal values have been published: Shay et al. conducted a multicenter study of 60 healthy volunteers and found that the upper limits of normal for total, acidic, weakly acidic, and non-acidic reflux were 73, 55, 26, and 1, respectively.[42] Zerbib et al. found similar numbers in normal adults with the upper limit of normal for healthy adults for total, acidic, weakly acidic, and non-acidic reflux being 75, 50, 33, and 15, respectively. [40]

Normal values that have been reported among preterm infants vary substantially than the values noted for the adult population. Lopez-Alonso et al. studied 21 asymptomatic preterm infants and found that the upper limit for total number of reflux events was 100 of which up to 52% can be acidic and up to 98% can be non-acidic.[28] In contrast, we studied older children with eosinophilic esophagitis ($n = 10$) and control patients ($n = 10$, patients with normal pH recording and normal esophageal biopsies and no gastrointestinal symptoms) and found that the 95th percentile for total events in patients with EE and control patients, respectively, was 80 and 69, which is very similar to adult data.[43] Larger studies are needed to confirm the range of normal values in children. Because normal cutoff values are not available in pediatrics, the main role of impedance is to correlate symptoms with reflux events since this does not require an absolute cutoff.

Symptom Association

Given the lack of normative data to determine normal MII-pH in children, the most important use of the technique has been to study the temporal association between symptoms and reflux. There is significant debate in the adult literature about the optimal way to correlate reflux with symptoms but the literature is clear that MII-pH is superior to pH probe alone when looking for symptom correlation.[16,32,44,45] The rates of SI, SSI, and the SAP positivity have been studied using MII-pH. In the adult literature, the SAP and the SSI were most reproducible indices in patients that had two impedance studies separated by a minimum of 1 week. Similarly, Bredenoord et al. found that the SAP was the most frequently positive index followed by the SI and then the SSI. They also found that the addition of MII-pH over a standard pH probe increased the number of patients with a positive SI and SAP but did not increase the number of patients with a positive SSI.[44]

We similarly studied 28 children taking acid-suppression therapy for intractable respiratory symptoms; in these patients, more patients had a positive SI for respiratory symptoms using MII-pH than pH probe alone but there was no difference in the number of patients with a positive SSI when MII-pH was used compared to a standard pH probe.[16] In contrast, Thilmany et al. found that the rate of positivity for the SI was higher for acidic reflux episodes, whereas the rate of positivity of SSI was higher for non-acidic reflux episodes suggesting that the value of MII-pH may differ depending on what SI is used.[46]

One symptom that has been studied using MII-pH in the pediatric literature is the association between apnea and reflux events; MII-pH has successfully been used with sleep studies to elucidate the relationship between reflux and sleep disordered breathing. Again, one of the primary limitations to the earlier studies is the inability of a standard pH probe to detect non-acidic reflux episodes that can account for up to 89% of the total reflux episodes in infants.[34,47] Several infant studies have focused on apnea alone and none have shown a correlation between acidic or non-acidic reflux and apnea events.[48,49] Nevertheless, there are a small number of reported cases suggesting that for some particular infants with apnea and associated reflux symptoms, transpyloric feeding or fundoplication may be beneficial as a diagnostic, in the former case, or therapeutic trial in the latter case.[50,51] With the addition of MII-pH to sleep studies, clinicians may be able to better define the relationship between GERD and apnea so that therapy can be better targeted to patients with a clear association between acidic and non-acidic reflux and apnea.

One of the limitations of symptom indices is that they only represent a significant temporal relationship rather than a true cause and effect relationship. The cutoff values, therefore, represent statistical definitions and are not tied to clinical outcomes. For example, if a patient has a SI >50%, one would expect, if this means reflux is causing symptoms, that the patient will have a favorable outcome to acid-suppression therapy, or more definitively, to fundoplication. Unfortunately, the normal values of 50% for the SI, 10% for the SSI, and 95% for the SAP were not generated by looking at clinical outcomes. Rosen et al. looked at the value of the SI and the SSI in predicting fundoplication outcome; they found that neither a positive SI nor SSI predicted fundoplication outcome and, using ROC curves, there was no clear cutoff value for either index that predicted fundoplication outcome.[52] These data suggest that a temporal association alone does not prove causality that is the key limitation to all of the symptom indices.

A second limitation of the symptom indices is the time lag between when a symptom occurs and when the

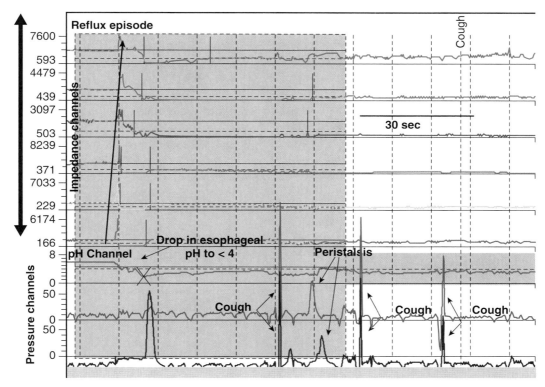

FIGURE 11–10 ■ Impedance tracing that shows the association between reflux and cough with the use of a cough catheter that detects simultaneous increase in intrathoracic pressure. The six upper channels are the impedance measurements (in ohms), and the lower ones the ph tracing (in pH units). There are also two distal pressure channels that capture coughs and peristalsis. This tracing shows an acidic reflux event that precedes coughing.

patient actually records the symptom. In a study by Sifrim et al., there was an average delay of 28 seconds between the time when a patient coughed and when they actually recorded a cough on the symptom log.[53] Furthermore, patients only record, on average, 38% of coughs on the log.[53] To address this limitation, impedance sensors can be paired with pressure sensors, the latter of which measures esophageal pressure spikes that occur when a patient coughs. Coughs appear as simultaneous high-pressure spikes in the esophagus (Figure 11–10) and this allows for precise correlation between reflux and cough without the possibility for recording error. The utility of this technology is currently limited because two catheters need to be placed simultaneously that, in the pediatric population, is a significant consideration.

Proximal Reflux

The importance of full-column reflux (Figure 11–6) in the genesis of symptoms is being clarified. Rosen and Nurko found that, in children with intractable respiratory symptom, full-column reflux is more highly associated with respiratory symptoms than distal reflux.[16] The importance of full-column reflux in the generation of

symptoms is further supported by Jadcherla et al. who looked at the association between acidic reflux, as detected by impedance, and respiratory symptoms in preterm and term infants. The authors found that acidic reflux events reaching the proximal esophagus were four times more likely to be associated with symptoms than reflux events reaching the distal esophagus.[54] In contrast, Thilmany et al. found that, in children with pulmonary disease, desaturations were much more likely to be temporally associated with distal reflux than proximal reflux but they did not look at the correlation of proximal reflux with any of the other reported symptoms during the study.[46] Condino et al. found that, in asthmatic children, proximal reflux was not a predictor of symptom generation.[45] Currently, the literature is limited by diversity of symptoms and diseases that are studied so that it may not be a reasonable assumption to compare the symptom indices of all patients with respiratory disease as patients with cough may be very different from patients with apnea or asthma.

Because of the ability of MII-pH to measure proximal reflux (Figure 11–6), the tool will likely be a gold standard tool to measure reflux in the evaluation of extraesophageal symptoms that may be caused by proximal reflux.

Role of Assessing Therapy

One of the most helpful uses of MII-pH is to objectively determine the efficacy of both pharmacologic and non-pharmacologic reflux therapies. Impedance has been used to study the effect of different non-invasive therapies in children. Wenzl et al. used MII-pH to study 14 infants who received thickened and thin feeds in an alternating fashion. The authors found that the amount of formula that was regurgitated out of the mouth was reduced with thickened feeds, but that the number of reflux events and the height of the reflux events were not statistically different between the two groups.[55] Similarly, Corvaglia et al. studied, using MII-pH, five preterm infants who received alternating thin mother's breast milk (MBM) and MBM thickened with starch and found that thickened feeds did not reduce the amount of total, acidic, or non-acidic reflux.[56]

Several studies in infants have been performed to determine the impact of positioning on reflux.[57–59] Omari et al. studied preterm infants in the right and left lateral decubitus positions amount and found that, in the postprandial period, there is significantly more reflux in the right lateral decubitus position and that the primary mechanism for this increase in reflux is an increase in the numbers of transient LES relaxations.[59]

Peter et al. studied the impact of nasogastric feeding on GER. The authors fed preterm infants orally with an impedance probe in the esophagus, or after it was advanced into the stomach. The authors found that by simply advancing the probe into the stomach, the amount of reflux increases by 70% due to stenting open of the LES.[60] Another method for treatment of reflux is transpyloric feeds. Rosen et al. studied the rates of reflux when the feeds were running compared to when they were off and found that the rate of esophageal reflux was doubled while transpyloric feeds were running compared to when they were not.[61] Further studies to understand why transpyloric feedings are beneficial are needed, but these preliminary findings indicate that acid suppression must continue while the patients are being fed transpylorically.

Another important study using MII-pH studies was conducted by Vela et al. who conducted MII-pH studies before and during a trial of omeprazole; the authors found that omeprazole converted acidic reflux to non-acidic reflux but did not change the total number of reflux episodes.[31] Others studies have confirmed what Vela et al. had shown, that acid suppression does not reduce the total amount of reflux. Impedance has also been used to study the effect of baclofen. Vela et al. assessed the effect of baclofen, a GABA agonist, on postprandial reflux. The authors found that baclofen reduced acidic, non-acidic, and total reflux events but the rate of side effects from the medication was high.[62]

Finally, MII-pH has been used as a tool to predict clinical response to fundoplication. Mainie et al. found that fundoplication is an effective therapy for patients with extraesophageal symptoms that correlate with non-acidic reflux.[63] Similarly Gruebel et al. found that abnormal preoperative MII-pH testing predicts a positive post-fundoplication outcome.[64]

Unfortunately, the pediatric experience is less favorable. We have retrospectively examined the outcomes of children who underwent fundoplication and who had a preceding MII-pH study. We found that the amount of reflux preoperatively did not predict post-fundoplication outcome. We also found that a positive SI did not predict outcome.[52] This suggests that there are other variables that determine outcome after fundoplication, and that at this point impedance testing in children cannot be the sole tool to predict success after a fundoplication.[52]

Clinical Indications

There is no question that impedance allows the detection of more episodes of reflux, as it detects non-acidic reflux episodes. It has not been shown that in untreated patients the use of impedance will alter the outcome over the findings provided by pH monitoring, and it is not clear that, in most patients, the additional information on the number of non-acidic reflux events changes therapy or outcome. Our own preliminary data show that impedance testing may change clinical management in <25% of the patients. Further studies to validate the impact of impedance testing on clinical outcome are needed.

At this time, given the lack of normal pediatric values, impedance should to be used to associate reflux with symptoms, and not to determine patterns of normal versus abnormal reflux.

Another important role is to assess the efficacy of therapy in patients who continue to experience symptoms. In these patients, the studies can be performed while the patient is taking acid-suppression therapy to determine how well the patient is blocked on their medication. This will also allow the clinician to correlate reflux events (which may be non-acidic while taking acid-suppression therapy) with symptoms. Finally, in the pediatric population, MII-pH is useful in evaluating patients who have postprandial symptoms or symptoms during continuous or frequent tube feeding. Finally the biggest use of impedance in pediatrics continues to be in research applications, and the technique has been invaluable in studying the pathophysiology of reflux, and in establishing the effectiveness of different therapies or interventions in children.

CONCLUSIONS

Twenty-four-hour esophageal pH monitoring is a valid and reliable measure of acidic reflux in children that can be performed to establish the presence of abnormal acidic reflux, determine the temporal relationship between acidic reflux episodes and frequently occurring symptoms, and assess the efficacy of acid-suppression therapy in patients who remain symptomatic despite treatment. Traditional catheter-based pH monitoring has several limitations, however, including issues of sensitivity and specificity for the diagnosis of GERD in the absence of erosions as well as for extraesophageal manifestations, tolerability of an intranasal catheter, and the inability to record non-acidic reflux events.

To address those limitations, the introduction of wireless pH monitoring in recent years has provided the ability to perform accurate and long-term studies while allowing patients to continue with their daily activities. Wireless pH monitoring has been shown to be a safe and effective way to study children. Disadvantages include the requirement for endoscopic placement in most cases as well as age and size limitations for its use. Normative data using wireless capsules, which may be different compared to catheter-based monitoring, are not available for children. Finally, it is not clear how having longer periods of study may affect outcome, especially when there are discrepancies between the first and second days of recording.

MII-pH has allowed for the detection of non-acidic reflux. This technique has led to improved symptom correlation in the evaluation of patients who have not responded to medical therapy or in those who need to be fed continuously. MII-pH testing continues to be limited, however, by the lack of normative data in children, time-consuming manual data analysis, and the lack of evidence that it changes clinical outcomes.

ACKNOWLEDGMENTS

This work was supported in part by grants DK77678-2 and DK082792-01 (SN) and DK073713 (RR).

REFERENCES

1. Rudolph C, Mazur L, Liptak G, et al. Guidlines for evaluation and treatment of gastroesophageal reflux in infants and children: recommendations of the North American Society for Pediatric Gastroenterology and Nutrition. *J Pediatr Gastroenterol Nutr.* 2001;32:S1–S31.
2. Hirano I, Richter J. ACG practice guidelines: esophageal reflux testing. *Am J Gastroenterol.* 2007;102:668–685.
3. Vandenplas Y, Belli D, Boige N. A standardized protocol for the methodology of esophageal pH monitoring and interpretation of the data for the diagnosis of gastro-esophageal reflux. *J Pediatr Gastroenterol Nutr.* 1992;14:467–471.
4. Strobel C, Byrne W, Ament M, Euler A. Correlation of esophageal lengths in children with height: application to the Tuttle test without prior esophageal manometry. *J Pediatr.* 1979;94:81–84.
5. Vandenplas Y. *Oesophageal pH Monitoring for Gastroesophageal Reflux in Infants and Children.* London: John Wiley & Sons; 1992.
6. Tuttle S, Grossman M. Detection of gastroesophageal reflux by simultaneous measurements of intraluminal pressure and pH. *Proc Soc Exp Biol.* 1958;98:224.
7. van Wijk MP, Benninga MA, Omari TI. Role of the multichannel intraluminal impedance technique in infants and children. *J Pediatr Gastroenterol Nutr.* 2009;48:2–12.
8. Johnson L, DeMeester T. Development of the 24-hour intraesophageal pH monitoring composite scoring system. *J Clin Gastroenterol.* 1986;8:52–58.
9. Jolley S, Johnson D, Herbst J, et al. As assessment of gastroesophageal reflux in children by extended pH monitoring of the distal esophagus. *Surgery.* 1978;84:16–24.
10. Vandenplas Y, Goyvaerts H, Helven R, et al. Gastroesophageal reflux, as assessed by 24-hour pH monitoring, in 509 healthy infants screened for SIDS-risk. *Pediatrics.* 1991;88:834–840.
11. Boix-Ochoa J, Lafuenta J, Gil-Vernet J. Twenty-four hour esophageal pH monitoring in gastroesophageal reflux. *J Pediatr Surg.* 1980;15:74–78.
12. Cucchiara S, Santamaria F, Minella R, et al. Simultaneous prolonged recordings of proximal and distal intraesophageal pH in children with gastroesophageal reflux disease and respiratory symptoms. *Am J Gastroenterol.* 1995;90:1791–1796.
13. Vandenplas Y, Helven R, Goyvaerts H, et al. Reproducibility of continuous 24 hour oesophageal pH monitoring in infants and children. *Gut.* 1990;31:374–377.
14. Mahajan L, Wyllie R, Oliva L, et al. Reproducibility of 24-hour intraesophageal pH monitoring in pediatric patients. *Pediatrics.* 1998;101:260–263.
15. Nielsen R, Kruse-Andersen S, Husby S. Low reproducibility of 2 × 24-hour continuous esophageal pH monitoring in infants and children: a limiting factor for interventional studies. *Dig Dis Sci.* 2003;48:1495–1502.
16. Rosen R, Nurko S. The importance of multichannel intraluminal impedance in the evaluation of children with persistent respiratory symptoms. *Am J Gastroenterol.* 2004;99:2452–2458.
17. Diaz S, Aymerich R, Clouse RE, et al. The symptom association probability (SAP) is superior to the symptom index (SI) for attributing symptoms to gastroesophageal reflux: validation using outcome from laparoscopic antireflux surgery (LARS). *Gastroenterology.* 2002;122:A75.
18. Toila V, Vandenplas Y. Systematic review: the extra-oesophageal symptoms of gastro-oesophageal reflux disease in children. *Aliment Phamacol Ther.* 2009;29:258–272.
19. Patterson N, Mainie I, Rafferty G, et al. Nonacid reflux episodes reaching the pharynx are important factors associated with cough. *J Clin Gastroenterol.* 2009;43:414–419.
20. Croffie J, Fitzgerald J, Molleson J, et al. Accuracy and tolerability of the Braco catheter-free pH capsule in patients

between the ages of 4 and 18 years. *J Pediatr Gastroenterol Nutr.* 2007;45:559–563.

21. Pandolfino J, Kahrilas P. Prolonged pH monitoring: Bravo capsule. *Gastrointest Endosc Clin N Am.* 2005;15:307–318.

22. Souza AL, Morley-Fletcher A, Nurko S, Rodriguez L. BRAVO wireless pH in children: is there an effect of anesthesia? *Gastroenterology.* 2009;136:A-510.

23. Gunnarsdottir A, Stenstrom P, Arnbjornsson E. 48-hour wireless oesophageal pH-monitoring in children: are two days better than one? *Eur J Pediatr Surg.* 2007;17:378–381.

24. Hochman J, Favaloro-Sabatier J. Tolerance and reliability of wireless pH monitoring in children. *J Pediatr Gastroenterol Nutr.* 2005;41:411–415.

25. Gunnarsdottir A, Stenstrom P, Arnbjornsson E. Wireless esophageal pH monitoring in children. *J Laparoendosc Adv Surg Tech.* 2008;18:443–447.

26. Ahlawat S, Novak D, Williams D, et al. Day-to-day variability in acid reflux patterns using the Bravo pH monitoring system. *J Clin Gastroenterol.* 2006;40:20–24.

27. Fajardo NR, Wise JL, Locke GR, Murray JA, Talley NJ. Esophageal perforation after placement of wireless Bravo pH probe. *Gastrointest Endosc.* 2006;63:184–185.

28. Lopez-Alonso M, Moya MJ, Cabo JA, et al. Twenty-four-hour esophageal impedance–pH monitoring in healthy preterm neonates: rate and characteristics of acid, weakly acidic, and weakly alkaline gastroesophageal reflux. *Pediatrics.* 2006;118:e299–e308.

29. Mitchell DJ, McClure BG, Tubman TR. Simultaneous monitoring of gastric and oesophageal pH reveals limitations of conventional oesophageal pH monitoring in milk fed infants. *Arch Dis Child.* 2001;84:273–276.

30. Sifrim D, Holloway R, Silny J, Tack J, Lerut A, Janssens J. Composition of the postprandial refluxate in patients with gastroesophageal reflux disease. *Am J Gastroenterol.* 2001;96:647–655.

31. Vela MF, Camacho-Lobato L, Srinivasan R, Tutuian R, Katz PO, Castell DO. Simultaneous intraesophageal impedance and pH measurement of acid and nonacid gastroesophageal reflux: effect of omeprazole. *Gastroenterology.* 2001;120:1599–1606.

32. Hemmink GJ, Bredenoord AJ, Weusten BL, Monkelbaan JF, Timmer R, Smout AJ. Esophageal pH–impedance monitoring in patients with therapy-resistant reflux symptoms: 'on' or 'off' proton pump inhibitor? *Am J Gastroenterol.* 2008;103:2446–2453.

33. Peter CS, Wiechers C, Bohnhorst B, Silny J, Poets CF. Detection of small bolus volumes using multiple intraluminal impedance in preterm infants. *J Pediatr Gastroenterol Nutr.* 2003;36:381–384.

34. Rosen R, Lord C, Nurko S. The sensitivity of multi-channel intraluminal impedance (MII) compared to pH probe in the detection of gastroesophgeal reflux in children. *Clin Gastroenterol Hepatol.* 2006;4:167–172.

35. Shay S, Richter J. Direct comparison of impedance, manometry, and pH probe in detecting reflux before and after a meal. *Dig Dis Sci.* 2005;50:1584–1590.

36. Hila A, Agrawal A, Castell DO. Combined multichannel intraluminal impedance and pH esophageal testing compared to pH alone for diagnosing both acid and weakly acidic gastroesophageal reflux. *Clin Gastroenterol Hepatol.* 2007;5:172–177.

37. Aanen MC, Bredenoord AJ, Samsom M, Smout AJ. Reliability of oesophageal pH recording for the detection of gastro-oesophageal reflux. *Scand J Gastroenterol.* 2008;43:1442–1447.

38. Wenzl TG, Moroder C, Trachterna M, et al. Esophageal pH monitoring and impedance measurement: a comparison of two diagnostic tests for gastroesophageal reflux. *J Pediatr Gastroenterol Nutr.* 2002;34:519–523.

39. Aanen MC, Bredenoord AJ, Numans ME, Samson M, Smout AJ. Reproducibility of symptom association analysis in ambulatory reflux monitoring. *Am J Gastroenterol.* 2008;103:2200–2208.

40. Zerbib F, des Varannes SB, Roman S, et al. Normal values and day-to-day variability of 24-h ambulatory oesophageal impedance–pH monitoring in a Belgian–French cohort of healthy subjects. *Aliment Pharmacol Ther.* 2005;22:1011–1021.

41. Roman S, Bruley des Varannes S, Pouderoux P, et al. Ambulatory 24-h oesophageal impedance–pH recordings: reliability of automatic analysis for gastro-oesophageal reflux assessment. *Neurogastroenterol Motil.* 2006;18:978–986.

42. Shay S, Tutuian R, Sifrim D, et al. Twenty-four hour ambulatory simultaneous impedance and pH monitoring: a multicenter report of normal values from 60 healthy volunteers. *Am J Gastroenterol.* 2004;99:1037–1043.

43. Rosen R, Furuta G, Fritz J, Donovan K, Nurko S. Role of acid and nonacid reflux in children with eosinophilic esophagitis compared with patients with gastroesophageal reflux and control patients. *J Pediatr Gastroenterol Nutr.* 2008;46:520–523.

44. Bredenoord AJ, Weusten BL, Timmer R, Conchillo JM, Smout AJ. Addition of esophageal impedance monitoring to pH monitoring increases the yield of symptom association analysis in patients off PPI therapy. *Am J Gastroenterol.* 2006;101:453–459.

45. Condino AA, Sondheimer J, Pan Z, Gralla J, Perry D, O'Connor JA. Evaluation of gastroesophageal reflux in pediatric patients with asthma using impedance–pH monitoring. *J Pediatr.* 2006;149:216–219.

46. Thilmany C, Beck-Ripp J, Griese M. Acid and non-acid gastro-esophageal refluxes in children with chronic pulmonary diseases. *Respir Med.* 2007;101:969–976.

47. Wenzl TG, Silny J, Schenke S, Peschgens T, Heimann G, Skopnik H. Gastroesophageal reflux and respiratory phenomena in infants: status of the intraluminal impedance technique. *J Pediatr Gastroenterol Nutr.* 1999;28:423–428.

48. Mousa H, Woodley F, Metheney M, Hayes J. Testing the association betweeen gastroesophageal reflux and apnea in infants. *J Pediatr Gastroenterol Nutr.* 2005;41:169–177.

49. Peter CS, Sprodowski N, Bohnhorst B, Silny J, Poets CF. Gastroesophageal reflux and apnea of prematurity: no temporal relationship. *Pediatrics.* 2002;109:8–11.

50. Dimarino AJ Jr, Banwait KS, Eschinger E, et al. The effect of gastro-oesophageal reflux and omeprazole on key sleep parameters. *Aliment Pharmacol Ther.* 2005;22:325–329.

51. Misra S, Macwan K, Albert V. Transpyloric feeding in gastroesophageal-reflux-associated apnea in premature infants. *Acta Paediatr.* 2007;96:1426–1429.

52. Rosen R, Levine P, Lewis J, Mitchell P, Nurko S. Reflux events detected by pH-MII do not determine fundoplication outcome. *J Pediatr Gastroenterol Nutr.* 2009;50:215–255.

53. Sifrim D, Dupont L, Blondeau K, Zhang X, Tack J, Janssens J. Weakly acidic reflux in patients with chronic unexplained cough during 24 hour pressure, pH, and impedance monitoring. *Gut.* 2005;54:449–454.

54. Jadcherla SR, Gupta A, Fernandez S, et al. Spatiotemporal characteristics of acid refluxate and relationship to symptoms in premature and term infants with chronic lung disease. *Am J Gastroenterol.* 2008;103:720–728.

55. Wenzl TG, Schneider S, Scheele F, Silny J, Heimann G, Skopnik H. Effects of thickened feeding on gastroesophageal reflux in infants: a placebo-controlled crossover study using intraluminal impedance. *Pediatrics.* 2003;111:e355–e359.

56. Corvaglia L, Ferlini M, Rotatori R, et al. Starch thickening of human milk is ineffective in reducing the gastroesophageal reflux in preterm infants: a crossover study using intraluminal impedance. *J Pediatr.* 2006;148: 265–268.

57. Corvaglia L, Rotatori R, Ferlini M, Aceti A, Ancora G, Faldella G. The effect of body positioning on gastroesophageal reflux in premature infants: evaluation by combined impedance and pH monitoring. *J Pediatr.* 2007;151:591–596, 6 e1.

58. van Wijk MP, Benninga MA, Dent J, et al. Effect of body position changes on postprandial gastroesophageal reflux and gastric emptying in the healthy premature neonate. *J Pediatr.* 2007;151:585–590, 90 e1–e2.

59. Omari TI, Rommel N, Staunton E, et al. Paradoxical impact of body positioning on gastroesophageal reflux and gastric emptying in the premature neonate. *J Pediatr.* 2004;145:194–200.

60. Peter CS, Wiechers C, Bohnhorst B, Silny J, Poets CF. Influence of nasogastric tubes on gastroesophageal reflux in preterm infants: a multiple intraluminal impedance study. *J Pediatr.* 2002;141:277–279.

61. Rosen R, Levine P, Nurko S. Do jejunal feeds decrease gastroesophageal reflux as detected by pH-MII? *J Pediatr Gastroenterol Nutr.* 2007;40:e40.

62. Vela MF, Tutuian R, Katz PO, Castell DO. Baclofen decreases acid and non-acid post-prandial gastro-oesophageal reflux measured by combined multichannel intraluminal impedance and pH. *Aliment Pharmacol Ther.* 2003;17:243–251.

63. Mainie I, Tutuian R, Agrawal A, Adams D, Castell DO. Combined multichannel intraluminal impedance–pH monitoring to select patients with persistent gastro-oesophageal reflux for laparoscopic Nissen fundoplication. *Br J Surg.* 2006;93:1483–1487.

64. Gruebel C, Linke G, Tutuian R, et al. Prospective study examining the impact of multichannel intraluminal impedance on antireflux surgery. *Surg Endosc.* 2008;22:1241–1247.

65. Sondheimer J. Continuous monitoring of distal esophageal pH: a diagnostic test for gastroesophageal reflux in infants. *J Pediatr.* 1980;96:804–807.

66. Euler A, Byrne W. Twenty-four-hour esophageal intraluminal pH probe testing: a comparative analysis. *Gastroenterology.* 1981;80:957–961.

67. Vitale G, Cheadle W, Sadek S, Michel M, Cuschieri A. Computerized 24-hour ambulatory esophageal pH monitoring and esophagastroduodenoscopy in the reflux patient. *Ann Surg.* 1984;20:724–728.

68. Richter J, Bradley L, DeMeester T, Wu W. Normal 24-hr ambulatory esophageal pH values. Influence of study center, pH electrode, age, and gender. *Dig Dis Sci.* 1992;38:795–802.

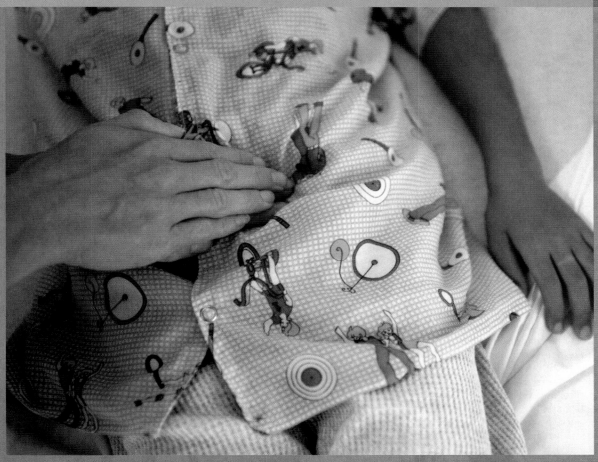

Disorders of the Stomach and Intestine

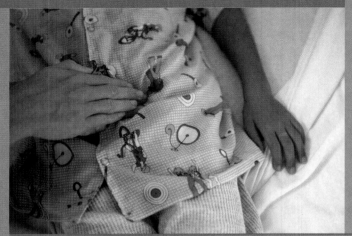

CHAPTER 12

Gastroesophageal Reflux Disease

Benjamin D. Gold

KEY CONCEPTS

- Gastroesophageal reflux (GER) frequently resolves most commonly by 1 year of age. However, gastroesophageal reflux disease (GERD) can become a chronic condition in some children.
- Regurgitation is the predominant symptom in infantile GERD. In older children, abdominal pain predominates. Both groups can present with extraesophageal symptoms (e.g., respiratory manifestations).
- GERD is optimally diagnosed by clinical suspicion and a response to therapy (i.e., most frequently acid suppression), but diagnostic testing such as upper endoscopy may be indicated to assess for GERD-related complications and/or its mimics (e.g., eosinophilic esophagitis).
- Conservative and lifestyle measures may be adequate to treat uncomplicated, mild GERD in infants, and should be employed in older children and adolescents with GERD, even in the face of pharmacological and/or surgical therapy.

DEFINITIONS AND EPIDEMIOLOGY

Gastroesophageal reflux (GER) refers to the passage of gastric contents into the esophagus or oropharynx, with or without vomiting.[1,2] GER can be a daily, normal physiological occurrence in infants, children, and adolescents. Most episodes of GER in healthy individuals last <3 minutes, occur in the postprandial period, and cause few or no troublesome symptoms. *Regurgitation* or "spitting up" is the most obviously visible symptom. It is characterized by effortless emesis and is seen particularly in a very young child, occurring daily in about 50% of infants <3 months of age. Regurgitation resolves spontaneously in most healthy infants by 12–14 months of age.[3,4] Reflux episodes sometimes trigger *vomiting*: the forceful expulsion of gastric contents from the mouth. Vomiting associated with GER is thought to be the result of stimulation of pharyngeal sensory afferents by refluxed gastric contents. *Rumination* refers to the effortless regurgitation of recently ingested food into the mouth with subsequent mastication and re-swallowing. *Rumination syndrome* is a distinct clinical entity with regurgitation of ingested food within minutes following meals due to the voluntary contraction of the abdominal muscles.

Gastroesophageal reflux disease (GERD) refers to the symptoms and complications that may develop secondary to persistent GER.[1,2] Differentiating GER from GERD is critical for the clinician in order to avoid unnecessary diagnostic testing and exposure to medications. Recently, there have been three critically important publications[1,2,5] that offer the clinician a complete characterization of the evidence-based definitions of GER and GERD, particularly GERD-related complications as well as the diagnostic and therapeutic approach to the child with GERD. Complications of GERD in children include esophagitis, growth disturbance, and feeding aversion as well as extraesophageal disease such as respiratory disorders. The first of the two "definition" publications was the Montreal definition of GERD in adults published by Vakil et al. in 2006,[5] and the second, using similar methodology for the establishment of the definitions, was the Global evidence-based consensus on the definition of GERD in children (Figures 12–1 and 12–2)[1] Shortly thereafter, a joint committee of the North American Society for Pediatric Gastroenterology, Hepatology and Nutrition (NASPGHAN) and the European Society for Gastroenterology, Hepatology and Nutrition (ESPGHAN) published recommendations for the management of children with reflux.[2]

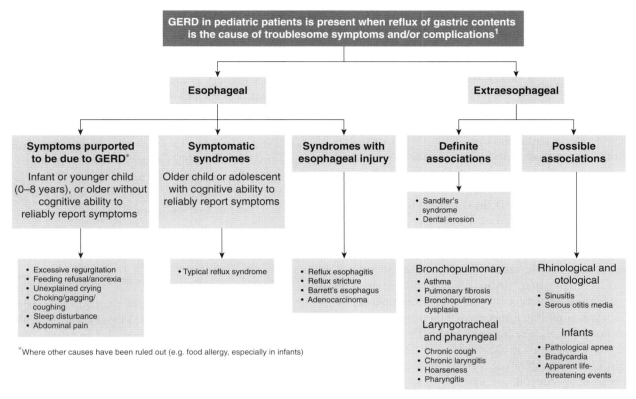

FIGURE 12–1 ■ Global Consensus definition of pediatric GERD. The diagram depicts the overall definition of GERD in children as determined by the Global Consensus Committee. In addition, the diagram provides the designated groups of esophageal and extraesophageal diseases that the Global Consensus Committee determined to be most likely associated with GERD. In specific, the Global Consensus definitions subdivide the esophageal GERD manifestations into symptoms purported to be due to GERD, symptomatic GERD syndromes, and syndromes associated with esophageal injury, as well as those extraesophageal manifestations that are definitively associated with GERD and those with possible association. Adapted by permission from Ref.[1] (Macmillan Publishers Ltd).

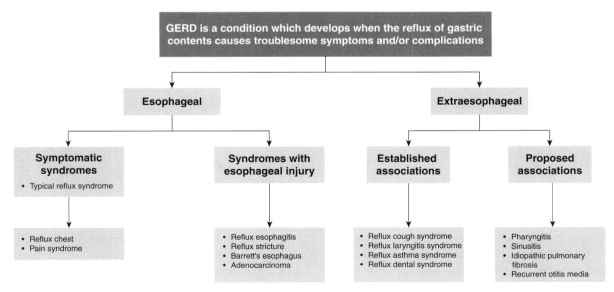

FIGURE 12–2 ■ Montreal definition and classification of GERD (adults). The diagram depicts the overall Montreal definition and classification of GERD in adults as determined by the Global Consensus Committee of experts in adult reflux-related disease. In addition, the diagram provides the designated groups of esophageal and extraesophageal diseases that the Montreal Classification committee determined to be most likely associated with GERD. In specific, the Montreal classification subdivides GERD into symptomatic syndromes and syndromes associated with esophageal injury. Moreover, the Montreal classification subdivides the extraesophageal manifestations into those with established associations and proposed associations.

GERD in Adults versus Children

The committee that developed the Montreal definition of GERD in adults used a *patient-centered, symptom-based* definition of symptoms that have a measurable impact on the patient's quality of life.[5] For children, the Global Consensus Definition Committee incorporated both development criteria and reports of troublesome symptoms. In particular, the Global Consensus Committee operated under the assumption that child development and communicative abilities mandate an age group-specific approach to GER and GERD definitions. Thus, unlike adult GERD, the definition of when reflux-related symptoms become troublesome in children depends on age.[1,5] Although the verbal child can communicate pain, descriptions of the intensity, location, and severity may be unreliable until at least 8 years old, and sometimes later.[6,7] Also, younger children are generally more suggestible, so that queries from parents or clinicians regarding a specific symptom may be biased toward affirmative responses. Thus, self-reporting cannot reliably be used as a component of a GERD definition until the individual is more than approximately 8 years of age. In younger patients, reliance on a parent or caregiver is generally necessary, but reporting of reflux-related symptoms by these surrogates may decrease the validity of diagnosis. Validated symptom questionnaires are currently lacking.[6,8]

In adults[5] and adolescents,[5,9,10] heartburn and regurgitation are the characteristic symptoms of GERD. In infants, the issue is clearly more complicated. During the development of a GERD questionnaire, differences were identified in the prevalence of regurgitation, food refusal, and crying between a healthy cohort and infants with abnormal esophageal pH studies and/or esophatitis.[11] However, these symptoms do not respond to proton pump inhibitor (PPI) therapy and improve with non-pharmacological therapy, raising questions about the causative role of acid reflux.[12,13]

PATHOGENESIS

Altered Motor Function

The patterns of normal physiological reflux change as a child ages, that is, in particular, the frequency and quantity of normal reflux are greater in the very young compared to older children, adolescents, and adults. The increase in normal physiological reflux in infants and young children is due primarily to a number of factors, namely: (1) higher frequency of feeds in infants (i.e., thus increased time over the 24-hour day that the stomach is full), (2) a shorter esophagus and wide angle between the esophagus and stomach in the ≤24-month-old population, thereby allowing reflux to occur more readily, and (3) the increased amount of time infants spend in the supine rather than upright position. Mechanisms for GERD in age groups have been carefully studied and characterized, and are similar across age groups, whether comparing infants, older children or adolescents, and adults (even those that are premature) with GERD to those subjects of similar age that have no GERD. Aerodigestive reflexes (oral, pharyngeal, and esophageal coordinated functions) are fully developed in most children before delivery, by an estimated 38 weeks of gestational age. If there is dysfunction of motility, troublesome GER-related symptoms can ensue. These mechanisms include:

- transient relaxation of the lower esophageal sphincter (LES);
- inhibition of esophageal body peristalsis;
- persistent decrease or absence of LES resting tone.[14–18]

Reflux episodes occur most often during transient LES relaxations unaccompanied by swallowing, which permit gastric contents to flow upward into the esophagus. A minor proportion of reflux episodes occur when the LES fails to increase pressure during a sudden increase in intra-abdominal pressure, or when LES resting pressure is chronically reduced.

Alterations in protective mechanisms allow physiological GER to become GERD. These include:

- insufficient clearance and buffering of refluxate;
- delayed gastric emptying;
- abnormalities in esophageal epithelial repair;
- decreased protective reflexes;
- hiatal hernia.

In hiatal hernia, the anti-reflux barriers at the LES (including the crural support, intra-abdominal segment, and angle of His) are compromised and transient LES relaxations also occur with greater frequency. Erosive esophagitis by itself may promote esophageal shortening and cause hiatal herniation. Hiatal hernia is prevalent in adults and children with severe reflux complications, and hernia size is a major determinant of GERD severity.

Genetic Factors

Significant clustering of reflux symptoms, hiatal hernia, erosive esophagitis, Barrett esophagus, and esophageal adenocarcinoma can occur in families, suggesting heritability of GERD and its complications. A large Swedish Twin Registry study found increased concordance for reflux in monozygotic, compared to dizygotic, twins. In another more recent study, collagen type III alpha I was determined to be a GERD susceptibility gene and a male risk factor for hiatus hernia in adults. Therefore, it is important for the clinician who is evaluating the child with suspected GERD to obtain a detailed family history.

Several other pediatric patient populations appear to be at higher risk of GERD symptoms.

Other Risk Factors for GERD in Children

High-risk groups include individuals with neurologic impairment (NI) or developmental impairment, obesity, many genetic syndromes, esophageal atresia, chronic lung diseases, and those with a history of premature birth. Persistent GERD also occurs in children who have none of these risk factors.[3,19,20] A significant proportion of adults with endoscopically proven GERD have a history of GERD-related symptoms in childhood, compared to adults without GERD.[19] Once GERD is clinically or endoscopically evident in a child or adolescent, it continues as chronic lifelong condition in a substantial percentage of these patients.[20,21] Although no population-based epidemiological studies have been performed, it is apparent that GERD is being increasingly recognized in children in both the United States and abroad.[22] There also appears to be a rising preva-

lence of severe GERD-related outcomes such as erosive esophagitis and Barrett esophagus.

DIFFERENTIAL DIAGNOSIS

Vomiting

Normal regurgitation appears to peak at 2–4 months of age and resolves soon after 1 year of age (Figure 12–3). It is typically effortless, although it may appear more forceful in some infants.[11,24,25] Regurgitation is distinguished from vomiting physiologically by the absence of the following factors: (1) a central nervous system emetic reflex, (2) retrograde upper intestinal contractions, (3) nausea, and (4) retching.[11,25] It is also important to note that parents and even medical practitioners may confuse vomiting with regurgitation, or use other terms for regurgitation (i.e., "spitting up" or "spilling").

Rumination refers to the effortless regurgitation of recently ingested food into the mouth with subsequent mastication and re-swallowing of food. *Rumination syndrome* has been more frequently recognized

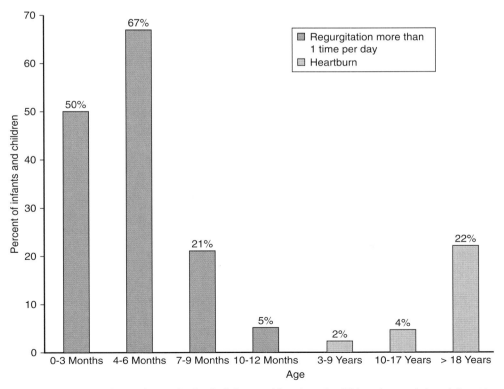

FIGURE 12–3 ▨ Prevalence of regurgitation in infants and heartburn in children, by age (adapted from the Gold[328] and Nelson et al.[4,329]).The figure on the left demonstrates the increase in normal regurgitation episodes over the first 4–6 months of life, as reported by mothers of almost 1000 infants in the metropolitan Chicago area. Moreover, the figure on the left demonstrates that regurgitation disappears in up to 95% by 12 months of age. Conversely, the figure on the right demonstrates that the primary symptom of GERD, that is, heartburn increases over the age of the child.

among older children, especially adolescent females, and is considered by some to lie within the spectrum of eating disorders.[26] Features of rumination that distinguish it from GERD include onset of regurgitation early during the process of eating or drinking. In addition, rumination is associated with an absence of nocturnal symptoms, does not occur when lying down, fails to respond to prokinetics or acid suppression, and has a female preponderance.[27,28] Infant rumination syndrome is a rare disorder that is characterized by voluntary, habitual regurgitation of stomach contents into the mouth for self-stimulation, and may be a sign of social deprivation or severe psycho-social dysfunction in the family.[29] The Rome III criteria[26,29] for rumination syndrome require that GERD be eliminated from the differential diagnosis.

Anatomic Lesions

Bilious vomiting or projectile vomiting are alarm signals that warrant further investigations to rule out anatomic abnormalities, such as intestinal malrotation, pyloric stenosis, or other causes of intestinal obstruction.

CLINICAL FEATURES IN INFANTS

Heartburn, a cardinal symptom of GERD in adults, generally does not manifest until adolescence. Heartburn is defined as an uncomfortable burning sensation behind the sternum that can often reach a painful quality.[5] Table 12–1 lists manifestations that should raise concern for GERD and alarm signals that could indicate other etiologies.

Crying and Sleep Disturbances

Infantile GERD can present with frequent regurgitation, vomiting, poor weight gain, feeding refusal, and irritability. Unfortunately, irritability is not very specific and often is a poor indicator of pathologic acid reflux. Crying is a normal feature of infancy, with an average daily duration that peaks in the second month of life at 2–2.5 hours/day.[30,31] Distinguishing normal crying from crying as a disease-related symptom is complicated. Consequently, in infants, the combined presence of both normal regurgitation and normal crying may be mistaken for GERD.[32,33] As with crying, sleeping patterns of normal infants show great individual and maturational variation as do parental expectations for sleep behavior.

The concept that irritability and sleep disturbances are manifestations of GER is largely extrapolated from descriptions of heartburn and sleep disturbances due to GERD in adult patients. Although

Table 12–1.

Clinical Manifestations of GERD in Children

Symptoms	Recurrent regurgitation with/without vomiting
	Weight loss or poor weight gain
	Irritability in infants
	Ruminative behavior
	Heartburn or chest pain
	Hematemesis
	Dysphagia, odynophagia
	Wheezing
	Stridor
	Cough
	Hoarseness
Signs	Esophagitis
	Esophageal stricture
	Barrett's esophagus
	Laryngeal/pharyngeal inflammation
	Recurrent pneumonia
	Anemia
	Dental erosion
	Feeding refusal
	Dystonic neck posturing (Sandifer syndrome)
	Apnea spells
	Apparent life-threatening events (ALTE)

Red flags in infants

Bilious vomiting	Fever
Gastrointestinal (GI) bleeding	Lethargy
■ Hematemesis	Hepatosplenomegaly
■ Hematochezia	Bulging fontanelle
Consistently forceful vomiting	Macro/microcephaly
Onset of vomiting after 6 months of life	Seizures
Failure to thrive	Abdominal tenderness or distension
Diarrhea	Documented/suspected genetic/ metabolic syndrome
Constipation	

one study in infants showed a correlation between infant grimacing and episodes of GER, multiple other studies have shown no relationship between crying and GERD, as determined by esophageal pH testing or the presence of esophagitis on endoscopy[34,35]. Recently, a study of colicky infants found abnormal pH test results only in those with excessive regurgitation or feeding difficulties.[36] Taken these data together, the correlation between crying, night-time awakening, and GER as based on a "diagnostic" test remains unclear.

One way to sort this out is to look at the response to acid-blocker therapy. An early study showed a greater decrease in crying time in infants treated with a 1.0 mg/kg dose of famotidine than in infants given 0.5 mg/kg.[37] The authors concluded that famotidine is effective in treating infant crying. However, this study had significant methodological shortcomings, including lack of a placebo control.[37] A placebo-controlled study of infants with irritability and normal esophageal pH tests found that combined ranitidine and cisapride treatment was not superior to placebo or parent-directed counseling for persistent crying.[38] A double-blind, placebo-controlled trial of a PPI (i.e., omeprazole) in irritable infants with proven GERD (esophagitis or abnormal pH probe study) found no difference in crying between treated and placebo groups.[39] However, the study design was flawed in that the PPI dose was low, there was a brief wash-out period, and the parameters used to define abnormal esophageal acidification were actually normal.[39] More recently, a larger, double-blind study of 162 infants randomized to 4 weeks of placebo or lansoprazole showed an identical response rate in each group (54%).[13] Thus, it appears that acid blockers have a limited role in distinguishing crying caused by GERD.

Although they have limited efficacy in stopping fussiness, PPIs do have efficacy against acid reflux in infants. Another recent study sought to characterize the pharmacodynamics and clinical effects of esomeprazole in 26 preterm infants and term neonates with symptoms of GER and abnormal pH probe studies.[40] Study patients received oral esomeprazole 0.5 mg/kg once daily for 7 days. As expected, acid reflux episodes were reduced on therapy. More importantly, in contrast to the previously mentioned study, the number of GER symptoms recorded over 24 hours was lower on therapy.[40] It seems clear that research is critically needed to determine and validate both diagnosis and treatment outcomes in the infant with suspected GERD, and in particular, study designs that (1) include validated symptom-based diagnosis in infants and (2) appropriately defined case and placebo/control groups with sufficient sample size to achieve adequate power.

CLINICAL FEATURES IN OLDER CHILDREN

Beyond infancy, a variety of symptoms can be attributed to GERD, and many of these symptoms change with age. In one study of 1–17-year olds, cough, anorexia/food refusal, and regurgitation/vomiting were more common and more severe in children 1–5 years of age, compared with older children[10] (in this study, toddlers and young children). In contrast, the predominant

symptoms in older children (6–17 years) included epigastric pain or heartburn.[10,41] These become increasing predominant with increasing age.[9,10] In addition, per the Global Consensus definition, epigastric pain in older children and adolescents can be a major symptom of GERD.[1] Overall, for 1–11-year olds, there are relatively few data on presenting symptoms, and no standardized definitions for reporting.[10] For example, some studies allow reporting of abdominal pain, or epigastric pain, or both.[10,41,42] In addition, the combination of arching of the back, torsion of the neck, and lifting of the chin suggests Sandifer syndrome.[43–46] This GERD-associated condition has its peak occurrence at 18–36 months of age and is a specific manifestation of GERD in pediatric patients. Table 12–1 lists age-specific GERD signs and symptoms and warning/alarm signs that indicate other diseases.

EXTRAESOPHAGEAL MANIFESTATIONS OF GERD

Head and neck manifestations that have been associated with GERD include dental erosions, otitis media, pharyngitis, and vocal cord disorders such as laryngitis. However, the Global Consensus Definition Committee determined that, at present, there is insufficient evidence that GERD causes or exacerbates sinusitis, pulmonary fibrosis, pharyngitis, or serous otitis media in children.[1] Placebo-controlled treatment trials in children with GERD and otolaryngologic manifestations (e.g., chronic otitis media), that are sufficiently powered (i.e., adequate cohort size), and include standard case definitions and clearly defined outcomes, are needed to support a cause-and-effect relationship.[47,48]

Lower respiratory manifestations that have been described include nocturnal cough or wheezing, reactive airway disease, asthma, and recurrent pneumonias.[49–51] Per the Global Consensus definition, chronic cough, chronic laryngitis, hoarseness, and asthma may be associated with GERD.[1] One study of 1037 children followed from birth to 26 years of age for respiratory symptoms and lung function found an association between symptoms of GERD (heartburn and regurgitation) and asthma, wheezing, and nocturnal cough. However, this association was only found in patients with late-onset asthma (teenage and adult), and not in childhood-onset asthma.[52]

Asthma

Proposed mechanisms by which GER might aggravate asthma have compelling supporting evidence. These mechanisms include the following: airway hyper-responsiveness triggered by aspiration of small amounts of acid, airway inflammation elicited by aspirated gastric contents, vagally mediated bronchial or laryngeal spasm, and neurally mediated inflammation.[53,54] Interestingly, esophageal acidification in healthy adults has minimal effect on pulmonary function, but in asthmatic patients can produce airway hyper-responsiveness and airflow obstruction.

In addition, similar to GERD as a cause for asthma, biological plausibility for the converse relationship is also strong.[55–58] Chronic hyperinflation caused by asthma can flatten the diaphragms, alter crural function, and displace the LES into the negative atmosphere of the chest, effectively reducing resting LES pressure and causing disappearance of the acute esophagogastric angle of His.[57–59] Lung hyperinflation and airflow obstruction may produce increased negative intrathoracic pressure, promoting GER. Theophylline (now rarely used in clinical practice) and β-receptor agonists cause a reduction of resting LES pressure.[60,61] However, to date, these drugs have not been associated with the development of GERD in treated asthmatics.

An association between asthma and measurements of GER by pH probe or pH probe plus multichannel intraluminal impedance (MII) has been recently demonstrated. These studies found that 60–80% of children with asthma have GER.[48,62–64] A study of 77 children aged 3–14 years old with difficult-to-control asthma found that 66% had an abnormal reflux index on pH testing. In a study of 84 otherwise healthy infants with daily wheezing, 64% had abnormal 24-hour pH studies, and 44% of these had no overt symptoms of GERD. In addition, in clinical practice and descriptive reports, nocturnal wheezing appears particularly related to GERD.[65,66] One study used combined esophageal pH and MII monitoring and demonstrated a tighter association between reflux episodes and respiratory symptoms than pH monitoring alone. Unfortunately, no studies to date demonstrate that pH/MII studies are useful in identifying those patients whose asthma might respond to anti-reflux therapy.

Apnea

A causal relationship between reflux and apnea has been postulated and instituted in clinical practice for many years, especially in newborns and young infants.[67] However, the GERD–apnea association could simply be attributed to both conditions being common at this stage in life. In addition, a recent study demonstrated no association between abnormal esophageal pH monitoring and apnea.[68–70] Moreover, the literature on the relationship between apnea, respiratory pauses, apparent life-threatening events (ALTEs), or sudden infant death syndrome (SIDS) and GER is quite conflicting. The confusion in the literature is due in part to the use of different criteria to define breath stoppage, varying methods used to measure GER and respiratory pauses, and the study of different populations.[1,71] MII and pH monitoring studies have both been used to demonstrate a relationship between short episodes of physiological apnea and reflux in infants.[72] Overall, GERD and apnea do not appear temporally related in "asymptomatic convalescent" preterm babies,[73] despite strong physiological evidence that stimulation of laryngeal afferents elicits central apnea and laryngeal adduction.[74] However, in a subpopulation of infants with neurodevelopmental impairment, there may be an increased incidence of both apnea and GER.[75] Despite the controversy, and the difficulty in "doing nothing" in clinical practice, many centers still treat all infants presenting with apnea with anti-reflux therapies.

Acute life-threatening events (ALTEs) are characterized by a combination of apnea, color change (cyanosis, pallor, and plethora), abnormal muscle tone (limpness and stiffness), choking, and gagging that require intervention by the observer. As might be expected, GERD is a frequent diagnostic consideration in infants following an ALTE.[76] Typically, these occur between 1 and 8 months of age. ALTEs may recur, and infants with an ALTE are felt to be at slightly increased risk for a subsequent sudden death. ALTEs may be associated with infection, child abuse, upper airway obstruction, and cardiac, respiratory, metabolic, and neurologic disorders. ALTEs associated with GERD may not be pathologic; some may be an exaggeration of normal protective reflexes that inhibit breathing while the infant retches or while the pharynx is filled with gastric contents. However, there are no compelling data available at present that reliably define the prevalence of GERD in ALTE. In fact, one study, reflux of gastric acid, appears to be related in <5% of infants with ALTE.[77]

DIAGNOSIS

A thorough history and physical examination can be the key to diagnosis of GERD, with specific attention to the child's age, as well as the character and frequency of GERD-related symptoms. The original NASPGHAN clinical practice guidelines for GERD in children recommended that a trial of acid suppression should be considered, based on history and physical examination.[78] This "PPI test" has been effective in adults, with resolution of symptoms being the diagnostic test for GERD.[79–81]

In the United States, a random sample of members of the American Academy of Pediatrics recently revealed that 82% of the respondents would initiate therapy solely based on clinical suspicion (i.e., history and physical exam).[82]

The PPI Test: Empiric Trial of Acid Suppression

In adults, a trial of empiric treatment with acid suppression using a defined dose, defined duration of therapy, and clear endpoints has been called the PPI test. This has particularly been used to differentiate cardiac from non-cardiac chest pain.[79,83] The PPI test has also been used for GERD-related complaints of heartburn, chronic cough, and dyspepsia.[80,84–86] Empiric therapy has variable sensitivity and specificity as a diagnostic test for GERD, depending on the comparative gold standard used (endoscopy, pH monitoring, or symptom questionnaires).[87] The appropriate duration of a diagnostic trial of acid suppression has not been determined. A meta-analysis evaluating pooled data from three large treatment trials among adults with non-erosive reflux disease showed that 85% of patients who had symptom resolution after 1 week of PPI treatment remained well for the entire 4 weeks of PPI treatment, thus "confirming" the diagnosis.[88] However, 22% of patients who had no improvement after 1 week of treatment did improve by the fourth week of treatment. An uncontrolled trial of esomeprazole therapy in adolescents with heartburn, epigastric pain, and acid regurgitation showed complete resolution of symptoms in 30–43% by 1 week, but the responders increased to 65% following 8 weeks of treatment.[89] Another uncontrolled treatment trial of pantoprazole in children aged 5–11 years reported greater symptom improvement at 1 week with a 40-mg dose compared to a 10- or 20-mg dose.[90] Interestingly, all treatment groups improved after 8 weeks. Similar improvement in symptoms over time has been observed in adults with erosive esophagitis.[91,92]

The treatment period required to achieve uniform therapeutic responses with PPI therapy probably varies with disease severity, treatment dose, and specific symptoms or complications.[93] A 2-week "PPI test" lacks adequate specificity and sensitivity for use in clinical practice, particularly in the pediatric patient. In an older child or adolescent with symptoms suggesting GERD, an empiric PPI trial is justified for up to 4 weeks. Nevertheless, improvement following treatment does not absolutely confirm a diagnosis of GERD, since symptoms may improve spontaneously or due to the placebo effect. Finally, data suggest there is no evidence to support an empiric trial of pharmacological treatment in infants ≤12 months of age with symptoms suggestive of GERD.

Barium Contrast Radiography

Although the above-mentioned American Academy of Pediatrics survey revealed that the upper gastrointestinal (GI) series is the preferred test of pediatricians for children with suspected GERD, this diagnostic approach is neither sensitive nor specific for diagnosing this condition.[82] The upper GI series is useful to detect anatomic abnormalities such as esophageal stricture, hiatal hernia, achalasia, tracheoesopahgeal fistula, intestinal malrotation, or pyloric stenosis that may be considered in the differential diagnosis. The sensitivity, specificity, and positive predictive value of the upper GI series range from 29% to 86%, 21% to 83%, and 80% to 82%, respectively, when compared to esophageal pH monitoring.[94–96] The brief duration of the upper GI series produces false-negative results, while the frequent occurrence of non-pathologic reflux during the examination produces false-positive results. Therefore, routine performance of upper GI series to diagnose GER and GERD is not justified.[97]

Scintigraphy

In gastroesophageal scintigraphy, food or formula labeled with [99]technitium is introduced into the stomach, following which the stomach, esophagus, and lungs are continuously imaged for evidence of GER and aspiration. The nuclear scan evaluates postprandial reflux and demonstrates reflux independent of the gastric pH. Scintigraphy can also provide information about gastric emptying, which may be delayed in children with GERD.[98] A lack of standardized techniques and the absence of age-specific norms limit the value of this test. Sensitivity and specificity of a 1-hour scintigraphy for the diagnosis of GERD are 15–59% and 83–100%, respectively, when compared to 24-hour esophageal pH monitoring.[99] Late postprandial acid exposure detected by pH monitoring may be missed with scintigraphy.[100] Comparisons of scintigraphy to MII, pH monitoring, and with symptom-based diagnosis are lacking. Gastroesophageal scintigraphy scanning can detect GER episodes and aspiration of gastric contents occurring during or shortly after meals, but its reported sensitivity for microaspiration is relatively low.[101] Evidence of pulmonary aspiration may be detected during a 1-hour scintigraphic study or on images obtained up to 24 hours after administration of the radionuclide. A negative test does not exclude the possibility of infrequently occurring aspiration. One study of children with refractory respiratory symptoms found that half had scintigraphic evidence of pulmonary aspiration.[101] However, aspiration of both gastric contents and saliva also occurs in healthy adults during deep sleep.[102] At present, there is no role for nuclear scintigraphy in the diagnosis and management of GERD in pediatric patients.

Ultrasonography

Ultrasonography is a relatively new technique for diagnosing gastroesophageal disease in adults. At present, although there is potential for utility as the technology and methodology become more refined,[103] ultrasound is not recommended as a test for pediatric GERD. Ultrasonography of the GE junction can detect fluid movements over short periods of time and thereby can detect non-acid reflux events. Ultrasound can also detect hiatal hernia, measure the length and position of the LES relative to the diaphragm, and demonstrate the gastroesophageal angle of His. When compared to the results of 24-hour esophageal pH testing as a diagnostic test for GERD, the sensitivity of color Doppler ultrasound performed for 15 minutes postprandially is about 95% with a specificity of only 11%, and there is no correlation between reflux frequency detected by ultrasound and reflux index detected by pH monitoring.[104]

Esophageal pH Monitoring

Intraluminal esophageal pH monitoring measures the frequency and duration of acid esophageal reflux episodes reaching the distal esophagus.[105–109] Most commercially available systems include a catheter for nasal insertion with one or more pH electrodes (antimony, glass, or ion-sensitive field effect) arrayed along its length and a system for data capture, analysis, and reporting. Slow electrode response times (antimony being the slowest) do not substantially alter the assessment of total reflux time, but may affect the accuracy of correlation between symptoms and reflux episodes.[110–112] Recently, wireless sensors that can be clipped to the esophageal mucosa during endoscopy (i.e., Bravo™ capsule) have allowed pH monitoring without a nasal cannula for up to 48 hours of monitoring.[113,114] Placement of wireless electrodes requires upper endoscopy, and the accompanying sedation or anesthesia, and comfort has been an issue in some studies.[113,114] The size of current wireless electrodes precludes their use in small infants. Benefits, risks, and indications for wireless electrode monitoring have also not been fully defined in children.

By convention, a drop in intraesophageal pH below 4.0 for >5 seconds is considered an acid reflux episode. This cut-off was initially chosen because heartburn induced by acid perfusion of the esophagus in adults generally occurs at pH <4.0. However, the duration of esophageal acidification necessary to cause symptoms or induce mucosal injury has not been clearly established, particularly in the pediatric patient population. Although interpretation of pH monitoring data is simplified by computerized analysis, visual inspection of the tracing is required to detect artifacts and evaluate clinical correlations.[115,116] Common parameters obtained from pH monitoring include the total number of reflux episodes, the number of reflux episodes lasting >5 minutes, the duration of the longest reflux episode, and the reflux index or RI (percentage of the entire

record that esophageal pH <4.0)[23]. The RI is the most commonly used summary score.

More recently, the value of esophageal pH-metry for diagnosis and management of pediatric GERD has been questioned as having a lack of utility overall.[69,117,118] Esophageal pH-metry is insensitive to weakly acid and non-acid reflux events, and the response times of the most widely used electrodes are slow. These barriers are overcome by multichannel intraluminal impedance (MII) monitoring and/or by the use of ion-sensitive field-effect electrodes. Esophageal pH monitoring can correlate poorly with symptom severity and with response to therapy in pediatric patients.[70] In infants with suspected GERD, an abnormal pH study (RI > 10%) was associated only with pneumonia, apnea with fussing, defecation less than once a day, and constipation.[70] An abnormal RI is more frequently observed in adults with erosive esophagitis than in normals or those with non-erosive reflux disease, but there is substantial overlap among groups.[119] In pediatric patients, the calculated area under the pH 4.0 curve has been associated with erosive esophagitis (Gold et al., unpublished data). Esophageal pH monitoring may be abnormal in patients with other disorders, including gastric outlet obstruction, motility disorders, and esophagitis due to other disorders, including eosinophilic esopahgitis.[77,120,121]

Esophageal pH monitoring may be useful for evaluating the efficacy of anti-secretory therapy. In children with esophagitis, normal esophageal pH monitoring suggests a diagnosis other than GERD.[122,123]

Multichannel Intraluminal Esophageal Impedance

MII is a procedure for measuring the movement of fluids, solids, and air in the esophagus.[124–126] It is a relatively new technology that, in comparison to pH monitoring, provides a more detailed description of substances within the esophageal lumen and correlation with symptoms.[125,127–131] MII measures changes in the electrical impedance (i.e., resistance) between multiple electrodes located along an esophageal catheter.[132] Esophageal impedance tracings are analyzed for the typical changes in impedance caused by the passage of liquid, solid, gas, or mixed boluses.[124] If the impedance changes of a liquid bolus appear first in the distal channels and proceed sequentially to the proximal channels, they indicate retrograde bolus movement, that is, GER.[132] The direction and velocity of a bolus can be calculated using the defined distance between electrodes and the time between alterations in the impedance pattern of sequential electrode pairs. The upward extent of the bolus and the physical length of the bolus can also be evaluated.[124–126] MII can detect very small bolus volumes.[133]

For improved performance, MII and pH electrodes can be combined on a single catheter. The combined measurement of pH and impedance (pH/MII) provides additional information as to whether a refluxed material is acid, weakly acidic, or non-acidic.[124,127,134] Recent studies have found variable reproducibility of MII studies in pediatric patients. However, more recently, evaluation of MII recordings is aided by automated analysis tools[135,136] that may improve accuracy. Until the currently available automatic analysis software has been validated, a visual reading of the data is still required. Normal values for all age groups have not yet been established.

The combination of pH/MII with simultaneous monitoring of other parameters using video polysomnography or manometry has proven useful for the evaluation of correlations between reflux episodes and apnea, cough, other respiratory symptoms, and behavioral symptoms.[18,137,138] The technology is especially useful, compared to the pH-only study, when gastric contents are non-acidic, as in the postprandial period or when patients are taking acid blockers. Whether this new technology will provide measurements that vary directly with disease severity, prognosis, and response to therapy has yet to be determined.

Invasive Diagnostic Approaches to GERD and Extraesophageal GERD

There are a number of invasive approaches to support the diagnosis of clinically suspected GERD in the pediatric patient. Clinicians employ laryngoscopy, bronchoscopy and alveolar lavage, endoscopy, esophageal and laryngeal biopsies, pH monitoring in the hypopharynx, and MII monitoring to diagnose GERD in pediatric patients presenting with extraesophageal symptoms.[47,139–142] However, none of these tools independently establishes the diagnosis of GERD with extraesophageal symptoms.[143–145] Hypopharyngeal pH-metry has been evaluated in children with symptoms suggestive of extraesophageal manifestation of GERD.[144] In a prospective study of 222 children (1 day to 16 years old) divided into subgroups by symptoms (laryngeal, pulmonary, recurrent emesis, and non-respiratory), 78 had pharyngeal acid reflux in spite of normal distal esophageal pH tracings.[145] Children with emesis, pulmonary symptoms, and laryngeal symptoms had more pharyngeal reflux episodes, compared with children with GI-related symptoms. The same method was applied in another prospective study of 105 children with symptoms suggestive of GERD, aged 4 months to 12 years, but in this instance hypopharynx-pH-metry did not differentiate between children with and without abnormal esophageal pH tracings, irrespective of presenting clinical symptoms.[144]

A blinded comparison of videomacrolaryngoscopy, laryngeal and esophageal biopsies, and dual pH-metry (of distal esophagus and hypopharynx) was performed in 39 consecutive children operated on for airway reconstruction.[143] The upper probe pH did not correlate with any of the other assessed parameters.[143] The definition of pathologic hypopharyngeal reflux is uncertain, because pharyngeal reflux also occurs in healthy controls.[146–149] It is also unknown how much acid reflux is needed to cause pathology of the larynx. The same issues probably also apply for MII. So far, normative data from different pediatric age groups are not available.[150] Therefore, additional carefully controlled studies are needed to define which diagnostic tool will best diagnose extraesophageal GERD.

When hematemesis or occult bleeding occurs in the face of GERD symptoms, esophagogastroduodenoscopy (EGD) or upper GI endoscopy may be indicated to assess for the presence and severity of GERD. EGD can also detect erosive (macroscopic) or histologic (microscopic) esophagitis, strictures, Barrett's esophagus, and eosinophilic esophagitis (EoE), a potential GERD masquerader.[120,151,152] EGD allows the pediatric gastroenterologist to have direct visual assessment of the esophageal mucosa, giving the clinician a macroscopic perspective. Random or targeted biopsies enable evaluation of the microscopic anatomy.[153] Macroscopic abnormalities associated with GERD include esophagitis, erosions, ulcers, strictures, hiatal hernia, areas of possible suspected esophageal metaplasia, and polyps (Table 12–2). While endoscopy can detect strictures, subtle degrees of narrowing are better shown on barium contrast study. Unfortunately, anatomic abnormalities such as malrotation and achalasia cannot be diagnosed by endoscopy. These and other anatomic and motility disorders of the esophagus are better evaluated by barium radiology or motility studies.

Recent Global Consensus guidelines define reflux esophagitis as the presence of endoscopically visible breaks in the esophageal mucosa at or immediately above the GE junction.[1,5,154] Evidence from adult studies indicates that visible breaks in the esophageal mucosa are the endoscopic sign of greatest interobserver reliability.[155] Mucosal erythema or an irregular Z-line is not a reliable sign of reflux esophagitis. Grading the severity of esophagitis, using a recognized endoscopic classification system, is useful for evaluation of the severity of esophagitis and response to treatment. The Hetzel–Dent classification has been used in several pediatric studies,[156,157] and more recently, the Los Angeles classification,[154] which was generally used for adults, is also quite suitable for use in children. However, it is important to note that the presence of endoscopically normal esophageal mucosa does not exclude a diagnosis of non-erosive reflux disease or esophagitis of other etiologies.[158,159]

Table 12–2.	

Classification of Visual or Macroscopic Esophagitis in Children and Adults—Hetzel–Dent and LA Classification

Hetzel–Dent classification

Grade 0	Normal mucosa
Grade 1	Mucosal edema, hyperemia, and friability
Grade 2	Superficial erosions involving <10% of the distal 5 cm of the esophageal mucosal surface
Grade 3	Superficial erosions and ulcerations involving 10–50% of the distal esophagus
Grade 4	Deep peptic ulceration anywhere in the esophagus or confluent erosion of >50% of the distal esophagus

Los Angeles classification

Grade A	One (or more) mucosal break *no longer than 5 mm* that does not extend between the tops of two mucosal folds (fx1)
Grade B	One (or more) mucosal break *>5 mm* that does not extend between the tops of two mucosal folds (fx2)
Grade C	One (or more) mucosal break that is continuous between the tops of two mucosal folds but which involves <75% of the circumference (fx3)
Grade D	One (or more) mucosal break that involves *at least 75%* of the esophageal circumference (fx4)

The diagnostic yield of endoscopy is generally greater if multiple samples of good size and orientation are obtained from esophageal mucosal biopsy sites that are identified relative to major anatomic features.[153,160,161] Several variables impact on the validity of histology as a diagnostic tool for reflux-associated esophagitis, and/or the ability to rule out other etiologies of esophageal disease (e.g., EoE), including: (1) sampling errors due to the patchy distribution of inflammatory changes, (2) a lack in standardization of biopsy location, (3) variable methodologies for tissue processing, and (4) variable interpretation of morphometric parameters.[159,162] His-

tology may be normal even in some patients with erosive reflux esophagitis; conversely, it may be abnormal in non-erosive reflux disease. Moreover, symptom severity has not been shown to correlate with either macroscopic or endoscopic findings in the child who has undergone diagnostic upper endoscopy.

Histologic findings of eosinophilia, elongation of papillae (rete pegs), basal cell hyperplasia, and dilated intercellular spaces (DIS, or spongiosis) are neither sensitive nor specific for reflux esophagitis.[70,122,158,162,163] These are non-specific reactive changes that may be found in esophagitis of other causes. Recent studies have shown considerable overlap between the histology of reflux esophagitis and EoE.[120,121,158,164] Many histologic parameters are influenced by drugs used to treat esophagitis or other disorders.

GERD is likely the most common cause of esophagitis in children, but other disorders such as EoE, Crohn's disease, and infections also cause esophagitis.[158] EoE and GERD have very similar symptoms and signs, and can be best distinguished by endoscopy with biopsy. A key difference endoscopically is that EoE is not generally an erosive disease, but has its own typical endoscopic features such as speckled exudates, trachealization of the esophagus, or linear furrowing. In up to 30% of cases, however, the esophageal mucosal appearance is normal.[165,166] When EoE is considered as part of the differential diagnosis, it is advisable to take esophageal biopsies from the proximal, mid, and distal esophagus.[165] Mucosal eosinophilia may be present in the esophageal mucosa in asymptomatic infants <1 year of age[167] and in symptomatic infants eosinophilic infiltrate may be due to milk protein allergy.[166]

Thus, at present, although hotly debated by pediatric gastroenterologists, there is insufficient evidence to support the use of histology to diagnose or exclude GERD. Clearly, more multicenter studies need to be done, particularly those that utilize a standard approach to anatomic landmarks, biopsy collection, and histologic characterization in order to address this issue. Currently, the primary role for esophageal histology is to rule out other conditions in the differential diagnosis, such as EoE, Crohn's disease, Barrett esophagus, infection, and others.

MANAGEMENT

The primary goals of treatment are to resolve symptoms, improve overall quality of life, and resolve and prevent complications of GERD. In "uncomplicated" infantile GER, conservative measures such as thickening the formula, giving smaller feeds more frequently, and upright positioning for at least 30 minutes after feeds may be sufficient to decrease regurgitation. In addition, thickening can increase the caloric density of the

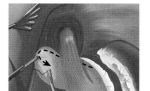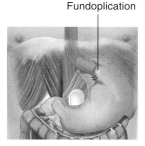

Fundoplication

FIGURE 12–4 ■ Anti-reflux surgery—Nissen fundoplication. The figure on the left demonstrates the anatomy as depicted via a laparoscopic surgical view of the abdomen. Note the surgical instruments grasping the gastric fundus and wrapping this around the distal or abdominal portion of the esophagus, covering the LES. The vasculature and nerve supply of the stomach is left intact so that the wrapped stomach, that is, figure on the right, provides the mechanism to prevent vomiting, emesis and thereby reflux.

formula, which may benefit infants who have weight gain issues as a result of GER (one tablespoon of rice cereal per 2 ounces of formula increases the caloric density to 27 kcal/ounce). Prone positioning may decrease regurgitation but is not recommended due to the increased risk for SIDS. If milk protein intolerance or allergy is suspected, a 2–4-week trial of protein (partial whey or casein) hydrolysate formula should be considered (Figure 12–4).

LIFESTYLE CHANGES

Feeding Changes in Infants

About 50% of normal 3–4-month-old infants regurgitate at least once a day and up to 20% of caregivers in the United States seek medical help for this normal behavior.[3,4] Breast-fed and formula-fed infants have a similar frequency of physiological GER, although the duration of reflux episodes measured by pH probe may be shorter in breast-fed infants.[168–170]

A subset of infants with allergy to cow's milk protein experiences regurgitation and vomiting indistinguishable from that associated with GER.[77,171–173] In these infants, vomiting frequency decreases significantly (usually within 2 weeks) after the elimination of cow's milk protein from the diet, and re-introduction causes recurrence of symptoms.[174,175] Studies support a trial of up to 4 weeks of extensively hydrolyzed or amino acid formula in formula-fed infants with bothersome emesis.[12] Cow's milk protein passes into human breast milk in small quantities. Breast-fed infants with regurgitation and vomiting may therefore benefit from a trial of withdrawal of cow's milk and eggs from the maternal diet.[176] The symptoms of infant GER are almost never so severe that breast-feeding

should be discontinued. There are no studies specifically evaluating soy protein allergy in infants with regurgitation and vomiting, or the role of soy protein-based formula in the treatment of infants with regurgitation.

One small study in infants showed that large-volume feedings promote regurgitation, probably by increasing the frequency of transient LES relaxations, and reduced feeding volume decreased reflux frequency.[177] Severe reduction in feeding volume over an extended period may deprive the infant of needed calories and adversely affect weight gain. Infants with inadequate weight gain due to losses by regurgitation may benefit from increasing the caloric density of formula when volume or frequency of feedings is decreased as part of therapy.

Adding *thickening agents* such as rice cereal to formula or milk does not decrease the time with pH <4 (reflux index) measured by esophageal pH studies, but does decrease the frequency of overt regurgitation.[177,178] Studies with combined pH/MII show that the height of reflux in the esophagus is decreased with thickened formula.[179] One study reported an improvement in esophageal pH parameters with cornstarch-thickened formula.[180] Another study showed no change in esophageal impedance parameters of premature infants receiving cornstarch-thickened human milk.[181]

In the United States, *rice cereal* is the most commonly used thickening agent for formula.[178] Rice cereal-thickened formula decreases the volume of regurgitation but may increase coughing during feedings.[182] Formula with added rice cereal usually requires using a nipple with an enlarged hole to allow adequate flow. Excessive calorie intake is a potential problem with long-term use of feedings thickened with rice cereal or cornstarch.[183] Thickening a 20 kcal/oz infant formula with one tablespoon of rice cereal per ounce increases the caloric density to 34 kcal/oz. Thickening with one tablespoon per 2 ounces of formula increases the caloric density to 27 kcal/oz.

Commercial anti-regurgitant (AR) formulas containing processed rice, corn or potato starch, guar gum, or locust bean gum are available in Europe, Asia, and the United States. These formulas decrease overt regurgitation and vomiting frequencies compared with unthickened formulas or formulas thickened with rice cereal.[180,183–186] A potential advantage of AR formulas over formula with added cereal or starch is that the former are designed to contain a caloric density, osmolarity, protein, calcium, and fatty acid content appropriate to an infant's nutritional needs when taken in normal volume. A largely untested potential advantage of AR formulas is that, because they thicken in the stomach, they do not require a large bore nipple hole and do not substantially increase sucking effort. In vitro studies have shown a decrease in the absorption of minerals and micronutrients from formulas commercially thickened with indigestible but not digestible carbohydrates.[186] The clinical significance of this is unclear.

The use of AR formulas and formulas with added thickener results in a decrease of observed regurgitation, although the difference may be small.[187] Although the actual number of reflux episodes detected by pH-metry of MII may not decrease, the reduction in regurgitation is often welcomed as an improvement in quality of life for caregivers and possibly the infant. The impact of thickened formula on the natural history of physiological GER or GERD has not been studied. The allergenicity of commercial thickening agents is uncertain and the possible nutritional risks of long-term use require further study.

Tube Feedings

There are rare infants with GERD who are unable to gain weight despite conservative measures in whom nasogastric or nasojejunal feeding may be beneficial. Similarly, nasojejunal feeding is occasionally useful in infants with recurrent GER-related pneumonia to prevent recurrent aspiration.[188] Although these approaches to therapy are widely utilized, there are no controlled studies comparing them to pharmacological or surgical treatments.

Positioning Therapy for Infants

Several studies in infants have demonstrated significantly decreased acid reflux in the flat prone compared to flat supine position.[73,189] There is conflicting evidence as to whether infants placed prone with the head elevated have less reflux than those kept prone but flat.[189,190] The amount of reflux in supine infants with head elevated is equal to or greater than in infants supine and flat.[189,191–193] The semi-supine positioning attained in an infant car seat actually has been shown by some studies to exacerbate GER in infants.[194] Although the full upright position appears to decrease measured reflux, studies have shown that using formula thickened with rice cereal is more effective in decreasing the frequency of regurgitation than upright positioning after feeds.[195]

In the 1980s, prone positioning was recommended for the treatment of GERD in infants because studies showed less reflux in this position. Interestingly, prone sleep positioning is associated with longer uninterrupted sleep periods, and supine sleep positioning with more frequent arousals and crying.[196] However, concerns regarding the association between prone positioning and SIDS required a reassessment of the benefits and risks of prone positioning for GERD treatment. A Scandinavian study (i.e., Nordic epidemiological SIDS study) demonstrated that the mortality from SIDS was >10 times higher in prone-sleeping infants and 3 times higher in side-sleeping infants than in supine infants.[197–199] Therefore, prone positioning is acceptable

if the infant is observed and awake, particularly in the postprandial period, but prone positioning during sleep can only be considered in infants with certain upper airway disorders where the risk of death from GERD outweighs the risk of SIDS. Prone positioning may be beneficial in children over 1 year of age with GER or GERD whose risk of SIDS is negligible.

Esophageal pH and combined pH/MII monitoring show that reflux is quantitatively similar in the left-side-down and prone positions. Measured reflux in these two positions is less than in the right-side-down and supine positions.[189,200,201] Additional, MII studies of preterm infants found that postprandial reflux was greater in the right-side-down than in the left-side-down position.[202] The impedance data prompted recommendations for infants to be placed right-side-down for the first hour after feeding, to promote gastric emptying and then switched to left-side-down thereafter to decrease GER. From a practical standpoint, it is important for parents and clinicians alike to note that side lying may end up changing unobserved into prone position during sleep. More importantly, using a propping pillow together to keep an infant in a side-lying position is not recommended.[203]

Lifestyle Changes in Children and Adolescents

Lifestyle changes often recommended for children and adolescents with GER and GERD include dietary modification, avoidance of alcohol, weight loss, positioning changes, and cessation of smoking. Most studies investigating these recommendations have been performed in adults; thus, their applicability to children of all ages is uncertain. A review of lifestyle changes in adults with GERD concluded that only weight loss improved pH profiles and symptoms. Although alcohol, chocolate, and high-fat meals reduce LES pressure, only a few studies have evaluated the impact of these factors on symptoms. Tobacco smoke exposure is associated with increased GER symptoms, yet neither tobacco nor alcohol cessation has been shown to improve esophageal pH profiles or symptoms. One uncontrolled study found that a very-low-carbohydrate diet reduced distal esophageal acid exposure and improved symptoms in obese individuals with GERD.[204] Gastric bypass surgery significantly improved symptoms of GERD in obese adults.[205] Another study detected more overnight reflux in adults eating a late evening meal than in adults eating an earlier evening meal. The difference was especially obvious in overweight adults.[206]

Current evidence generally does not support (or refute) the use of dietary changes to treat GER beyond infancy. Expert opinion suggests that children and adolescents with GERD should avoid caffeine, chocolate, alcohol, and spicy foods if they provoke symptoms.[207–210] Based on the current epidemic of obesity in the United States, and the concordant increase in GERD, at least in adults, it is logical that reducing or eliminating obesity likely decreases GER. Exposure to tobacco should be avoided because, among many reasons, it has been linked to adenocarcinoma of the esophagus in adults, and more importantly, to esophagitis development in children.[211] Although it is recommended that lifestyle changes should be implemented, irrespective of additional therapeutic interventions (i.e., medication), it is not known whether any lifestyle changes have an additive benefit in pediatric patients receiving pharmacological therapy.

The effectiveness of positioning for treatment of GERD in children over 1 year of age has not been comprehensively evaluated. It is unclear whether the benefits of positional therapy identified in adults and in infants <1 year can be extrapolated to children in general.[212] Some investigations demonstrated that adults who sleep with the head of the bed elevated have fewer, shorter episodes of reflux, and fewer reflux symptoms.[213] It is likely therefore that adolescents, and potentially older children, similar to their adult counterparts, may benefit from the left lateral decubitus-sleeping position with elevation of the head of the bed.

PHARMACOLOGICAL INTERVENTION

The major pharmacological agents currently used for treating GERD in children are gastric acid buffers, mucosal surface barriers, and gastric anti-secretory agents. Since the withdrawal of cisapride from commercial availability in most countries, prokinetic agents have been less frequently used, though domperidone is commercially available in Canada and Europe.

Comparisons between pharmacological agents for GERD in children have been impaired by small sample size, absence of controls, and use of unreliable endpoints such as esophageal histology.

Buffering Agents

Antacids directly buffer gastric contents, thereby reducing heartburn and potentially healing esophagitis. On-demand use of antacids may provide rapid symptom relief in some children and adolescents with non-erosive reflux disease. Although this commonly used practice appears to carry little risk, it has not been formally studied in children.[82] Intensive, high-dose antacid regimens (e.g., magnesium hydroxide and aluminum hydroxide; 700 mmol/1.73 m^2/day) are as effective as cimetidine for treating peptic esophagitis in children aged 2–42 months.[214] No studies of antacids to date have employed combined esophageal pH/MII to assess outcome. Prolonged treatment with aluminum-containing antacids significantly increases plasma aluminum in infants, and some studies report plasma aluminum concentrations close to those that have been associated with osteopenia, microcytic anemia, and neurotoxicity.[215] Milk-alkali syndrome, a triad of hypercalcemia, alkalosis, and renal failure, can occur due to chronic or high-dose ingestion of calcium carbonate. Although this is much less common than it was in the era before acid-suppressive drugs, all antacid buffering agents should be used with particular caution in infants and young children. Because safe, convenient alternatives are available that are more acceptable to patients, chronic antacid therapy is generally not recommended for patients with GERD.

Most *surface-protective agents* contain either alginate or sucralfate. Alginates are insoluble salts of alginic acid, a component of algal cell walls. In older studies of alginic acid therapy in pediatric patients with GERD, the liquid preparations used also contained buffering agents, making it difficult to isolate the effect of the surface-protective agent itself.[216] Efficacy in these studies has varied widely. In one clinical study, a commercial liquid preparation containing only sodium/magnesium alginate significantly decreased the mean frequency and severity of vomiting in infants compared to placebo.[217,218] Another placebo-controlled study of this preparation in infants showed that although symptoms improved with therapy, the only objective change on combined pH/MII evaluation was a marginal decrease in the height of reflux in the esophagus.[219] Alginate is also available as tablets, and is useful for on-demand treatment of symptoms.

Sucralfate is a compound of sucrose, sulfate, and aluminum that, in an acid environment, forms a gel that binds to the exposed mucosa of peptic erosions. In adults, sucralfate (1 g po QID) decreased symptoms and promoted healing of non-erosive esophagitis.[220] The only randomized comparison study in children demonstrates that sucralfate was as effective as cimetidine for treatment of esophagitis.[221] The available data are less than adequate for evidence-based guidelines that provide recommendations on safety or efficacy of sucralfate in the treatment of GERD in infants and children, particularly the risk of aluminum toxicity with long-term use.

None of the surface agents is recommended as sole treatment for severe symptoms or erosive esophagitis. Moreover, the long-term or prolonged use of the surface agents, even as adjunctive therapy for GERD-related symptoms and esophageal disease, is not advised.

Histamine-2 Receptor Antagonists (H$_2$RAs)

H$_2$RAs decrease acid secretion by inhibiting histamine-2 receptors on gastric parietal cells. One dose of ranitidine (5 mg/kg) has been shown to increase gastric pH for 9–10 hours in infants.[222] Pharmacokinetic studies in 4–11-year-old children suggest that peak plasma ranitidine concentration occurs 2.5 hours after dosing with a half-life of 2 hours. Gastric pH begins to increase within 30 minutes of administration and the effect lasts for 6 hours.[223] In an infant study, ranitidine (2 mg/kg per dose orally) reduced the time that gastric pH was below 4.0 by 44% when given twice daily and by 90% when given three times per day.[224] Tachyphylaxis to intravenous ranitidine has been observed after 6 weeks, and tolerance to oral H$_2$RAs in adults is well recognized.[225–227] A number of placebo-controlled, randomized adult trials demonstrated that cimetidine, ranitidine, and famotidine are all superior to placebo for relief of symptoms and healing of esophageal mucosa.[228–230] However, the efficacy of H$_2$RAs in achieving mucosal healing is much greater in mild esophagitis than in severe esophagitis.[231] In infants and children with erosive esophagitis, significant improvement in clinical and histopathology scores was demonstrated in the cimetidine-treated group compared to the placebo group.[232] More recently, a randomized controlled trial of 24 children with mild to moderate esophagitis demonstrated that nizatidine (10 mg/kg/day) was more effective than placebo for the healing of esophagitis and symptom relief.[233] No randomized controlled studies in children demonstrate the efficacy of ranitidine or famotidine for the treatment of esophagitis; however, clinical practice guidelines suggest that these agents are as effective as cimetidine and nizatidine.[2] Extrapolation of the results of a large number of adult studies to older children and adolescents suggests that H$_2$RAs may be used in these patients for the treatment of GERD symptoms and for healing esophagitis, although H$_2$RAs are less effective than PPI for both symptom relief and healing of esophagitis.[216,228,234]

The fairly rapid tachyphylaxis that develops with H$_2$RAs is a drawback to chronic use. In some infants, H$_2$RA therapy causes a number of side effects including: irritability, head banging, headache, and somnolence. These symptoms often can be interpreted as ongoing symptoms of GERD and could result in an inappropriate increase in dosage. Other side effects include liver disease and gynecomastia.[235–237] Other adverse effects of suppression of gastric acid are discussed in the section "Proton Pump Inhibitors."

Proton Pump Inhibitors

PPIs inhibit acid secretion by blocking Na$^+$,K$^+$-ATPase, the final common pathway of parietal cell acid secretion, often called the proton pump. Studies in adults have shown that PPI therapy produces higher and faster healing rates for erosive esophagitis than H$_2$RAs. Although there have been no head-to-head clinical trials in children comparing the H$_2$RAs to PPIs, data strongly suggest that PPIs are superior (see Figure 12–5). The superior efficacy of PPIs is largely due to their ability to maintain intragastric pH at or above 4 for longer periods and to inhibit meal-induced acid secretion, a characteristic not shared by H$_2$RAs. In contrast with H$_2$RAs, the effect of PPIs does decrease with chronic or long-term use. The potent suppression of acid secretion by PPIs also results in decrease of 24-hour intragastric volumes, thereby facilitating gastric emptying and decreasing the volume of reflux.[238]

PPIs currently approved for use in children in North America are omeprazole, lansoprazole, esomeprazole, pantoprazole, and rabeprazole. In Europe, omeprazole, lansoprazole, and esomeprazole are approved. To date, no PPI has been approved for use in infants <1 year of age in either North America or Europe.

Children 1–10 years of age appear to have a greater metabolic capacity, due to their hepatic functionality, for some PPIs than adolescents and adults. Studies demonstrated that pediatric patients ≤10 years of age require higher per kilogram doses to attain the same acid-blocking effect, or area under the curve.[239–241] However, these observations may not apply to each of the PPIs.[242] There are few pharmacokinetic data for PPIs in infants, but studies indicate that infants <6 months may have a *lower* per kilogram dose requirement than older children and adolescents.[243,244]

Interestingly, there is a great debate among pediatric gastroenterologists and pediatricians about the pros and cons of pharmacological management in the <12-month-old population with suspected GERD. The number of PPI prescriptions written for infants has increased many-fold in recent years despite the absence of evidence for acid-related disorders in the great majority.[33,245,246] The Global Consensus Committee wrestled with this area enthusiastically but without final definitive decisions due to the lack of data. Infant responses to many stimuli, including GER, are nonspecific and need to be characterized with careful, thoughtful, and sensitive questioning by the healthcare provider.[32] Two recently published double-blind, randomized, placebo-controlled trials of PPI efficacy in infants with GERD-like symptoms showed opposite findings—one study demonstrated that PPI and placebo produced similar improvement in crying and the other showed a significant reduction in GERD-related symptoms including crying over the study duration.[13,40] Thus, to date, placebo-controlled treatment trials with PPIs in which enrollment was based on "typical" GERD symptoms have demonstrated conflicting outcomes when evaluating symptom improvement in infants.

Erosive esophagitis healing rates of H₂RAs and PPIs in children

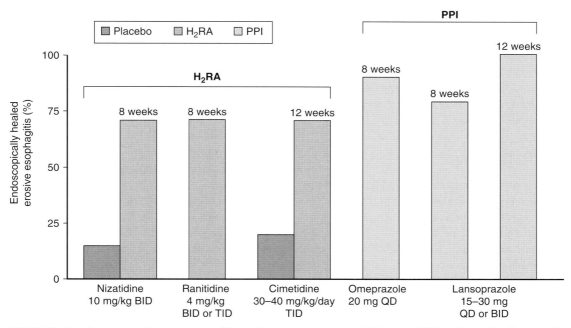

FIGURE 12–5 ■ Comparison of erosive esophagitis healing rates comparing an H₂RA versus PPI in children. The figure on the left demonstrates that the H₂RAs heal erosive esophagitis in up to 75% of patients, and are clearly superior to placebo, that is, nizatidine and cimetidine, in placebo-controlled trials of 8–12-week duration. However, the PPIs omeprazole or lansoprazole heal the esophageal mucosa (resolve erosions) in up to 100% of patients by 12-week duration.

This result may be due to a lack of specificity of symptom-based diagnosis of GERD, especially with esophagitis, in this age group (see above discussion on history). However, this may also be due the quality of the case selection, the dose of the PPI, the study duration, and the outcome variables. More research in this infant population with suspect GERD is clearly indicated.

Side effects occur in up to 14% of children taking PPIs.[247,248,161] The most common are headache, diarrhea, constipation, and nausea, each occurring in 2–7%. These often resolve with decreased dose or change to a different PPI. Parietal cell hyperplasia and occasional fundic gland polyps are benign changes that result from PPI-induced acid suppression and hypergastrinemia.[249–251] Enterochromaffin-like cell hyperplasia also occurs as a function of acid suppression. A prospective study monitoring treated patients for up to 2 years, and retrospective studies of patients treated for up to 11 years, has found only milder grades of enterochromaffin-like cell hyperplasia.[252–254] A more recent retrospective study using more sensitive staining techniques showed ECL hyperplasia in the gastric body in almost half of children receiving long-term PPI continuously for a median of 2.84 years (up to 10.8 years); the hyperplasia was of the lowest two grades (not clinically significant), and no patient developed atrophic gastritis, or carcinoid tumors.[161,252]

Increasing evidence suggests that acid suppression by H₂RA or PPI may increase rates of community-acquired pneumonia in adults and children, gastroenteritis in children, and candidemia and necrotizing enterocolitis in preterm infants.[255–260] In one study, PPI use was associated with bacterial enterocolitis in adults; doubling of the PPI dose increased the risk.[261] PPIs have been shown to alter the gastric and intestinal bacterial flora of adults, but this has only rarely been shown to cause clinical disease.[262] The effect of PPI therapy on the GI flora of infants and children, or the consequences of any alteration in flora, has not been evaluated fully and critically requires studies to address this potential risk.

Deficiency of vitamin B₁₂ has been found in adults over 65 years of age chronically treated with PPI, probably as a result of gastric achlorhydria.[263] A recent study of adults in the United Kingdom showed a significantly increased incidence of hip fractures that was related to dose and duration of acid suppression.[264] It is important to note that this observation, or for that matter any evidence of bone demineralization, has not yet been documented in pediatric patients. In retrospective case review, 18 cases of biopsy-proven PPI-induced acute interstitial nephritis causing acute renal failure were reported, and the authors suggest this entity may go unrecognized as "unclassified acute renal failure".[265] Despite the small sizes of the studies, and lack of prospective data, PPIs are considered one of the most common causes of acute interstitial nephritis in adults.[266] This adverse effect is considered to be an idiosyncratic reaction, more frequent in the elderly, for unclear reasons. Animal studies suggest that acid suppression may predispose to the development of food allergy, but this remains to be confirmed by human studies.[267] None of these adverse events have been demonstrated in pediatric patients receiving PPIs.

Prokinetic Therapy

Cisapride is a mixed serotonergic agent that facilitates the release of acetylcholine at synapses in the myenteric plexus, thus increasing gastric emptying and improving esophageal and intestinal peristalsis.[268–274] After cisapride was found to produce prolongation of the QTc interval on electrocardiogram, a finding increasing the risk for sudden death, its use was restricted to limited-access programs supervised by a pediatric gastroenterologist and to patients in clinical trials, safety studies, or registries.

Domperidone and metoclopramide are antidopaminergic agents that facilitate gastric emptying. A recent systematic review of studies on domperidone identified only four RCTs in children, none providing "robust evidence" for efficacy of domperidone in pediatric GERD.[275] Domperidone occasionally causes extrapyramidal central nervous system side effects and rarely produces QTc prolongation on electrocardiogram.[276,277] Metoclopramide has cholinergic and mixed serotonergic effects. A meta-analysis of seven randomized controlled trials of metoclopramide in developmentally normal children 1 month to 2 years of age with symptoms of GER found that metoclopramide reduced daily symptoms and the RI in children 1 month to 2 years of age but was associated with significant side effects.[212] Another study found that metoclopramide and placebo equally reduced symptom scores of infants with GER. However, metoclopramide did reduce the RI on 24-hour pH probe monitoring but did not normalize it.[278] Metoclopramide commonly produces adverse side effects in infants and children, particularly lethargy, irritability, gynecomastia, and extrapyramidal reactions and has caused permanent tardive dyskinesia.[279–282]

Bethanechol, a direct cholinergic agonist, studied in a few controlled trials has uncertain efficacy and a high incidence of side effects in children with GERD.[281,283,284] Erythromycin, a dopamine receptor antagonist, is sometimes used in patients with gastroparesis to hasten gastric emptying. Its role in therapy of GER and GERD has not been investigated. Baclofen is a gamma-amino-butyric-acid receptor agonist that reduces both acid and non-acid reflux in healthy adults and in adults with GERD (Table 12–3).[285] In children, it was shown to accelerate gastric emptying for 2 hours after dosing, without any deleterious effect on LES resting pressure or esophageal peristalsis.[286] In a small group of children with GERD and NI, it was reported to decrease the frequency of emesis.[287] Although no side effects were noted in one study, baclofen is known to cause dyspeptic symptoms, drowsiness, dizziness, and fatigue, and to lower the threshold for seizures.

Table 12–3.

Baclofen Reduces Both TLESRs and Acid Reflux in Children with GERD*

Esophageal Motility and Acid GER	Placebo Group		Baclofen Group	
	Control Period	Test Period	Control Period	Test Period
Number of TLESRs	6.0 ± 0.8	5.3 ± 0.6	7.3 ± 1.5	3.6 ± 1.2[†]
Change (%)	−6 [−38%, −18%]		−67 [−95%, −33%][†]	
Number of TLESRs + acid GER	1.9 ± 0.4	1.9 ± 0.4	4.2 ± 0.7[‡]	1.7 ± 1.0[†]
Change (%)	0 [−38%, +63%]		−83 [−100%, −75%][†]	

Data expressed as mean ± standard error of mean, or median (interquartile range). Patients intubated with manometric/pH assembly and given 250 mL cow's milk. Esophageal motility and pH measured for 2 hours (control period). Baclofen or placebo administered. Measurements performed for another 2 hours (test period). N = 30 (18 males, 12 females; mean age 10.0 ± 0.8 years). The table demonstrates that in a placebo-controlled trial, baclofen was able to significantly reduce transient lower esophageal sphincter relaxations (TLESRs) compared to control, that is, placebo group. In addition, the table further demonstrates that Baclofen significantly decreases TLESRs and acid reflux compared to placebo in this small cohort of children.
Randomized, double-blind, placebo-controlled trial.
[†]*p < 0.05.*
[‡]*p < 0.01.*

At present, although the "class of agents" holds much promise for new reflux inhibitors, the present side effect profile may preclude its routine use.[2,288,289] Thus, despite the ongoing widespread use of prokinetics in the pediatric provider community, the combined NASPGHAN and ESPGHAN committee proposed that there is insufficient evidence to justify the routine use of domperidone, baclofen, cisapride, metoclopramide, erythromycin, or bethanechol for GERD in pediatric patients.[2]

Anti-reflux Surgery

Fundoplication prevents GER by increasing the LES baseline pressure, decreasing the number of TLESRs and the nadir pressure during swallow-induced relaxation, increasing the length of the esophagus that is intra-abdominal, accentuating the angle of His, and reducing a hiatal hernia if present.[290] Fundoplication usually eliminates GER, including physiological reflux.[291] However, surgery does not correct poor esophageal clearance or improve gastric emptying.[17,292,293]

Most of the literature on surgical therapy in children with GERD consists of retrospective case series in which documentation of the diagnosis of GERD and details of previous medical therapy are deficient, making it difficult to assess the indications for and responses to surgery.[294–296] Children with underlying conditions predisposing to the most severe GERD comprise a large percentage of most surgical series, further confounding efforts to determine the benefits versus risks of surgical anti-reflux procedures in specific patient populations. The absence of systematic postoperative evaluation, including objective testing with pH or impedance studies and endoscopy, further complicates the assessment of surgical outcomes in most series.[290,293,297]

In general, outcomes of anti-reflux surgery have been more carefully evaluated in adults than in children. In one study, at a mean of 20 months after surgery, 61% of adults were satisfied with their outcome; 32% were taking medications for heartburn, 11% required esophageal dilatation, and 7% had repeat surgery.[298,299] This study found that a substantial number of patients underwent fundoplication for questionable reasons. In another study of patients relieved of typical reflux symptoms postoperatively, up to two-thirds developed new symptoms postoperatively, including excessive gas, abdominal bloating, increased flatus, dysphagia, difficulty with eructation, and vomiting.[299,300] In a large multicenter controlled study, 62% of adults were taking PPIs for reflux symptoms 7 years after anti-reflux surgery.[300] In another study, 37% of adults were taking anti-reflux medications at a mean of 5.9 years following anti-reflux surgery.[301] Another study showed a similarly high surgical failure rate.

A large open randomized controlled trial compared the efficacy and safety of laparoscopic fundoplication versus esomeprazole (20 mg qd) for treatment of adults with GERD.[302] Short-term outcomes were reported in an interim analysis of data at 3 years. Over 90% of both the surgically and medically treated adults showed good to excellent symptom control; 10% of the surgical group had dysphagia while dysphagia was uncommon in the medically treated group. Quality of life measures were similar in both groups.[302] Death related to open or laparoscopic surgery occurs. In adults, the mortality of the first operation is reported to be between 1 in 1000 and 1 in 330.[303]

In operated children, those with NI have more than twice the complication rate, three times the morbidity, and four times the re-operation rate of children without NI.[304] Other studies show similar data.[305–308] One case series with a follow-up period of 3.5 years reported that over 30% of NI children had major complications or died within 30 days of anti-reflux surgery.[307,308] Twenty-five percent of those patients had operative failure and 71% had a return of one or more preoperative symptoms within a year of surgery.

Children with repaired esophageal atresia also have a high rate of operative failure, though not as high as those with NI.[309,310] Recurrence of GER after anti-reflux surgery in children with NI or EA may not be obvious and detection often requires a high index of suspicion, repeated evaluation over time, and use of more than one test.[307,310] In a recent retrospective review of 198 children, 74% of whom had underlying disorders, two-thirds had GERD symptoms or required medical treatment for GERD within 2 months of anti-reflux surgery.[294] Fundoplication in early infancy has a higher failure rate than fundoplication performed later in childhood and appears to be more frequent in children with associated anomalies.[311,312]

The impact of anti-reflux surgery on hospitalization for reflux-related events, especially adverse respiratory events, was reviewed using a large administrative database.[313] A significant reduction in the number of adverse respiratory events was observed in the year following surgery in those operated at <4 years of age (1.95 events/year versus 0.67 events/year). However, in older children, no benefit in the rate of hospitalization for adverse respiratory events was found. In fact, children with developmental delay were hospitalized more frequently in the year following anti-reflux surgery than before surgery.[313] In a recent pediatric study, Nissen fundoplication did not decrease hospital admissions for pneumonia, respiratory distress/apnea, or failure to thrive, even in those with underlying NI.[314]

Complications following anti-reflux surgery may be due to alterations in gastric volume and to altered gastric compliance and sensory responses that may persist from months to years. Symptoms include gas bloat syndrome, early satiety, dumping syndrome, and postoperative retching and gagging. In a postoperative study of otherwise healthy children, that is, with no underlying disorders, 36% had mild-moderate gas bloat symptoms, 32% were "very slow" to finish most meals, 28% were unable to burp or vomit, and 25% choked on some solids. Early and late operative failure may result from disruption of the wrap or slippage of the wrap into the chest.[306–308,315] In otherwise healthy children evaluated at a mean of 10 months (1–35 months) following anti-reflux surgery, 67% had "no complaints" but one-third had objective evidence of operative failure.[316] Operative complications include splenic or esophageal laceration, each of which occurs in about 0.2% of pediatric cases.[317] In children, those with underlying disorders, such as NI, are at a substantially greater risk for surgical mortality as are those in early infancy.[304,318] Mortality due to surgery in children without NI is difficult to assess because of the heterogeneous population in most surgical studies.

Laparoscopic Nissen fundoplication (LNF) has largely replaced open Nissen fundoplication (ONF) as the preferred anti-reflux surgery for adults and children, due to its decreased morbidity, shorter hospital stays, and fewer perioperative problems.[296,297,312,315,319,320] However, LNF is attended by as high a failure rate as open surgery in adults.[297,315] In a randomized study of ONF versus LNF in adults, LNF patients had a higher incidence of disabling dysphagia.[321] In a series of 456 children undergoing surgery <5 years of age, Diaz et al.[312] reported that those with LNF had a higher re-operation rate than those with ONF. Average time to re-operation with LNF was 11 months versus 17 months for ONF. In children with one to three co-morbidities, the probability of re-operation was 18–24% after LNF, compared with 6–16% for ONF.[312]

Total esophagogastric dissociation is an operative procedure that is useful in selected children with NI or other conditions causing life-threatening aspiration during oral feedings. The operation has been used either after failed fundoplication or as a primary procedure.[322,323] The esophagogastric disconnection eliminates all GER while allowing tube feedings oral supplementation up to the patient's tolerance. This is a technically demanding operation, and because of the fragile nature of the children involved—most of whom have histories of aspiration and pulmonary compromise—it carries significant morbidity.[322,323]

Endoluminal endoscopic gastroplication has been described in children as an alternative to surgical fundoplication. When a group of 16 children with GERD refractory to or dependent on medical therapy was evaluated after endoluminal gastroplication, 4 had recurrent

symptoms requiring a repeat procedure 2–24 months postoperatively. Three years after surgery, nine patients (56%) were taking no anti-reflux medication. Longer term studies in adults have shown little or no difference in procedure time or failure rate between endoluminal and surgical anti-reflux procedures.[324,325] In some studies, sham-operated patients have done as well as operated patients.[326,327] Other endoscopic GERD treatments have not been studied in children.[290]

The annual number of anti-reflux operations has been on the increase in the United States, especially in children under 2 years of age.[318] In contrast, in adults, rates of fundoplication are declining in the United States and have dropped 30% from their peak in 1999.[297] The greatest decline is in teaching hospitals and in young adult patients.

Anti-reflux surgery may be of benefit in children with confirmed GERD who have failed optimal medical therapy, are dependent on medical therapy over a long period of time, are significantly non-adherent with medical therapy, or have life-threatening complications of GERD. Children with respiratory complications including asthma and recurrent aspiration related to GERD are generally considered most likely to benefit from anti-reflux surgery when medical therapy fails, but further study is required to confirm this. Children with underlying disorders predisposing to the most severe GERD are at the highest risk for operative morbidity and operative failure. Prior to surgery, it is essential to rule out non-GERD causes of symptoms, and ensure that the diagnosis of chronic, relapsing GERD is firmly established. It is important to provide families with appropriate education and a realistic understanding of the potential complications of surgery, including symptom recurrence.

When pharmacotherapy is required, H$_2$RAs may be effective for mild GERD in children. However, tachyphylaxis develops quickly with symptom recurrence within days to a few weeks of treatment. Therefore, PPIs are becoming the preferred treatment for GERD in infants and children. PPIs have been shown in pediatric studies to be safe and effective. Omeprazole at doses ranging from 0.5 to 4 mg/kg has been shown to decrease GERD symptoms in children after only 14 days.[157] Lansoprazole given at doses of 15 or 30 mg once or twice daily, based on weight, resulted in resolution of erosive esophagitis after 3 months of treatment in one study.[248] Recently, esomeprazole has been shown to improve GERD-related symptoms and resolve extraesophageal manifestations after 8–12 weeks of therapy in children 12–17 years of age.[89] In general, studies have suggested beginning PPI treatment with a dose of 1 mg/kg/day divided in one or two doses. Prokinetics such as metoclopramide are effective in approximately 50% of children with GERD; however,

Table 12–4.

Drugs Demonstrated to be Effective in Gastroesophageal Reflux Disease*

Type of Medicine	Recommended Oral Dosage	Adverse Effects/Precautions
Histamine-2 receptor antagonists		
Cimetidine (Tagamet)	Safety and effectiveness have not been established in children <16 years (adult dose: 800 mg BID or 400 mg QID)	Breast development in men, headache, diarrhea, dizziness; less commonly, agitation, anxiety, confusion, depression, disorientation, and hallucinations
Famotidine (Pepcid)	<3 months: 0.5 mg/kg/dose QD 3 months to <1 year: 0.5 mg/kg/dose BID 1–16 years: 1.0 mg/kg/day BID up to 40 mg BID (adult dose: 20 or 40 mg, BID)	Headache, dizziness, constipation, diarrhea, agitation (<1 year)
Nizatidine (Axid)	≥12 years:150 mg BID (adult dose: 150 mg BID)	Pyrexia (i.e., fevers), nasopharyngitis, diarrhea, vomiting, irritability, nasal congestion, cough
Ranitidine (Zantac)	1 month to 16 years: 5–10 mg/kg/day, divided BID (adult dose: 150 mg, BID or QID)	Headache, irregular heartbeats, dizziness, liver problems, rash, changes in the counts of blood cells in your blood, constipation, nausea, vomiting, possible allergic reaction including anaphylaxis
Proton pump inhibitors		
Esomeprazole (Nexium)	1–11 years: 10 or 20 mg, QD 12–17 years: 20 or 40 mg, QD (adult dose 20 or 40 mg, QD)	Headache, diarrhea, abdominal pain, nausea, somnolence
Lansoprazole (Prevacid)	1–11 years: ≤30 kg = 15 mg QD >30 kg = 30 mg QD (adult dose: 15 or 30 mg, QD)	Diarrhea, abdominal pain, nausea, constipation
Omeprazole (Prilosec)	1–16 years: 5 to < 10 kg = 5 mg QD 10 to < 20 kg = 10 mg QD ≥20 kg = 20 mg QD (adult dose 20 mg QD)	Respiratory system events, fever, headache, abdominal pain, nausea, diarrhea, vomiting, flatulence
Pantoprazole (Protonix)	No pediatric dose available (adult dose: 40 mg QD)	Headache, abdominal pain, liver function tests abnormal, nausea, vomiting
Rabeprazole (Aciphex)	≥12 years = 20 mg QD (adult dose: 20 mg QD)	Pain, pharyngitis, flatulence, infection, constipation

Sources:
1. Drugs@FDA. Food and Drug Administration. Available at http://www.accessdata.fda.gov/scripts/cder/drugsatfda/index.cfm?fuseaction=Search.SearchResults_Browse&DrugInitial=Z.
2. PDRhealth Prescription Drugs. Available at http://www.pdrhealth.com/drugs/drugs-index.as.
*Drug information updated October 2009.

they can be associated with neurologic side effects. Thus, usage should be limited to children with regurgitation-predominant symptoms. Finally, anti-reflux surgery should be considered in children with complications of GERD such as aspiration (with or without oral–pharyngeal function), Barrett esophagus, and esophageal strictures. Predictors of fundoplication success are response to medical therapy and surgeon experience (Table 12–4).[78]

CONCLUSIONS

GERD:

- Is less easily diagnosed under 1 year of age wherein GER may occur instead.
- Can resolve in many children, particularly those <1 year of age, but tends to persist in older patients.
- Is diagnosed based on clinical suspicion (thorough history and physical examination) followed by a

course of empiric therapy, which often resolves symptoms. Diagnostic testing such as a GI series to rule out anatomic abnormalities or endoscopy for GI bleeding and refractory symptoms should be utilized as needed to rule out alternative diagnoses, complications, and predisposing conditions.

■ Is often treatable conservatively when mild. Suspected milk protein intolerance, which can masquerade as GERD in infancy, necessitates a trial of protein hydrolysate formula.

■ PPIs are superior for symptomatic relief and mucosal healing, and are safe for long-term use, with an adverse event profile similar to adults.

REFERENCES

1. Sherman PM, Hassall E, Fagundes-Neto U, et al. A global, evidence-based consensus on the definition of gastroesophageal reflux disease in the pediatric population. *Am J Gastroenterol.* 2009;104:1278–1295 [quiz 96].

2. Vandenplas Y, Rudolph CD, Di Lorenzo C, et al. Pediatric gastroesophageal reflux clinical practice guidelines: joint recommendations of the North American Society of Pediatric Gastroenterology, Hepatology, and Nutrition and the European Society of Pediatric Gastroenterology, Hepatology, and Nutrition. *J Pediatr Gastroenterol Nutr.* 2009;49: 498–547.

3. Martin AJ, Pratt N, Kennedy JD, et al. Natural history and familial relationships of infant spilling to 9 years of age. *Pediatrics.* 2002;109:1061–1067.

4. Nelson SP, Chen EH, Syniar GM, Christoffel KK. Prevalence of symptoms of gastroesophageal reflux during infancy. A pediatric practice-based survey. Pediatric Practice Research Group. *Arch Pediatr Adolesc Med.* 1997;151:569–572.

5. Vakil N, van Zanten SV, Kahrilas P, Dent J, Jones R. The Montreal definition and classification of gastroesophageal reflux disease: a global evidence-based consensus. *Am J Gastroenterol.* 2006;101:1900–1920 [quiz 43].

6. Kleinman L, Revicki DA, Flood E. Validation issues in questionnaires for diagnosis and monitoring of gastroesophageal reflux disease in children. *Curr Gastroenterol Rep.* 2006;8:230–236.

7. Stanford EA, Chambers CT, Craig KD. The role of developmental factors in predicting young children's use of a self-report scale for pain. *Pain.* 2006;120:16–23.

8. Deal L, Gold BD, Gremse DA, et al. Age-specific questionnaires distinguish GERD symptom frequency and severity in infants and young children: development and initial validation. *J Pediatr Gastroenterol Nutr.* 2005;41:178–185.

9. Gunasekaran TS, Dahlberg M, Ramesh P, Namachivayam G. Prevalence and associated features of gastroesophageal reflux symptoms in a Caucasian-predominant adolescent school population. *Dig Dis Sci.* 2008;53:2373–2379.

10. Gupta SK, Hassall E, Chiu YL, Amer F, Heyman MB. Presenting symptoms of nonerosive and erosive esophagitis in pediatric patients. *Dig Dis Sci.* 2006;51:858–863.

11. Orenstein SR, Shalaby TM, Cohn JF. Reflux symptoms in 100 normal infants: diagnostic validity of the infant gastroesophageal reflux questionnaire. *Clin Pediatr (Phila).* 1996;35:607–614.

12. Orenstein SR, McGowan JD. Efficacy of conservative therapy as taught in the primary care setting for symptoms suggesting infant gastroesophageal reflux. *J Pediatr.* 2008;152:310–314.

13. Orenstein SR, Hassall E, Furmaga-Jablonska W, Atkinson S, Raanan M. Multicenter, double-blind, randomized, placebo-controlled trial assessing the efficacy and safety of proton pump inhibitor lansoprazole in infants with symptoms of gastroesophageal reflux disease. *J Pediatr.* 2009;154:514–520 e4.

14. Jadcherla SR, Duong HQ, Hoffmann RG, Shaker R. Esophageal body and upper esophageal sphincter motor responses to esophageal provocation during maturation in preterm newborns. *J Pediatr.* 2003;143:31–38.

15. Jadcherla SR. Manometric evaluation of esophageal-protective reflexes in infants and children. *Am J Med.* 2003;115(suppl 3A):157S–160S.

16. Kawahara H, Dent J, Davidson G. Mechanisms responsible for gastroesophageal reflux in children [see comments]. *Gastroenterology.* 1997;113:399–408.

17. Kawahara H, Imura K, Yagi M, et al. Mechanisms underlying the antireflux effect of Nissen fundoplication in children. *J Pediatr Surg.* 1998;33:1618–1622.

18. Omari TI, Rommel N, Staunton E, et al. Paradoxical impact of body positioning on gastroesophageal reflux and gastric emptying in the premature neonate. *J Pediatr.* 2004;145:194–200.

19. Waring JP, Feiler MJ, Hunter JG, Smith CD, Gold BD. Childhood gastroesophageal reflux symptoms in adult patients. *J Pediatr Gastroenterol Nutr.* 2002;35:334–338.

20. El-Serag HB, Richardson P, Pilgrim P, Gilger MA. Determinants of gastroesophageal reflux disease in adults with a history of childhood gastroesophageal reflux disease. *Clin Gastroenterol Hepatol.* 2007;5:696–701.

21. El-Serag HB, Gilger M, Carter J, Genta RM, Rabeneck L. Childhood GERD is a risk factor for GERD in adolescents and young adults. *Am J Gastroenterol.* 2004;99: 806–812.

22. Chan FKL, Gold BD. Issues in acid-related disorders in children in Asian countries. *Aliment Pharmacol Ther.* 2007;3:15–19.

23. Vandenplas Y, Goyvaerts H, Helven R, Sacre L. Gastroesophageal reflux, as measured by 24-hour pH monitoring, in 509 healthy infants screened for risk of sudden infant death syndrome. *Pediatrics.* 1991;88:834–840.

24. Orenstein SR. Tests to assess symptoms of gastroesophageal reflux in infants and children. *J Pediatr Gastroenterol Nutr.* 2003;37(suppl 1):S29–S32.

25. Orenstein SR, Cohn JF, Shalaby TM, Kartan R. Reliability and validity of an infant gastroesophageal reflux questionnaire. *Clin Pediatr (Phila).* 1993;32:472–484.

26. Rasquin A, Di Lorenzo C, Forbes D, et al. Childhood functional gastrointestinal disorders: child/adolescent. *Gastroenterology.* 2006;130:1527–1537.

27. Chial HJ, Camilleri M, Williams DE, Litzinger K, Perrault J. Rumination syndrome in children and adolescents: diagnosis, treatment, and prognosis. *Pediatrics.* 2003;111:158–162.

28. Khan S, Hyman PE, Cocjin J, Di Lorenzo C. Rumination syndrome in adolescents. *J Pediatr.* 2000;136:528–531.

29. Hyman PE, Milla PJ, Benninga MA, Davidson GP, Fleisher DF, Taminiau J. Childhood functional gastrointestinal disorders: neonate/toddler. *Gastroenterology.* 2006;130:1519–1526.

30. Barr RG. Crying behavior and its importance in psychosocial development in children. In: Tremblay R, ed. *Encyclopedia of Early Childhood Development.* Montreal, Que.: Centre for Excellence for Early Childhood Development; 2006:1–10.

31. St James-Roberts I, Halil T. Infant crying patterns in the first year: normal community and clinical findings. *J Child Psychol Psychiatry.* 1991;32:951–968.

32. Hassall E. Talk is cheap, often effective: symptoms in infants often respond to non-pharmacologic measures. *J Pediatr.* 2008;152:301–303.

33. Orenstein SR, Hassall E. Infants and proton pump inhibitors: tribulations, no trials. *J Pediatr Gastroenterol Nutr.* 2007;45:395–398.

34. Ghaem M, Armstrong KL, Trocki O, Cleghorn GJ, Patrick MK, Shepherd RW. The sleep patterns of infants and young children with gastro-oesophageal reflux. *J Paediatr Child Health.* 1998;34:160–163.

35. Douglas PS. Excessive crying and gastro-oesophageal reflux disease in infants: misalignment of biology and culture. *Med Hypotheses.* 2005;64:887–898.

36. Omari T. Gastroesophageal reflux in infants: can a simple left side positioning strategy help this diagnostic and therapeutic conundrum? *Minerva Pediatr.* 2008;60:193–200.

37. Orenstein SR, Shalaby TM, Devandry SN, et al. Famotidine for infant gastro-oesophageal reflux: a multi-centre, randomized, placebo-controlled, withdrawal trial. *Aliment Pharmacol Ther.* 2003;17:1097–1107.

38. McKenna CJ, Mills JG, Goodwin C, Wood JR. Combination of ranitidine and cisapride in the treatment of reflux oesophagitis. *Eur J Gastroenterol Hepatol.* 1995;7:817–822.

39. Omari TI, Haslam RR, Lundborg P, Davidson GP. Effect of omeprazole on acid gastroesophageal reflux and gastric acidity in preterm infants with pathological acid reflux. *J Pediatr Gastroenterol Nutr.* 2007;44:41–44.

40. Omari T, Lundborg P, Sandstrom M, et al. Pharmacodynamics and systemic exposure of esomeprazole in preterm infants and term neonates with gastroesophageal reflux disease. *J Pediatr.* 2009;155:222–228.

41. Ashorn M, Ruuska T, Karikoski R, Laippala P. The natural course of gastroesophageal reflux disease in children. *Scand J Gastroenterol.* 2002;37:638–641.

42. Hassall E. Decisions in diagnosing and managing chronic gastroesophageal reflux disease in children. *J Pediatr.* 2005;146:S3–S12.

43. Deskin RW. Sandifer syndrome: a cause of torticollis in infancy. *Int J Pediatr Otorhinolaryngol.* 1995;32:183–185.

44. Frankel EA, Shalaby TM, Orenstein SR. Sandifer syndrome posturing: relation to abdominal wall contractions, gastroesophageal reflux, and fundoplication. *Dig Dis Sci.* 2006;51:635–640.

45. Theodoropoulos DS, Flockey RF, Boyce HW Jr. Sandifer's syndrome and gastro-oesophageal reflux disease [letter; comment]. *J Neurol Neurosurg Psychiatry.* 1999;66:805–806.

46. Tokuhara D, Yamano T, Okano Y. A case of Sandifer's syndrome: significance in the differential diagnosis of growth retardation. *J Paediatr Child Health.* 2008;44:311–312.

47. Stavroulaki P. Diagnostic and management problems of laryngopharyngeal reflux disease in children. *Int J Pediatr Otorhinolaryngol.* 2006;70:579–590.

48. Gilger MA. Pediatric otolaryngologic manifestations of gastroesophageal reflux disease. *Curr Gastroenterol Rep.* 2003;5:247–252.

49. Chang AB, Lasserson TJ, Gaffney J, Connor FL, Garske LA. Gastro-oesophageal reflux treatment for prolonged non-specific cough in children and adults. *Cochrane Database Syst Rev.* 2005:CD004823.

50. Chang AB, Lasserson TJ, Gaffney J, Connor FL, Garske LA. Gastro-oesophageal reflux treatment for prolonged non-specific cough in children and adults. *Cochrane Database Syst Rev.* 2005;18:CD004823.

51. Chang AB, Lasserson TJ, Kiljander TO, Connor FL, Gaffney JT, Garske LA. Systematic review and meta-analysis of randomised controlled trials of gastro-oesophageal reflux interventions for chronic cough associated with gastro-oesophageal reflux. *BMJ.* 2006;332:11–17.

52. Hancox RJ, Poulton R, Taylor DR, et al. Associations between respiratory symptoms, lung function and gastro-oesophageal reflux symptoms in a population-based birth cohort. *Respir Res.* 2006;7:142.

53. Cinquetti M, Micelli S, Voltolina C, Zoppi G. The pattern of gastroesophageal reflux in asthmatic children. *J Asthma.* 2002;39:135–142.

54. Eid NS. Gastroesophageal reflux is a major cause of lung disease-pro. *Pediatr Pulmonol Suppl.* 2004;26:194–196.

55. Gibson PG, Henry RL, Coughlan JL. Gastro-oesophageal reflux treatment for asthma in adults and children. *Cochrane Database Syst Rev.* 2003;(2):CD001496.

56. Gold BD. Asthma and gastroesophageal reflux disease in children: exploring the relationship. *J Pediatr.* 2005;146:S13–S20.

57. Harding SM. Acid reflux and asthma. *Curr Opin Pulm Med.* 2003;9:42–45.

58. Harding SM. Gastroesophageal reflux: a potential asthma trigger. *Immunol Allergy Clin North Am.* 2005;25:131–148.

59. Everett CF, Kastelik JA, Mulrennan SA, Morice AH. Predictors of therapy resistant asthma. *Thorax.* 2004;59:270–271 [author reply 1].

60. Dimarino M, Banwait K, Rattan S, Cohen S, DiMarino AJ. Beta3 adrenergic stimulation inhibits the opossum lower esophageal sphincter. *Gastroenterology.* 2002;123:1508–1515.

61. Abbasi S, Bhutani VK, Gerdes JS. Long-term pulmonary consequences of respiratory distress syndrome in preterm infants treated with exogenous surfactant. *J Pediatr.* 1993;122:446–452.

62. Debley JS, Carter ER, Redding GJ. Prevalence and impact of gastroesophageal reflux in adolescents with asthma: a population-based study. *Pediatr Pulmonol.* 2006 May;41(5):475–481

63. Khoshoo V, Haydel R Jr. Effect of antireflux treatment on asthma exacerbations in nonatopic children. *J Pediatr Gastroenterol Nutr.* 2007;44:331–335.

64. Malagelada JR. Review article: supra-oesophageal manifestations of gastro-oesophageal reflux disease. *Aliment Pharmacol Ther.* 2004;19(suppl 1):43–48.

65. Harding SM. Nocturnal asthma: role of nocturnal gastroesophageal reflux. *Chronobiol Int.* 1999;16:641–662.

66. Sontag SJ, O'Connell S, Miller TQ, Bernsen M, Seidel J. Asthmatics have more nocturnal gasping and reflux symptoms than nonasthmatics, and they are related to bedtime eating. *Am J Gastroenterol.* 2004;99:789–796.

67. Herbst JJ, Minton SD, Book LS. Gastroesophageal reflux causing respiratory distress and apnea in newborn infants. *J Pediatr.* 1979;95:763–768.

68. Mousa H, Woodley FW, Metheney M, Hayes J. Testing the association between gastroesophageal reflux and apnea in infants. *J Pediatr Gastroenterol Nutr.* 2005;41:169–177.

69. Kohelet D, Boaz M, Serour F, Cohen-Adad N, Arbel E, Gorenstein A. Esophageal pH study and symptomatology of gastroesophageal reflux in newborn infants. *Am J Perinatol.* 2004;21:85–91.

70. Salvatore S, Hauser B, Vandemaele K, Novario R, Vandenplas Y. Gastroesophageal reflux disease in infants: how much is predictable with questionnaires, pH-metry, endoscopy and histology? *J Pediatr Gastroenterol Nutr.* 2005;40:210–215.

71. Slocum C, Hibbs AM, Martin RJ, Orenstein SR. Infant apnea and gastroesophageal reflux: a critical review and framework for further investigation. *Curr Gastroenterol Rep.* 2007;9:219–224.

72. Wenzl TG, Schenke S, Peschgens T, Silny J, Heimann G, Skopnik H. Association of apnea and nonacid gastroesophageal reflux in infants: investigations with the intraluminal impedance technique. *Pediatr Pulmonol.* 2001;31:144–149.

73. Bhat RY, Rafferty GF, Hannam S, Greenough A. Acid gastroesophageal reflux in convalescent preterm infants: effect of posture and relationship to apnea. *Pediatr Res.* 2007;62:620–623.

74. Thach BT. Maturation of cough and other reflexes that protect the fetal and neonatal airway. *Pulm Pharmacol Ther.* 2007;20:365–370.

75. Molloy EJ, Di Fiore JM, Martin RJ. Does gastroesophageal reflux cause apnea in preterm infants? *Biol Neonate.* 2005;87:254–261.

76. McGovern MC, Smith MB. Causes of apparent life threatening events in infants: a systematic review. *Arch Dis Child.* 2004;89:1043–1048.

77. Semeniuk J, Kaczmarski M, Wasilewska J, Nowowiejska B. Is acid gastroesophageal reflux in children with ALTE etiopathogenetic factor of life threatening symptoms? *Adv Med Sci.* 2007;52:213–221.

78. Rudolph CD, Mazur LJ, Liptak GS, et al. Guidelines for evaluation and treatment of gastroesophageal reflux in infants and children: recommendations of the North American Society for Pediatric Gastroenterology and Nutrition. *J Pediatr Gastroenterol Nutr.* 2001;32: S1–S31.

79. Faybush EM, Fass R. Gastroesophageal reflux disease in noncardiac chest pain. *Gastroenterol Clin North Am.* 2004;33:41–54.

80. Cremonini F, Wise J, Moayyedi P, Talley NJ. Diagnostic and therapeutic use of proton pump inhibitors in non-cardiac chest pain: a metaanalysis. *Am J Gastroenterol.* 2005;100:1226–1232.

81. Wang WH, Huang JQ, Zheng GF, et al. Is proton pump inhibitor testing an effective approach to diagnose gastroesophageal reflux disease in patients with noncardiac chest pain? A meta-analysis. *Arch Intern Med.* 2005;165:1222–1228.

82. Diaz DM, Winter HS, Colletti RB, et al. Knowledge, attitudes and practice styles of North American pediatricians regarding gastroesophageal reflux disease. *J Pediatr Gastroenterol Nutr.* 2007;45:56–64.

83. Richter JE. Chest pain and gastroesophageal reflux disease. *J Clin Gastroenterol.* 2000;30:S39–S41.

84. Irwin RS. Chronic cough due to gastroesophageal reflux disease: ACCP evidence-based clinical practice guidelines. *Chest.* 2006;129:80S–94S.

85. Ours TM, Kavuru MS, Schilz RJ, Richter JE. A prospective evaluation of esophageal testing and a double-blind, randomized study of omeprazole in a diagnostic and therapeutic algorithm for chronic cough. *Am J Gastroenterol.* 1999;94:3131–3138.

86. Talley NJ, Vakil N. Guidelines for the management of dyspepsia. *Am J Gastroenterol.* 2005;100:2324–2337.

87. Numans ME, Lau J, de Wit NJ, Bonis PA. Short-term treatment with proton-pump inhibitors as a test for gastroesophageal reflux disease: a meta-analysis of diagnostic test characteristics. *Ann Intern Med.* 2004;140: 518–527.

88. Talley NJ, Locke GR, Lahr BD, et al. Predictors of the placebo response in functional dyspepsia. *Aliment Pharmacol Ther.* 2006;23:923–936.

89. Gold BD, Gunasekaran T, Tolia V, et al. Safety and symptom improvement with esomeprazole in adolescents with gastroesophageal reflux disease. *J Pediatr Gastroenterol Nutr.* 2007;45:520–529.

90. Tolia V, Bishop PR, Tsou VM, Gremse D, Soffer EF, Comer GM. Multicenter, randomized, double-blind study comparing 10, 20 and 40 mg pantoprazole in children (5–11 years) with symptomatic gastroesophageal reflux disease. *J Pediatr Gastroenterol Nutr.* 2006;42: 384–391.

91. Kahrilas PJ, Falk GW, Johnson DA, et al. Esomeprazole improves healing and symptom resolution as compared with omeprazole in reflux oesophagitis patients: a randomized controlled trial. The Esomeprazole Study Investigators. *Aliment Pharmacol Ther.* 2000;14: 1249–1258.

92. Richter JE, Kahrilas PJ, Sontag SJ, Kovacs TO, Huang B, Pencyla JL. Comparing lansoprazole and omeprazole in onset of heartburn relief: results of a randomized, controlled trial in erosive esophagitis patients. *Am J Gastroenterol.* 2001;96:3089–3098.

93. Vakil N. Review article: how valuable are proton-pump inhibitors in establishing a diagnosis of gastro-oesophageal reflux disease? *Aliment Pharmacol Ther.* 2005;22(suppl 1):64–69.

94. Stephen TC, Younoszai MK, Massey MP, Fellows RA. Diagnosis of gastroesophageal reflux in pediatrics. *J Ky Med Assoc.* 1994;92:188–191.

95. Meyers WF, Roberts CC, Johnson DG, Herbst JJ. Value of tests for evaluation of gastroesophageal reflux in children. *J Pediatr Surg.* 1985;20:515–520.

96. Aksglaede K, Pedersen JB, Lange A, Funch-Jensen P, Thommesen P. Gastro-esophageal reflux demonstrated by radiography in infants less than 1 year of age. Comparison with pH monitoring. *Acta Radiol.* 2003;44:136–138.

97. Simanovsky N, Buonomo C, Nurko S. The infant with chronic vomiting: the value of the upper GI series. *Pediatr Radiol.* 2002;32:549–550 [discussion 51].

98. Di Lorenzo C, Piepsz A, Ham H, Cadranel S. Gastric emptying with gastro-oesophageal reflux. *Arch Dis Child.* 1987;62:449–453.

99. Tolia V, Kauffman RE. Comparison of evaluation of gastroesophageal reflux in infants using different feedings during intraesophageal pH monitoring. *J Pediatr Gastroenterol Nutr.* 1990;10:426–429.

100. Vandenplas Y, Derde MP, Piepsz A. Evaluation of reflux episodes during simultaneous esophageal pH monitoring and gastroesophageal reflux scintigraphy in children. *J Pediatr Gastroenterol Nutr.* 1992;14:256–260.

101. Ravelli AM, Panarotto MB, Verdoni L, Consolati V, Bolognini S. Pulmonary aspiration shown by scintigraphy in gastroesophageal reflux-related respiratory disease. *Chest.* 2006;130:1520–1526.

102. Gleeson K, Eggli DF, Maxwell SL. Quantitative aspiration during sleep in normal subjects. *Chest.* 1997;111:1266–1272.

103. Farina R, Pennisi F, La Rosa M, et al. Contrast-enhanced colour-Doppler sonography versus pH-metry in the diagnosis of gastro-oesophageal reflux in children. *Radiol Med.* 2008. Jun;113:591–598. Epub 2008.

104. Jang HS, Lee JS, Lim GY, Choi BG, Choi GH, Park SH. Correlation of color Doppler sonographic findings with pH measurements in gastroesophageal reflux in children. *J Clin Ultrasound.* 2001;29:212–217.

105. Adhami T, Richter JE. Twenty-four hour pH monitoring in the assessment of esophageal function. *Semin Thorac Cardiovasc Surg.* 2001;13:241–254.

106. Ahmed T, Vaezi MF. The role of pH monitoring in extraesophageal gastroesophageal reflux disease. *Gastrointest Endosc Clin N Am.* 2005;15:319–331.

107. Badriul H, Vandemaele K, Vandenplas Y. Esophageal pH monitoring in infants: elimination of gastric buffering does not modify reflux index [letter; in process citation]. *J Pediatr Gastroenterol Nutr.* 1999;29:627.

108. Colletti RB, Christie DL, Orenstein SR. Statement of the North American Society for Pediatric Gastroenterology and Nutrition (NASPGN). Indications for pediatric esophageal pH monitoring. *J Pediatr Gastroenterol Nutr.* 1995;21:253–262.

109. Colletti RB. Esophageal pH monitoring in infants and children. *Pediatrics.* 1996;98:515.

110. Vandenplas Y, de Roy C, Sacre L. Cisapride decreases prolonged episodes of reflux in infants. *J Pediatr Gastroenterol Nutr.* 1991;12:44–47.

111. Vandenplas Y, Bury F, Cadranel S, et al. Draft protocol for oesophageal pH monitoring. pH Monitoring Working-group of the Belgian Group of Paediatric Gastroenterology and Nutrition. *Acta Gastroenterol Belg.* 1991;54:195–200.

112. Vandenplas Y, Diericx A, Blecker U, Lanciers S, Deneyer M. Esophageal pH monitoring data during chest physiotherapy. *J Pediatr Gastroenterol Nutr.* 1991;13:23–26.

113. Gunnarsdottir A, Stenstrom P, Arnbjornsson E. 48-Hour wireless oesophageal pH-monitoring in children: are two days better than one? *Eur J Pediatr Surg.* 2007;17:378–381.

114. Hochman JA, Favaloro-Sabatier J. Tolerance and reliability of wireless pH monitoring in children. *J Pediatr Gastroenterol Nutr.* 2005;41:411–415.

115. Fass R, Fennerty MB, Johnson C, Camargo L, Sampliner RE. Correlation of ambulatory 24-hour esophageal pH monitoring results with symptom improvement in patients with noncardiac chest pain due to gastroesophageal reflux disease. *J Clin Gastroenterol.* 1999;28:36–39.

116. Fass R, Hell R, Sampliner RE, et al. Effect of ambulatory 24-hour esophageal pH monitoring on reflux-provoking activities. *Dig Dis Sci.* 1999;44:2263–2269.

117. Jolley SG. Reproducibility of 24-hour intraesophageal pH monitoring [letter]. *Pediatrics.* 2000;105:1371–1372.

118. Nielsen RG, Kruse-Andersen S, Husby S. Low reproducibility of 2 × 24-hour continuous esophageal pH monitoring in infants and children: a limiting factor for interventional studies. *Dig Dis Sci.* 2003;48:1495–1502.

119. Wenner J, Johansson J, Johnsson F, Oberg S. Optimal thresholds and discriminatory power of 48-h wireless esophageal pH monitoring in the diagnosis of GERD. *Am J Gastroenterol.* 2007;102:1862–1869.

120. Furuta GT, Liacouras CA, Collins MH, et al. Eosinophilic esophagitis in children and adults: a systematic review and consensus recommendations for diagnosis and treatment. *Gastroenterology.* 2007;133:1342–1363.

121. Spechler SJ, Genta RM, Souza RF. Thoughts on the complex relationship between gastroesophageal reflux disease and eosinophilic esophagitis. *Am J Gastroenterol.* 2007;102:1301–1306.

122. Steiner SJ, Gupta SK, Croffie JM, Fitzgerald JF. Correlation between number of eosinophils and reflux index on same day esophageal biopsy and 24 hour esophageal pH monitoring. *Am J Gastroenterol.* 2004;99:801–805.

123. Sant'Anna AM, Rolland S, Fournet JC, Yazbeck S, Drouin E. Eosinophilic esophagitis in children: symptoms, histology and pH probe results. *J Pediatr Gastroenterol Nutr.* 2004;39:373–377.

124. Wenzl TG, Moroder C, Trachterna M, et al. Esophageal pH monitoring and impedance measurement: a comparison of two diagnostic tests for gastroesophageal reflux. *J Pediatr Gastroenterol Nutr.* 2002;34:519–523.

125. Rosen R, Lord C, Nurko S. The sensitivity of multichannel intraluminal impedance and the pH probe in the evaluation of gastroesophageal reflux in children. *Clin Gastroenterol Hepatol.* 2006;4:167–172.

126. Wenzl TG, Silny J, Schenke S, Peschgens T, Heimann G, Skopnik H. Gastroesophageal reflux and respiratory phenomena in infants: status of the intraluminal impedance technique. *J Pediatr Gastroenterol Nutr.* 1999;28:423–428.

127. Rosen R, Nurko S. The importance of multichannel intraluminal impedance in the evaluation of children with persistent respiratory symptoms. *Am J Gastroenterol.* 2004;99:2452–2458.

128. Bove MJ, Rosen C. Diagnosis and management of laryngopharyngeal reflux disease. *Curr Opin Otolaryngol Head Neck Surg.* 2006;14:116–123.

129. DiMarino AJ Jr, Cohen S. Clinical relevance of esophageal and gastric pH measurements in patients with gastro-esophageal reflux disease (GERD). *Curr Med Res Opin.* 2005;21:27–36.

130. Hirano I, Richter JE. ACG practice guidelines: esophageal reflux testing. *Am J Gastroenterol.* 2007;102:668–685.

131. Loots CM, Benninga MA, Davidson GP, Omari TI. Addition of pH-impedance monitoring to standard pH monitoring increases the yield of symptom association analysis in infants and children with gastroesophageal reflux. *J Pediatr.* 2009;154:248–252.

132. Roman S, Serraj I, Damon H, Mion F. Correlation between gastric pH and gastro-oesophageal reflux contents: ambulatory pH-impedance monitoring results. *Neurogastroenterol Motil.* 2007;19:562–568.

133. Peter CS, Wiechers C, Bohnhorst B, Silny J, Poets CF. Influence of nasogastric tubes on gastroesophageal reflux in preterm infants: a multiple intraluminal impedance study. *J Pediatr.* 2002;141:277–279.

134. Skopnik H, Silny J, Heiber O, Schulz J, Rau G, Heimann G. Gastroesophageal reflux in infants: evaluation of a new intraluminal impedance technique. *J Pediatr Gastroenterol Nutr.* 1996;23:591–598.

135. Salvatore S, Hauser B, Devreker T, et al. Esophageal impedance and esophagitis in children: any correlation? *J Pediatr Gastroenterol Nutr.* 2009.

136. Sharma N, Agrawal A, Freeman J, Vela MF, Castell D. An analysis of persistent symptoms in acid-suppressed patients undergoing impedance-pH monitoring. *Clin Gastroenterol Hepatol.* 2008;6:521–524.

137. van Wijk MP, Benninga MA, Omari TI. Role of the multichannel intraluminal impedance technique in infants and children. *J Pediatr Gastroenterol Nutr.* 2009;48:2–12.

138. Tutuian R, Castell DO. Combined multichannel intraluminal impedance and manometry clarifies esophageal function abnormalities: study in 350 patients. *Am J Gastroenterol.* 2004;99:1011–1019.

139. Rosen R, Fritz J, Nurko A, Simon D, Nurko S. Lipid-laden macrophage index is not an indicator of gastroesophageal reflux-related respiratory disease in children. *Pediatrics.* 2008;121:e879–e884.

140. Stapleton A, Brodsky L. Extra-esophageal acid reflux induced adenotonsillar hyperplasia: case report and literature review. *Int J Pediatr Otorhinolaryngol.* 2008;72:409–413.

141. Teissier N, Kaguelidou F, Couloigner V, Francois M, Van Den Abbeele T. Predictive factors for success after transnasal endoscopic treatment of choanal atresia. *Arch Otolaryngol Head Neck Surg.* 2008;134:57–61.

142. Willging JP, Thompson DM. Pediatric FEESST: fiberoptic endoscopic evaluation of swallowing with sensory testing. *Curr Gastroenterol Rep.* 2005;7:240–243.

143. McMurray JS, Gerber M, Stern Y, et al. Role of laryngoscopy, dual pH probe monitoring, and laryngeal mucosal biopsy in the diagnosis of pharyngoesophageal reflux. *Ann Otol Rhinol Laryngol.* 2001;110:299–304.

144. Ramaiah RN, Stevenson M, McCallion WA. Hypopharyngeal and distal esophageal pH monitoring in children with gastroesophageal reflux and respiratory symptoms. *J Pediatr Surg.* 2005;40:1557–1561.

145. Little JP, Matthews BL, Glock MS, et al. Extraesophageal pediatric reflux: 24-hour double-probe pH monitoring of 222 children. *Ann Otol Rhinol Laryngol Suppl.* 1997;169:1–16.

146. Chung JH, Tae K, Lee YS, et al. The significance of laryngopharyngeal reflux in benign vocal mucosal lesions. *Otolaryngol Head Neck Surg.* 2009;141:369–373.

147. Johnston N, Wells CW, Samuels TL, Blumin JH. Pepsin in nonacidic refluxate can damage hypopharyngeal epithelial cells. *Ann Otol Rhinol Laryngol.* 2009;118:677–685.

148. Richter JE. Role of the gastric refluxate in gastroesophageal reflux disease: acid, weak acid and bile. *Am J Med Sci* 2009;338:89–95.

149. Vanderhal AL, Berci G, Simmons CF Jr, Hagiike M. A videolaryngoscopy technique for the intubation of the newborn: preliminary report. *Pediatrics.* 2009;124:e339–e346.

150. Nurko S, Rosen R. Use of multi-channel intraluminal impedance (MII) in the evaluation of children with respiratory symptoms: a new phenomenon? *J Pediatr Gastroenterol Nutr.* 2005;41:166–168.

151. Aceves SS, Newbury RO, Dohil R, Schwimmer J, Bastian JF. Distinguishing eosinophilic esophagitis in pediatric patients: clinical, endoscopic, and histologic features of an emerging disorder. *J Clin Gastroenterol.* 2007;41:252–256.

152. Liacouras CA. Eosinophilic esophagitis: treatment in 2005. *Curr Opin Gastroenterol.* 2006;22:147–152.

153. Gillett P, Hassall E. Pediatric gastrointestinal mucosal biopsy. Special considerations in children. *Gastrointest Endosc Clin N Am.* 2000;10:669–712, vi–vii.

154. Lundell LR, Dent J, Bennett JR, et al. Endoscopic assessment of oesophagitis: clinical and functional correlates and further validation of the Los Angeles classification. *Gut.* 1999;45:172–180.

155. Bytzer P, Havelund T, Hansen JM. Interobserver variation in the endoscopic diagnosis of reflux esophagitis. *Scand J Gastroenterol.* 1993;28:119–125.

156. Boccia G, Manguso F, Miele E, Buonavolonta R, Staiano A. Maintenance therapy for erosive esophagitis in children after healing by omeprazole: is it advisable? *Am J Gastroenterol.* 2007;102:1291–1297.

157. Hassall E, Israel D, Shepherd R, et al. Omeprazole for treatment of chronic erosive esophagitis in children: a multicenter study of efficacy, safety, tolerability and dose requirements. International Pediatric Omeprazole Study Group. *J Pediatr.* 2000;137:800–807.

158. Dahms BB. Reflux esophagitis: sequelae and differential diagnosis in infants and children including eosinophilic esophagitis. *Pediatr Dev Pathol.* 2004;7:5–16.

159. Dent J. Microscopic esophageal mucosal injury in nonerosive reflux disease. *Clin Gastroenterol Hepatol.* 2007;5:4–16.

160. Hassall E. Esophageal metaplasia: definition and prevalence in childhood. *Gastrointest Endosc.* 2006;64:676–677.

161. Hassall E, Kerr W, El-Serag HB. Characteristics of children receiving proton pump inhibitors continuously for up to 11 years duration. *J Pediatr.* 2007;150:262–267, 7 e1.

162. van Malenstein H, Farre R, Sifrim D. Esophageal dilated intercellular spaces (DIS) and nonerosive reflux disease. *Am J Gastroenterol.* 2008;103:1021–1028.

163. Heine RG, Cameron DJ, Chow CW, Hill DJ, Catto-Smith AG. Esophagitis in distressed infants: poor diagnostic agreement between esophageal pH monitoring and histopathologic findings. *J Pediatr.* 2002;140:14–19.

164. Ravelli AM, Villanacci V, Ruzzenenti N, et al. Dilated intercellular spaces: a major morphological feature of esophagitis. *J Pediatr Gastroenterol Nutr.* 2006;42:510–515.

165. Furuta GT, Nurko S, Bousvaros A, Antonioli D, Badizadegan K. The spectrum of pediatric gastroesophageal reflux. *JAMA.* 2000;284:3125–3126.

166. Heine RG. Allergic gastrointestinal motility disorders in infancy and early childhood. *Pediatr Allergy Immunol.* 2008;19:383–391.

167. Orenstein SR, Shalaby TM, Kelsey SF, Frankel E. Natural history of infant reflux esophagitis: symptoms and morphometric histology during one year without pharmacotherapy. *Am J Gastroenterol.* 2006;101:628–640.

168. Osatakul S, Sriplung H, Puetpaiboon A, Junjana CO, Chamnongpakdi S. Prevalence and natural course of gastroesophageal reflux symptoms: a 1-year cohort study in Thai infants. *J Pediatr Gastroenterol Nutr.* 2002;34:63–67.

169. Heine RG, Jordan B, Lubitz L, Meehan M, Catto-Smith AG. Clinical predictors of pathological gastro-oesophageal reflux in infants with persistent distress. *J Paediatr Child Health.* 2006;42:134–139.

170. Nevo N, Rubin L, Tamir A, Levine A, Shaoul R. Infant feeding patterns in the first 6 months: an assessment in full-term infants. *J Pediatr Gastroenterol Nutr.* 2007;45:234–239.

171. Iacono G, Merolla R, D'Amico D, et al. Gastrointestinal symptoms in infancy: a population-based prospective study. *Dig Liver Dis.* 2005;37:432–438.

172. Nielsen RG, Bindslev-Jensen C, Kruse-Andersen S, Husby S. Severe gastroesophageal reflux disease and cow milk hypersensitivity in infants and children: disease association and evaluation of a new challenge procedure. *J Pediatr Gastroenterol Nutr.* 2004;39:383–391.

173. Hill DJ, Heine RG, Cameron DJ, et al. Role of food protein intolerance in infants with persistent distress attributed to reflux esophagitis. *J Pediatr.* 2000;136:641–647.

174. Iacono G, Carroccio A, Cavataio F, et al. Gastroesophageal reflux and cow's milk allergy in infants: a prospective study. *J Allergy Clin Immunol.* 1996;97:822–827.

175. Hill DJ, Cameron DJ, Francis DE, Gonzalez-Andaya AM, Hosking CS. Challenge confirmation of late-onset reactions to extensively hydrolyzed formulas in infants with multiple food protein intolerance. *J Allergy Clin Immunol.* 1995;96:386–394.

176. Vance GH, Lewis SA, Grimshaw KE, et al. Exposure of the fetus and infant to hens' egg ovalbumin via the placenta and breast milk in relation to maternal intake of dietary egg. *Clin Exp Allergy.* 2005;35:1318–1326.

177. Khoshoo V, Ross G, Brown S, Edell D. Smaller volume, thickened formulas in the management of gastroesophageal reflux in thriving infants. *J Pediatr Gastroenterol Nutr.* 2000;31:554–556.

178. Orenstein SR, Magill HL, Brooks P. Thickening of infant feedings for therapy of gastroesophageal reflux. *J Pediatr.* 1987;110:181–186.

179. Wenzl TG, Schneider S, Scheele F, Silny J, Heimann G, Skopnik H. Effects of thickened feeding on gastroesophageal reflux in infants: a placebo-controlled crossover study using intraluminal impedance. *Pediatrics.* 2003;111:e355–e359.

180. Xinias I, Mouane N, Le Luyer B, et al. Cornstarch thickened formula reduces oesophageal acid exposure time in infants. *Dig Liver Dis.* 2005;37:23–27.

181. Corvaglia L, Ferlini M, Rotatori R, et al. Starch thickening of human milk is ineffective in reducing the gastroesophageal reflux in preterm infants: a crossover study using intraluminal impedance. *J Pediatr.* 2006;148:265–268.

182. Orenstein SR, Shalaby TM, Putnam PE. Thickened feedings as a cause of increased coughing when used as therapy for gastroesophageal reflux in infants. *J Pediatr.* 1992;121:913–915.

183. Chao HC, Vandenplas Y. Comparison of the effect of a cornstarch thickened formula and strengthened regular formula on regurgitation, gastric emptying and weight gain in infantile regurgitation. *Dis Esophagus.* 2007;20:155–160.

184. Vandenplas Y, Hachimi-Idrissi S, Casteels A, Mahler T, Loeb H. A clinical trial with an "anti-regurgitation" formula. *Eur J Pediatr.* 1994;153:419–423.

185. Miyazawa R, Tomomasa T, Kaneko H, Arakawa H, Morikawa A. Effect of formula thickened with reduced concentration of locust bean gum on gastroesophageal reflux. *Acta Paediatr.* 2007;96:910–914.

186. Bosscher D, Van Caillie-Bertrand M, Deelstra H. Do thickening properties of locust bean gum affect the amount of calcium, iron and zinc available for absorption from infant formula? In vitro studies. *Int J Food Sci Nutr.* 2003;54:261–268.

187. Hegar B, Boediarso A, Firmansyah A, Vandenplas Y. Investigation of regurgitation and other symptoms of gastroesophageal reflux in Indonesian infants. *World J Gastroenterol.* 2004;10:1795–1797.

188. DiSario JA. Endoscopic approaches to enteral nutritional support. *Best Pract Res Clin Gastroenterol.* 2006;20:605–630.

189. Tobin JM, McCloud P, Cameron DJ. Posture and gastro-oesophageal reflux: a case for left lateral positioning. *Arch Dis Child.* 1997;76:254–258.

190. Vandenplas Y, Sacre-Smits L. Seventeen-hour continuous esophageal pH monitoring in the newborn: evaluation of the influence of position in asymptomatic and symptomatic babies. *J Pediatr Gastroenterol Nutr.* 1985;4:356–361.

191. Meyers WF, Herbst JJ. Effectiveness of positioning therapy for gastroesophageal reflux. *Pediatrics.* 1985;69:768–772.

192. Jeske HC, Borovicka J, von Goedecke A, Meyenberger C, Heidegger T, Benzer A. The influence of postural changes on gastroesophageal reflux and barrier pressure in nonfasting individuals. *Anesth Analg.* 2005;101:597–600 [table of contents].

193. Bagucka B, De Schepper J, Peelman M, Van de Maele K, Vandenplas Y. Acid gastro-esophageal reflux in the 10 degrees-reversed-Trendelenburg-position in supine sleeping infants. *Acta Paediatr Taiwan.* 1999;40:298–301.

194. Orenstein SR, Whitington PF, Orenstein DM. The infant seat as treatment for gastroesophageal reflux. *N Engl J Med.* 1983;309:760–763.

195. Chao HC, Vandenplas Y. Effect of cereal-thickened formula and upright positioning on regurgitation, gastric emptying, and weight gain in infants with regurgitation. *Nutrition.* 2007;23:23–28.

196. Vandenplas Y, Hauser B. Gastro-oesophageal reflux, sleep pattern, apparent life threatening event and sudden infant death. The point of view of a gastro-enterologist. *Eur J Pediatr.* 2000;159:726–729.

197. Oyen N, Markestad T, Skaerven R, et al. Combined effects of sleeping position and prenatal risk factors in sudden infant death syndrome: the Nordic Epidemiological SIDS Study. *Pediatrics.* 1997;100:613–621.

198. Skadberg BT, Morild I, Markestad T. Abandoning prone sleeping: effect on the risk of sudden infant death syndrome. *J Pediatr.* 1998;132:340–343.

199. Adams EJ, Chavez GF, Steen D, Shah R, Iyasu S, Krous HF. Changes in the epidemiologic profile of sudden infant death syndrome as rates decline among California infants: 1990–1995. *Pediatrics.* 1998;102:1445–1451.

200. Katz LC, Just R, Castell DO. Body position affects recumbent postprandial reflux. *J Clin Gastroenterol.* 1994;18:280–283.

201. Khoury RM, Camacho-Lobato L, Katz PO, Mohiuddin MA, Castell DO. Influence of spontaneous sleep positions on nighttime recumbent reflux in patients with gastroesophageal reflux disease. *Am J Gastroenterol.* 1999;94:2069–2073.

202. Corvaglia L, Rotatori R, Ferlini M, Aceti A, Ancora G, Faldella G. The effect of body positioning on gastroesophageal reflux in premature infants: evaluation by combined impedance and pH monitoring. *J Pediatr.* 2007;151:591–596, 6 e1.

203. Task Force on Sudden Infant Death Syndrome. The Changing Concept of Sudden Infant Death Syndrome: Diagnostic Coding Shifts, Controversies Regarding the Sleeping Environment, and New Variables to Consider in Reducing Risk. *Pediatrics* 2005;116:1245–1255.

204. Austin GL, Thiny MT, Westman EC, Yancy WS Jr, Shaheen NJ. A very low-carbohydrate diet improves gastroesophageal reflux and its symptoms. *Dig Dis Sci.* 2006;51:1307–1312.

205. Peluso L, Vanek VW. Efficacy of gastric bypass in the treatment of obesity-related comorbidities. *Nutr Clin Pract.* 2007;22:22–28.

206. Piesman M, Hwang I, Maydonovitch C, Wong RK. Nocturnal reflux episodes following the administration of a standardized meal. Does timing matter? *Am J Gastroenterol.* 2007;102:2128–2134.

207. Festi D, Scaioli E, Baldi F, et al. Body weight, lifestyle, dietary habits and gastroesophageal reflux disease. *World J Gastroenterol.* 2009;15:1690–1701.

208. Fox M, Barr C, Nolan S, Lomer M, Anggiansah A, Wong T. The effects of dietary fat and calorie density on esophageal acid exposure and reflux symptoms. *Clin Gastroenterol Hepatol.* 2007;5:439–444.

209. Mulholland HG, Cantwell MM, Anderson LA, et al. Glycemic index, carbohydrate and fiber intakes and risk of reflux esophagitis, Barrett's esophagus, and esophageal adenocarcinoma. *Cancer Causes Control.* 2009;20:279–288.

210. Zheng Z, Nordenstedt H, Pedersen NL, Lagergren J, Ye W. Lifestyle factors and risk for symptomatic gastroesophageal reflux in monozygotic twins. *Gastroenterology.* 2007;132:87–95.

211. Shabib SM, Cutz E, Sherman PM. Passive smoking is a risk factor for esophagitis in children. *J Pediatr.* 1995;127:435–437.

212. Craig WR, Hanlon-Dearman A, Sinclair C, Taback S, Moffatt M. Metoclopramide, thickened feedings, and positioning for gastro-oesophageal reflux in children under two years. *Cochrane Database Syst Rev.* 2004:CD003502.

213. Meining A, Classen M. The role of diet and lifestyle measures in the pathogenesis and treatment of gastro-esophageal reflux disease. *Am J Gastroenterol.* 2000;95:2692–2697.

214. Cucchiara S, Staiano A, Romaniello G, Capobianco S, Auricchio S. Antacids and cimetidine treatment for gastro-oesophageal reflux and peptic oesophagitis. *Arch Dis Child.* 1984;59:842–847.

215. Tsou VM, Young RM, Hart MH, Vanderhoof JA. Elevated plasma aluminum levels in normal infants receiving antacids containing aluminum. *Pediatrics.* 1991;87:148–151.

216. Khan M, Santana J, Donnellan C, Preston C, Moayyedi P. Medical treatments in the short term management of reflux oesophagitis. *Cochrane Database Syst Rev.* 2007:CD003244.

217. Millar AJ, Numanoglu A, Mann M, Marven S, Rode H. Detection of caustic oesophageal injury with technetium 99m-labelled sucralfate. *J Pediatr Surg.* 2001;36:262–265.

218. Candelli M, Carloni E, Armuzzi A, et al. Role of sucralfate in gastrointestinal diseases. *Panminerva Med.* 2000;42:55–59.

219. Del Buono R, Wenzl TG, Ball G, Keady S, Thomson M. Effect of Gaviscon Infant on gastro-oesophageal reflux in infants assessed by combined intraluminal impedance/pH. *Arch Dis Child.* 2005;90:460–463.

220. Donnellan C, Sharma N, Preston C, Moayyedi P. Medical treatments for the maintenance therapy of reflux oesophagitis and endoscopic negative reflux disease. *Cochrane Database Syst Rev.* 2005:CD003245.

221. Arguelles-Martin F, Gonzalez-Fernandez F, Gentles MG. Sucralfate versus cimetidine in the treatment of reflux esophagitis in children. *Am J Med.* 1989;86:73–76.

222. Mallet E, Mouterde O, Dubois F, Flipo JL, Moore N. Use of ranitidine in young infants with gastro-oesophageal reflux. *Eur J Clin Pharmacol.* 1989;36:641–642.

223. Orenstein SR, Blumer JL, Faessel HM, et al. Ranitidine, 75 mg, over-the-counter dose: pharmacokinetic and pharmacodynamic effects in children with symptoms of gastro-oesophageal reflux. *Aliment Pharmacol Ther.* 2002;16:899–907.

224. Sutphen JL, Dillard VL. Effect of ranitidine on twenty-four-hour gastric acidity in infants. *J Pediatr.* 1989;114:472–474.

225. Hyman PE, Garvey TQ 3rd, Abrams CE. Tolerance to intravenous ranitidine. *J Pediatr.* 1987;110:794–796.

226. Nwokolo CU, Smith JT, Gavey C, Sawyerr A, Pounder RE. Tolerance during 29 days of conventional dosing with cimetidine, nizatidine, famotidine or ranitidine. *Aliment Pharmacol Ther.* 1990;4(suppl 1):29–45.

227. Wilder-Smith CH, Ernst T, Gennoni M, Zeyen B, Halter F, Merki HS. Tolerance to oral H2-receptor antagonists. *Dig Dis Sci.* 1990;35:976–983.

228. Chiba N, De Gara CJ, Wilkinson JM, Hunt RH. Speed of healing and symptom relief in grade II to IV

gastroesophageal reflux disease: a meta-analysis. *Gastroenterology*. 1997;112:1798–1810.

229. McCarty-Dawson D, Sue SO, Morrill B, Murdock RH Jr. Ranitidine versus cimetidine in the healing of erosive esophagitis. *Clin Ther*. 1996;18:1150–1160.

230. Stacey JH, Miocevich ML, Sacks GE. The effect of ranitidine (as effervescent tablets) on the quality of life of GORD patients. *Br J Clin Pract*. 1996;50:190–194, 196.

231. Sabesin SM, Berlin RG, Humphries TJ, Bradstreet DC, Walton-Bowen KL, Zaidi S. Famotidine relieves symptoms of gastroesophageal reflux disease and heals erosions and ulcerations. Results of a multicenter, placebo-controlled, dose-ranging study. USA Merck Gastroesophageal Reflux Disease Study Group. *Arch Intern Med*. 1991;151:2394–2400.

232. Cucchiara S, Gobio-Casali L, Balli F, et al. Cimetidine treatment of reflux esophagitis in children: an Italian multicentric study. *J Pediatr Gastroenterol Nutr*. 1989;8:150–156.

233. Simeone D, Caria MC, Miele E, Staiano A. Treatment of childhood peptic esophagitis: a double-blind placebo-controlled trial of nizatidine. *J Pediatr Gastroenterol Nutr*. 1997;25:51–55.

234. van Pinxteren B, Numans ME, Bonis PA, Lau J. Short-term treatment with proton pump inhibitors, H2-receptor antagonists and prokinetics for gastro-oesophageal reflux disease-like symptoms and endoscopy negative reflux disease. *Cochrane Database Syst Rev*. 2006;3:CD002095.

235. Garcia Rodriguez LA, Wallander MA, Stricker BH. The risk of acute liver injury associated with cimetidine and other acid-suppressing anti-ulcer drugs. *Br J Clin Pharmacol*. 1997;43:183–188.

236. Ribeiro JM, Lucas M, Baptista A, Victorino RM. Fatal hepatitis associated with ranitidine. *Am J Gastroenterol*. 2000;95:559–560.

237. Garcia Rodriguez LA, Jick H. Risk of gynaecomastia associated with cimetidine, omeprazole, and other anti-ulcer drugs. *BMJ*. 1994;308:503–506.

238. Champion G, Richter JE, Vaezi MF, Singh S, Alexander R. Duodenogastroesophageal reflux: relationship to pH and importance in Barrett's esophagus. *Gastroenterology*. 1994;107:747–754.

239. Litalien C, Theoret Y, Faure C. Pharmacokinetics of proton pump inhibitors in children. *Clin Pharmacokinet*. 2005;44:441–466.

240. Zhao J, Li J, Hamer-Maansson JE, et al. Pharmacokinetic properties of esomeprazole in children aged 1 to 11 years with symptoms of gastroesophageal reflux disease: a randomized, open-label study. *Clin Ther*. 2006;28:1868–1876.

241. Andersson T, Hassall E, Lundborg P, et al. Pharmacokinetics of orally administered omeprazole in children. International Pediatric Omeprazole Pharmacokinetic Group. *Am J Gastroenterol*. 2000;95:3101–3106.

242. Gremse D, Winter H, Tolia V, et al. Pharmacokinetics and pharmacodynamics of lansoprazole in children with gastroesophageal reflux disease. *J Pediatr Gastroenterol Nutr*. 2002;35(suppl 4):S319–S326.

243. Omari TI, Davidson GP. Multipoint measurement of intragastric pH in healthy preterm infants. *Arch Dis Child Fetal Neonatal Ed*. 2003;88:F517–F520.

244. Zhang W, Kukulka M, Witt G, Sutkowski-Markmann D, North J, Atkinson S. Age-dependent pharmacokinetics of lansoprazole in neonates and infants. *Paediatr Drugs*. 2008;10:265–274.

245. Barron JJ, Tan H, Spalding J, Bakst AW, Singer J. Proton pump inhibitor utilization patterns in infants. *J Pediatr Gastroenterol Nutr*. 2007;45:421–427.

246. Khoshoo V, Edell D, Thompson A, Rubin M. Are we overprescribing antireflux medications for infants with regurgitation? *Pediatrics*. 2007;120:946–949.

247. Li J, Zhao J, Hamer-Maansson JE, et al. Pharmacokinetic properties of esomeprazole in adolescent patients aged 12 to 17 years with symptoms of gastroesophageal reflux disease: a randomized, open-label study. *Clin Ther*. 2006;28:419–427.

248. Tolia V, Fitzgerald J, Hassall E, Huang B, Pilmer B, Kane R 3rd. Safety of lansoprazole in the treatment of gastroesophageal reflux disease in children. *J Pediatr Gastroenterol Nutr*. 2002;35:S300–S307.

249. Raghunath AS, O'Morain C, McLoughlin RC. Review article: the long-term use of proton-pump inhibitors. *Aliment Pharmacol Ther*. 2005;22(suppl 1):55–63.

250. Drut R, Altamirano E, Cueto Rua E. Omeprazole-associated changes in the gastric mucosa of children. *J Clin Pathol*. 2008;61:754–756.

251. Pashankar DS, Israel DM. Gastric polyps and nodules in children receiving long-term omeprazole therapy. *J Pediatr Gastroenterol Nutr*. 2002;35:658–662.

252. Humphries TJ. On gastric polyps, proton pump inhibitors and long-term risks. *Aliment Pharmacol Ther*. 2001;15:559–560.

253. Graham DY, Genta RM. Long-term proton pump inhibitor use and gastrointestinal cancer. *Curr Gastroenterol Rep*. 2008;10:543–547.

254. Carmack SW, Genta RM, Schuler CM, Saboorian MH. The current spectrum of gastric polyps: a 1-year national study of over 120,000 patients. *Am J Gastroenterol*. 2009;104:1524–1532.

255. Canani RB, Cirillo P, Roggero P, et al. Therapy with gastric acidity inhibitors increases the risk of acute gastroenteritis and community-acquired pneumonia in children. *Pediatrics*. 2006;117:e817–e820.

256. Guillet R, Stoll BJ, Cotten CM, et al. Association of H2-blocker therapy and higher incidence of necrotizing enterocolitis in very low birth weight infants. *Pediatrics*. 2006;117:e137–e142.

257. Pulsifer-Anderson E, Guillet R. National Institutes of Health recommends the routine use of H2 blockers in preterm infants be carefully evaluated. *Neonatal Netw*. 2006;25:223–224.

258. Saiman L, Ludington E, Dawson JD, et al. Risk factors for *Candida* species colonization of neonatal intensive care unit patients. *Pediatr Infect Dis J*. 2001;20:1119–1124.

259. Dial S, Delaney JA, Barkun AN, Suissa S. Use of gastric acid-suppressive agents and the risk of community-acquired *Clostridium difficile*-associated disease. *JAMA*. 2005;294:2989–2995.

260. Laheij RJ, Sturkenboom MC, Hassing RJ, Dieleman J, Stricker BH, Jansen JB. Risk of community-acquired pneumonia and use of gastric acid-suppressive drugs. *JAMA*. 2004;292:1955–1960.

261. Garcia Rodriguez LA, Ruigomez A, Panes J. Use of acid-suppressing drugs and the risk of bacterial gastroenteritis. *Clin Gastroenterol Hepatol.* 2007;5:1418–1423.

262. Williams C, McColl KE. Review article: proton pump inhibitors and bacterial overgrowth. *Aliment Pharmacol Ther.* 2006;23:3–10.

263. Valuck RJ, Ruscin JM. A case–control study on adverse effects: H2 blocker or proton pump inhibitor use and risk of vitamin B12 deficiency in older adults. *J Clin Epidemiol.* 2004;57:422–428.

264. Yang YX, Lewis JD, Epstein S, Metz DC. Long-term proton pump inhibitor therapy and risk of hip fracture. *JAMA.* 2006;296:2947–2953.

265. Geevasinga N, Coleman PL, Webster AC, Roger SD. Proton pump inhibitors and acute interstitial nephritis. *Clin Gastroenterol Hepatol.* 2006;4:597–604.

266. Brewster UC, Perazella MA. Acute kidney injury following proton pump inhibitor therapy. *Kidney Int.* 2007;71:589–593.

267. Untersmayr E, Jensen-Jarolim E. The role of protein digestibility and antacids on food allergy outcomes. *J Allergy Clin Immunol.* 2008;121:1301–1308 [quiz 9–10].

268. Rode H, Stunden RJ, Millar AJ, Cywes S. Esophageal pH assessment of gastroesophageal reflux in 18 patients and the effect of two prokinetic agents: cisapride and metoclopramide. *J Pediatr Surg.* 1987;22:931–934.

269. Hegar B, Alatas S, Advani N, Firmansyah A, Vandenplas Y. Domperidone versus cisapride in the treatment of infant regurgitation and increased acid gastro-oesophageal reflux: a pilot study. *Acta Paediatr.* 2009;98:750–755.

270. Khorana M, Chankajorn W, Kanjanapattanakul W, et al. Effect of cisapride on corrected QT interval in neonates. *J Med Assoc Thai.* 2003;86(suppl 3):S590–S595.

271. Wang SJ, La JL, Chen DY, Chen YH, Hsieh TY, Lin WY. Effects of cisapride on oesophageal transit of solids in patients with progressive systemic sclerosis. *Clin Rheumatol.* 2002;21:43–45.

272. Vandenplas Y, Badriul H, Salvatore S, Hauser B. Pharmacotherapy of gastro-oesophageal reflux disease in children: focus on safety. *Expert Opin Drug Saf.* 2002;1:355–364.

273. Vandenplas Y. Cisapride: the black sheep. *J Pediatr Gastroenterol Nutr.* 2002;35:5–6.

274. Sharma MP. Cisapride controversy. *Trop Gastroenterol.* 2002;23:188–189.

275. Pritchard DS, Baber N, Stephenson T. Should domperidone be used for the treatment of gastro-oesophageal reflux in children? Systematic review of randomized controlled trials in children aged 1 month to 11 years old. *Br J Clin Pharmacol.* 2005;59:725–729.

276. Shafrir Y, Levy Y, Ben-Amitai D, Nitzan M, Steinherz R. Oculogyric crisis due to domperidone therapy. *Helv Paediatr Acta.* 1985;40:95.

277. Rocha CM, Barbosa MM. QT interval prolongation associated with the oral use of domperidone in an infant. *Pediatr Cardiol.* 2005;26:720–723.

278. Tolia V, Calhoun J, Kuhns L, Kauffman RE. Randomized, prospective double-blind trial of metoclopramide and placebo for gastroesophageal reflux in infants. *J Pediatr.* 1989;115:141–145.

279. Machida HM, Forbes DA, Gall DG, Scott RB. Metoclopramide in gastroesophageal reflux of infancy. *J Pediatr.* 1988;112:483–487.

280. Shafrir Y, Levy Y, Beharab A, Nitzam M, Steinherz R. Acute dystonic reaction to bethanechol—a direct acetylcholine receptor agonist. *Dev Med Child Neurol.* 1986;28:646–648.

281. Madani S, Tolia V. Gynecomastia with metoclopramide use in pediatric patients. *J Clin Gastroenterol.* 1997;24: 79–81.

282. Putnam PE, Orenstein SR, Wessel HB, Stowe RM. Tardive dyskinesia associated with use of metoclopramide in a child. *J Pediatr.* 1992;121:983–985.

283. Euler AR. Use of bethanechol for the treatment of gastroesophageal reflux. *J Pediatr.* 1980;96:321–324.

284. Levi P, Marmo F, Saluzzo C, et al. Bethanechol versus antiacids in the treatment of gastroesophageal reflux. *Helv Paediatr Acta.* 1985;40:349–359.

285. Vela MF, Tutuian R, Katz PO, Castell DO. Baclofen decreases acid and non-acid post-prandial gastro-oesophageal reflux measured by combined multichannel intraluminal impedance and pH. *Aliment Pharmacol Ther.* 2003;17:243–251.

286. Omari TI, Benninga MA, Sansom L, Butler RN, Dent J, Davidson GP. Effect of baclofen on esophagogastric motility and gastroesophageal reflux in children with gastroesophageal reflux disease: a randomized controlled trial. *J Pediatr.* 2006;149:468–474.

287. Kawai M, Kawahara H, Hirayama S, Yoshimura N, Ida S. Effect of baclofen on emesis and 24-hour esophageal pH in neurologically impaired children with gastroesophageal reflux disease. *J Pediatr Gastroenterol Nutr.* 2004;38:317–323.

288. Hibbs AM, Lorch SA. Metoclopramide for the treatment of gastroesophageal reflux disease in infants: a systematic review. *Pediatrics.* 2006;118:746–752.

289. Di Lorenzo C. Gastroesophageal reflux: not a time to "relax". *J Pediatr.* 2006;149:436–438.

290. Lobe TE. The current role of laparoscopic surgery for gastroesophageal reflux disease in infants and children. *Surg Endosc.* 2007;21:167–174.

291. Berquist WE, Rachelefsky GS, Kadden M, et al. Effect of theophylline on gastroesophageal reflux in normal adults. *J Allergy Clin Immunol.* 1981;67:407–411.

292. Di Lorenzo C, Orenstein S. Fundoplication: friend or foe? *J Pediatr Gastroenterol Nutr.* 2002;34:117–124.

293. Hassall E. Outcomes of fundoplication: causes for concern, newer options. *Arch Dis Child.* 2005;90:1047–1052.

294. Gilger MA, Yeh C, Chiang J, Dietrich C, Brandt ML, El-Serag HB. Outcomes of surgical fundoplication in children. *Clin Gastroenterol Hepatol.* 2004;2:978–984.

295. Fonkalsrud EW. Nissen fundoplication for gastroesophageal reflux disease in infants and children. *Semin Pediatr Surg.* 1998;7:110–114.

296. Mathei J, Coosemans W, Nafteux P, et al. Laparoscopic Nissen fundoplication in infants and children: analysis of 106 consecutive patients with special emphasis in neurologically impaired vs. neurologically normal patients. *Surg Endosc.* 2008;22:1054–1059.

297. Vakil N. Review article: the role of surgery in gastro-oesophageal reflux disease. *Aliment Pharmacol Ther.* 2007;25:1365–1372.

298. Jackson PG, Gleiber MA, Askari R, Evans SR. Predictors of outcome in 100 consecutive laparoscopic antireflux procedures. *Am J Surg.* 2001;181:231–235.

299. Vakil N, Shaw M, Kirby R. Clinical effectiveness of laparoscopic fundoplication in a U.S. community. *Am J Med.* 2003;114:1–5.

300. Spechler SJ, Lee E, Ahnen D, et al. Long-term outcome of medical and surgical therapies for gastroesophageal reflux disease: follow-up of a randomized controlled trial. *JAMA.* 2001;285:2331–2338.

301. Wijnhoven BP, Lally CJ, Kelly JJ, Myers JC, Watson DI. Use of antireflux medication after antireflux surgery. *J Gastrointest Surg.* 2008;12:510–517.

302. Lundell L, Attwood S, Ell C, et al. Comparing laparoscopic antireflux surgery with esomeprazole in the management of patients with chronic gastro-oesophageal reflux disease: a 3-year interim analysis of the LOTUS trial. *Gut.* 2008;57:1207–1213.

303. Rantanen TK, Salo JA, Sipponen JT. Fatal and life-threatening complications in antireflux surgery: analysis of 5,502 operations. *Br J Surg.* 1999;86:1573–1577.

304. Pearl RH, Robie DK, Ein SH, et al. Complications of gastroesophageal antireflux surgery in neurologically impaired versus neurologically normal children. *J Pediatr Surg.* 1990;25:1169–1173.

305. Spitz L, Roth K, Kiely EM, Brereton RJ, Drake DP, Milla PJ. Operation for gastro-oesophageal reflux associated with severe mental retardation. *Arch Dis Child.* 1993;68:347–351.

306. Smith CD, Othersen HB Jr, Gogan NJ, Walker JD. Nissen fundoplication in children with profound neurologic disability. High risks and unmet goals. *Ann Surg.* 1992;215:654–658 [discussion 8–9].

307. Martinez DA, Ginn-Pease ME, Caniano DA. Recognition of recurrent gastroesophageal reflux following antireflux surgery in the neurologically disabled child: high index of suspicion and definitive evaluation. *J Pediatr Surg.* 1992;27:983–988 [discussion 8–90].

308. Martinez DA, Ginn-Pease ME, Caniano DA. Sequelae of antireflux surgery in profoundly disabled children [see comments]. *J Pediatr Surg.* 1992;27:267–271 [discussion 71–73].

309. Curci MR, Dibbins AW. Problems associated with a Nissen fundoplication following tracheoesophageal fistula and esophageal atresia repair. *Arch Surg.* 1988;123:618–620.

310. Wheatley MJ, Coran AG, Wesley JR. Efficacy of the Nissen fundoplication in the management of gastroesophageal reflux following esophageal atresia repair. *J Pediatr Surg.* 1993;28:53–55.

311. Kubiak R, Spitz L, Kiely EM, Drake D, Pierro A. Effectiveness of fundoplication in early infancy. *J Pediatr Surg.* 1999;34:295–299.

312. Diaz DM, Gibbons TE, Heiss K, Wulkan ML, Ricketts RR, Gold BD. Antireflux surgery outcomes in pediatric gastroesophageal reflux disease. *Am J Gastroenterol.* 2005;100:1844–1852.

313. Goldin AB, Sawin R, Seidel KD, Flum DR. Do antireflux operations decrease the rate of reflux-related hospitalizations in children? *Pediatrics.* 2006;118:2326–2333.

314. Lee SL, Shabatian H, Hsu JW, Applebaum H, Haigh PI. Hospital admissions for respiratory symptoms and failure to thrive before and after Nissen fundoplication. *J Pediatr Surg.* 2008;43:59–63 [discussion -5].

315. Carlson MA, Frantzides CT. Complications and results of primary minimally invasive antireflux procedures: a review of 10,735 reported cases. *J Am Coll Surg.* 2001;193:428–439.

316. van der Zee DC, Arends NJ, Bax NM. The value of 24-h pH study in evaluating the results of laparoscopic antireflux surgery in children. *Surg Endosc.* 1999;13:918–921.

317. Dijkman KP, van Heurn LW, Leroy PL, Vos GD. Vanishing spleen after Nissen fundoplication: a case report. *Eur J Pediatr.* 2009;168:355–357.

318. Lasser MS, Liao JG, Burd RS. National trends in the use of antireflux procedures for children. *Pediatrics.* 2006;118:1828–1835.

319. Capito C, Leclair MD, Piloquet H, Plattner V, Heloury Y, Podevin G. Long-term outcome of laparoscopic Nissen–Rossetti fundoplication for neurologically impaired and normal children. *Surg Endosc.* 2008;22:875–880.

320. Luostarinen ME, Isolauri JO. Surgical experience improves the long-term results of Nissen fundoplication. *Scand J Gastroenterol.* 1999;34:117–120.

321. Bais JE, Bartelsman JF, Bonjer HJ, et al. Laparoscopic or conventional Nissen fundoplication for gastro-oesophageal reflux disease: randomised clinical trial. The Netherlands Antireflux Surgery Study Group. *Lancet.* 2000;355:170–174.

322. Lall A, Morabito A, Dall'Oglio L, et al. Total oesophagogastric dissociation: experience in 2 centres. *J Pediatr Surg.* 2006;41:342–346.

323. Morabito A, Lall A, Lo Piccolo R, et al. Total esophagogastric dissociation: 10 years' review. *J Pediatr Surg.* 2006;41:919–922.

324. Rothstein RI. Endoscopic therapy of gastroesophageal reflux disease: outcomes of the randomized-controlled trials done to date. *J Clin Gastroenterol.* 2008;42:594–602.

325. Pace F, Costamagna G, Penagini R, Repici A, Annese V. Review article: endoscopic antireflux procedures—an unfulfilled promise? *Aliment Pharmacol Ther.* 2008;27:375–384.

326. Hogan WJ. Clinical trials evaluating endoscopic GERD treatments: is it time for a moratorium on the clinical use of these procedures? *Am J Gastroenterol.* 2006;101:437–439.

327. Corley DA, Katz P, Wo JM, et al. Improvement of gastroesophageal reflux symptoms after radiofrequency energy: a randomized, sham-controlled trial. *Gastroenterology.* 2003;125:668–676.

328. Gold BD. Gastroesophageal reflux disease: could intervention in childhood reduce the risk of later complications? *Am J Med.* 2004;117(suppl 5A):23S–29S.

329. Nelson SP, Chen EH, Syniar GM, Christoffel KK. Prevalence of symptoms of gastroesophageal reflux during childhood: a pediatric practice-based survey. Pediatric Practice Research Group. *Arch Pediatr Adolesc Med.* 2000;154:150–154.

CHAPTER 13

Gastritis and Peptic Ulcer Disease

Aliye Uc and Bharani Pandrangi

DEFINITIONS AND EPIDEMIOLOGY

Gastritis is an inflammatory process associated with gastric mucosal injury. It is usually classified by histologic features (atrophic or non-atrophic, chemical, granulomatous, eosinophilic, lymphocytic, etc.), time course (acute versus chronic), etiology (*Helicobacter pylori*, bile, non-steroidal anti-inflammatory drugs (NSAIDs), Crohn's disease, etc.), and proposed pathophysiology. *Peptic ulcers* are deep mucosal ulcerations that penetrate into the muscularis mucosa of the stomach or duodenum. *Peptic erosions* are superficial mucosal lesions; they do not involve the muscularis mucosa. Peptic ulcers and erosions are relatively uncommon in children, found in less than 25% of children undergoing upper gastrointestinal endoscopy for abdominal pain.[1] *H. pylori* is by far the most common etiology for gastritis and peptic ulcer disease (PUD) in the pediatric age group.

The Role of *H. pylori* in Peptic Disease

H. pylori is a Gram-negative spiral organism that colonizes the gastric mucosa of humans. The bacteria live in the gastric mucus and cause chronic gastritis, duodenal ulcers, and, to a lesser extent, gastric ulcers. Infection with *H. pylori* is strongly associated with gastric adenocarcinoma and mucosal-associated lymphomas (MALT) in humans.[4]

H. pylori is almost always acquired in childhood (usually before 10 years of age), and if untreated, infection is lifelong.[2] It is estimated that 50% of the world's population is infected with this organism. Infection with *H. pylori* is prevalent in developing countries where about 80% of children are colonized. The highest rates of *H. pylori* prevalence are in Eastern Europe, Asia, and many developing countries. The organism is also prevalent in selected populations in the United States (e.g., Native Americans, African Americans, and Hispanics). Lifetime risk of developing PUD from *H. pylori* infection is 10–15%, while gastric cancer develops in less than 1%.[3]

The route of transmission of *H. pylori* remains incompletely defined. Infection is thought to result from direct human-to-human contact via fecal–oral, oral–oral, or gastro-oral routes.[4] Contaminated water can also be a reservoir. Low socioeconomic status, poverty, crowding, and poor hygiene are considered as major risk factors for this infection. Twenty-one percent of children whose mothers are infected with *H. pylori* acquire the infection, compared to 3% of children whose mothers are not infected, confirming that *H. pylori*-infected mothers are a key source of infection.[5] *H. pylori* infection is uncommon in children from developed countries (10%) and the number of symptomatic cases seems to be decreasing.

PATHOGENESIS

Pathogenesis of *H. pylori*-associated Peptic Disease

Adherence of *H. pylori* to gastric epithelial cells facilitates access to nutrients and delivery of effector molecules that are essential for the development of the disease.[6] The main virulence determinant of *H. pylori* is a 40-kb genomic "pathogenicity island" called cytotoxin-associated gene or *cag*. *Cag*-positive strains are closely associated with PUD and gastric cancer[7]; patients infected with *cag*-negative strains tend to have less severe disease. Genes in the *cag* pathogenicity island encode a type IV secretion system through which an effector protein, CagA, is translocated into the epithelial cell cytoplasm. Once inside the epithelial cell, CagA can disrupt signaling pathways, leading to abnormal proliferation, motility, and cytoskeletal changes. These changes may increase the predisposition to gastric cancer.

Other virulence factors also play a role in *H. pylori* infections. *VacA* is a protein encoded by the gene, *vacA*, which is thought to facilitate colonization by *H. pylori*.[8] All strains of *H. pylori* possess the *vacA* gene, but only about 50% express the mature protein. VacA possibly helps increase intracellular permeability, which would make nutrients more available to the organism. *BabA2* is another important pathogenetic factor. It is an adhesin that recognizes the blood group antigen A and allows *H. pylori* to adhere to gastric epithelial cells. *H. pylori* can cause cytotoxicity and stimulate the release of cytokines via its cell wall lipopolysaccharides (*LPS*). Exposure of the gastric mucosa to *H. pylori* LPS leads to loss of mucosal integrity, inhibition of mucin synthesis, and stimulation of pepsinogen secretion, all creating an environment favoring mucosal injury. *H. pylori* is a powerful producer of *urease*, an enzyme that generates ammonia from urea. Although urease is probably not essential for colonization and virulence, it helps bacteria survive in the stomach by creating a less acidic environment.

Children have much lower gastritis scores and an intact epithelium when compared to adults with a similar bacterial load. This is probably related to increased activity of regulatory T cells (Tregs) that down-regulate the inflammatory response to *H. pylori* in children.[9]

Pathogenesis of non-*H. pylori* Peptic Disease

Any agent that disrupts the delicate balance between potentially injurious gastric acid and pepsin and the gastric mucosal protective mechanisms (mucus and bicarbonate secretion, and gastric blood flow) can result in gastric ulcers or gastritis. NSAIDs, alcohol, caustic agents, bilious refluxate from the duodenum, pancreatic enzymes, hemodynamic shock, and a variety of ingested irritants can all upset the balance and result in gastritis or ulcer.

CLINICAL PRESENTATION

Gastritis and peptic ulcers, regardless of etiology, may present with a wide variety of symptoms, or may be completely asymptomatic, until complications (i.e.,

Table 13–1.

Clinical Manifestations of Gastritis and Peptic Ulcer Disease

Abdominal pain (epigastric, worse after meals, awakens from sleep)
Dyspepsia
Nausea
Vomiting
Nocturnal awakening
Anorexia
Early satiety
Weight loss
Hematemesis
Melena
Iron deficiency anemia
Asymptomatic

(Table 13–1). Therefore, the differential diagnosis may be quite broad (Table 13–2). Abdominal pain, poor appetite, nausea, vomiting, nocturnal awakening, and weight loss may be symptoms of severe gastric inflammation and/or PUD.

In the majority of patients, abdominal pain from peptic injury is experienced in the epigastrium, but may occasionally localize to the right or left upper quadrants or even the hypochondrium. Radiation of pain to the back may occur, but primary back pain is unusual. Although the pain is often burning or hunger-like in quality, it may also be vague and non-specific. Onset may be acute or chronic. Anorexia and weight loss may occur. Recurrent and intractable vomiting may be manifestations of gastritis and PUD. Hematemesis and/or melena may be seen if peptic ulcers are present.

Table 13–2.

Differential Diagnosis of Gastritis and Peptic Ulcer Disease

Functional abdominal pain
Non-ulcer dyspepsia
Irritable bowel syndrome
Gastroesophageal reflux
Gallstones
Crohn's disease
Celiac disease
Acute/chronic pancreatitis

Table 13–3.

Physical Exam Findings in Gastritis and Peptic Ulcer Disease

Epigastric tenderness
Right–left upper quadrant tenderness
Pallor
Rebound abdominal tenderness and guarding if perforation of ulcer
Signs of hemorrhagic shock if child is acutely bleeding

Physical exam findings are usually non-specific (Table 13–3). Children may have some tenderness in the epigastrium and/or right and left upper quadrants. Rebound tenderness is present in a rare incident of perforated ulcer. Pallor may be seen if the patient has iron deficiency anemia secondary to chronic gastrointestinal blood loss. In an acutely bleeding child, signs of hemorrhagic shock (tachycardia, hypotension, prolonged capillary refill, etc.) may predominate.

Clinical Features Specific to *H. pylori* Infection

Acute H. pylori infection is typically associated with a transient mild illness characterized by epigastric pain and nausea. Transient hypochlorhydria and neutrophilic gastritis are usually seen with the acute infection. Over the several months, acid secretion returns to near-baseline levels and severity of gastritis improves. It is not known how often the acute infection occurs with *H. pylori* and it spontaneously clears.

Chronic H. pylori infection symptoms run the entire spectrum from none at all to severe abdominal pain and bleeding from ulcers. The association between recurrent abdominal pain/non-ulcer dyspepsia (see Chapter 1 for definitions) and *H. pylori* infection continues to be debated. RAP and NUD are commonly of functional origin in children. Despite this, the Maastricht III Consensus Report recommends testing children with upper gastrointestinal symptoms for *H. pylori* infection, after exclusion of other causes of the symptoms.[10]

H. pylori infection may increase predisposition to gastroesophageal reflux disease (GERD), probably by increasing gastric acid secretion. Although some studies support an association between *H. pylori* and reflux esophagitis,[11] some report no difference in the prevalence of esophagitis in *H. pylori*-positive and -negative patients.[12]

H. pylori infection has been reported in children with iron deficiency anemia, short stature, growth delay, immune thrombocytopenic purpura (ITP), and migraines. A relationship between these manifestations and *H. pylori* remains controversial. In children with refractory iron deficiency anemia, testing for *H. pylori* may be indicated.[13]

DIFFERENTIAL DIAGNOSIS

The differential diagnosis for gastritis and PUD includes functional gastrointestinal disorders (functional abdominal pain, non-ulcer dyspepsia, and irritable bowel syndrome), gastroesophageal reflux, gallstones, pancreatitis, Crohn's disease, and celiac disease (Table 13–2). Other etiologies of gastritis and PUD are collagenous gastritis, eosinophilic gastroenteritis (EGE), Crohn's disease, lymphocytic gastritis (LG), chronic NSAID use, bile-induced gastritis, and Menetrier disease (Table 13–4).

Functional Gut Disorders

Ten to 20% of school age children complain of recurrent abdominal pain that is commonly of functional origin. In general, these children do not have alarm symptoms (vomiting, weight loss, nocturnal awakening, hematemesis, or melena). If in doubt, an upper gastrointestinal endoscopy will help determine the diagnosis.

Gastroesophageal Reflux Disease

GERD usually manifests with effortless regurgitation, heartburn, and sometimes with chest pain and dysphagia. In infants, GER is benign with a high chance of spontaneous remission by 12 months of age, thus rarely needing any treatment. If children have typical GERD symptoms in the absence of alarming symptoms (hematemesis, melena, weight loss, and dysphagia), a trial of a histamine 2 (H2) blocker or a proton pump inhibitor (PPI) is a reasonable approach. Children with alarm symptoms or no response to acid suppression have to be evaluated by a pediatric gastroenterologist.

Table 13–4.

Etiology of Gastritis and PUD in Children

Helicobacter pylori
Collagenous gastritis
Lymphocytic gastritis
Chemical gastropathy (NSAIDs, bile)
Eosinophilic
Granulomatous (Crohn's disease)

Acute–Chronic Pancreatitis

Children with acute and chronic pancreatitis can present with upper abdominal/epigastric pain, nausea, and vomiting. Epigastric tenderness is commonly found if the pancreas is inflamed. Serum amylase and lipase measurement will be helpful in distinguishing pancreatitis from peptic disease. Imaging studies (ultrasound or CT scan) can be used when the distinction is in doubt.

Gallstones

Gallstones may be asymptomatic or cause dyspepsia, epigastric pain, or right upper quadrant pain. Pain is usually postprandial. The cardinal symptom of gallstones is biliary colic. Biliary colic is a moderately severe, crescendo-type pain in the right upper quadrant radiating to the back and right shoulder, which may be accompanied by nausea. Pain may be brought on after ingestion of fatty foods. A right quadrant ultrasound will be helpful in making the differential diagnosis.

Celiac Disease

Celiac disease can present with abdominal pain, chronic or recurrent diarrhea, anorexia, weight loss, failure to thrive, vomiting, constipation, and irritability. Serologic tests, including endomysial and tissue transglutaminase antibodies, are highly sensitive and specific and will be helpful in differential diagnosis.

Chemical Gastropathy/NSAIDs

Chemical gastropathy, also known as chemical or reactive gastritis, is characterized by foveolar cell (gastric surface epithelium) hyperplasia, vascular congestion, lamina propria edema, and prominent mucosal smooth muscle fibers in the absence of mucosal inflammation.[14] Common presenting symptoms are epigastric pain and vomiting. Duodenogastric bile reflux and NSAIDs are established causes of chemical gastropathy.

NSAIDs may also cause gastritis and PUD in children, much less frequently than adults. NSAIDs are normally used for the short-term relief of pain and fever in children and are well tolerated. Chronic NSAID therapy may be associated with significant gastric injury: more than 75% of children with abdominal pain while taking NSAIDs have gastritis, antral erosions, or ulcers.[15,16]

Crohn's Disease

Crohn's disease is an inflammatory disorder of the gastrointestinal tract that can involve any portion of the gastrointestinal tract from mouth to anus. Although the most commonly involved areas are the terminal ileum and the colon, the involvement of the stomach is being recognized with increasing frequency. Children with gastric Crohn's disease may present with epigastric pain, vomiting, weight loss, hematemesis, and melena. Endoscopically, erythema, erosions, and ulcers can be seen in the stomach and the duodenum. Histologically, noncaseating epithelioid granulomas, mild focal acute, and chronic gastritis can be seen.[17]

Eosinophilic Gastroenteritis

Stomach and duodenum can also be involved in EGE. Children can present with abdominal pain, vomiting, weight loss, and diarrhea. There may be a history of other atopic conditions (asthma, allergic rhinitis, etc.), peripheral eosinophilia, and elevated serum IgE. Predominance of eosinophils within glandular gastric epithelium usually helps EGE from other gastritides.

Collagenous Gastritis

Collagenous gastritis is a very rare disorder characterized by the deposition of a subepithelial collagen and accompanying inflammatory infiltrate of the stomach.[18] Diagnosis is made by histologic examination of the stomach tissue. The natural history and pathogenesis remain unclear. The majority of adult patients with collagenous gastritis have accompanying autoimmune diseases (Hashimoto thyroiditis and polymyositis) or other intestinal diseases (celiac disease and collagenous colitis).

Lymphocytic Gastritis

LG is a rare form of gastritis (0.8–1.6% of cases) with an unclear pathogenesis. According to the updated Sydney classification system, it is characterized by a dense lymphocytic infiltration ($\geq$25 lymphocytes/100 epithelial cells) of the gastric foveolar and pit epithelium, together with a variable increase in chronic inflammatory cells in the lamina propria of the gastric mucosa.[19] There is scanty information about the etiopathogenesis, clinical significance, and evolution of LG. There may be an association between LG and gluten sensitivity or *H. pylori* infection.[20]

Menetrier Disease

Menetrier disease is a rare form of hypertrophic gastropathy characterized by the replacement of gastric acid and pepsin-producing cells (parietal and chief cells) with gastric mucous cells. This leads to excessive mucous secretion and subsequent loss of excessive amounts of protein in the mucus, resulting in hypoalbuminemia. Gastric folds are grossly enlarged in a cerebriform pattern, secondary to mucosal hypertrophy. Diagnosis can be made with contrast radiography, as barium fills the pockets of the dramatically enlarged gastric folds, creating a characteristic image. Children with Menetrier disease present with vomiting, abdominal pain, anorexia, pleural effusions, and ascites. There is an association between cytomegalovirus (CMV) infection and Menetrier disease.[21] Treatment with anticholinergics or H2 receptor antagonists can help relieve symptoms of protein loss by decreasing mucous secretion. CMV infection should be treated with appropriate antiviral drugs. Menetrier disease appears to run a benign course in children, contrary to the adult disease.

DIAGNOSIS

PPI treatment can result in false-negative invasive and non-invasive diagnostic tests for *H. pylori* (Table 13–5). Therefore, PPI should be stopped, when clinically feasible, for at least 2 weeks before testing.[10] The algorithm in Figure 13–1 summarizes the strategy for the diagnosis of gastritis and PUD in children.

Endoscopy

Upper gastrointestinal endoscopy is the best technique to investigate symptoms associated with gastritis and PUD.[22] Endoscopically, peptic ulcers have a round shape with a white base that is composed of debris and fibrin

(Figure 13–2). The border of the ulcer may be elevated and hyperemic. Gastric hyperemia may be present but it is not always concordant with the histologic diagnosis of gastritis. Grossly thickened gastric folds suggest the diagnosis of Menetrier disease (Figure 13–3). Nodules in the gastric antrum with a cobblestone appearance are associated with *H. pylori* gastritis (Figure 13–4). While the presence of antral nodularity has a high specificity for this infection, it has poor sensitivity.

Gastric and duodenal tissue samples are obtained via the endoscope's biopsy channel and submitted for histopathology. Samples sent for histopathologic studies are usually formalin-fixed, paraffin-embedded, and stained with hematoxylin and eosin (H&E). Special stains (Giemsa and silver impregnation stains such as Genta and Steiner) can be used to better visualize *H. pylori* in the mucosa. *H. pylori* is diagnosed when the spiral organisms (Figure 13–5a) are noted on histologic sections of the inflamed gastric mucosa (Figure 13–5b). A rapid urease test can be done by placing a gastric biopsy specimen in a growth medium containing urea and phenolphthalein, resulting in a color change as the bacteria grow and hydrolyze urea (Figure 13–6). The test can be read within 24 hours, and it may be positive sooner if the *H. pylori* bacteria load is high. False-negative results can occur in patients taking antisecretory drugs.

Culturing *H. pylori* from the biopsy specimen can be done, but the bacteria are difficult to grow. Bacterial culture has 100% specificity, but sensitivity varies

Table 13–5.

Diagnostic Tests for *H. pylori*[35]

Test	Sensitivity (%)	Specificity (%)	Usefulness
Invasive tests			
Endoscopy with biopsy	>95	100	Sensitivity reduced by PPIs, antibiotics, and bismuth-containing compounds
Rapid urease test	93–97	>95	Sensitivity reduced by PPIs, antibiotics, bismuth-containing compounds, active bleeding
Culture	70–80	100	Technically difficult
Non-invasive tests			
Serology	85	79	Positive result may persist for months after eradication; not recommended
Urea breath test	95–100	91–98	Sensitivity reduced by PPIs, antibiotics, and bismuth-containing compounds; reliable test for cure; high false-positive rates <6 y/o
HpSA	91–98	94–99	Test for cure 7 days after therapy is accurate; sensitivity reduced by PPIs, antibiotics, and bismuth-containing compounds, easy to do, monoclonal antibody-based test most reliable

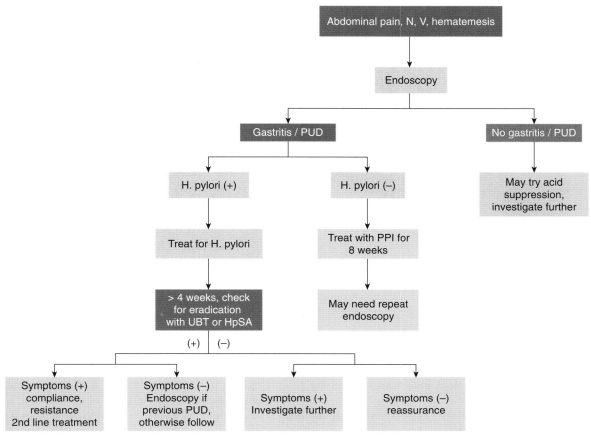

FIGURE 13–1 ■ Algorithm for the diagnosis of gastritis–PUD.

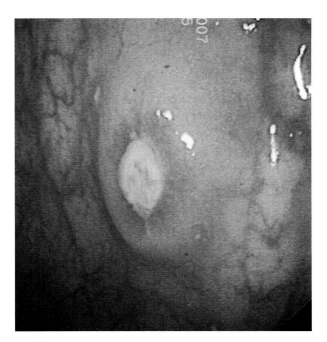

FIGURE 13–2 ■ Gastric ulcer. Figure shows a gastric ulcer viewed during endoscopy. Note the white base of the ulcer. Border of the ulcer is elevated and hyperemic.

depending on the experience of the laboratory. In children, endoscopy and biopsy remain the gold standard, as they offer the advantage of directly examining the gastrointestinal mucosa, obtaining tissue for histology and rapid urease test and culture if needed.[13]

Non-invasive Testing

^{13}C-urea breath test (UBT)

UBT is a simple, safe, and non-invasive test that can be used for the diagnosis of *H. pylori* infection. The test involves drinking a solution of ^{13}C-labeled urea, an important substrate for the *H. pylori* metabolism. If *H. pylori* is present in the stomach, the bacteria's urease hydrolyzes the urea into ammonia and CO_2:

$$(NH2)_2{}^{13}CO + H_2O \rightarrow {}^{13}CO_2 + 2NH_3$$

$^{13}CO_2$ diffuses into the bloodstream and is then measured in the exhaled breath specimen using mass spectrometry. UBT can be used for the diagnosis of *H. pylori* as well as confirming eradication of the bacteria after therapy. PPIs and/or antibiotics should be discontinued at least 4 weeks before the test to avoid a

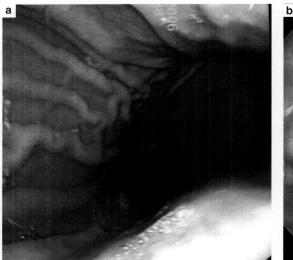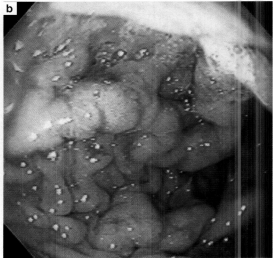

FIGURE 13–3 ▪ (a) Normal gastric folds for comparison. (b) Menetrier disease. Figure shows visibly thickened gastric folds that are typically seen in Menetrier disease.

false-negative UBT. This test has been shown to be safe (it uses a non-radioactive stable isotope of carbon) and accurate in older children with high sensitivity (93%) and specificity (95%).[23,24]

There are several different protocols available for children over 6 years of age (variety of ^{13}C-urea doses and test meals). The test is commercially available in the United States, but it has not been used extensively in pediatrics. Although the UBT has been studied in children, its diagnostic ability, especially in those younger than 3 years of age, may be limited by several factors. For example, performance of the test requires rapidly swallowing the solution to avoid contamination with urease-producing organisms from the oropharynx.

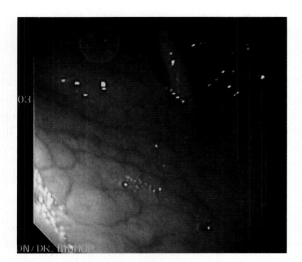

FIGURE 13–4 ▪ Gastric lymphoid nodular hyperplasia. Nodules in the gastric antrum give a cobblestone appearance. This finding is commonly associated with *H. pylori* gastritis.

Young children who resist swallowing the unfamiliar drink may therefore have false-positive test results. Being able to exhale into a straw is also critical for test reliability and accuracy. False-negative results may occur in those who have recently taken gastric acid antisecretory agents, bismuth compounds, or antibiotic agents. Although the ^{13}C-labeled UBT has been used in children and appears promising, reliability and determination of threshold values have not been adequately validated in multiple, large multicenter, randomized, controlled trials. UBT has the additional drawback, compared to endoscopy, of not being able to determine gastroduodenal pathology.

H. pylori stool antigen (HpSA)

H. pylori antigen stool EIA testing is a cheap and easy method for the diagnosis of the *H. pylori* infection. Keeping the stool samples at room temperature for up to 5 days or freezing them for months/years does not seem to influence the accuracy of this test. Stool antigen test seems to be reliable at all ages (93% sensitivity and 98% specificity) but it must be noted that only a small number of children below 6 years of age have been studied. In adults, PPIs decrease the sensitivity of the stool *H. pylori* antigen test. Although likely, it is not known if this restriction applies to pediatric patients as well. Monoclonal antibody-based tests are preferred because of their higher sensitivity compared to those using polyclonal antibodies (95% versus 83%). Alternatively, several commercially available 10-minute one-step kits using immunochromatography with monoclonal antibody capture and detection can also be done in stool specimens. These are convenient to perform in the office. However, the occurrence

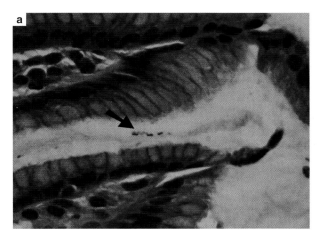 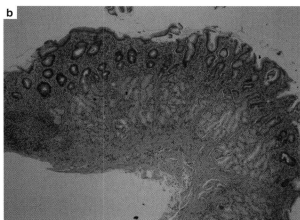

FIGURE 13–5 ■ Histologic diagnosis of *Helicobacter pylori* infection. Gastric antral biopsy at lower magnification shows inflammatory cell infiltrates in the superficial layer of the lamina propria (b), confirming gastritis; silver stain show spiral-shaped microorganisms in gastric pits (a). (Photo courtesy of Dr. Chris Jensen, University of Iowa.)

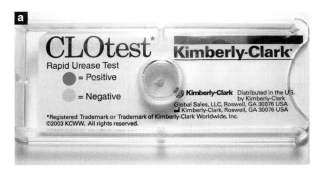

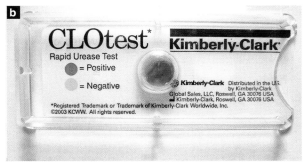

FIGURE 13–6 ■ Rapid urease test. Figure shows a negative (a) and a positive (b) urease test. Presence of *Helicobacter* organisms alkalinize urea containing medium and cause the color change from yellow to red.

of equivocal results remains a major problem with these tests.

Studies with *H. pylori* antigen in North American children are limited. Most of the studies are conducted at specialized referral centers; therefore, it is not known how this test will perform in a community practice setting. Perhaps because the test is not yet validated in different populations, it is generally not used in North America as a diagnostic tool for children infected with *H. pylori*, but nevertheless seems promising, based on the available adult studies.

Serologic tests

Serologic tests are available for the diagnosis of *H. pylori* infection. The sensitivity and the specificity of these antibodies (IgG or IgA) against *H. pylori* vary widely in children.[22] Serologic assays should not be used solely for the diagnosis of *H. pylori* infection or to monitor response to therapy because a positive IgG test can be found several months or even years after the infection. We do not recommend this test for the diagnosis of *H. pylori* or the response to therapy.

Stool PCR for H. pylori detection

A biprobe real-time PCR method (*Helicobacter pylori* ClariRes assay® (Ingenetix, Vienna, Austria)) is designed for the detection of *H. pylori* infection and the simultaneous clarithromycin susceptibility testing of *H. pylori* isolates in stool samples.[25] The specificity of PCR is 100%, while the sensitivity is ~60%. The test may give false-positive results after treatment, because DNA may persist in the stool up to 4–8 weeks after eradication. Stool PCR test is currently not recommended for routine use, but may be a helpful method for the detection of clarithromycin resistance of *H. pylori*, which is an emerging problem in pediatrics.

TREATMENT

Treatment of *H. pylori*-related Gastritis and PUD

North American Society for Pediatric Gastroenterology, Hepatology and Nutrition (NASPGHAN) recommends eradication therapy in children with an endoscopically proven duodenal or gastric ulcer with *H. pylori* documented via histopathology. Another indication is documentation of *H. pylori* in patients with previous ulcer

Table 13–6.

H. pylori Eradication Regimens

Triple therapies	
PPI	
Omeprazole, lansoprazole	1–2 mg/kg/day
Antibiotics	
Amoxicillin	50 mg/kg day, given twice a day
Plus	
Clarithromycin	15 mg/kg/day, given twice a day
Amoxicillin	50 mg/kg/day, given twice a day
Plus	
Metronidazole	20 mg/kg/day, given twice a day
Clarithromycin	15 mg/kg/day, given twice a day
Plus	
Metronidazole	20 mg/kg/day, given twice a day
Regimen includes 1 PPI plus a combination antibiotic regimen for 7–14 days	
Quadruple therapies	
Bismuth subsalicylate	8 mg/kg/day
Tetracycline (>8 y/o)	25–50 mg/kg/day
Regimen includes PPI+metronidazole+bismuth+tetracycline for 7–14 days	

disease or iron deficiency anemia. This guideline does not support eradication therapy or withholding treatment in children with gastritis, even if positive for *H. pylori*, because of a lack of data demonstrating that eradication prevents PUD. Nevertheless, the clinical trend is to treat symptomatic children who are *H. pylori*-positive.

PPI-based triple therapy is the treatment of choice for *H. pylori* infection. This includes a combination of PPI, clarithromycin, and amoxicillin or metronidazole, all given twice a day (Table 13–6). There is some controversy over the most effective length of treatment for this regimen. The duration of treatment varies from 7 to 14 days with eradication rates at 60–85%. Although 7–10 days have been proven to be effective, 14-day duration is preferred to better eradicate the organism.[13] Bacterial resistance and poor compliance are the main reasons of treatment failure in *H. pylori* infection. In an era of increasing clarithromycin resistance and declining eradication rates, triple therapy may not be effective in all cases. *Quadruple therapies* comprising PPI, metronidazole, tetracycline, and bismuth are effective alternative first-line treatments that may be advocated in areas of high antibiotic resistance. However, this regime requires the administration of four drugs at frequent intervals and may be associated with a high incidence of side effects. The most commonly reported adverse events are nausea, vomiting, and diarrhea. A bitter or metallic taste in the mouth is associated with eradication regimens

containing clarithromycin. Bismuth subsalicylate may cause a temporary grayish-black discoloration of the stool.

Collecting data on the success of various treatment regimens for childhood *H. pylori* is difficult because of the small number of infected children in each individual center. A pediatric European register for treatment of *H. pylori* (PERTH) was established to collect data on treatment of *H. pylori* in children.[26] Overall eradication rate was 65.6%, and was significantly higher in children with ulcer than without. Omeprazole-containing triple therapies were the most commonly used, although their efficacy was low. Bismuth-containing therapies resulted in higher eradication rate. The most promising new treatment regime for *H. pylori* in children has been reported from Russia, where Nijevitch et al. observed eradication rates of 86% with bismuth subcitrate (8 mg/kg/day), nifuratel (30 mg/kg/day), and amoxicillin (50 mg/kg/day) for 10 days.[27] At the present time, quadruple therapy possibly offers the best second-line treatment option in children.

There are reports showing successful eradication of *H. pylori* with sequential treatment strategies (omeprazole plus amoxicillin for 5 days, followed by omeprazole plus clarithromycin plus tinidazole for another 5 days).[28] Children with persistent *H. pylori* despite treatment with a triple therapy regimen should be assessed for several predictors of treatment failure, in particular, treatment compliance. Antimicrobial resistance is the other main reason for treatment failures, and thus should also be considered in a child with persistent infection.

Follow-up After Treatment

Non-invasive tests should be employed for confirmation of eradication unless otherwise an endoscopy is indicated. UBT or monoclonal HpSA are reasonable options. Confirmation of *H. pylori* eradication should be performed at least 4 weeks after treatment.

Antibiotic Resistance

Antibiotic resistance to *H. pylori* is an emerging problem and an important cause of treatment failure. In the United States, clarithromycin resistance rates have reached 10–12.5%.[29] Resistance to metronidazole is much more common than resistance to macrolides, ~30–40%. There is some concern about the reliability of current methods for testing *H. pylori* resistance to metronidazole in both children and adults, and routine testing for metronidazole resistance is not recommended.[30]

Prevention

Immunization with vaccines containing the *H. pylori* VacA, CagA, and neutrophil-activating protein (NAP), alone or in combination, have been shown to prevent experimental infection in animals. A phase I study with an intramuscular *H. pylori* vaccine in non-infected volunteers demonstrated safety and immunogenicity.[31] *H. pylori* vaccine will not be one of the childhood vaccines in the near future, but this study holds promise for the future.

Treatment of Non-*H. pylori*-related Gastritis and PUD

H2 receptor antagonists

These agents may be used for the healing of gastritis and PUD. They inhibit acid secretion, competing with the H2 receptors of parietal cells, and reduce pepsinogen secretion. Ranitidine, 5–10 mg/kg/day, divided in two doses, heals ulcers in 80–100% of cases after 8 weeks of treatment.[32]

Proton pump inhibitors

PPIs (omeprazole, lansoprazole, pantoprazole, esomeprazole, and rabeprazole) are the most potent acid-secretion blockers available on the market. They specifically block the H^+–K^+-ATPase on the apical membrane of the parietal cell, with consequent, almost complete suppression of acid secretion. They are most effective if given 15–20 minutes before meals, in one or two divided doses per day. With a dose range of 0.7–3.3 mg/kg/day,[33] PPIs will promote healing of up to 100% of cases after 6 weeks. For NSAID-induced gastritis and PUD, PPIs remain the best choice for therapy.[34]

Sucralfate has no effect on gastric acid secretion; however, it can contribute to the healing of ulcers by increasing the blood flow in the mucosa, as well as bicarbonate secretion and gastric mucus.

REFERENCES

1. Egbaria R, Levine A, Tamir A, Shaoul R. Peptic ulcers and erosions are common in Israeli children undergoing upper endoscopy. *Helicobacter*. 2008;13:62–68.
2. Czinn SJ. *Helicobacter pylori* infection: detection, investigation, and management. *J Pediatr*. 2005;146:S21–S26.
3. Drumm B, Day AS, Gold B, et al. *Helicobacter pylori* and peptic ulcer: Working Group report of the second World Congress of Pediatric Gastroenterology, Hepatology, and Nutrition. *J Pediatr Gastroenterol Nutr*. 2004;39(suppl 2):S626–S631.
4. Gold BD, Colletti RB, Abbott M, et al. *Helicobacter pylori* infection in children: recommendations for diagnosis and treatment. *J Pediatr Gastroenterol Nutr*. 2000;31:490–497.
5. Fujimoto Y, Furusyo N, Toyoda K, Takeoka H, Sawayama Y, Hayashi J. Intrafamilial transmission of *Helicobacter pylori* among the population of endemic areas in Japan. *Helicobacter*. 2007;12:170–176.
6. Maeda S, Mentis AF. Pathogenesis of *Helicobacter pylori* infection. *Helicobacter*. 2007;12(suppl 1):10–14.
7. Basso D, Zambon CF, Letley DP, et al. Clinical relevance of *Helicobacter pylori* cagA and vacA gene polymorphisms. *Gastroenterology*. 2008;135:91–99.
8. Cover TL, Blanke SR. *Helicobacter pylori* VacA, a paradigm for toxin multifunctionality. *Nat Rev Microbiol*. 2005;3:320–332.
9. Harris PR, Wright SW, Serrano C, et al. *Helicobacter pylori* gastritis in children is associated with a regulatory T-cell response. *Gastroenterology*. 2008;134:491–499.
10. Malfertheiner P, Megraud F, O'Morain C, et al. Current concepts in the management of *Helicobacter pylori* infection: the Maastricht III Consensus Report. *Gut*. 2007;56:772–781.
11. Daugule I, Rumba I, Alksnis J, Ejderhamn J. *Helicobacter pylori* infection among children with gastrointestinal symptoms: a high prevalence of infection among patients with reflux oesophagitis. *Acta Paediatr*. 2007;96:1047–1049.
12. Elitsur Y, Durst P, Lawrence Z, Rewalt M. Does *Helicobacter pylori* protect children from reflux disease? *J Clin Gastroenterol*. 2008;42:215–216.
13. Bourke B, Ceponis P, Chiba N, et al. Canadian *Helicobacter* Study Group Consensus Conference: update on the approach to *Helicobacter pylori* infection in children and adolescents—an evidence-based evaluation. *Can J Gastroenterol*. 2005;19:399–408.
14. Pashankar DS, Bishop WP, Mitros FA. Chemical gastropathy: a distinct histopathologic entity in children. *J Pediatr Gastroenterol Nutr*. 2002;35:653–657.
15. Mulberg AE, Linz C, Bern E, Tucker L, Verhave M, Grand RJ. Identification of nonsteroidal antiinflammatory drug-induced gastroduodenal injury in children with juvenile rheumatoid arthritis. *J Pediatr*. 1993;122:647–649.
16. Ashorn M, Verronen P, Ruuska T, Huhtala H. Upper endoscopic findings in children with active juvenile chronic arthritis. *Acta Paediatr*. 2003;92:558–561.
17. Pascasio JM, Hammond S, Qualman SJ. Recognition of Crohn disease on incidental gastric biopsy in childhood. *Pediatr Dev Pathol*. 2003;6:209–214.
18. Leung ST, Chandan VS, Murray JA, Wu TT. Collagenous gastritis: histopathologic features and association with other gastrointestinal diseases. *Am J Surg Pathol*. 2009;33:788–798.
19. Dixon MF, Genta RM, Yardley JH, Correa P. Classification and grading of gastritis. The updated Sydney system. International workshop on the histopathology of gastritis, Houston, 1994. *Am J Surg Pathol*. 1996;20:1161–1181.
20. Prasad KK, Thapa BR, Lal S, Sharma AK, Nain CK, Singh K. Lymphocytic gastritis and celiac disease in Indian children: evidence of a positive relation. *J Pediatr Gastroenterol Nutr*. 2008;47:568–572.
21. Occena RO, Taylor SF, Robinson CC, Sokol RJ. Association of cytomegalovirus with Menetrier's disease in childhood: report of two new cases with a review of literature. *J Pediatr Gastroenterol Nutr*. 1993;17:217–224.

22. Guarner J, Kalach N, Elitsur Y, Koletzko S. *Helicobacter pylori* diagnostic tests in children: review of the literature from 1999 to 2009. *Eur J Pediatr.* 2010;169:15–25. Epub 2009.

23. Elitsur Y, Tolia V, Gilger MA, et al. Urea breath test in children: the United States prospective, multicenter study. *Helicobacter.* 2009;14:134–140.

24. Dondi E, Rapa A, Boldorini R, Fonio P, Zanetta S, Oderda G. High accuracy of noninvasive tests to diagnose *Helicobacter pylori* infection in very young children. *J Pediatr.* 2006;149:817–821.

25. Lottspeich C, Schwarzer A, Panthel K, Koletzko S, Russmann H. Evaluation of the novel *Helicobacter pylori* ClariRes real-time PCR assay for detection and clarithromycin susceptibility testing of *H. pylori* in stool specimens from symptomatic children. *J Clin Microbiol.* 2007;45:1718–1722.

26. Oderda G, Shcherbakov P, Bontems P, et al. Results from the pediatric European register for treatment of *Helicobacter pylori* (PERTH). *Helicobacter.* 2007;12:150–156.

27. Nijevitch AA, Sataev VU, Akhmadeyeva EN, Arsamastsev AG. Nifuratel-containing initial anti-*Helicobacter pylori* triple therapy in children. *Helicobacter.* 2007;12:132–135.

28. Francavilla R, Lionetti E, Castellaneta SP, et al. Improved efficacy of 10-day sequential treatment for *Helicobacter pylori* eradication in children: a randomized trial. *Gastroenterology.* 2005;129:1414–1419.

29. Egan BJ, Katicic M, O'Connor HJ, O'Morain CA. Treatment of *Helicobacter pylori*. *Helicobacter.* 2007;12(suppl 1): 31–37.

30. Daugule I, Rowland M. *Helicobacter pylori* infection in children. *Helicobacter.* 2008;13(suppl 1):41–46.

31. Malfertheiner P, Schultze V, Rosenkranz B, et al. Safety and immunogenicity of an intramuscular *Helicobacter pylori* vaccine in noninfected volunteers: a phase I study. *Gastroenterology.* 2008;135:787–795.

32. Bittencourt PF, Rocha GA, Penna FJ, Queiroz DM. Gastroduodenal peptic ulcer and *Helicobacter pylori* infection in children and adolescents. *J Pediatr (Rio J).* 2006;82:325–334.

33. Hassall E, Israel D, Shepherd R, et al. Omeprazole for treatment of chronic erosive esophagitis in children: a multicenter study of efficacy, safety, tolerability and dose requirements. International Pediatric Omeprazole Study Group. *J Pediatr.* 2000;137:800–807.

34. Goldstein JL, Johanson JF, Suchower LJ, Brown KA. Healing of gastric ulcers with esomeprazole versus ranitidine in patients who continued to receive NSAID therapy: a randomized trial. *Am J Gastroenterol.* 2005;100:2650–2657.

35. Ables AZ, Simon I, Melton ER. Update on *Helicobacter pylori* treatment. *Am Fam Physician.* 2007;75:351–358.

CHAPTER 14

Abdominal Wall Defects

Steven Elliott and Anthony Sandler

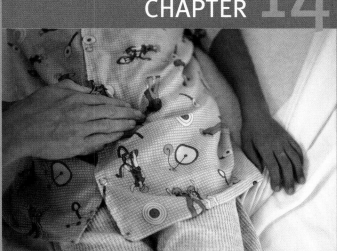

DEFINITIONS AND EPIDEMIOLOGY

Abdominal wall defects in children present as a range of anomalies, from minor hernias of the umbilical or inguinal region to major protrusions of the abdominal wall, such as omphaloceles and gastroschisis. The range of care for these defects spans elective outpatient surgery to emergent care with extended stays in the neonatal intensive care unit. Advances in medical care have greatly improved the survival of infants born with congenital abdominal wall defects such as gastroschisis and omphalocele. Advances include parenteral nutrition, perinatal care, and surgical techniques when primary closure is not possible. However, after the perinatal period challenges for these children with abdominal wall defects may continue for some time.

Hernias and Embryologic Remnants

Abdominal wall hernias are very common in the pediatric population, and the surgical treatments are among the most common procedures performed by pediatric surgeons. Hernias are defined by location as well as reducibility. Reducibility will dictate treatment management of a hernia. A *reducible hernia* allows the patient or examiner to place the abdominal contents back into the abdominal cavity with palpation. An *incarcerated hernia* is one in which reduction of the abdominal contents is not possible. A *strangulated hernia* is an incarcerated hernia that is being rendered ischemic by loss of blood supply, a true surgical emergency.

Epigastric hernias are small midline protrusions located between the umbilicus and the xiphoid process. These hernias have no sac and consist of preperitoneal fat protruding through a small fascial defect. Although small, epigastric defects do not close spontaneously and operative closure is recommended to avoid symptomatic fat entrapment. Umbilical hernias develop when the umbilical ring is unsupported, and the rectus muscles fail to approximate in the midline and close the fascial ring through which the umbilical cord protrudes.[1]

The most common hernia treated by pediatric surgeons is an inguinal hernia. Inguinal hernias are formed by failure of the processus vaginalis to completely close, leaving a potential peritoneal diverticulum into which abdominal viscera may herniate or into which fluid can accumulate and form a cystic fluid-filled cavity (hydrocele). In males, persistent patency of all or part of the processus vaginalis may result in various anomalies, including an inguinal hernia (Figure 14–1), a scrotal hernia (Figure 14–2), a communicating hydrocele, a hydrocele of the spermatic cord (Figure 14–3), and a scrotal hydrocele. In females, inguinal hernias and hydroceles can present as a protrusion or mass in the labia majora but arise far less commonly due to the absence of gonadal descent (Figure 14–4).

Urachal remnants involve the embryologic urachus, a cord-like structure that extends from the dome of the bladder to the inferior border of the umbilical ring, which has failed to obliterate. An embryologic remnant, the omphalomesenteric duct is a normal developmental structure that connects the fetal gut with the yolk sac and subsequently obliterates. Failure of obliteration may result in the formation of a polyp, fistula, cyst, fibrous band, sinus, or Meckel's diverticulum.

Congenital Defects of the Abdominal Wall

Gastroschisis is a defect of the anterior abdominal wall in which the viscera extrude and are not covered by

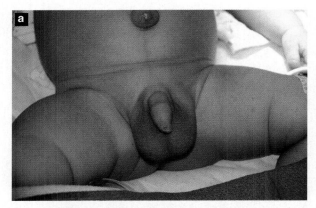

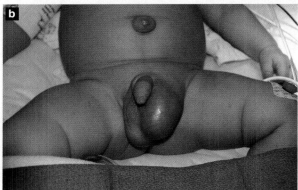

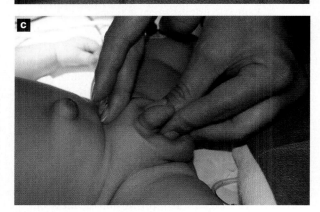

FIGURE 14–1 ■ Inguinal hernia with reduction (a–c).

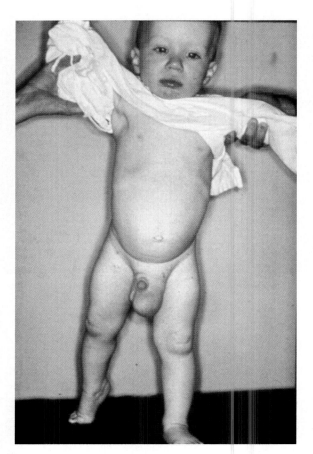

FIGURE 14–2 ■ Scrotal hernia.

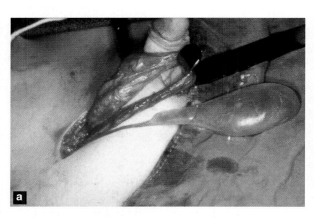

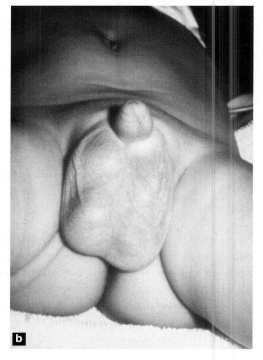

FIGURE 14–3 ■ Operative image of the hydrocele (a) and hydrocele of the spermatic cord (b).

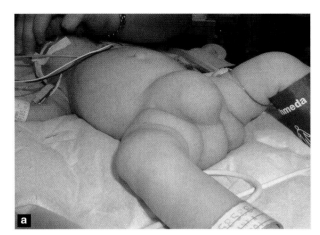
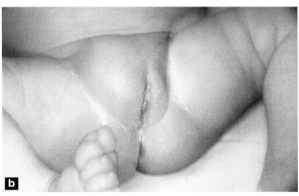
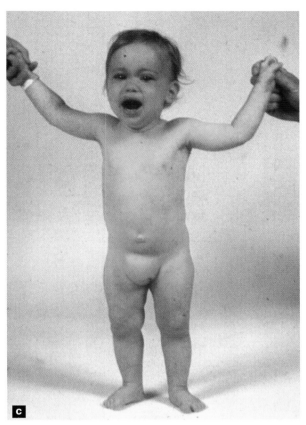

FIGURE 14–4 ■ Female hernia (a) and female inguinal hernia (b and c).

amnion or a peritoneal membrane. This defect almost always occurs to the right of the umbilical cord (Figure 14–5). Gastroschisis is not usually associated with other anomalies and chromosomal syndromes as is the case in omphalocele; however, intestinal atresia may be present in 10% of patients with gastroschisis.[2]

Omphalocele is a herniation of abdominal contents through the umbilical ring (Figure 14–6). The herniation (also known as exomphalos) is covered by a sac composed of an outer layer of amnion and an inner layer of peritoneum. Approximately 50% of patients with omphalocele will have anomalies of the cardiovascular, alimentary, genitourinary, musculoskeletal, and/or CNS. Various defined syndromes and trisomies are associated with omphaloceles.[2–4]

Abdominal wall defects can be associated with other organ system anomalies beyond the GI tract, including pentalogy of Cantrell (ectopia cordis, pericardial and diaphragmatic defects, cardiac defects, cleft sternum, and omphalocele) (Figure 14–7) and cloacal exstrophy (imperforate anus, omphalocele, exstrophy of the bladder, and lower neural tube defects) (Figure 14–8). A less dramatic abdominal wall defect is an umbilical cord hernia. This is a small (<4 cm) anomaly with a thin membrane and usually only contains the midgut.

This occurs because the midgut fails to completely return to the abdominal cavity at 10–12 weeks gestation. This defect can almost always be closed primarily, via a simple closure following reduction of the prolapsed bowel. Unlike simple umbilical hernias, these do not usually close spontaneously.

The overall prevalence of abdominal wall defects is 4–5 per 10,000 live births; with the increased use of prenatal ultrasound this has been reported to be as high as 1 in 2500 fetuses. The incidence of omphalocele is historically reported as 1 in 4000 births and gastroschisis as 1 in 6000–10,000 births. The incidence of gastroschisis is increasing in reports from both the United Kingdom and the United States and gastroschisis is becoming more frequently encountered than omphalocele in clinical practice. Male and female infants are equally affected.[2,3,6]

Embryology of the Abdominal Wall

A basic understanding of the embryology of the anterior abdominal wall is necessary to understand the pathogenesis of abdominal wall defects. During the first 3 weeks of gestation, the body is a disc-like structure between the chorion and the amnion. Around the fourth week of

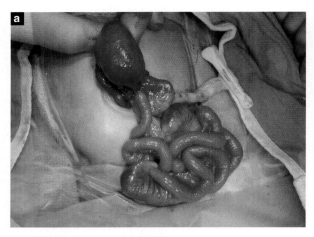 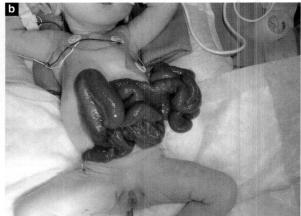

FIGURE 14–5 ■ Gastroschisis (a) and gastroschisis with atresia (b).

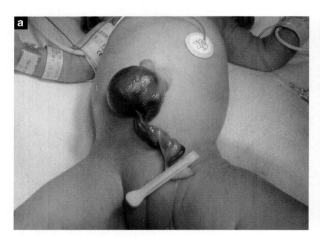 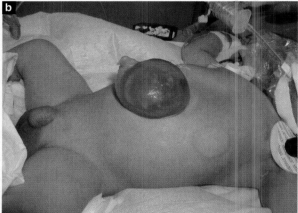

FIGURE 14–6 ■ Epigastric omphalocele (a) and small omphalocele (b).

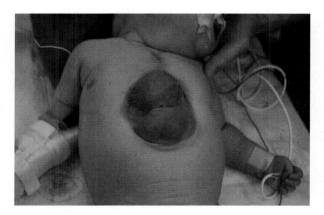

FIGURE 14–7 ■ Pentalogy of Cantrell.

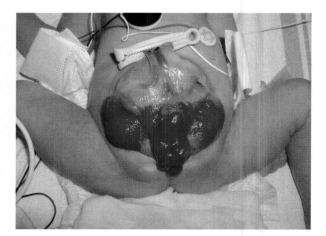

FIGURE 14–8 ■ Cloacal exstrophy.

gestation, the formation of a body cavity begins with the inversion of the lateral edges of the body disk. The division of thoracic and abdominal cavities is performed by the descent of the cephalic fold, which brings the embryologic heart downward, as the septum transversum. The cephalic fold components will contribute to the thoracic and epigastric walls. Failure of these mesodermal myotomes in the upper midline to fuse leads to the defect known as pentalogy of Cantrell. The caudad fold moves upward to form the infraumbilical abdominal wall and bringing the bladder (allantois) upward, additionally contributing to the hindgut and hypogastric wall. Failure of the urorectal septum to rise and separate will result in cloacal exstrophy. The lateral folds will develop into the midgut and lateral abdominal wall.[2–6]

At this point, the primitive gut is a straight tube in continuity with the yolk sac, which will diminish, leaving a solid umbilical stalk. The fifth to sixth weeks of gestation marks the rapid growth of the midgut (a.k.a. primary intestinal loop) and a physiologic herniation occurs through the umbilical ring into the umbilical coelom. The formation of the umbilical/extraembryonic coelom is formed (5–6 weeks gestation) by coalescence of vacuoles of Wharton's jelly within the umbilical stalk. At the 10–12th weeks of gestation, the embryonic gut returns to the abdominal cavity and undergoes a 270° (counter-clockwise) rotation around the superior mesenteric artery.[2,6]

During the development of the anterior abdominal wall, the anatomic structures of the umbilical ring include: the allantois, four umbilical vessels (two arteries and two veins), the vitelline duct, vitelline vessels, and the umbilical/extraembryonic coelom. At the fifth week of gestation the right umbilical vein resorbs, leaving the left umbilical vein to return placental blood to the heart. This involution may create a weakness on the right side of the umbilical cord. When the midgut returns to the abdominal wall, the allantois, vitelline duct, and vitelline vessels are obliterated. This process leaves the paired umbilical arteries and left umbilical vein remaining in the umbilical ring.

PATHOGENESIS

Hernias and Embryologic Remnants

The development of a patent processus vaginalis and subsequent inguinal hernia is based on descent of the testis. Under typical conditions, the internal inguinal ring closes and the lumen of the processus vaginalis, an outpouching of the peritoneal cavity, obliterates above the testis (Figure 14–9).

Urachal remnants are formed if the mucosa-lined urachus does not obliterate. One of the following five uncommon anomalies can occur: (1) congenital persistence of a *patent urachus*, causing a fistulous tract joining the bladder lumen and the umbilicus. Surgical repair consists of urachal tract excision and ligation at the bladder junction. (2) A remnant *urachal sinus* opens to the umbilicus, while a (3) *urachal diverticulum* opens to the bladder. (4) A *urachal cyst* forms anywhere along the urachal tract but does not communicate with either the umbilicus or the bladder. (5) An *alternating sinus* is a cyst-like struc-

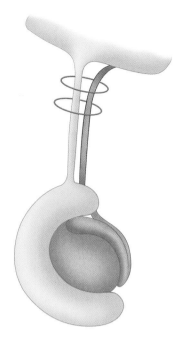

FIGURE 14–9 ■ Diagram of inguinal hernia anatomy.

ture that can drain into either the bladder or the umbilicus. Diagnosis and differentiation of these anomalies is aided by fistulography, ultrasound, and/or CT scan.[7]

Congenital Defects of the Abdominal Wall

The earlier the embryologic abnormality manifests, the more complex and usually devastating the anomaly (Table 14–1). Abdominal wall defects can occur because of: (1) failed mesoderm migration and decreased apoptosis, (2) failure of the yolk sac and body stalk to approximate with the amnion, (3) lack of the umbilical ring development, and (4) abnormal neuronal differentiation.

Gastroschisis develops between the sixth and seventh weeks of gestation, believed to be caused by vascular compromise to the right-sided abdominal wall. The gestational timing of gastroschisis coincides with the obliteration of the right umbilical vein. Early obliteration of the right umbilical vein or persistence of the vessel, interfering with the development of collateral circulation, has been used to explain this ischemic event. Another unproven, but possible, explanation is that simple separation of the cord occurs from the umbilical ring on the right side of its attachment. Indirect evidence of this may be encountered from the clinical observation of spontaneous closure of the umbilical port with simple reduction of the bowel without fascial repair. Normal abdominal wall development is present. A rare occurrence is prenatal rupture of an omphalocele. The infant presents with an abdominal wall defect with the appearance of gastroschisis, but with abnormal abdominal wall development.

Table 14–1.

Embryologic Timeline

Gestational Age	Embryology Development	Defect	Anomaly
3–4 weeks	Development of four folds to form body cavities		
4–6 weeks	Anterior abdominal wall development, development of umbilical coelom	Failure of folds to develop	Body stalk defect
	Umbilical coelom develops, atrophy of right umbilical vein	Failure of coelom development or vascular accident	Gastroschisis
7–8 weeks	Myotome fusions in midline	Defective fusion of midline cranial fold	Pentalogy of Cantrell
		Defective fusion of midline caudal fold	Bladder or cloacal exstrophy
	Development of cloacal membrane and urorectal septum	Abnormal development of urorectal septum	Imperforate anus
7–12 weeks	Herniation of bowel and return to abdominal cavity	Failure of lateral folds to fuse	Omphalocele
	Bowel undergoes rotation and fixation	Failure of appropriate rotation and fixation	Malrotation

Adapted from Klein MD. Congenital abdominal wall defects. In: Ashcraft KW, ed. Pediatric Surgery. 4th ed. Saunders; 2004:chap 46; and Minkes RK. In: Oldham KT, ed. Principles and Practice of Pediatric Surgery. 2nd ed. Lippincott Williams and Wilkins; 2004:chap 69.

Omphalocele is believed to develop from failure of the lateral folds to migrate and fuse appropriately at the umbilical ring, resulting in continued herniation of the midgut. The fascial defect can vary widely from small (i.e., congenital hernia of the umbilical cord) to large (>12 cm). Giant omphaloceles can present with the entire gastrointestinal system, liver, spleen, bladder, and gonads outside of the abdominal cavity. These cases are extremely difficult to treat because without intra-abdominal organs the abdominal cavity loses domain and fails to grow.

Multiple studies have been performed to address possible maternal and environmental factors that may attribute to the development of abdominal wall defects. Epidemiologic and animal models suggest possible causal factors, including use of cyclooxygenase inhibitors (ibuprofen and aspirin) during gestation, and recreational and illicit drugs (nicotine and cocaine), and are also associated in children of women with multiple children who have different fathers.[8–11] Maternal obesity has been shown to increase the risk of omphalocele; however, a recent meta-analysis suggests that obesity reduces the risk of gastroschisis.[12,13] Gastroschisis is associated with young maternal age.[14] Additional medications producing vasoconstriction early in pregnancy increase the risk of gastroschisis; this includes common medications for colds, cough, and pain.[15] Omphalocele can present either independently or with other associated anomalies. There are no environmental factors or teratogens identified that are associated with isolated omphalocele. In a single study, preconceptional multivitamin use was associated with a 60% reduction in the risk for non-syndromic omphalocele.[16]

CLINICAL PRESENTATION

Umbilical Hernias

Umbilical hernias most commonly present during the early months of infancy and occur more frequently in Black, low-birth-weight, and premature infants. Most umbilical hernias are isolated findings, but some are associated with other disorders including Beckwith–Wiedemann syndrome (omphalocele–macroglossia–gigantism), hypothyroidism, mucopolysaccharidosis, and Down's syndrome (trisomy 21).[17] Concomitant inguinal hernias are noted in about 15% of children with umbilical hernias.[18] Umbilical hernias are rarely symptomatic and infants are commonly brought for medical evaluation because of family concern. Palpation of the umbilicus reveals a well-defined rim that surrounds the umbilical defect.

Inguinal Hernias

Premature infants

The clinical presentation of inguinal hernias can vary between premature infants and children. Inguinal hernias arise in about 10% of preterm infants. Bilateral inguinal hernias also occur more commonly in preterm infants.[19] The risk of incarceration of a hernia in a preterm infant is two to five times greater than the risk in older children (30% versus 6–15%).[20] Repair of incarcerated hernias and large hernias in preterm infants can be very difficult due to the inflammatory changes and tissue-paper consistency of structures in the inguinal region.

Infant and childhood hernias

Approximately 4% of term infants are born with a congenital indirect inguinal hernia. Inguinal hernias occur on the right in 60%, on the left in 30%, and bilaterally in 10% of cases. The increased incidence of right-sided hernias may be related to later descent of the right testis and delayed obliteration of the processus vaginalis.[21] Inguinal hernias in boys usually present as a bulge in the groin that is more apparent with crying or straining and may extend into the hemiscrotum. Inguinal hernias may reduce spontaneously when the child relaxes, or be reduced manually with gentle pressure. Once the hernia is reduced, digital pressure on the external ring will prevent re-herniation of the viscus. Inguinal hernias in females present as a bulge in the superior aspect of the labia majora. A palpable mass may represent a herniated ovary. If gonads are palpable bilaterally in female patients, one should suspect androgen insensitivity syndrome (formerly known as testicular feminization syndrome).

Incarceration is the most common complication of inguinal hernias and occurs in up to 10% of children overall. In the first year of life, the incidence is higher and incarceration is reported to occur in as many as 31% of children with hernias.[22] Presenting symptoms of an incarcerated inguinal hernia include irritability, pain, abdominal distension, and vomiting. Small bowel obstruction may occur if the entrapped mass becomes edematous. Examination of an incarcerated hernia usually reveals a tender, firm, erythematous mass in the inguinal region (Figure 14–10). Edema of the groin and scrotal skin may also be present. In girls, a palpable, irreducible ovary occurs in 15% of inguinal hernias and despite possible incarceration and strangulation of the ovary, intestinal symptoms will be absent in these children. A bimanual technique should be used when attempting reduction. Digital manipulation with one hand compresses the hernia, while the other hand, placed over the external ring, guides the hernia through it.

Congenital Defects of the Abdominal Wall

Abdominal wall defects can present either at birth or with prenatal diagnosis from a maternal screening ultrasound. Pregnant women may present with an elevated

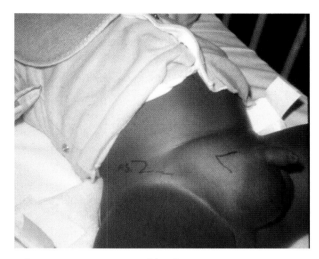

FIGURE 14–10 ■ Incarcerated hernia.

alpha-fetoprotein (maternal serum alpha-fetoprotein (msAFP)) on a maternal triple-screen evaluation. The sensitivity of msAFP for gastroschisis is higher than for omphalocele, but a majority of omphaloceles do have an elevated msAFP.[23] Additionally, elevated msAFP is an indication to proceed with a fetal ultrasound. A maternal ultrasound after 12 weeks gestation can identify abdominal wall defects because, at this point in gestation, the midgut has usually returned to the abdominal cavity.[24] Detailed description of ultrasound and triple screen will be addressed in the section "Diagnostic Tests."

Infants who are diagnosed at delivery with an abdominal wall defect must be assessed for the type of defect by working through the differential diagnosis (discussed in the following section). Infants diagnosed with an omphalocele require ultrasound examination to identify other congenital abnormalities prior to proceeding with definitive repair, as these abnormalities may affect anesthesia. The clinical presentations of other abdominal wall defects such as pentology of Cantrell and cloacal exstrophy are similar to omphalocele and gastroschisis but require a multidisciplinary approach with cardiothoracic surgery for pentology of Cantrell and urology and orthopedic surgery for cloacal exstrophy.

DIFFERENTIAL DIAGNOSIS

Hernias and Embryologic Remnants

Umbilical hernias

The differential diagnosis is listed in Table 14–2. Umbilical hernias are usually quite straightforward to diagnose on exam; however, masses and discharges from the umbilicus may be incorrectly referred as an umbilical hernia.

Table 14–2.

Differential Diagnosis of Umbilical Masses in Infants and Children

Condition	Frequency
Umbilical hernia	Common
Omphalocele	Common
Lipoma	Common
Inclusion cysts	Uncommon
Nevi	Uncommon
Hamartomas	Uncommon
Umbilical polyp	Uncommon
Umbilical pyogenic granuloma	Uncommon
Patient urachus	Uncommon
Hemangiomas	Uncommon
Dermatofibromas	Uncommon
Omphalomesenteric duct remnant	Rare
Urachal adenocarcinoma	Rare

Inguinal hernias

The differential diagnosis involves any entity that may appear as a groin mass (Table 14–3).

Congenital Defects of the Abdominal Wall

The differential diagnosis of abdominal wall defects includes any of the developmental abnormalities of the anterior abdominal wall defined in Table 14–4. Though abdominal wall defects occur in 4–5/10,000 live births, the more common defects include umbilical cord hernia,

Table 14–3.

Differential Diagnosis of an Inguinal Mass

Condition	Frequency
Incarcerated hernia	Common
Inguinal hernia	Common
Varicocele	Common
Hydrocele	Common
Retractile testis	Common
Inguinal lymphadenitis	Common
Spermatocele	Common
Testicular torsion	Uncommon
Torsion of the appendix testis	Uncommon
Femoral hernia	Rare

Table 14–4.

Differential Diagnosis of Abdominal Wall Defects

Disorder	Frequency
Gastroschisis	Common
Omphalocele	Common
Umbilical cord hernia	Uncommon
Pentalogy of Cantrell	Rare
Cloacal exstrophy	Rare

gastroschisis, and omphalocele.[2] Rare conditions are cloacal exstrophy, pentalogy of Cantrell, ectopic cordis, and body stalk deformities.

A physician may be requested to differentiate between an umbilical cord hernia and an umbilical hernia in an infant. They are located at the same anatomic site, but are separate entities. An *umbilical cord hernia* is a small (<4 cm) defect with midgut inside the cord, in which the cord often takes an on abnormal appearance and can be both membrane and/or skin covered. The abdominal wall superior to the defect is normal and these patients by definition have malrotation due to failure of the midgut to return to the abdominal cavity. *Umbilical hernias* are defects in the anterior abdominal wall but are not usually considered a congenital abdominal wall defect. On evaluation, umbilical hernias are easily distinguished from the umbilical cord hernias as the area is *covered by normal skin* and the hernia does not usually present at birth.[3]

Table 14–5 illustrates the differentiating features between gastroschisis and omphalocele. Initial evaluation for the presence of a membrane covering the viscera can distinguish between gastroschisis and omphalocele. However, this salient feature can be complicated if the membrane of omphalocele has ruptured in utero or during delivery. The location of the umbilicus in relation to viscera and the appearance of the viscera differ between gastroschisis and omphalocele. The gastroschisis defect is usually to the right of the umbilicus and the bowel may appear entirely normal, but more frequently edematous and inflamed. In omphalocele, the defect lies in the center of the umbilicus and the bowel will appear normal, due to the covering of the membrane. The umbilical cord may be identified at the apex of the membranous defect. The size of the abdominal wall defect also may vary between the three abdominal wall defects. Gastroschisis is 2–5 cm in size while a broader range from 2 to 15 cm exists for omphalocele. There are cases of giant omphaloceles in which the entire abdominal contents are outside of the abdominal wall (Figure 14–11).

Other features distinguishing gastroschisis and omphalocele are not immediately obvious on clinical

Table 14–5.

Different Features of Omphalocele and Gastroschisis

Feature	Omphalocele	Gastroschisis
Embryology	Malformation of abdominal wall	Disruption of a normal structure (?)
Location	Umbilical ring	Right side of cord
Cord	Inserts in sac	Normal insertion
Size	Large	Small
Sac	Present	None
Contents	Frequently liver, bowel	Bowel, occasionally bladder, ovaries, testes
Bowel	Normal	Matted and inflamed
Malrotation	Present	Present
GI function	Normal	Prolonged ileus
Associated anomalies	Common, 30–70%	Unusual (intestinal atresia 10–15%)
Associated syndromes	Common	None
Fluid requirements	Maintenance (unless membrane ruptures)	2–3 times normal

exam and include gastrointestinal function and the presence or absence of other anomalies. Feeding tolerance differs between gastroschisis and omphalocele, as intestinal injury due to exposure typically causes initially impaired motility in patients with gastroschisis. Alimentation in patients with omphalocele is usually normal and is attributed to protection by the covering membrane. Gastroschisis is also associated with intestinal atresia in approximately 10% of patients and may present once feeding has been initiated and feeding intolerance occurs.

Associated anomalies with omphalocele are reported to be as high as 60%, while these are present in only 10% of gastroschisis infants.[3] Infants with omphalocele require thorough investigation, if not previously done, to identify other potential anomalies. Table 14–6 represents associated anomalies in infants born with omphalocele. Addressing these anomalies requires a systematic approach that can be addressed in the prenatal period or after delivery. Chromosomal

analysis performed during pregnancy or after delivery will identify trisomies and other chromosomal abnormalities, such as Turner, Klinefelter, and triploidy syndromes. Perinatal ultrasound is a powerful tool for identifying other anomalies such as cardiac, genitourinary, head and neck, musculoskeletal, and maternal/fetal abnormalities. After delivery, these anomalies may be confirmed or identified with ultrasound technologies (i.e., cardiac and genitourinary) or on initial physical examination (musculoskeletal and head and neck abnormalities).

There are numerous distinct syndromes associated with omphalocele including Beckwith–Wiedemann; omphalocele, exstrophy, imperforate anus, and spinal anomalies (OEIS); and prune belly syndromes. Beckwith–Wiedemann syndrome is associated with omphalocele, macroglossia, and visceromegaly.[3,25] Additionally, these infants with Beckwith–Wiedemann syndrome will require regular surveillance (U/S and alpha-fetoprotein monitoring) during childhood for specific tumors including Wilms tumor and hepatoblastomas.[26]

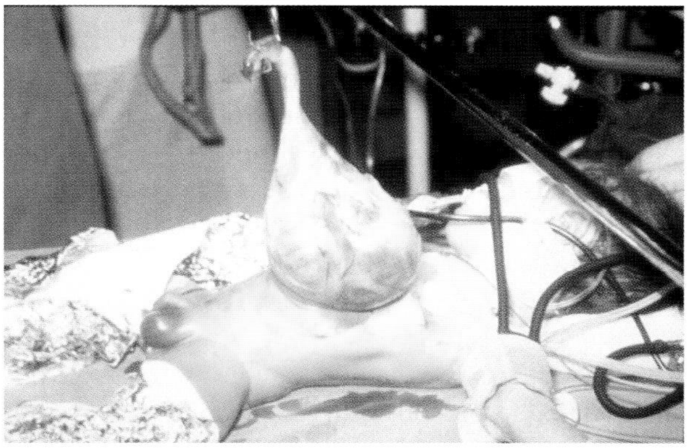

DIAGNOSIS

Congenital Defects of the Abdominal Wall

Prenatal diagnosis of an abdominal wall defect should initiate a multidisciplinary approach (involving genetic counseling, radiology, obstetrics, neonatal, and pediatric surgery) with the parents, to assist with education and decision making. Prenatal counseling should begin once the diagnosis is made; this will assist the family if lethal anomalies are identified as well as prepare the

FIGURE 14–11 ■ Giant omphalocele.

Table 14-6.	
Associated Anomalies with Omphalocele	
Cardiac defects (20–40%)	**Maternal/fetal developmental anomalies**
Septal defects (atrial and/or ventricular)	IUGR
Tetrology of Fallot	Oligohydramnios
Pulmonary artery stenosis	Polyhydramnios
Pulmonary hypoplasia	Single umbilical artery
Transposition of the great vessels	Placental chorioangioma
Coarctation of the aorta	Allantoic cysts
Ectopia cordis	**Musculoskeletal anomalies**
Absence of inferior vena cava	Scoliosis
Chromosomal anomalies	Hemivertebra
Trisomies: 13, 18, and 21	Camptomelic dwarfism
Triploidy syndromes	Syndactyly
Turner and Klinefelter syndromes	Clubfeet
Gastrointestinal anomalies (as high as 40%)	**Neural tube anomalies**
Diaphragmatic hernia	Neural tube defects
Malrotation	Holoprosencephaly
Intestinal duplications	Encephalocele
Atresias	Cerebellar hypoplasia
Tracheoesophageal fistula	**Respiratory insufficiency with giant omphalocele**
Imperforate anus	**Syndromes**
Genitourinary anomalies (as high as 40%)	Beckwith–Wiedemann syndrome
Ureteropelvic junction obstruction	OEIS syndrome (omphalocele, exstrophy, imperforate anus, and spinal anomalies)
Cloacal exstrophy	Gershoni-Baruch syndrome (omphalocele, diaphragmatic hernia, cardiovascular anomalies, and radial ray defects)
Bladder exstrophy	Donnai–Barrow syndrome (omphalocele, diaphragmatic hernia, absent corpus callosum, hypertelorism, myopia, and sensorineural deafness)
Renal malpositioning	
Head/neck anomalies	Prune belly syndrome
Cleft lip	
Facial clefts	
Micrognathia	
Cystic hygroma	

expectations of the family. Chromosomal karyotyping is indicated with the diagnosis of omphalocele or other congenital abnormalities; some centers perform karyotyping for gastroschisis. Once thorough imaging and chromosomal studies are performed, a review of the results with the parents is essential to explain the expected treatment and outcome.

Serial ultrasonography is performed over the course of the pregnancy. Omphaloceles may diminish in size due to fetal growth and intrauterine rupture of the omphalocele is a poor prognosis, leading to growth retardation and pulmonary hypoplasia. Monitoring gastroschisis for size and character of the eviscerated bowel may be useful to plan delivery. There is no advantage in delivering infants with small or moderately large omphaloceles by cesarean section. It is prudent to deliver infants with giant omphaloceles and exteriorized livers by cesarean section to avoid hepatic injury.

ALGORITHM (ABDOMINAL WALL DEFECTS)

Diagnostic Tests

Ultrasound

Prenatal ultrasound is a useful modality for diagnosing abdominal wall defects. After the 12th gestational week, eviscerated bowel contents identified by sonography may be considered an abdominal wall defect. Specific measurements associated with abdominal wall defects involve the length of herniation (>7 mm) or if herniation is visible once the crown rump length is 45 mm.[27–29] Differentiating between gastroschisis and omphalocele with this study is important, given the high rate of concomitant malformations with the latter. Identification of omphalocele should therefore prompt further investigation. Identification of the umbilical cord insertion distinguishes between gastroschisis and omphalocele. The umbilical cord insertion site will be the apex of the eviscerated components in a central omphalocele.[28] With gastroschisis, the insertion of the umbilical cord usually appears normal with the defect located to the right. Ultrasound can be used to identify the rarer abdominal wall defects, that is, pentalogy of Cantrell and cloacal exstrophy. Pentalogy of Cantrell will show exteriorization of the heart and usually a large omphalocele located in the upper abdomen. Prenatal identification of cloacal exstrophy is made by failure to identify a normal urinary bladder and the presence of pubic diastasis.

Prenatal sonographic studies are used in a retrospective manner to determine if any predictive information can be established with abdominal wall defects. Infants with giant omphalocele can have significant morbidity from pulmonary hypoplasia. Prenatal sonographic measurements of chest/trunk ratio and lung/thorax transverse area measurement can detect this problem.[30] In infants with gastroschisis, prenatal evaluation of intestinal dilatation and/or bowel wall thickness has not shown to predict complications such as atresia and bowel perforations.[31] Ultrasound technology is continuing to advance, with three-dimensional imaging using multiplanar and orthogonal plane modes. Despite these advancements, no current studies show a diagnostic advantage over two-dimensional ultrasound.[32] Over the past decade, fetal MRI has been used to diagnose congenital disorders. Utilization of this technology for abdominal wall defects is limited; however, certain situations, that is, maternal obesity or oligohydramnios, may justify its use.[33,34]

Maternal serum screening

The quadruple serum screen is recommended for all pregnancies, and is performed during the second trimester between 15 and 20 weeks gestation. Maternal serum screening evaluates the following components: msAFP, unconjugated estriol (uE3), human chorionic gonadotropin (hCG), and inhibin A. Inhibin A was added to the "triple screen" to increase sensitivity for diagnosing Down's syndrome. There is an association with these serum markers and various fetal and chromosomal abnormalities, including Down's syndrome, neural tube defects, and abdominal wall defects.[35] Elevated msAFP is present in virtually all cases of gastroschisis and a majority of omphaloceles. Ultrasound examination is recommended in any pregnant women found to have abnormalities on maternal serum screening.

Genetic tests

A genetic role in gastroschisis is considered low, though a population-based registry found approximately 5% of patients with gastroschisis had a relative with a similar

diagnosis when extended pedigrees were evaluated.[36] Some have hypothesized a disruption in the endothelial nitric oxide pathway and vasculogenesis by either environmental or genetic factors, and this may represent a pathogenetic model of gastroschisis.[37]

Though no specific gene is identified with abdominal wall defects, there are rare reports of omphaloceles occurring in families. Autosomal recessive syndromes where omphalocele is a component include: Donnai–Barrow syndrome (absent corpus callosum, myopia, sensorineural defects, diaphragmatic hernia, omphalocele, and hypertelorism) and Gershoni-Baruch syndrome (cardiovascular anomalies, diaphragmatic hernia, omphalocele, and radial ray defects).[3]

TREATMENT

Hernias

The treatment for hernias is surgical repair; however, the timing of the procedure will vary with type of hernia and age of the patient. Usually these surgeries are performed on an outpatient basis, but some patients do require admission based on their gestational age (varies per center but ranges between 55 and 60 weeks).

Umbilical hernias

Over 90% of umbilical hernias close spontaneously by 2–3 years of age, so during the first few years of life, no treatment, other than parental reassurance, is recommended.[38] Surgical repair is reserved for those umbilical hernias that fail to close spontaneously prior to school age. Hernias that are large and protruding or become symptomatic also need surgical repair. Parents of children with very large defects will often appropriately request early surgical intervention as such hernias seldom close spontaneously or if they do, the cosmetic skin anomaly is pronounced. Umbilical herniorraphy is usually performed under general anesthesia in an outpatient setting. A curvilinear infraumbilical or supraumbilical incision is made and the fascia is closed in a transverse direction. Large umbilical hernias may require an umbilicoplasty for closure.[39] Following skin closure, a light pressure dressing is applied for 48 hours to avoid a wound hematoma or seroma.

Inguinal hernias

Inguinal hernias identified in the hospitalized preterm infant can be electively repaired prior to the infant's discharge. There is a high incidence (20%) of post-anesthetic apnea within the first 12 hours after a general anesthetic in premature infants whose post-conceptual age is less than 45 weeks, so careful postoperative monitoring for apnea, bradycardia, and periodic breathing is

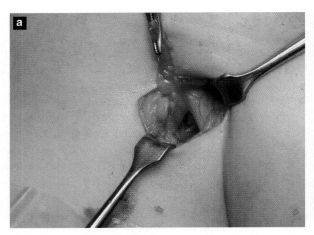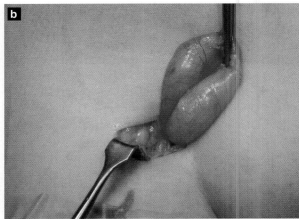

FIGURE 14–12 ■ Infant hernia repair—femoral hernia repair in an infant and high ligation of the sac (a and b).

indicated. Additionally, children under 60 weeks post-conceptional age with a history of apnea, lung disease, or other comorbidities should be monitored after surgery.[39] Repair of hernias identified in the preterm infant after hospital discharge can be delayed until the patient is well past 45 weeks gestational age (Figure 14–12).

Most cases of inguinal hernia and hydrocele can be safely and effectively repaired in an outpatient surgical setting. Hydroceles usually close within the first year of life. The exception to this is when an inguinal component is present or the hydrocele is enlarging. This suggests an abdominoscrotal hydrocele that usually does not resolve spontaneously and will need closure after the first year of life. Surgical repair is performed with a high ligation of the hernia sac through a groin incision. Whether to perform a contralateral groin exploration in children with unilateral inguinal hernias remains a subject of great debate. Although the processus vaginalis is often patent in children under 2 years of age, it usually closes spontaneously. Only 6% of patients undergoing herniorraphy develop a contralateral hernia and require a second surgical procedure. This small percentage of patients does not appear to warrant routine exploration in the absence of a clinically apparent hernia.[40] Assessing the contralateral processus vaginalis with a laparoscope, introduced through the ipsilateral open sac, is proposed as a method to identify patients who will benefit from contralateral repair.[41] The utilization of a laparoscope for inspection of the contralateral side has not resolved this debate among pediatric surgeons that may only be surpassed in controversy, with the topic of performing laparoscopic ligation of inguinal hernias in children.

Hernia Complications

Intraoperative complications of hernia repair include injury to the ilioinguinal nerve, the spermatic vessels, or the vas deferens. If inadvertently divided, the vas defer-

ens can be repaired with fine monofilament absorbable sutures. Postoperative complications include formation of a hydrocele, scrotal hematoma, recurrent inguinal hernia, or wound infection in about 1% of cases.[42] Nonviable bowel is encountered in 1–2% of incarcerated hernias and in 5% of irreducible hernias. Testicular infarction occurs in 2% of incarcerated hernias, and in 10% of all irreducible cases.[43]

ALGORITHM (MANAGEMENT OF INGUINAL HERNIAS)

Congenital Defects of the Abdominal Wall

Resuscitation and immediate care

As previously mentioned, delivery of most infants with abdominal wall defects can be safely accomplished via vaginal or cesarean section and should be based on obstetrical parameters and not solely on the presence of an abdominal wall defect. On delivery, common principles of newborn resuscitation apply to these infants. Immediate goals are to prevent evaporative fluid loss, hypothermia, and infection. These goals are achieved by placing the infant in a warm aseptic environment and covering the exteriorized viscera, with warm saline-soaked gauze or a "bowel bag." The bowel bag is a commercially available plastic/cellophane bag in which the lower half of the infant, including the viscera, is placed, to avoid evaporative losses. Special care should be taken when positioning the exposed viscera, to avoid vascular compromise. The infant should be placed in a lateral position with bowel contents supported. If the infant is transferred to another facility with compromised blood flow to the exposed viscera, a devastating ischemic complication can occur. A nasogastric or oral–gastric tube should be placed for decompression of the stomach and viscera. Vascular access should be achieved to provide intravascular support and administer broad-spectrum antibiotics. Infants with an abdominal wall defect may require mechanical ventilation based on their pulmonary status but this should not be based on a default pathway due to an abdominal wall defect. The next step will be to transfer the patient to a neonatal intensive care unit with pediatric surgical support. If prenatal assessment of the infant's cardiac and renal systems is incomplete, then this too should be addressed. The goal of surgical intervention is to return the eviscerated abdominal contents back to the abdominal cavity. The surgical options for abdominal wall defects differ between gastroschisis and omphalocele and will be discussed individually.

Gastroschisis

The timing of surgical treatments for gastroschisis and omphalocele are different. Infants with omphalocele can proceed first with further diagnostic work-up to identify additional abnormalities. In gastroschisis, the exposed viscera place the infant at an increased risk for infections and are a continual source of evaporative fluid loss. After initial evaluation, operative intervention for gastroschisis is warranted in an attempt for visceral reduction. Primary reduction is considered the procedure of choice for both omphalocele and gastroschisis if the eviscerated contents can be placed back in the abdominal cavity without causing undue increased intra-abdominal pressure.

Primary closure of gastroschisis has a reported success rate between 50% and 83%, depending on the published study.[44,45] During the attempted closure, the bowel is inspected for intestinal atresia and placed back into the abdominal cavity. Thorough evaluation may not be possible if the bowel is inflamed and matted together and no attempt should be made to separate the matted bowel. Careful reduction of the edematous abdominal contents is required. If successful, the fascial defect can be closed followed by skin closure, with or without reconstruction of the umbilicus. An alternative method is to reduce the bowel and cover the defect with umbilical cord and a watertight dressing. To facilitate this technique, it is beneficial for the obstetrician to leave the cord long in a child with gastroschisis. This technique allows for spontaneous closure and an attempt at minimizing the increase in intra-abdominal pressure[46] (Figure 14–13). Monitoring

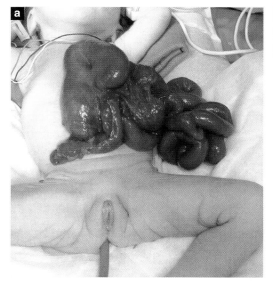
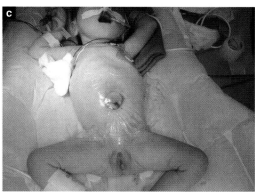
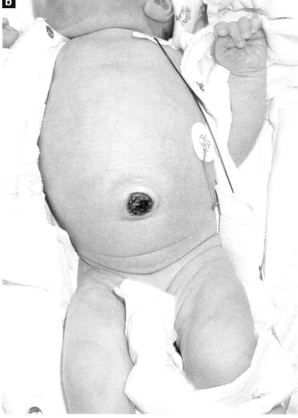

FIGURE 14–13 ▪ Abdominal wall closure with watertight dressing and umbilical cord (a–c).

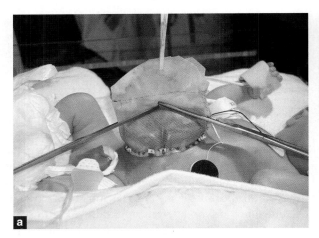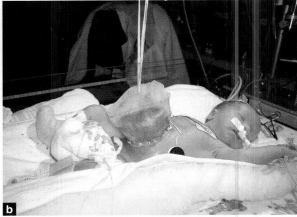

FIGURE 14–14 ■ Abdominal wall closure with Silo (a) and with gradual reduction (b).

for increased intra-abdominal pressure is very useful and if noted, primary closure should be abandoned and staged closure with a silo should be performed. Some institutions attempt reduction of abdominal contents on the ward with or without general anesthesia and mechanical ventilation.[47] In 2002, a Cochrane review on this topic could not identify any evidence from randomized control trials to support or refute this practice.[48]

Staged closure for gastroschisis involves using a variety of synthetic materials and fabricated spring-loaded silos, to contain and protect exteriorized bowel, with or without suturing into the fascia. This silo approach allows for gradual reduction of the eviscerated abdominal contents until adequate abdominal volume is achieved (Figure 14–14). Gradual reduction of the silo contents can be done with suturing or stapling devices in the NICU. Once the abdominal con-

tents are reduced, fascial closure can be attempted, with the same principles of primary closure in avoiding increased abdominal pressure. Alternatively, the technique described for primary closure with umbilical cord covering and a dressing can also be used secondarily after silo placement and removal.[46] Many pediatric surgeons prefer the preformed spring-loaded silastic silo for staged closure (Figure 14–15). This technique does not require sutures to be placed into the fascia because the silo is kept in place by a spring-loaded ring beneath the fascia. Recently, a small multicenter randomized control trial reported using a silastic spring showed similar outcomes to primary repair, allowing for closure in a more elective setting.[49] Some pediatric surgeons prefer the staged closure citing a lower complication rate, that is, infection and abdominal compartment syndrome, and accept subsequently longer hospital stays.[50]

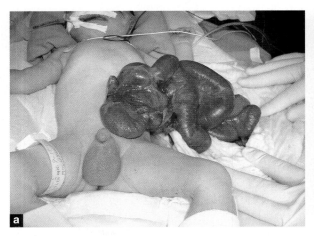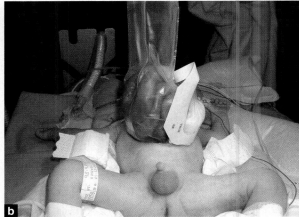

FIGURE 14–15 ■ Large gastroschisis (a) treated with silastic silo (b).

Omphalocele

Primary closure for omphaloceles has a lower success rate than with gastroschisis. While primary closure is usually feasible with small- to medium-sized defects, large omphaloceles will require staged closure. Primary closure of omphaloceles requires careful removal of the covering membrane (membrane adherent to an eviscerated liver is left in place to avoid unnecessary and hard-to-control bleeding) and ligation of the umbilical vessels is performed. The abdominal contents are carefully reduced and may be facilitated by the following techniques: developing skin flaps, extending the fascial defect cephalad and caudad, and stretching the abdominal wall. If closure is not possible, synthetic mesh may be used to cover the defect and the skin should be used to cover the mesh.

The treatment of giant omphaloceles deserves special mention due to the difficult nature of these cases, high complication rates, and significant mortality. Giant omphaloceles are omphaloceles that are not amendable to primary or standard delayed closure techniques. There is no ideal treatment for these infants. Attempted closure usually requires a prosthetic patch or irritant covering, such as silver sulfadiazine or Aquacel Ag to induce eschar formation and subsequent epithelialization. If these infants survive, they will ultimately require an attempted fascial closure at a much later date with prosthesis to gain abdominal domain and close the large ventral defect.[51] This too is staged with progressive excision of the prosthesis until primary fascial closure is achieved.

Umbilical cord hernias

The defect with umbilical cord hernias is easily reducible, usually performed by elevating the sac upward and reducing the bowel into the peritoneal cavity. The fascia can be approximated and a cosmetic umbilicoplasty performed. Though the midgut has not been fixed in the appropriate position and malrotation is present, intestinal obstruction in these patients usually does not occur. Although these hernias are relatively simple, occasionally the appendix or an omphalomesenteric duct remnant is entrapped and attached to the cord. Careful separation during closure is needed to avoid injury.

Postoperative care of Congenital Defects of the Abdominal Wall

The foundation of postoperative management includes wound care, respiratory support, and nutritional support. Initially after the operation, abdominal wall edema and erythema may develop, and intravenous antibiotics should be continued until this erythema resolves. Respiratory support is usually necessary for a few days (recent

reports of gastroschisis range from 2.5 to 8 days) after surgery.[45,47–49,52] Respiratory support may be long term for infants with large defects due to chronic respiratory failure and these infants may require tracheostomy. For a limited time, paralysis and heavy sedation may be used to avoid increased intra-abdominal pressure, but this can lead to deleterious effects. Total parental nutrition (TPN) is needed for these infants and central venous access should be established early, as either a PICC line or tunneled central line. Continued gastric decompression is needed in the postoperative period.

Nutritional support during the perioperative period is provided with TPN until bowel activity begins. Signs of increased bowel activity include clearing of gastric aspirate and bowel movements, allowing for the initiation of enteral feedings. Bowel function usually returns to infants with omphalocele faster than with gastroschisis, provided other congenital anomalies are not present. Kitchanan reported a 10-year review showing a statistically significant difference in TPN use between infants with gastroschisis and omphalocele. TPN was required for a median length of 23 and 6 days, respectively.[53] In infants with gastroschisis treated with primary closure, there is a significant decrease in length of TPN treatment compared to those treated with delayed closure.[54] This observation is self-selecting, as the patients needing delayed closure more frequently have complex gastroschisis associated with inflamed and matted intestine. The impetus to transition infants with gastroschisis and delayed intestinal function to full oral feeds is strong given the risk of cholestatic liver disease and infectious morbidity and mortality associated with TPN use. TPN-associated cholestasis causes jaundice and cirrhosis, and can eventually lead to liver failure, requiring liver transplantation.[55]

Complications with Congenital Defects of the Abdominal Wall

Atresias

Intestinal atresias occur in approximately 10% of infants with gastroschisis and the management is usually individualized based on location and time of discovery. Proximal atresias discovered during initial reduction should be reduced with the bowel and decompressed with nasogastric suction. The abdomen can be explored as soon as 2 weeks (2–4 weeks) following reduction with a plan for definitive repair once the bowel inflammation has decreased. Intestinal atresias may not be identified during the initial closure due to intestinal inflammation and should be considered in those infants with prolonged feeding intolerance. Diagnosis is complicated by the impaired intestinal motility seen in these infants. Intestinal atresia should be investigated with contrast studies if coordinated peristalsis does not occur within 4 weeks of abdominal closure.[2,3]

Abdominal compartment syndrome

After abdominal closure, bowel ischemia can ensue if the abdominal closure is too tight or if positioning causes vascular compromise. Intra-operative assessment of ventilation pressures following bowel reduction is useful to determine whether closure is safe. Monitoring intra-abdominal pressure in the postoperative period can be done with a variety of methods including NG or intravesical manometry. Postoperatively, if abdominal pressure is too high (>20 mm Hg), the treatment is surgical, and relieving the pressure is a priority. If primary closure was initially attempted, then placement of a silo should be performed and followed by staged closure. If the patient has a silo in place and there is elevated abdominal pressure or signs of intestinal ischemia (usually visible through clear silo), widening the fascial defect or eviscerating more intestine is beneficial. When intestinal necrosis is discovered, the treatment is resection and stoma formation. Short bowel syndrome can occur in infants with abdominal compartment syndrome, causing significant morbidity and mortality.[56]

Associated anomalies, respiratory complications, and necrotizing enterocolitis

Additional complications often occur with these infants, related to prematurity and associated anomalies. These patients benefit from an experienced NICU prepared to treat the problems of prematurity. Management issues include: heat loss, pulmonary hypoplasia/respiratory failure, hyperbilirubinemia, electrolyte and fluid imbalances (exacerbated by abdominal wall defect), and extremes of blood glucose level.

Pulmonary complications in infants with omphalocele can lead to significant morbidity and mortality. Infants with giant omphaloceles are at increased risk for pulmonary complications due to the deformation of the thoracic cage.[57] Pulmonary hypoplasia, resulting in respiratory insufficiency, impacts morbidity and mortality of infants with large omphaloceles, and ventilatory dependence may continue beyond the neonatal period.[58] Respiratory distress at birth was found to be predictive of mortality in infants with omphalocele. The authors concluded initial conservative management in infants who present at birth in respiratory distress, until improvement in respiratory status occurs.[59]

Additional complications that can affect the recovery of these infants and possibly require re-exploration in the perioperative or postoperative period include: necrotizing enterocolitis, malrotation, and adhesive disease. Necrotizing enterocolitis is reported to be as high as 18.5% in infants with gastroschisis who have undergone repair.[60] This form of necrotizing enterocolitis is usually benign and operative intervention is unusual. Maternal breast milk may help decrease the high incidence of NEC in infants with gastroschisis.[61] Infants with abdominal wall defects have intestinal malrotation, as the bowel has not undergone the appropriate rotation and subsequent fixation of the mesentery. The dreaded complication of midgut volvulus is considered low in this population, probably as the result of adhesions from operations or from the non-rotated position of the bowel. A review of patients with malrotation found that 1.2% of patients with abdominal wall defects who were not treated with a Ladd's procedure developed midgut volvulus.[62] Reoperation for obstructive adhesions after treatment of gastroschisis and omphaloceles in neonates is reported to be the highest within the first year. Analysis of this population showed an increase in clinically significant adhesions if the initial operation was complicated with sepsis or fascial dehiscence.[63,64]

Outcomes

Approximately 50 years ago infant survival with abdominal wall defects was rare, whereas current series suggest survival rates between 90% and 100% in gastroschisis and 70% and 92% in patients with omphalocele. The mortality is generally related to associated cardiac or chromosomal anomalies.[65–68] Long-term follow-up of these infants usually report satisfactory quality of life with decreased physical ability and stature as compared to peers. Surgical treatment for small bowel obstruction, scar revision, umbilicoplasty, and hernia treatment ranges between 10% and 35%.[69,70] Although we have come a long way in the management of abdominal wall defects, significant morbidity still exists in some of these children. The future goals for the treatment of these children will be focused on optimizing outcomes, especially in the complicated or high-risk subsets of these patients.

REFERENCES

1. Skandalakis JE, Gray SW, Philadelphia. *Anterior Abdominal Wall. Embryology for Surgeons*. 2nd ed. Williams and Wilkins; 1994:567.
2. Minkes RK. Abdominal wall defect. In: Welch KJ, et al., eds. *Pediatric Surgery*. 4th ed. Chicago: Year Book Medical Publishers, 1986.
3. Klein MD. Congenital defects of the abdominal wall. In: Grosfeld JL, Oneill JA, Fonkalsrud EW, Coran AG, eds. *Pediatric Surgery*. Philadelphia: Mosby Elsevier; 2006:1157–1171.
4. Nicolaides KH, Snijders RS, Cheng HH, et al. Fetal gastrointestinal and abdominal wall defects: associated malformations and chromosomal abnormalities. *Fetal Diagn Ther*. 1992;(7):102–115.
5. Stovroff MA, Teague WG. Omphalocele and gastroschisis. In: Ziegler MM, Azizkhan RG, Weber TR, eds. *Operative Pediatric Surgery*. McGraw Hill; New York. 2003:525–535.

6. Sadler TW. *Body Cavities and Digestive System in Langman's Medical Embryology.* Baltimore: Lippincott Williams & Wilkin; 2000:197–207, 270–303.

7. Suita S, Nagasaki A. Urachal remnants. *Semin Pediatr Surg.* 1996;5(2):107–115.

8. Draper ES, Rankin J, Tonks AM, et al. Recreational drug use: a major risk factor for gastroshisis? *Am J Epidemiol.* 2007;167:485–491.

9. Torfs CP, Katz EA, Bateson TF, et al. Maternal medications and environmental exposures as risk factors for gastroschisis. *Teratology.* 1996;54(2):84–92.

10. Drongowski RA, Smith RK Jr, Coran AG, et al. Contribution of demographic and environmental factors to the etiology of gastroschisis: a hypothesis. *Fetal Diagn Ther.* 1991;6(1–2):14–27.

11. Chambers CD, Chen BH, Kalla K, et al. Novel risk factor in gastroschisis: change of paternity. *Am J Med Genet A.* 2007;143(7):653–659.

12. Watkins ML, Rasmussen SA, Honein MA. Maternal obesity and risk for birth defects. *Pediatrics.* 2003;111(5 part 2):1152–1158.

13. Stothard KJ, Tennant PW, Bell R, et al. Maternal overweight and obesity and the risk of congenital anomalies: a systematic review and meta-analysis. *JAMA.* 2009; 301(6):636–650.

14. Rasmussen SA, Frias JL. Non-genetic risk factors for gastroschisis. *Am J Med Genet C Semin Med Genet.* 2008;148C(3):199–212.

15. Werler MM, Sheehan JE, Mitchell AA. Association of vasoconstrictive exposures with risks of gastroschisis and small intestinal atresia. *Epidemiology.* 2003;14(3): 349–354.

16. Botto LD, Mulinare J, Erickson JD. Occurrence of omphalocele in relation to maternal multivitamin use: a population-based study. *Pediatrics.* 2002;109:904–908.

17. Jones KL. Abdominal wall. In Jones KL, ed. *Smith's Recognizable Patterns of Human Malformation.* 4th ed. WB Saunders, *Philadelphia*; 1988:753–754.

18. Lassaletta L, Fonkalsrud EW, Tovar J, et al. The management of umbilical hernias in infancy and childhood. *J Pediatr Surg.* 1975;10:405–409.

19. Grosfeld JL. Current concepts in inguinal hernia in infants and children. *World J Surg.* 1989;13(5):506–515.

20. Rescorla FG, Grosfeld JL. Inguinal hernia repair in the perinatal period and early infancy. *J Pediatr Surg.* 1984;19(6):832–837.

21. Rowe M, O'Neill J, Grosfeld J, Fonkalsrud E, Coran A. Inguinal and scrotal disorders. In: *Essentials of Pediatric Surgery.* Mosby; 1995:446.

22. Jeri P, Ginney EJ, Odonnell B. Inguinal hernia in infants: the fate of the testis following incarceration. *J Pediatr Surg.* 1984;19(1):44–46.

23. Palomaki GE, Hill LE, Knight GJ, et al. Second-trimester maternal serum alpha-fetoprotein levels in pregnancies associated with gastroschisis and omphalocele. *Obstet Gynecol.* 1988;71(1):906–909.

24. Fong KW, Toi A, Salem S, et al. Detection of fetal structural abnormalities with US during early pregnancy. *Radiographics.* 2004;24(1):157–174.

25. Islam S. Clinical care outcomes in abdominal wall defects. *Curr Opin Pediatr.* 2008;20:305–310.

26. Rao A, Rothman J, Nichols KE. Genetic testing and tumor surveillance for children with cancer predisposition syndromes. *Curr Opin Pediatr.* 2008;20(1):1–7.

27. Castro-Aragon I, Levine D. Ultrasound detection of first trimester malformations: a pictorial essay. *Radiol Clin North Am.* 2003;41:681–693.

28. Fong KW, Toi A, Salem S, et al. Detection of fetal structural abnormalities with US during early pregnancy. *Radiographics.* 2004;24(1):157–174.

29. Emanuel PG, Garcia GI, Anqtuaco TL. Prenatal detection of anterior abdominal wall defects with US. *Radiographics.* 1995;15(3):517–530.

30. Kamata S, Usui, N, Sawai T, Nose K, et al. Prenatal detection of pulmonary hypoplasia in giant omphalocele. *Pediatr Surg Int.* 2008;24(1):107–111.

31. Davis RP, Treadwell MC, Drongowski RA, Teitelbaum DH, et al. Risk stratification in gastroschisis; can prenatal evaluation or early postnatal factors predict outcome. *Pediatr Surg Int.* 2009;25(4):319–325.

32. Bonilla-Musoles F, Machado LE, Bailao LA, et al. Abdominal wall defects: two- versus three-dimensional ultrasonographic diagnosis. *J Ultrasound Med.* 2001;20(4): 379–389.

33. Hill MC, Lande IM, Larsen JW Jr. Prenatal diagnosis of fetal anomalies using ultrasound and MRI. *Radiol Clin North Am.* 1988;26(2):287–307.

34. Pugash D, Brugger PC, Bettelheim D, et al. Prenatal ultrasound and fetal MRI: the comparative value of each modality in prenatal diagnosis. *Eur J Radiol.* 2008;68(2): 214–226.

35. Simpson JL, Otano L. Prenatal genetic diagnosis. In: Gabbe SG, Niebyl JR, Simpson SL, eds. *Obstetrics: Normal and Problem Pregnancies.* Philadelphia: Churchill Livingstone Elsevier; 2007:153–177.

36. Torfs CP, Curry CJ. Familial cases of gastroschisis in a population-based registry. *Am J Med Genet.* 1993;45(4):465–467.

37. Lammer EJ, Iovannisci DM, Tom L, et al. Gastroschisis: a gene–environmental model involving the VEGF–NOS3 pathway. *Am J Med Genet C Semin Med Gene.* 2008;148C(3):213–218.

38. Heifetz CJ, Bilsel ZT, Gaus WW. Observations on the disappearance of umbilical hernias of infancy and childhood. *Surg Gynecol Obstet.* 1963;116:467–473.

39. Brandt ML. Pediatric hernias. *Surg Clin North Am.* 2008;88:27–43.

40. Fonkalsrud EW. Is routine contralateral exploration advisable for children with unilateral inguinal hernias. *Am J Surg.* 1995;169(3):285.

41. Holcomb GW, Morgan WM, Brock JW. Laparoscopic evaluation for contralateral patent processus vaginalis. Part II. *J Pediatr Surg.* 1996;31(8):1170–1173.

42. Grosfeld JL, Minnick K, West KW, et al. Inguinal hernias in children: factors affecting recurrence in 62 cases. *J Pediatr Surg.* 1991;26(3):283–287.

43. Jeri P, Ginney EJ, Odonnell B. Inguinal hernia in infants: the fate of the testis following incarceration. *J Pediatr Surg.* 1984;19(1):44–46.

44. Henrich K, Huemmer HP, Reingruber B, et al. Gastroschisis and omphalocele; treatments and long-term outcomes. *Pediatr Surg Int.* 2008;24:167–173.

45. Driver CP, Bianchi BA, Doig CM, et al. The contemporary outcome of gastroschisis. *J Pediatr Surg.* 2008;35:1719–1723.

46. Sandler A, Lawrence J, Meehan J, et al. A "plastic" sutureless abdominal wall closure in gastroschisis. *J Pediatr Surg.* 2004;39(5):738–741.

47. Owen A, Marveen S, Jackson L, et al. Experience of bedside preformed silo staged reduction and closure for gastroschisis. *J Pediatr Surg.* 2006;41:1830–1835.

48. Davies MW, Kimble RM, Woodgate PG. Ward reduction without general anesthesia versus reduction and repair under general anaesthesia for gastroschisis in newborn infants. *Cochrane Database Syst Rev.* 2002;(3):CD003671.

49. Pastor AC, Phillips JD, Fenton SJ, et al. Routine use of a SILASTIC spring-loaded silo for infants with gastroschisis: a multicenter randomized controlled trial. *J Pediatr Surg.* 2008;43:1807–1812.

50. Kidd JN Jr, Jackson RJ, Smith SD, et al. Evolution of staged versus primary closure of gastroschisis. *Ann Surg.* 2003;237(6):759–765.

51. Lee, SL, Beyer TD, Kim SS, et al. Initial nonoperative management and delayed closure for treatment of giant omphaloceles. *J Pediatr Surg.* 2006;41(11):1846–1849.

52. Vegunta RK, Wallace LJ, Leonardi MR, et al. Perinatal management of gastroschisis: analysis of a newly established clinical pathway. *J Pediatr Surg.* 2005;40(3):528–534.

53. Kitchanan S, Patole SK, Muller R, Whitehall JS. Neonatal outcome of gastroschisis and exomphalos: a 10-year review. *J Paediatr Child Health.* 2000;36:428–430.

54. Skarsgard ED, Claydon J, Bouchard S, et al. Canadian Pediatric Surgical Network: a population-based pediatric surgery network and database for analyzing surgical birth defects. The first 100 cases of gastroschisis. *J Pediatr Surg.* 2008;43(1):30–34.

55. Kelly DA. Liver complications of pediatric parenteral nutrition—epidemiology. *Nutrition.* 1998;14(1):153–157.

56. Thakur A, Chiu C, Quiros-Tejeira RE, et al. Morbidity and mortality of short-bowel syndrome in infants with abdominal wall defects. *Am Surg.* 2002;68(1):75–79.

57. Argyle JC. Pulmonary hypoplasia in infants with giant omphalocele. *Pediatr Pathol.* 1989;9(1):43–55.

58. Edwards EA, Broome S, Green S, et al. Long-term respiratory support in children with giant omphalocele. *Anaesth Intensive Care.* 2007;35(1):94–98.

59. Tsakayannis DE, Zurakowski D, Lillehei CW. Respiratory insufficiency at birth: a predictor of mortality for infants with omphalocele. *J Pediatr Surg.* 1996;31(8):1088–1090.

60. Oldman KT, Coran AG, Drongowski RA, et al. The development of necrotizing enterocolitis following repair of gastroschisis: a surprisingly high incidence. *J Pediatr Surg.* 1988;23(10):945–949.

61. Jayanthi S, Seymour P, Puntis JW, et al. Necrotizing enterocolitis after gastroschisis repair: a preventable complication? *J Pediatr Surg.* 1998;33(5):705–707.

62. Rescoria FJ, Shedd FJ, Grosfeld JL, et al. Anomalies of intestinal malrotation in childhood: analysis of 447 cases. *Surgery.* 1990;108(4):710–715.

63. Grant HW, Parker MC, Wilson MS, et al. Population-based analysis of the risk of adhesion-related readmissions after abdominal surgery in children. *J Pediatr Surg.* 2006;41(8);1453–1456.

64. Van Eijck FC, Wijnen RMH, Van Goor H. The incidence and morbidity of adhesions after treatment of neonates with gastroschisis and omphalocele: a 30 year review. *J Pediatr Surg.* 2008;43(3): 479–483.

65. Salihu HM, Pierre-Luis BJ, Druschell CM, et al. Omphalocele and gastroschisis in the state of New York, 1992–1999. *Birth Defects Res (Part A).* 2003;67:630–636.

66. Forrester MB, Merz ER. Epidemiology of abdominal wall defects, Hawaii 1986–1997. *Teratology.* 1999;60:117–123.

67. Henrick K, Huemmer HP, Reingruber B, et al. Gastroschisis and omphalocele: treatments and long-term outcomes. *Pediatr Surg Int.* 2008;24:167–173.

68. Baerg J, Kaban G, Tonita J, et al. Gastroschisis: a sixteen-year review. *J Pediatr Surg.* 2003;38:771–774.

69. Davies BW, Stringer MD. The survivors of gastroschisis. *Arch Dis Child.* 1997;77(2):158–160.

70. Tunell WP, Puffinbarger NK, Tuggle DW, et al. Abdominal wall defects in infants. Survival and implications for adult life. *Ann Surg.* 1995;221(5):525–528.

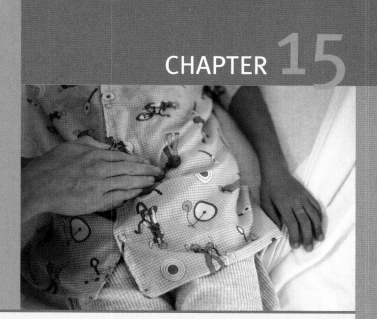

CHAPTER 15

Atresias, Webs, and Duplications

*Joel Shilyansky and
Graeme Pitcher*

DEFINITIONS

Intestinal *atresia* (from Greek meaning "non-perforated") denotes a complete obliteration of the intestinal lumen and is commonly used to describe congenital conditions. Intestinal *webs*, which are thin intraluminal diaphragms that are lined with mucosa, are a form of atresia. Webs may be stretched out to give the appearance of a windsock. *Stenosis* is a narrowing of the intestinal lumen. Intestinal atresias and webs may be subclassified based on anatomical location. They may occur in the esophagus, stomach, duodenum, jejunum, ileum, colon, or anus.[1]

The underlying pathophysiology in all children with atresias and webs is obstruction to the flow of intestinal contents. The mode of presentation can be acute, with obvious features of regurgitation, vomiting, abdominal pain, and abdominal distension. Neglected cases may present with systemic decompensation and shock. Presentation can also be subtle especially when the obstruction is incomplete as may be seen with intestinal stenosis. Patients may have chronic intermittent abdominal pain, intermittent vomiting, and distension. They may have long-standing nutritional compromise or weight loss; however, some children will present with normal weight as they adjust their diet to minimize symptoms. Early diagnosis can be prompted by careful evaluation of clinical findings as well as antenatal history, and subsequent accurate interpretation of radiographic findings. Initial care should include appropriate resuscitation and identification of associated anomalies in preparation of the child for definitive therapy. It is critical that early in the course of the work-up, conditions that threaten the child's life or lead to loss of intestinal length, such as heart disease, malrotation, or intestinal perforation, are identified and treated. Secondary investigation could then be performed safely. Treatment of intestinal atresia is surgical. The goal of the surgical treatment is relief of intestinal obstruction while preserving intestinal length and function. Prior to the advent of safe pediatric anesthesia and intensive care, as many as 50% of the children did not survive treatment.[1–3] Mortality declined sharply starting in the 1950s, and currently acute mortality is less than 4–8%. Most patients can expect a good quality of life after surgical correction but a significant burden of disease is borne by those with inadequate intestinal length.

ESOPHAGUS

Congenital Esophageal Atresia

Definitions and epidemiology

Esophageal atresia (EA) is a congenital malformation in which the esophagus is interrupted. Congenital EA occurs approximately in 1 in 3000 live births.[4] The embryological basis for esophageal anomalies is still poorly understood. The esophagus and trachea separate 28–37 days following fertilization. Failure of the tracheal bud to separate from the primordial foregut is thought to result in EA. EA is often associated with other congenital anomalies, most commonly cardiac, and can be a component of vertebral, anorectal, cardiac, tracheoesophageal, renal, and limb anomalies (VACTERL) complex of anomalies (Table 15–1).

The primary finding in EA is an interrupted esophagus that ends in a blind pouch proximally, usually at the level of the thoracic outlet.[5] In addition, a tracheoesophageal fistula (TEF) is associated with EA in

Table 15–1.

Associated Anomalies in Babies with Esophageal Atresia

Anomaly	Incidence (%)
Cardiac	30
VSD	10
Tetralogy of Fallot	5
ASD	4
Aortic coarctation	2.5
Single ventricle physiology	2.5
Non-cardiac	33
VACTERL	18
Chromosomal (18, 21)	9
Duodenal atresia	2.5

Babies may have more than one associated anomaly.[20]

Table 15–2.

History, Physical, and Radiological Findings in Patients with Esophageal Atresia

History
Polyhydramnios
Feeding intolerance
Sputtering with feeds
Cyanosis with feeds
Drooling

Physical
Inability to pass naso- or orogastric tube
Drooling

Radiological
CXR: air in proximal pouch contrasts with soft tissues in mediastinum
CXR: naso/orogastric tube in proximal esophageal pouch, does not advance
AXR: air in stomach if TEF present
AXR: air in duodenum but not in the rest of intestinal tract if associated DA
Contrast swallow: contrast in upper esophageal pouch, not in stomach

TEF = tracheoesophageal fistula; DA = duodenal atresia.

greater than 85% of babies (Figure 15–1). In these children, the distal esophagus has a fistulous connection to the posterior trachea at or above the carina. Air entering the airway can pass through the fistula into the intestinal tract. Gastric contents can also reflux into the trachea through the fistula. A pure atresia with a short distal esophagus without communication to the trachea accounts for 5–7% of esophageal anomalies. Other subtypes including the H-type, where the esophagus has normal patency but communicates to the trachea via a TEF, and the even more rare variant with a fistula between the proximal pouch and the trachea are occasionally seen.

Clinical presentation

The diagnosis of EA may be suspected antenatally based on the presence of polyhydramnios and a small stomach, but often the diagnosis is not made until after the child is born. Newborn children often sputter and spit up or may experience cyanotic episodes due to aspiration of feeds. Babies characteristically drool because they are

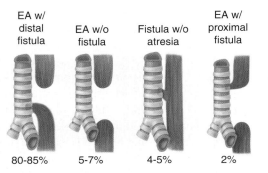

EA w/ distal fistula	EA w/o fistula	Fistula w/o atresia	EA w/ proximal fistula
80-85%	5-7%	4-5%	2%

FIGURE 15–1 ■ Classification of esophageal atresia and tracheoesophageal fistula.

unable to swallow saliva. Since the esophagus is interrupted, a naso- or orogastric tube cannot be passed (Table 15–2).

The clinical course of babies with EA can be complicated by aspiration, pneumonia, and respiratory compromise. Aspiration pneumonitis can occur due to reflux of gastric contents through the TEF as well as from aspiration of excessive saliva from the upper pouch. Aspiration can lead to respiratory failure or pneumonia, necessitating mechanical ventilation. Specific complications can ensue in ventilated patients especially if the fistula is large or if high pressures are required for ventilation. Passage of air through the fistula can cause gastric and intestinal dilatation with diaphragmatic splinting, making ventilation inefficient. In cases where there is a distal intestinal obstruction (such as associated duodenal atresia), the stomach can distend enormously, leading to respiratory compromise and even gastric rupture, which presents with a very large pneumoperitoneum and acute clinical deterioration (Figure 15–2). Such patients will sometimes require life-saving emergent fistula interruption by either placement of a balloon catheter or surgery.

Differential diagnosis

The differential for EA is short. Conditions to consider include laryngo-tracheoesophageal cleft, tracheal agenesis, esophageal stenosis, gastroesophageal reflux

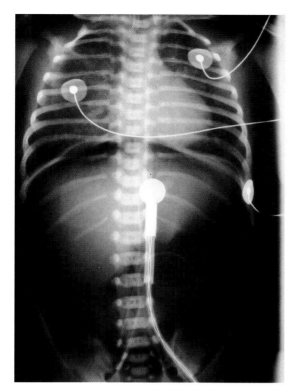

FIGURE 15–2 ■ Gastric perforation in esophageal atresia.

disease, and pharyngeal perforation. This latter iatrogenic condition typically occurs in premature very-low-birth-weight babies. The naso- or orogastric tube fails to pass because it perforates the pharynx and enters the mediastinum. The arrested passage of a tube in the mediastinum can give a false impression of EA.

Diagnosis

There are usually few findings on the physical exam that suggest the diagnosis of EA. However, the diagnosis needs to be strongly suspected if a naso- or orogastric tube cannot be advanced into the stomach in a newborn baby that experiences feeding difficulties, cyanosis with feeds, or excessive salivation. Chest auscultation may reveal signs of lobar atelectasis (especially on the right), or pneumonia. Few radiological studies are required to make the diagnosis of EA. A chest X-ray is usually sufficient, as it demonstrates the proximal esophagus filled with air contrasting against the soft tissues of the mediastinum, and the naso/orogastric tube stopping or curling in the upper esophageal pouch (Figure 15–3a). A chest X-ray is also valuable to assess the lung fields. An abdominal X-ray is mandatory to determine if there is air in the gastrointestinal tract, which suggests the presence of distal TEF. If the abdomen is gasless, a pure EA is likely (Figure 15–3b); if there is air in the stomach and duodenum but not beyond, duodenal atresia is likely to be present. Chest and abdominal films are also required as they reveal associated conditions such as vertebral and rib anomalies, which strongly support the diagnosis. In rare cases, if the diagnosis is in doubt, a contrast esophagram may be performed by an experienced practitioner (Figure 15–3c). As aspiration with severe pneumonitis is a significant risk, non-ionic contrast should be used judiciously. An alternative approach that can confirm the diagnosis and delineate the anatomy is bronchoscopy and esophagoscopy in the operating room.

The presence of other anomalies should be meticulously sought. Cardiac, renal, and chromosomal abnormalities have a great impact on the infant's perioperative course, morbidity, and mortality. An echocardiogram is

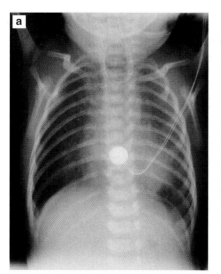 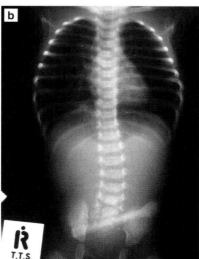 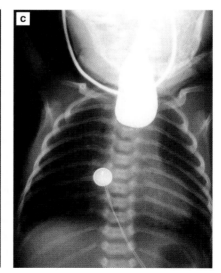

FIGURE 15–3 ■ Esophageal atresia: radiological findings. (a) Orogastric tube curled in the esophageal pouch (delta sign). (b) Gasless abdomen in a child with pure atresia. (c) Contrast study of the proximal esophageal pouch.

usually done to evaluate cardiac anomalies and to determine the location of the aortic arch. The patency of the anus should be established and duodenal atresia excluded and other features of the VACTERL association should be sought. To that end, ultrasound studies of the abdomen to evaluate renal anomalies, of the spine to rule out tethered cord, and of the head to assess for intracranial pathology are routinely performed. The studies need to be performed expeditiously but do not need to be performed emergently as long as the child is stable.

Treatment

The first step in treatment is resuscitation and cardiopulmonary support. To reduce the risk of aspiration of oral secretions, a Replogle-style orogastric suction tube (a double-lumen vented tube with suction openings near the tip) should be placed in the proximal esophageal pouch and connected to suction in order to evacuate saliva. The head of the bed needs to be elevated to minimize gastroesophageal reflux. Spontaneous ventilation without an endotracheal tube is preferred. If mechanical ventilation or airway control is required, strategies that minimize ventilator pressures should be used. Once the work-up is complete, surgical repair should be performed. The goal of surgery is two-fold: to divide and ligate the TEF in order to avoid pulmonary compromise from aspiration and abdominal distention, and to reconstruct the esophagus. Most children with EA and TEF can undergo successful surgical repair of the esophagus in the first few days of life. Babies that develop clinically significant abdominal distention or aspirate oral secretions may require emergent surgical intervention. Unstable babies that have severe pulmonary compromise or cyanotic heart disease, and babies whose esophagus cannot be reconstructed may benefit from delayed esophageal repair. Such babies may require gastrostomy tube placement to decompress the stomach and to provide access for enteral feeds. Non-cyanotic heart disease usually can be treated after repair of EA and TEF.

Successful repair of the esophagus depends on the length of the gap between the proximal dilated esophageal pouch and the distal esophagus. In children with EA and TEF, the esophagus usually can be repaired primarily. Isolated or pure EAs may be associated with a very small stomach and very long gap between the proximal and the distal ends. Children with long-gap EA are usually managed by delayed repair performed usually at 2–3 months of age. Innovative methods of placing traction on the esophageal ends in order to encourage growth and allow for primary anastomosis have been reported; however, long-term success and general acceptance has been difficult to achieve. If primary anastomosis is not possible, esophageal reconnection by "pulling up" the stomach into the mediastinum may be

Group	Risk	Weight (g)	Cardiac Anomalies	Survival (%)
I	Low	>2000	−	100
II	Moderate	<2000	−	81
III	Moderate	<2000	+	72
IV	high High	<2000	+	27

Table 15–3.
Survival Rates for Babies with Esophageal Atresia[20]

achieved. Early esophageal reconstruction, in the first few months of life, even if it requires a gastric pull-up procedure, has been favored recently with the hope of avoiding feeding aversion.

Outcome

Mortality following esophageal repair depends on birth weight, and the presence of major congenital heart disease. Babies with major heart anomalies weighing less than 2000 g have approximately 40% survival rate (Table 15–3). Such high-risk babies may be considered for delayed esophageal repair. Repair of EA may be complicated by anastomotic leak, recurrent tracheoesophageal fistula, sepsis, and stenosis. Early complications may result from technical errors, long gap between the esophageal ends, tension at the anastomosis, and ischemia. Late stenosis may be the result of gastroesophageal reflux disease. Patients often complain of difficulty eating and food sticking in the esophagus. Anastomotic stenoses often respond to treatment that includes control of acid reflux and dilatations. Balloon dilatation under direct endoscopic or fluoroscopic control appears safest. Few babies may eventually require esophageal replacement using stomach, colon, or jejunum as a conduit. In addition to complications related to the esophageal surgery, children may suffer from airway compromise due to tracheomalacia.

Congenital Esophageal Stenosis

Presentation and diagnosis

Embryologically, congenital esophageal stenosis is related to EA, and usually presents beyond the newborn period with difficulty swallowing solids and food sticking in the esophagus.[5] Contrast studies demonstrate a short narrow segment in the mid or distal third of the esophagus. Computed tomography (CT) imaging usually demonstrates ectopic cartilaginous rings. The differential includes esophageal stenosis secondary to previous surgery, esophagitis resulting from gastroesophageal reflux disease, and eosinophilic esophagitis.

Treatment and outcome

Congenital esophageal stenosis is treated with segmental esophageal resection and primary anastomosis. Resolution of symptoms is expected in most children.

STOMACH

Antral atresia and prepyloric web are rare congenital obstructions of the stomach, occurring in 1 in 20,000 live births.[6] Patients present with feeding intolerance and non-bilious vomiting. Investigation demonstrates a single bubble sign on radiographs: an air-filled stomach with no air in the distal intestine. Gastric outlet obstruction may be diagnosed antenatally by ultrasound, in which case no further work-up is unnecessary. The treatment is surgical correction of the obstruction in the neonatal period and there are usually few long-term complications.

Junctional epidermolysis pyloric atresia syndrome is a specific rare entity transmitted in an autosomal recessive fashion and associated with a form of epidermolysis bullosa.[6] Infants present with inability to feed due to gastric obstruction. Diagnosis is aided by genetic work-up. Surgical repair of the pyloric atresia can successfully relieve the obstruction; however, many patients continue to feed poorly, and suffer from malabsorption, failure to thrive, and sepsis eventually resulting in death in the first year of life. Because of poor prognosis, palliative care is usually offered to such children.

DUODENUM

Duodenal Atresia and Stenosis

Definitions and epidemiology

Congenital duodenal atresia and stenosis are the most common causes of duodenal obstruction in newborns and children. Duodenal atresia occurs in approximately 1 in 5000 live births.[1,3,7] Unlike jejunal or ileal atresias, duodenal atresias are commonly associated with other anomalies, including cardiac malformations, malrotation, jejunoileal atresia, vertebral anomalies, TEF, renal anomalies, anorectal malformation, and VACTERL (Table 15–4). Up to 30% of babies have Down's syndrome (trisomy 21) or other serious chromosomal anomalies.

Pathogenesis

Duodenal atresia is thought to be the result of abnormal recanalization during development. It is often associated with abnormalities in the anatomy of the common bile duct, including a bifid common bile duct, or with the presence of a preduodenal portal vein or annular pancreas. These findings suggest an embryological

Table 15–4.

Incidence of the Most Common Associated Anomalies in Duodenal and Jejunoileal Atresias[3]

Associated Anomaly	Duodenal (%)	Jejunoileal (%)
Cardiac	49	7
Trisomy 21	35	0
CNS	15	5
Pulmonary	10	13
Hypothyroidism	10	0
Esophageal	8	0
Musculoskeletal	8	3
Genitourinary	6	7

CNS = central nervous system.

origin distinct from other small intestinal atresias. Gray and Skandalakis classified duodenal atresias into three types (Table 15–5).[8,9]

Clinical features

The primary pathology is proximal intestinal obstruction, usually in the post-ampullary segment of duodenum. Babies present with feeding intolerance and bilious vomiting or bile-stained gastric tube output. The abdomen is scaphoid and is not tender.

Differential diagnosis

The differential for babies with scaphoid abdomen and bilious vomiting is short and is essentially limited to duodenal atresia and malrotation (Figure 15–4).

Diagnosis

The diagnostic work-up usually includes a history, physical exam, and plain radiographs of the chest and abdomen (Table 15–6). The history of a "double bubble" (enlarged, fluid-filled stomach and proximal duodenum) seen on *antenatal ultrasound* in association with *polyhydramnios* is highly suggestive of duodenal atresia

Table 15–5.

Classification of Duodenal Atresia After Gray and Skandalakis[8,9]

Morphology	Type
Intestinal wall in continuity; mucosal lined web or windsock	1
Fibrous chord connecting ends of duodenum	2
Complete separation of duodenal ends	3

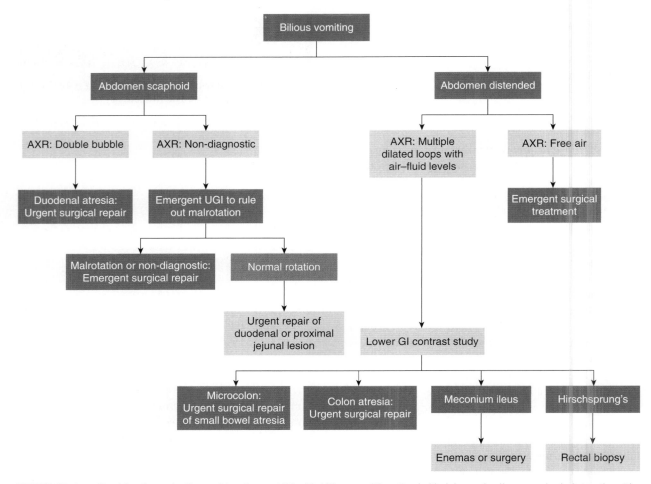

FIGURE 15–4 ■ Algorithm for evaluating and treating a child with bilious vomiting. Scaphoid abdomen implies a proximal obstruction. Distended abdomen implies distal obstruction.

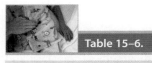

Table 15–6.

History, Physical, and Radiological Findings in Patients with Duodenal Atresia

History
Polyhydramnios on antenatal ultrasound
Double bubble on antenatal ultrasound
Feeding intolerance
Bilious vomiting

Physical
Abdomen scaphoid
Abdomen soft and not tender

Radiological
AXR: double bubble with no or minimal air beyond the
    duodenum
Contrast swallow: contrast in stomach and dilated duodenum,
    no contrast in jejunum, no malrotation

(Figure 15–5a). The classic finding of a double bubble on plain abdominal X-rays of a neonate in a baby with bilious vomiting and scaphoid abdomen is diagnostic

(Figure 15–5b). The X-ray findings are the result of air-filled dilated stomach and air-filled dilated duodenum. If an oro- or nasogastric tube is placed early and the stomach is emptied, one can reproduce the classic findings by instilling a small amount of air into the stomach and obtaining a plain radiograph.

A double bubble appearance associated with the presence of distal gas may suggest duodenal stenosis. In some cases, gas may enter the distal intestine through a bifid distal common bile duct communicating with the duodenal lumen proximal and distal to the obstruction. In the absence of classic double bubble appearance, contrast studies may be obtained with the objective of distinguishing stenosis and atresia from malrotation (Table 15–7). If malrotation cannot be ruled out definitively, emergent surgery should be performed in order to avoid the catastrophic consequences of midgut volvulus and intestinal necrosis. If malrotation can be clearly ruled out, surgical repair could be delayed until the remainder of the work-up is completed. Children with duodenal stenosis usually present with typical obstructive symptoms in the neonatal period, but can at times present months and even years

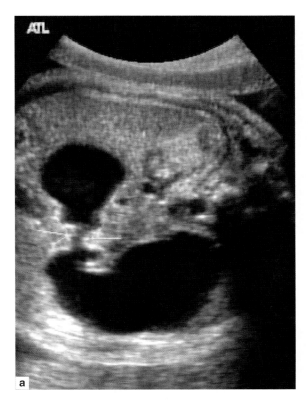 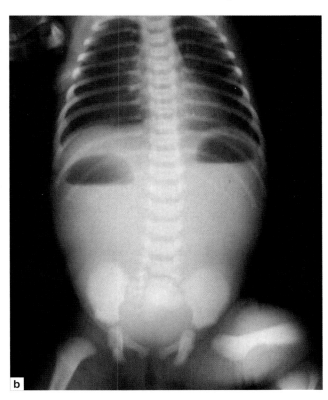

FIGURE 15–5 ■ Radiological findings in a child with duodenal atresia. (a) Antenatal ultrasound demonstrating double bubble sign. (b) Double bubble sign in a child with bilious vomiting.

Table 15–7.

The Relationship Between the Level of Intestinal Obstruction and Presenting Symptoms in a Neonate with Duodenal, Jejunoileal, and Colonic Atresia, Web or Duplication

Site of Obstruction	Antenatal Ultrasound		Bile in Emesis	Abdominal Distension	Differential	Radiological Studies
	Polyhydramnios	Dilated Loops				
Proximal (duodenum, proximal jejunum)	++	+	+	−	Malrotation	AXR UGI
Distal (distal jejunum, ileum, colon)	+/−	++	+	+	Hirschsprung's Meconium ileus	AXR Contrast Enema Rectal biopsy

later. In these cases, massive dilatation of the duodenum proximal to the obstruction is typically seen (Figure 15–6a and b).

Treatment

Babies with duodenal atresia and stenosis require surgical treatment. The duodenal obstruction is usually bypassed by performing a duodenoduodenostomy.[7] If a web is found it could be excised safely at times, but should be approached with caution as the bile duct often empties into the stenotic segment and could be injured. Excision of the lateral aspect of the web, which

is typically windsock-shaped, and a transverse duodenal closure is sufficient to relieve the obstruction. Surgical repair of the duodenum has traditionally been performed through a transabdominal incision. Use of a diamond-shaped anastomosis became popular in the 1990s following a report by Kimura et al.[10] More recently, successful laparoscopic repair of duodenum has been reported, although such approach has not been universally embraced to date. At least 1–2% of cases will have an associated downstream atresia, which should always be excluded at the time of operative repair.

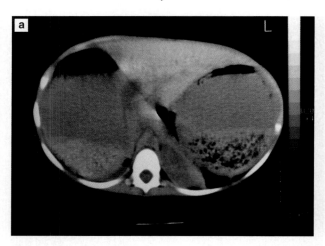
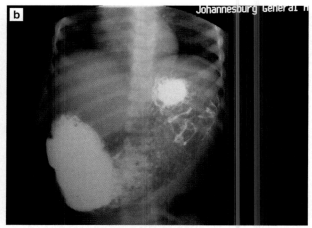

FIGURE 15–6 ■ Duodenal stenosis left untreated in a 4-year-old boy with long-standing intermittent bilious vomiting. (a) CT scan demonstrated an extremely dilated duodenum. (b) Barium meal and follow-through showing gross dilatation of the first portion of the duodenum in association with congenital duodenal stenosis.

Survival following duodenal atresia is greater than 96%, and deaths are usually the result of associated anomalies.[3,11] Following surgical repair, many babies continue to have bilious drainage out of the oro- or nasogastric tube lasting as long as 2 weeks. This is thought to be the result of poor motility and the chronically dilated thickened duodenum. Complications of surgical repair are related to anastomotic stenosis or leak. In cases where the duodenum is very dilated, it may require plication. Up to 10% of children who do well initially will come back over the following 2–4 years with recurrent episode of vomiting and poor oral intake and will be found to have very dilated proximal duodenum. Such children may benefit from surgical re-exploration, revision of duodenoduodenostomy, and duodenal plication, which could improve the mechanics of flow of enteral contents.

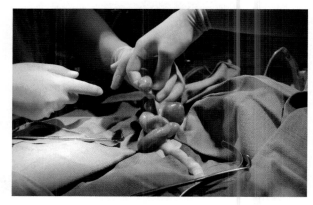

FIGURE 15–7 ■ Intestinal atresia in the context of gastroschisis. Dilated proximal small bowel ending in a blind loop.

SMALL INTESTINE

Jejunoileal Atresia and Stenosis

Definition and epidemiology

Jejunoileal intestinal atresias and stenoses occur in 1 in 6000 live births.[12] The most common site of atresia is in the jejunum.[2] In contrast to duodenal atresia, the incidence of associated non-intestinal anomalies is much lower in patients with jejunoileal atresia (Table 15–4).

Pathogenesis The etiology is thought to be in utero segmental occlusion of mesenteric vasculature due to emboli, malrotation with volvulus, gastroschisis with obstruction, Hirschsprung's disease, or cystic fibrosis (Figure 15–7).[12] In contrast to duodenal atresia,

Table 15–8.	
Classification of Intestinal Atresias According to Louw and Barnard[1,21]	
Morphology	Type
Intestinal wall in continuity; mucosal lined web or windsock	1
Fibrous string without mesenteric defect	2
Mesenteric defect with no fibrous string	3
Apple peel or Christmas tree deformity	3b
Multiple atresias	4

jejunoileal atresia is rarely associated with chromosomal abnormalities or cardiac anomalies. Jejunoileal atresias are classified based on their morphology (Table 15–8; Figure 15–8).[1]

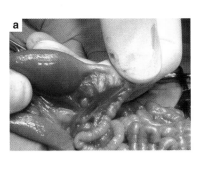
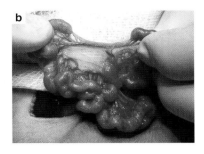
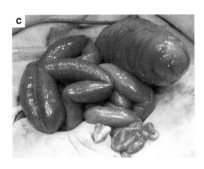
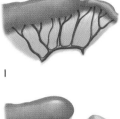
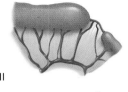
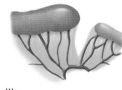
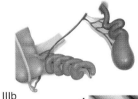
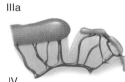
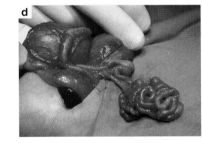
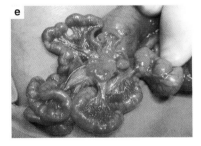

FIGURE 15–8 ■ Jejunoileal atresia: classification and operative findings. The central cartoon illustrates the findings in the adjacent operative photograph. (a) Type I, muscularis in continuity (b) Type II, muscularis interrupted but mesentery is intact (c) type IIIa, both intestine and mesentery are interrupted (d) Type IIIb, apple peel deformity. Bowel spirals around a tenuous blood supply which originates distally (e) Type IV, multiple atresias.

Clinical features

As in other sites of atresia, the primary pathology is intestinal obstruction. Increasingly the condition is being diagnosed prenatally with the recognition of gross bowel dilatation on prenatal ultrasound examinations. Polyhydramnios may not be prominent in the context of distal obstruction.[13,14] Newborns typically present with inability to feed, bilious vomiting, and abdominal distension (Table 15–9).

Differential diagnosis

The differential diagnosis for babies presenting with jejunal and ileal atresia is broad. Malrotation and duodenal atresia may be considered in babies with a flat abdomen. In babies with abdominal distention, sepsis, necrotizing enterocolitis, meconium ileus, Hirschsprung's disease, duplication cysts with volvulus,

Table 15–9.

History, Physical, and Radiological Findings in Patients with Jejunoileal or Colonic Atresia

History
+/− polyhydramnios on antenatal ultrasound
Dilated intestinal loops on antenatal ultrasound
Feeding intolerance
Bilious vomiting

Physical
Abdomen distended, visible and palpable loops
Abdomen may be tender if intestinal perforation or ischemia

Radiological
AXR: dilated loops on intestine with air–fluid levels
Contrast enema: may demonstrate colonic atresia or microcolon

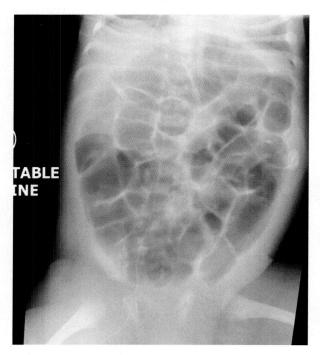

FIGURE 15–9 ■ Abdominal radiograph in a child with distal intestinal obstruction demonstrating multiple dilated loops of bowel.

omphalomesenteric duct, intestinal dysmotility, small left colon syndrome, meconium plug syndrome, and colonic atresia may be considered.

Diagnosis

The diagnosis is based on history, physical exam, plain radiographs, and contrast studies. The more distal the atresia, the more intestinal distension is observed. Abdominal radiographs show multiple dilated loops of small intestine and no air in the rectum (Figure 15–9). Air–fluid levels are characteristically seen on decubitus abdominal radiographs. The intestinal loops in congenital atresias are typically grossly dilated, indicating a long-standing duration of obstruction occurring during fetal life. Children who have a flat abdomen are likely to have a proximal obstruction and upper gastrointestinal contrast study may be helpful. Children who present with a distended abdomen suggesting a distal obstruction should be evaluated with a contrast enema study. The finding of microcolon is often associated with atresias.

Treatment

The management of atresia and stenosis includes naso- or orogastric decompression, resuscitation, and, once it is safe, surgical exploration and repair. Surgical repair should not be unduly delayed, as the obstructed dilated intestinal loop can become ischemic. If the baby is unstable, extremely small, or has associated anomalies, a diverting ostomy may be required. In most babies, however, primary repair can be performed. A functional end-to-end anastomosis can be fashioned between the intestine proximal to the atresia and the intestine distal to the atresia. The presence of additional atretic and stenotic segments has to be excluded. A challenge for surgical repair is the luminal size discrepancy between the proximal dilated end and the diminutive caliber of the distal unused intestine. When the discrepancy in the luminal diameter is great, the proximal dilated end may be resected, plicated, or tapered.[1,2] When the remaining intestinal length is a concern, bowel preservation techniques, such as serial tapered enteroplasty (STEP), may be considered, although these are usually delayed until the dilatation associated with adaptation has occurred and then performed as secondary procedures.

Early postoperative complications include anastomotic leak, anastomotic stenosis, prolonged ileus, and delayed feeding. Long-term complications include small bowel obstruction, poor feeding, malabsorption, and short gut syndrome. Historically, the reported mortality of children with jejunoileal atresia is between 11% and 16%. Mortality is the result of cardiorespiratory failure, sepsis, pneumonia, and liver failure, and is often related to co-morbidities or short bowel syndrome. Fifteen percent of the surviving patients may have short bowel syndrome and require prolonged parenteral nutrition to supplement enteral intake. It appears that mortality in children with jejunoileal atresia has decreased in the past decade, but complication rate has increased, possibly due to survival of children with short bowel syndrome who have a prolonged complicated course.

COLON

Colonic Atresias and Stenosis

Definition and epidemiology

Congenital colonic atresias and stenosis are obstructive congenital lesions of the colon.[1,3] Colonic atresias are rare and account for 5–8% of all intestinal atresias. They can occur in association with upstream small bowel atresias but also as isolated lesions.

Pathogenesis

As with jejunoileal atresias, vascular compromise during fetal life is thought to lead to colonic atresias. Additionally, Hirschsprung's disease and cystic fibrosis in association with colonic atresias have been reported. Colonic atresias may be described using the classification for jejunoileal atresias and fall into Type I, Type II, or Type IIIa.

Clinical features

Colonic atresias present with obstructive symptoms, including bilious vomiting, abdominal distention, and failure to pass meconium (Table 15–9). Since the obstruction is distal, symptoms may not be immediately obvious.

Differential

The differential diagnosis is that of a distal intestinal obstruction in a neonate. Sepsis, necrotizing enterocolitis, meconium ileus, Hirschsprung's disease, duplication cysts with volvulus, omphalomesenteric duct, intestinal dysmotility, small left colon syndrome, meconium plug syndrome, pelvic masses, and imperforate anus should be considered.

Diagnosis

The diagnosis is based on history, physical exam, plain radiographs, and contrast enema. The exact anomaly may not be apparent until surgery is performed. Plain abdominal radiographs demonstrate multiple dilated loops of intestine, absence of air in the rectum, and air–fluid levels. A contrast enema study is helpful to delineate the site of obstruction, rule out alternative diagnoses, and plan the surgical approach.

Treatment

Initial treatment includes gastric decompression, resuscitation, and evaluation for associated anomalies. Treatment is surgical (Figure 15–10). Resection of the atretic segment and primary repair may be performed in most babies. Similar to jejunoileal atresia, colonic atresia may present with dilated proximal segment and decompressed distal segment. The dilated segment may be resected, plicated, or tapered in order to perform a successful anastomosis. Postoperatively, patients may have prolonged ileus due to dysmotility in the proximal

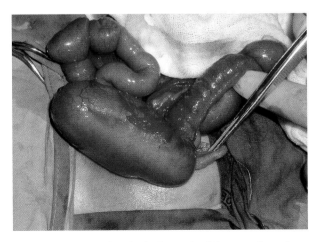

FIGURE 15–10 ■ Isolated colonic atresia of the ascending colon.

dilated segment. As with distal ileal atresias, the possibility of associated meconium ileus and Hirschsprung's disease has to be considered. In cases where the surgeon is not confident to anastomose due to caliber discrepancy or the inability to exclude Hirschsprung's disease, creation of a stoma is the safe option.

Anorectal Malformations

Definition and epidemiology

Anorectal malformations are spectrum of developmental anomalies affecting the formation of the distal rectum and anus. The anal opening is missing, displaced, or narrow. The incidence is approximately 1 in 5000 live births.[15,16] Anorectal malformations may be isolated or may be part of a spectrum of complex malformations, such as the VACTERL association, Currarino triad (anorectal malformation, sacral bony abnormality, and a presacral mass), and cloacal exstrophy.

Pathogenesis

Anorectal malformations can be divided into two general groups: low defects, which are characterized by a fistula to the perineum, and high defects, which are characterized by a fistula to the urinary tract or a blind-ending rectum.

Clinical features

Children with complete or near-complete obstruction present with feeding difficulties, bilious vomiting, and abdominal distention in the newborn period. Children with stenotic anus or anteriorly displaced anus may present later in life with constipation, overflow incontinence, and abdominal pain.

Differential diagnosis

The differential is narrow, and includes rare conditions such as rectal atresia and anal duplication. It is important to distinguish "simple" imperforate anus malformation from the rare and extremely complex cloacal anomalies.

Diagnosis

Careful examination of the perineum is critical and demonstrates absence of a normally positioned and normal caliber anus. The diagnosis could be missed if an inexperienced provider assumes that a perineal dimple is an anus; however, a more complete examination reveals the dimple is blind-ending (Figure 15–11). Repeat examination at 24–36 hours of life is required to look for meconium staining. Appearance of meconium along the median raphe in boys and in the posterior fourchette in girls strongly suggests a low defect. The identification of the cloacal malformation is critically

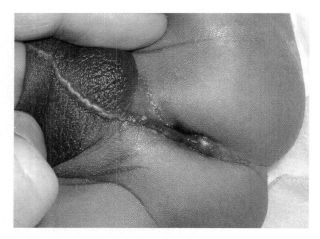

FIGURE 15–11 ■ String of pearls appearance on the median raphe of a patient suggests a low anorectal malformation that can be treated primarily in the newborn period.

important in girls. A large hydrocolpos, which frequently occurs with this lesion, may cause urinary tract obstruction and is at risk of rupture if not treated expeditiously. The appearance of a single perineal opening with foreshortened labia minora, absent hymen, and a prominent clitoris is typical. Plain radiographs should be performed to rule out associated anomalies. A cardiac echo and a renal ultrasound should be obtained to evaluate for cardiac and renal anomalies. A voiding cystourethrogram (VCUG) is essential since urinary tract anomalies are commonly associated with this malformation.

Treatment

Babies should be treated with oro- or nasogastric decompression, resuscitation, and evaluation of associated anomalies. Low anorectal malformations can be repaired primarily in the neonatal period. High anomalies require intestinal diversion and delayed reconstruction. If a hydrocolpos is present in the context of a cloaca, separate vaginal drainage with a tube vaginostomy is mandatory. Definitive repair is performed using a posterior sagittal anorectoplasty (PSARP) approach. Children with low defects have good prospects for continence, although they may require continuing treatment of constipation. The outcomes for children with high anorectal anomalies are varied. Social continence may be achieved in most children; however, true continence is achieved in only approximately 60% of children, depending on the severity of the malformation. Long-term follow-up is required for these children since they continue to be challenged with problems related to constipation, bowel management, and social acceptance. Procedures that provide access for antegrade enemas can help older children achieve independence and maintain social continence. The authors' experience is that properly reconstructed patients that are incontinent

as young children can develop greater degree of fecal continence as they get older, possibly as a result of improved levator muscle function.

Enteric Duplications

Definition and epidemiology

Enteric duplications occur in 1 in 6000–10,000 live births, and may be found anywhere along the gastrointestinal tract.[17,18] Duplications are found in the midgut 50% of the time, in the foregut approximately one-third of time, and the remainder are in the hindgut (Table 15–10). As the name implies, the intestinal lumen forms in duplicate resulting in cystic masses or rarely long tubular structures associated with the intestinal tract.

Pathogenesis

Duplications are thought to result from aberrant development of the intestinal tract. The duplicated portion of the intestine, which may be cystic or tubular, shares its blood supply and the muscular wall with the adjacent normal intestine. Enteric duplications are usually lined with intestinal epithelium, but could be lined with heterotopic epithelium. If gastric epithelium is present, bleeding ulcerations may occur. Duplications involving the small and large bowel are located in the mesentery. In most patients, the duplications are not in continuity with the primary intestinal lumen. In some cases, the duplication may occur ectopically. An example is gastric duplication in the pancreas causing recurrent pancreatitis. Since duplications are lined with intestinal mucosa,

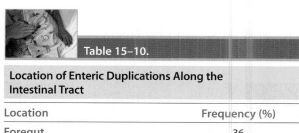

Table 15–10.

Location of Enteric Duplications Along the Intestinal Tract

Location	Frequency (%)
Foregut	36
Esophageal	19
Thoracoabdominal	4
Gastric	9
Duodenal	4
Midgut	50
Jejunal	10
Ileal	35
Appendeceal	2
Cecal	3
Hindgut	12
	7
	5

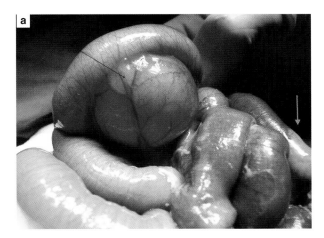

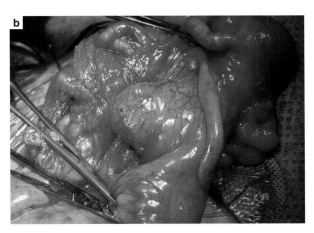

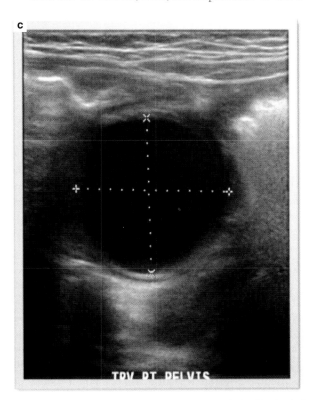

FIGURE 15–12 ■ Intestinal duplication. (a) Enteric duplication led to volvulus, bowel necrosis, and perforation in a newborn baby. (b) Enteric duplication found in the mesentery of the distal ileum and treated with segmental resection. (c) A cystic mass in the right lower quadrant examined using ultrasound.

mucus is produced and secreted into the cyst lumen. Without egress, the fluid accumulates resulting in slow but progressive enlargement of enteric duplications. If the mucosa ulcerates due to acid production, duplication may increase in size rapidly and even rupture. Associated anomalies are more common with complex long tubular duplications.

Presentation, differential, and diagnosis

Most enteric duplications present in the first year of life, but can be found at any age. Duplications may present with intestinal obstruction, volvulus (Figure 15–12a), gastrointestinal bleeding, or mass. Duplications may be asymptomatic and diagnosed incidentally on antenatal ultrasound or radiological studies performed after birth (Figure 15–12b). The specific complex of symptoms depends on the site of the duplication.

Esophageal duplications may present with dysphagia and difficulty swallowing. Duplications can also displace or impinge on the trachea leading to cough, dyspnea, and stridor. Respiratory symptoms may be exacerbated by viral illness. CT evaluation of the chest demonstrates a cystic mediastinal mass. The differential diagnosis includes neurenteric cysts, bronchogenic cysts, abscess, and lymphadenopathy.

Gastric duplications are often asymptomatic and may be identified during a work-up for abdominal pain. Large gastric duplications may present with difficulty eating, early satiety, reflux, or abdominal fullness. Isolated duplications containing purely antral-type mucosa may cause hypersecretion of acid with peptic ulceration of the stomach or duodenum. This is caused by overactivity of gastrin-producing G cells in the cyst, which are not subject to the usual feedback inhibition by gastric acid. Upper gastrointestinal contrast study or upper endoscopy demonstrates a submucosal mass in the wall of the stomach. CT scan may show a cystic gastric wall mass. The differential diagnosis includes hamartomatous polyps, lymphoma, leiomyoma, and leiomyosarcoma.

Duodenal duplications may be asymptomatic, or/ and present with a large retroperitoneal mass and symptoms of proximal intestinal obstruction. Duodenal duplications may also involve the pancreas or the common bile duct leading to jaundice and pancreatitis. Ultrasound and CT scan reveal a cystic mass in the right retroperitoneum or the head of the pancreas. Intrahepatic and extrahepatic bile duct dilatation may be seen if bile duct obstruction were present. The differential diagnosis includes retroperitoneal abscess, duodenal perforation, tumor, and pancreatic pseudocyst.

The midgut is the most common site to find enteric duplications. As they enlarge, duplications can produce intestinal obstruction or promote volvulus. Ultrasound and CT scan often demonstrate a cystic mass in the mesentery with a characteristic intestinal "signature." The differential includes mesenteric cysts, omental cysts, abscesses, lymphatic malformations, and tumors.

Duplications involving the anorectum present with a mass palpable on rectal exam.[19] Patients may complain of fullness, difficulty defecating, discharge, and pain. Ultrasound and CT scan demonstrate a cystic mass in the wall of the rectum. The differential includes perirectal abscess, tailgut cyst, and sacrococcygeal teratoma.

Treatment

Enteric duplications require surgical management. Even if duplications are identified incidentally, they are likely to become symptomatic during early childhood. The urgency and surgical approach are dictated by the anatomical location of the duplication. Since they share the blood supply and the muscular wall with the intestinal tract, cystic duplications in the midgut are treated with segmental intestinal resection and primary anastomosis (Figure 15–12c). Recovery is usually uneventful. Gastric duplications may be treated using simple wedge resection of the stomach wall. Duplications involving the esophagus, duodenum, rectum, and anus can be very challenging due to the complex anatomy. Large tubular duplications are also challenging, because they may involve long segments of the small or large intestine and are not amenable to segmental resection. Complex duplications may be treated by submucosal resection, leaving the muscularis in situ. Submucosal resection of smaller duplications is usually successful with relief of symptoms and minimal morbidity. If complete or submucosal resection cannot be performed safely, the duplicated segment may be drained into the primary intestinal lumen. Such procedures have variable outcome as children may have poor emptying of the duplication and poor intestinal motility. Gastrointestinal bleeding may persist if heterotopic gastric mucosa were present in the duplication.

REFERENCES

1. Hajivassiliou CA. Intestinal obstruction in neonatal/pediatric surgery. *Semin Pediatr Surg*. 2003;12:241–253.
2. Stollman TH, de Blaauw I, Wijnen MH, et al. Decreased mortality but increased morbidity in neonates with jejunoileal atresia; a study of 114 cases over a 34-year period. *J Pediatr Surg*. 2009;44:217–221.
3. Piper HG, Alesbury J, Waterford SD, Zurakowski D, Jaksic T. Intestinal atresias: factors affecting clinical outcomes. *J Pediatr Surg*. 2008;43:1244–1248.
4. Ioannides AS, Copp AJ. Embryology of oesophageal atresia. *Semin Pediatr Surg*. 2009;18:2–11.
5. Spitz L. Oesophageal atresia. *Orphanet J Rare Dis*. 2007;2:24.
6. Maclennan AC. Investigation in vomiting children. *Semin Pediatr Surg*. 2003;12:220–228.
7. Escobar MA, Ladd AP, Grosfeld JL, et al. Duodenal atresia and stenosis: long-term follow-up over 30 years. *J Pediatr Surg*. 2004;39:867–871 [discussion 71].
8. Androulakis J, Colborn GL, Skandalakis PN, Skandalakis LJ, Skandalakis JE. Embryologic and anatomic basis of duodenal surgery. *Surg Clin North Am*. 2000;80:171–199.
9. Colborn GL, Gray SW, Pemberton LB, Skandalakis LJ, Skandalakis JE. The duodenum. Part 3: pathology. *Am Surg*. 1989;55:469–473.
10. Kimura K, Tsugawa C, Ogawa K, Matsumoto Y, Yamamoto T, Asada S. Diamond-shaped anastomosis for congenital duodenal obstruction. *Arch Surg*. 1977;112:1262–1263.
11. Spigland N, Yazbeck S. Complications associated with surgical treatment of congenital intrinsic duodenal obstruction. *J Pediatr Surg*. 1990;25:1127–1130.
12. Hemming V, Rankin J. Small intestinal atresia in a defined population: occurrence, prenatal diagnosis and survival. *Prenat Diagn*. 2007;27:1205–1211.
13. Corteville JE, Gray DL, Langer JC. Bowel abnormalities in the fetus—correlation of prenatal ultrasonographic findings with outcome. *Am J Obstet Gynecol*. 1996;175:724–729.
14. Ruiz MJ, Thatch KA, Fisher JC, Simpson LL, Cowles RA. Neonatal outcomes associated with intestinal abnormalities diagnosed by fetal ultrasound. *J Pediatr Surg*. 2009;44:71–74 [discussion 4–5].
15. Levitt MA, Pena A. Outcomes from the correction of anorectal malformations. *Curr Opin Pediatr*. 2005;17:394–401.
16. Levitt MA, Pena A. Anorectal malformations. *Orphanet J Rare Dis*. 2007;2:33.
17. Bissler JJ, Klein RL. Alimentary tract duplications in children: case and literature review. *Clin Pediatr (Phila)*. 1988;27:152–157.
18. Stringer MD, Spitz L, Abel R, et al. Management of alimentary tract duplication in children. *Br J Surg*. 1995;82:74–78.
19. Kratz JR, Deshpande V, Ryan DP, Goldstein AM. Anal canal duplication associated with presacral cyst. *J Pediatr Surg*. 2008;43:1749–1752.
20. Okamoto T, Takamizawa S, Arai H, et al. Esophageal atresia: prognostic classification revisited. *Surgery*. 2009;145:675–681.
21. Louw JH, Barnard CN. Congenital intestinal atresia; observations on its origin. *Lancet*. 1955;269:1065–1067.

CHAPTER 16

Inflammatory Bowel Disease

Rebecca Scherr
and Subra Kugathasan

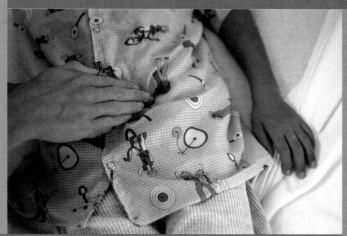

In a day-to-day practice, general pediatricians are expected to care for a wide variety of gastrointestinal disorders. Fortunately, most of the gastrointestinal ailments in childhood are not serious and self-limiting in nature and do not usually require a referral to a subspecialty such as pediatric gastroenterology with few exceptions. Inflammatory bowel disease (IBD) is an exception; consultation with a pediatric gastroenterologist is mandatory for adequate management. Crohn's disease (CD) and ulcerative colitis (UC) are the two most common chronic IBDs. For decades, CD and UC were considered totally different entities, since the clinical features, treatment options, and natural history of these diseases appeared to be quite different. However, recent developments and findings have made clinicians and scientists begin to think of IBD as one entity, with a spectrum of findings. Recent work has, for example, identified CD and UC occurring in the same families, common susceptibility genes and pathways between these two entities, and similar responses to emerging therapies to both conditions. Classic CD is found at one end of the spectrum and UC at the other, but many patients have features that overlap. In this chapter, we will try to approach CD and UC as one entity but differentiate CD from UC whenever necessary.

EPIDEMIOLOGY

Although a diagnosis of IBD can be made at any age, about one in every four new diagnoses of IBD is made before the age of 20 years. Population-based studies suggest that IBD is unevenly distributed throughout the world, with the highest disease rates occurring in Western or industrialized countries. Recent epidemiologic surveys have also suggested that IBD incidence rates have changed over the second half of the twentieth century, with a gradual increase in CD, but reaching a plateau in UC incidence.[1] Only a few systematic, population-based studies have been done in North America regarding the true incidence of childhood IBD to date, and estimate the incidence is about 7–12 per 100,000 children. Although the true impact of IBD in children is not entirely known, we estimate that about 100,000 children are suffering from IBD in North America at any given time.[2] This makes IBD one of the common chronic gastrointestinal disorders for which pediatricians and pediatric gastroenterologists provide care.

There are differences in the descriptive epidemiology of IBD when pediatric IBD is compared with adult-onset IBD. While CD and UC occur with equal distribution in adults, the incidence of CD is three times higher than UC in pediatric age groups.[2] In adult IBD, there is a nearly equal ratio of male to female disease, with a slight female predominance. In contrast, prepubertal children with CD exhibit a male preponderance of 1.5:1.[3] Currently there is no molecular explanation why children with IBD differ from adults in regard to gender ratio.

ETIOLOGY AND PATHOGENESIS

The etiology of IBD is not completely understood at present, although significant advances have been made over the last decade. It is becoming increasingly more evident that certain individuals have a genetic predisposition and that one or more environmental triggers can lead to the development of disease.

Environmental Factors

The well-documented increase in the incidence and prevalence of IBD is part of a world-wide emergence of chronic autoimmune and inflammatory diseases, a phenomenon closely linked to social and economic development. Initially noted in Northern Europe and North America, this increase has now been documented in the rest of Europe, Japan, and South America, and most recently in the Asia-Pacific region.[4] An explanation for the higher frequency of IBD has been known as the "hygiene hypothesis," which postulates that there has been a fundamental lifestyle change from one with high to one with low microbial exposure.[5] Exposure to fewer microbial antigens early in life would lead to a less robust immune system, ill prepared to tackle challenges later on in life, and mounting immune responses unable to eliminate offending agents resulting in chronic inflammation. Numerous other environmental factors and stimuli are considered risk factors for IBD, including smoking, diet (junk food), drugs, geography and social status, increased stress, the enteric flora, altered intestinal permeability, and appendectomy.[1,4]

Genetic Susceptibility

IBD is highly heritable. This concept is strongly supported by family, twin, and phenotype concordance studies and is now confirmed by the discoveries of many susceptibility genes.[6,7] A positive family history is a well-known risk factor for development of IBD. Recent research also shows that heritable factors have more influence in CD than in schizophrenia, asthma, and essential hypertension.[8] Initial family-based linkage studies of IBD implicated the *NOD2* gene in CD and the *MHC* region in UC for increased susceptibility.[7,9] Recently, genome-wide association scans (GWAS), which employ high-density single nucleotide polymorphism (SNP) array technology, have increased the number of possible genetic factors linked to IBD. To date, this method of broad, unbiased screening has provided as many as 30 susceptibility loci in CD and 17 loci in UC. However, the most surprising finding was that the vast majority of the new gene discoveries were common to both CD and UC, further reinforcing our belief that CD and UC stem from same pathogenic process, with a differing clinical spectrum.

Microbial Factors

The hypothesis that infectious agents cause IBD has been popular for many years. However, a multitude of studies have failed to confirm the presence of infectious agents by histological examination, culture of tissue homogenates, genomic identification, and serum antibodies. More recently an entero-adhesive/invasive strain of *E. coli* has been described as being associated with ileal CD, but its potential etiological role remains unclear. Instead of specific infectious agents, evidence continues to accumulate that the indigenous commensal gut flora is the target of the chronic immune response in IBD. The majority of IBD patients show an enhanced immunological reactivity against gut bacterial antigens. Bacterial flagellin has been recently reported as a dominant antigen in CD, apparently defining a population of patients with complicated CD. The discovery that CD is associated with mutations of the *NOD2/CARD15* gene, whose product is a bacteria-sensing cytoplasmic protein, suggests that the ability of the immune system to normally recognize the gut flora may be genetically altered in IBD.

Immune Factors

Inflammation is the most common type of reaction that the body mounts against external or internal offending agents. The gut is particularly susceptible to inflammation because, even under normal circumstances, a baseline "physiological inflammation" is present in the mucosa, representing a controlled immune response against dietary and microbial antigens. When this physiological response becomes excessive and chronic, it leads to injury, resulting in anatomical and functional abnormalities. Major advances during the past few decades have helped our understanding of the cellular and molecular mechanisms mediating mucosal immunity, as well as the alterations that lead to chronic gut inflammation.[10]

CLINICAL PRESENTATION

UC and CD are grouped together in this chapter due to many similarities in their clinical and epidemiologic features and therapeutic responses. They are both chronic, inflammatory diseases of the gastrointestinal tract with periods of remission and exacerbation. Although they share many similarities, they each have distinguishing characteristics. *UC* is chronic inflammation involving only the mucosa of the colon. The inflammation is *continuous*, starting in the rectum and extending proximally to varying extents. In contrast, *CD* has transmural inflammation and is not localized solely to the colon. CD can be found anywhere in the GI tract, from mouth to anus. The inflammatory process in CD is *patchy*, which can be helpful in distinguishing UC from colonic CD. The terminal ileum is the most common site of CD. Because disease activity often occurs in several areas, about 60% pediatric patients have ileocolonic involvement while 20–30% have isolated colonic disease.[3] In certain cases, if skip lesions, granulomas, and small bowel involvement, all hallmarks of CD, are absent, the diagnosis between UC and CD may be more difficult. If there is oral or perianal involvement, then CD is more likely. However, in approximately 10% of cases of colonic IBD, it is difficult to distinguish between CD and UC. These patients are given an interim diagnosis of *indeterminate colitis* or the newly coined term *inflammatory bowel disease-undetermined* (IBDU).[11]

The most common presentation of UC is diarrhea and rectal bleeding, while the "classic presentation" of CD consists of abdominal pain, diarrhea, poor appetite, and weight loss. Since CD presentation can be insidious and nonspecific, a delay in the diagnosis of CD is more common, compared with UC. The time from diagnosis to the onset of symptoms in CD can be anywhere from 5 months to a few years. In both UC and CD, approximately 30% of pediatric patients present with moderate signs of systemic illness. Another 10% present with severe colitis, defined as more than five bloody stools per day, anemia, fever, hypoalbuminemia, tachycardia, and weight loss.[12]

Although abdominal pain is the single most common presenting symptom in IBD, it can have several other less obvious presentations, such as growth failure, arthralgias, rashes, and iron deficiency anemia, without notable GI symptoms. Being aware of these other presentations can aid in early referral and initiation of treatment. In addition, since abdominal pain is a common symptom in a general pediatrician or family practitioner's office, and most of these children will not have IBD, not every child with abdominal pain needs to be referred to a gastroenterologist. Table 16–1 lists "red flags" in the history and physical examination that should raise suspicion for IBD in a patient and warrant further investigation.

Abdominal Pain

Abdominal pain is seen in 60–95% of patients presenting with CD and 30–70% of patients presenting with UC. Sometimes it can be difficult to distinguish between abdominal pain from IBD and functional abdominal pain. Location, chronicity, and severity may help determine if it is from IBD. Abdominal pain in CD can awaken the child at night, cause decreased appetite, and in the case of ileocecal disease, can be localized to the RLQ. Odynophagia and dysphagia can be seen in esophageal CD, which occurs in approximately 10% of CD patients.[13]

Diarrhea

Diarrhea is seen commonly in UC (70–90%). It is seen in 65–75% of CD patients, and can be intermittent, depending on the location of disease.[12] Distal colonic

Table 16–1.

"Red Flags" Suspicious for IBD

History	Physical Exam
Abdominal pain	Anemia
Abdominal pain distant from umbilicus	Decreased growth velocity
Pain that interferes with sleep	Delayed sexual maturation
Discrete episodes of pain that are acute in onset	Finger clubbing
Pain precipitated by eating	Oral ulcerations
Dysphagia, odynophagia	Abdominal tenderness
Involuntary weight loss	Abdominal mass
Rectal bleeding	Perianal fistula, fissures
Nocturnal diarrhea	
Extraintestinal manifestations	
Unexplained low-grade fevers	
Erythema nodosum, pyoderma gangrenosum	
Joint pain/swelling	
Jaundice	
Severe eye pain or persistent conjunctivitis	
Strong family history of IBD	

disease is typically associated with *tenesmus* (a sensation of incomplete evacuation) and *urgency*. Gross blood is usually seen with colonic involvement and may or may not be associated with abdominal pain. Nocturnal stooling is also common in colonic disease.

Hematochezia

Between 50% and 90% of UC patients and 20% and 60% in CD present with rectal bleeding.[12] The severity is dependent on location and severity of disease, and can be intermittent. In addition, CD can often have occult blood-positive stools without gross blood. Because of this, any child with iron deficiency anemia should have stool tested for blood and may require further GI work-up if positive.

Weight Loss

Weight loss is a major problem in CD; over 80% of patients have some degree of weight loss at presentation.[14] The cause is probably multifactorial, but is mostly due to poor nutritional intake. Many children have decreased appetite/intake due to pain or increased stools. Adding to this, they can have decreased nutritional absorption due to small bowel disease. A higher metabolic state due to chronic inflammation may have some contribution as well.

Growth Failure

Growth failure is a critical concern in childhood-onset IBD. It is important for physicians to know that growth impairment can be the only presenting sign of CD, even before GI symptoms manifest (Figure 16–1).[15] In a child with decreased height velocity or lack of growth, IBD should be on the differential diagnosis. About 30% of pediatric CD patients and 6% of UC patients will have growth failure at presentation.[16] It has been shown that the majority of early onset CD patients (onset prior to puberty) have reduced adult height.[17] Growth failure is more pronounced in boys than girls for unknown reasons.[14] The cause of persistent growth

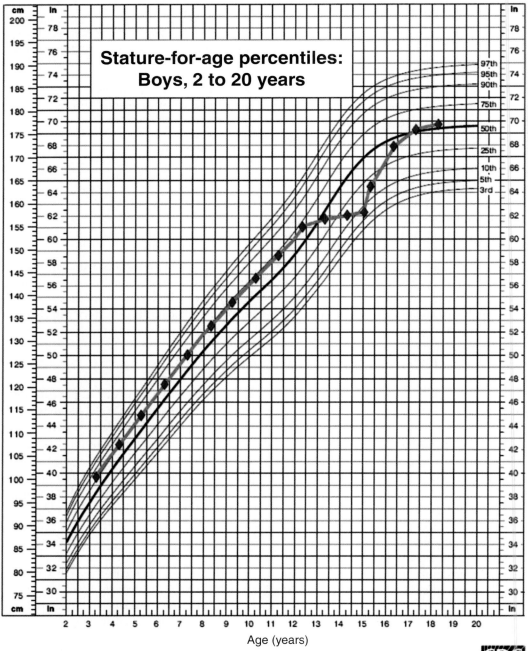

CDC Growth Charts: United States

Stature-for-age percentiles:
Boys, 2 to 20 years

Age (years)

Published May 30, 2000.
SOURCE: Developed by the National Center for Health Statistics in collaboration with
the National Center for Chronic Disease Prevention and Health Promotion (2000).

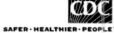

SAFER · HEALTHIER · PEOPLE™

FIGURE 16–1 ■ Growth chart of a patient with Crohn's disease. He had deceleration of height from the age of 12 years that continued for 2.5 years before the diagnosis of Crohn's disease.

failure is multifactorial, including nutritional deficits, malabsorption, increased metabolic demands, medications, and possibly other unknown mechanisms.

Delayed Puberty

Delayed puberty affects twice as many patients with CD compared to UC. Average age of menarche in healthy adolescents is 12.8 years; however, one study found that more than one-half of females with CD had delayed menarche to age 16 years if disease started before puberty. Duration of puberty might also be prolonged in patients due to frequent relapses of disease during puberty.[18] The role of endocrinologic mechanisms in the delay is not known. In evaluating a patient for delayed growth and puberty, bone age radiography can aid in determining if they will have time to catch up in those areas.

Perianal Disease

Perianal or perirectal disease is one of the features distinguishing between UC and CD, since it is not a feature of UC. Perianal disease can vary widely and can include multiple large anal tags (Figure 16–2), perirectal *abscesses*, nonhealing deep *fissures*, and *fistulas* (Figure 16–3). A single noninflamed anal skin tag at the midline position is not considered perianal disease. Most perianal disease is painless unless there is abscess formation. Approximately 80% of fistulas seen in CD are perianal/perirectal. One third of patients will develop a perianal fistula or abscess at some point in their disease course.

Extraintestinal Manifestations (EIM)

IBD is not a single-organ disease, but a systemic disease with many "extra"-intestinal features. Over 130 different EIM have been reported in the literature, with most

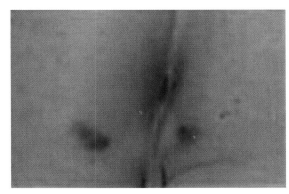

FIGURE 16–3 ■ Two discrete perianal fistula in Crohn's disease.

being very rare. However, between 25% and 30% of patients will exhibit some EIM in their lifetime.[19] These cause varying degrees of morbidity and mortality in IBD patients. The exact etiology of these conditions is unknown, but autoimmune reactions to bacteria, induction of immune complexes and associated inflammatory responses, and genetic factors are all possible explanations. EIM often correlate with GI symptoms, but some will be present even in remission. The most common EIM will be covered here.

Joint disease

Joint manifestations are the most common EIM in IBD. Up to 25% of IBD patients are affected by *arthralgias or arthritis*, and 20–40% patients have more than one episode.[20] These manifestations can precede intestinal symptoms, and some children will be referred to a rheumatologist before being seen by a gastroenterologist. Joint disease in IBD can be separated into two categories, axial and peripheral. *Axial forms* include ankylosing spondylitis and sacroiliitis. Asymptomatic sacroiliitis can be found in 10–52% of patients and is usually revealed by bone scans.[20] *Ankylosing spondylitis* occurs in <2% of patients and is also associated with HLA-B27 positivity.[21] Axial arthropathy does not usually parallel GI disease symptoms, and treatment consists of physical therapy and exercise. *Peripheral joint disease*, on the other hand, is less commonly seen in IBD and is often associated with large bowel disease. As the IBD is treated, the peripheral joint symptoms also decrease in most cases.[20]

Cutaneous manifestations

Skin involvement has been described in 10–15% of patients with IBD.[19] Cutaneous manifestations can be classified into three main groups: granulomatous, reactive, and nutritional. The two most common cutaneous manifestations of IBD are *erythema nodosum* (Figure 16–4) and *pyoderma gangrenosum* (Figure 16–5), which are reactive in nature.

Erythema nodosum is seen in CD more than UC with prevalence between 2% and 12%.[22] It presents as

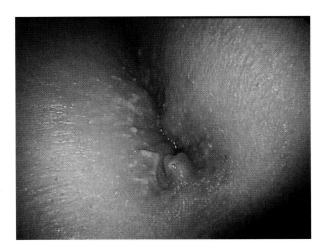

FIGURE 16–2 ■ Perianal disease.

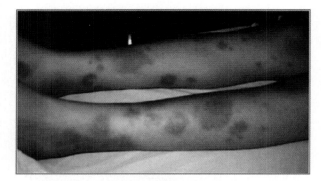

FIGURE 16–4 ■ Erythema nodosum.

a single or multiple tender red nodules typically on the extensor surface of the lower extremities that spreads rapidly to adjacent skin and develops into a burrowing ulcer with irregular violaceous edges. Over days to weeks, the nodules flatten and turn brown or gray. In addition, patients can have systemic symptoms such as fever. It usually *correlates with disease activity*, so treatment should focus on treating the underlying IBD.

Pyoderma gangrenosum is reported in 0.5–5% of patients with IBD but specific prevalence data in children are lacking.[22] Pyoderma gangrenosum may develop before bowel symptoms, during quiescent disease, or even following colectomy. About 40% of IBD patients with pyoderma gangrenosum also develop arthritis.[21] These ulcerated lesions are multiple in the majority of patients, and most appear below the knee.

Other skin manifestations are more rare. *Sweet syndrome*, an acute febrile neutrophilic dermatosis, is a rare manifestation of IBD and presents as tender, erythematous plaques or nodules involving the arms, legs, trunk, hands, or face. It may parallel the intestinal disease or may precede the diagnosis of IBD. Skin biopsies reveal a neutrophilic infiltrate. *Granulomatous skin*

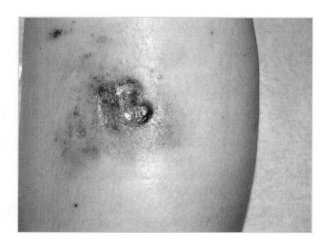

FIGURE 16–5 ■ Pyoderma gangrenosum.

lesions can occur as perianal and peristomal ulcers and fistulas, oral ulcers, and cutaneous granulomatous ulcers, all of which are commonly referred to as *metastatic CD*. The skin lesions have the same histological features as the bowel disease. The most frequent nutritional deficiency presenting with cutaneous manifestations is *acrodermatitis enteropathica*, caused by zinc deficiency. In addition, associations between autoimmune cutaneous diseases and IBD have been reported, including psoriasis.[22]

Ocular

Ocular manifestations occur in approximately 1% of patients with IBD.[21] These are seen more frequently in CD patients with colonic disease. Ocular diseases can mimic conjunctivitis, so it is important that the clinician be aware that these patients are at higher risk for serious eye disease. Acute anterior uveitis is an ophthalmological emergency and requires prompt intervention. Treatment of uveitis with systemic or topical steroids is essential to prevent progression to blindness. Patients with IBD can also develop eye disease, such as cataracts and glaucoma, secondary to corticosteroid use.

Bone Disease

Bone disease is being studied intensively since the recognition that up to 40% of adult IBD patients have osteoporosis. In one study, the relative risk for fractures in adult IBD patients was 1.4 times that of the general population.[23] This is extremely important in the pediatric population, since this is the time of skeletal growth and maturation. Multiple factors could contribute to decreased bone mass density (BMD) in these patients, including medications (corticosteroids), inflammatory responses, decreased physical activity, and nutritional deficiencies. Studies have used the DEXA scan to determine if IBD children do have lower bone mass and increased risk of fractures compared to their peers. It seems that they do have lower bone mass density but this may be in part due to smaller bone size, which may or may not cause an increased risk of fracture.[24] Currently, a DEXA scan is not indicated in all pediatric IBD patients. Until more studies are done, the most beneficial thing for these children is disease control (while trying to spare corticosteroids), nutrition (including vitamin D and calcium), and increased activity level. Bisphosphonates can be considered in certain patients, but should not be used without referral to endocrinology.

Oral Lesions

Oral *aphthous stomatitis* (Figure 16–6) is seen in at least 5–10% of patients with UC and 20–30% with CD.[22]

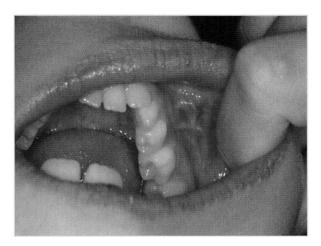

FIGURE 16–6 ■ Oral ulcerations.

Oral lesions may occur before the onset of intestinal symptoms of IBD or may parallel intestinal disease activity. Symptoms range from mild discomfort to severe debilitating pain. Biopsies of these lesions often reveal lymphedema and granulomata in patients with CD. Other oral lesions can include lip swelling, fissures (Figure 16–7), and gingivitis.

Hepatobiliary

The most common serious hepatobiliary complication among pediatric IBD patients is *primary sclerosing cholangitis* (PSC), a disorder of both intrahepatic and extrahepatic bile ducts. It affects patients with UC more than CD and males more than females. It is estimated that 3.5% of UC patients will develop cholangitis.[21] PSC should be suspected in an IBD patient with pruritus, jaundice, fatigue, and anorexia, although they can be

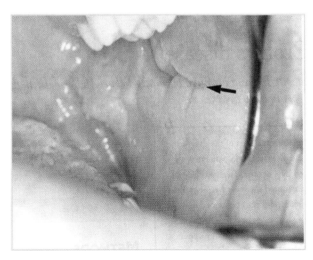

FIGURE 16–7 ■ Fissurea and cobblestoning of the mouth in Crohn's disease (black arrow).

asymptomatic. Laboratories show persistently increased alanine aminotransferase, gamma-glutamyl transpeptidase, and alkaline phosphatase levels. Diagnosis is confirmed with cholangiography and liver biopsy. Treatment with ursodeoxycholic acid improves liver tests but it does not change disease course.[21] IBD patients with PSC are also more likely to have other autoimmune manifestations.

Pancreatitis can also be an EIM, but it is more commonly due to duodenal CD, PSC, or drug reactions.[22] Cholelithiasis is usually a complication secondary to malabsorption of bile acids in small intestinal disease and is reported in approximately 10% of adults with CD.[22]

Thrombosis

Thrombosis has been reported in 1.8% of patients with UC and 3.1% of patients with CD, but is less frequently reported in pediatric patients. Reports in adults suggest that IBD patients have three-fold greater risk compared with subjects without IBD for developing deep venous thrombosis and pulmonary embolism.[25] The mechanism for a hypercoagulable state in IBD is unknown at this time but some of them are found to have high antiphospholipid antibodies. The IBD patients have several risk factors that put them at risk including inflammation, fluid depletion, immobilization, surgery, steroids, central venous lines, thrombocytosis, and an increase in acute-phase reactants during active inflammation. If a child (without the diagnosis of IBD) has a thromboembolism and the hematologic work-up is negative, they should be evaluated for IBD.

Renal

Nephrolithiasis, obstructive uropathy, and fistulous connections between the bowel and the urinary tract directly result from the underlying disease process. The reported incidence of genitourinary complications in pediatric IBD patients is 1–2%.[22] Nephrolithiasis from calcium oxalate stones due to hyperoxaluria is typically associated with either distal ileal CD or ileal resection (see Figure 20–2). Patients with an ileostomy are prone to uric-acid stones due to frequent dehydration.

DIAGNOSIS

Differential Diagnosis

Diagnosis of IBD is based on clinical presentation and subsequent imaging, laboratory, and endoscopic assessment. In a child with bloody diarrhea, bacterial infectious etiologies need to be ruled out first. Also in the differential are vasculitides (Henoch–Schönlein purpura), ischemic bowel, radiation colitis, and hemolytic-uremic syndrome. Causes of watery diarrhea alone can range from irritable bowel syndrome to lactose intolerance, giardiasis, viral enteritis, or laxatives. Rectal bleeding without diarrhea can be due to fissure, polyp, rectal ulcer syndrome, or Meckel diverticulum. Perirectal disease, while very suspicious for CD, can be the result of fissure or streptococcal infection. It should be noted that hemorrhoids are not common in children and therefore are rarely the cause of rectal bleeding or perianal/perirectal disease. Chronic abdominal pain located in the periumbilical or epigastric region is common in children, and is most likely due to irritable bowel syndrome, constipation, lactose intolerance, and occasionally peptic disease. However, localized pain, especially to the right lower quadrant, is a red flag for IBD. Etiologies that can mimic CD pain include appendicitis, although this would have an acute presentation, intussusception, mesenteric adenitis, Meckel diverticulum, ovarian cyst, or lymphoma. In addition, some infections, such as *Yersinia* and gastrointestinal tuberculosis, can cause similar radiographic and endoscopic findings as small bowel CD. Celiac disease can have some of the same clinical symptoms as CD including weight loss, diarrhea, growth retardation, anorexia, and protein-losing enteropathy. Arthritis can be due to rheumatologic or collagen vascular disease or infection. Table 16–2 shows the various systemic presentations of IBD and how many other sub-specialists can be involved in the work-up and management of IBD.

Laboratory

Laboratory studies can be helpful in a child suspected of having IBD if they are abnormal. However, up to 20% of children with IBD can also have normal laboratory values.

Tests should include complete blood count with white blood cell differential, sedimentation rate, total protein/albumin, aminotransferases, alkaline phosphatase, bilirubin, and C-reactive protein. The *four laboratory tests that are most commonly abnormal* and are therefore reasonably good indicators of the presence of IBD include:

- elevated ESR (>20 mm/hour);
- thrombocytosis (>400,000);
- decreased albumin level (2.0–3.5 g/dL);
- anemia (low hemoglobin).

In 2007, the Pediatric Inflammatory Bowel Disease Collaborative Research Group evaluated these laboratory values in newly diagnosed pediatric IBD patients.[26] The data showed that children with more severe IBD rarely have four normal laboratories. For example, in CD only 2% of those with severe disease had four normal laboratories as opposed to mild CD where 21% had four normal laboratories. If any of these laboratories are abnormal, referral to a specialist should be made in a timely manner. If a child has symptoms of mild abdominal pain, nonbloody diarrhea, and normal screening laboratories, then it is most likely functional abdominal pain, although not guaranteed. However, if a patient has hematochezia and normal laboratories, a referral is still warranted. A child with anemia should have a hemoccult of the stool performed to look for GI blood loss.

Serologic markers have recently been introduced as a possible tool to help diagnose IBD and also differentiate between UC and CD. Unfortunately, their use is still limited and should not be ordered by the general practitioner to rule out IBD. These markers are indirect and detect antibodies in the serum that have been found in patients with IBD. Several serologic tests have been developed and commercially available. One of the commonly ordered panels includes the following antibodies: atypical perinuclear anticytoplasmic antibodies

Table 16–2.

Medical Specialty Contributions to IBD Care

Specialists Referred and System Involvement	Reason for Referral/Clinical Presentation
Rheumatologists	Arthritis, back pain (sacroilitis), enthesitis
Dermatologists	Pyoderma gangrenosun, erythema nodosum
Hepatologists	Primary sclerosing cholangitis, cholelithiasis, fatty liver
Hematologists	Anemia (iron deficiency), thrombosis
Opthalmologists	Episcleritis, uveitis
Nephrologists/urologists	Stones, hydronephrosis
Endocrinologists	Growth failure, delayed puberty
Infectious disease	Fever of unknown origin
Orthopedists	Avascular necrosis, spinal fractures, enthesitis
Psychiatrists	Feeding and eating disorder, depression

(pANCA), antibodies to *Saccharomyces cerevisiae* (ASCA), *E. coli* outer membrane porin C antibodies (anti-OmpC), and antibodies to bacterial flagellin (anti-CBir1). Antibodies to a bacterial sequence from *Pseudomonas flourescens* (anti-I2) and anti-glycan antibodies are also being investigated for their possible use as serologic markers.[27] These tests have many limitations, especially in children. Seroconversion may depend on exposure and children may not have fully mature immune systems to produce these antibodies. Also, the tests have higher specificity than sensitivity and should not be used as a general screening tool.[28] Finally, a *positive antibody screen alone is not sufficient to make the diagnosis of IBD* and gastrointestinal work-up, including endoscopy, is still needed.

Radiology

The diagnosis of IBD is dependent on endoscopic, histological, and radiological findings. Radiography is necessary at diagnosis to determine extent, location, and severity of disease. In the past, upper gastrointestinal series (UGI) with small bowel follow-through (UGI-SBFT) was the "gold standard." However, technology has made great strides in the last decade, and other modalities such as magnetic resonance imaging (MRI), computed tomography scans (CT), and ultrasound (US) have been used with success.[29] A 2008 meta-analysis comparing US, MRI, CT, and scintigraphy (white blood cell scan) found that there was no significant difference in the yield among the imaging techniques.[30] In deciding which technique to choose, it is important to consider what information is needed from the study, the experience of the radiologist, and the available technology.

Plain abdominal X-rays can be abnormal in up to 60% patients with IBD. However, the findings are very nonspecific and can include colonic dilatation, small bowel distention, and "thumbprinting." Abdominal plain films have no indication in diagnosis but do become important in the acute abdomen when toxic megacolon or obstruction is suspected. In this case, plain films should be ordered before any contrast study. In toxic megacolon, abdominal X-rays will show marked colonic dilation and can be followed to monitor for possible bowel perforation.

Contrast enemas are rarely used secondary to patient discomfort and the increased availability of colonoscopy, which also has the benefit of providing biopsies. However, contrast enema can be used to evaluate extent of colonic disease if needed.

The *UGI-SBFT* has been considered the "gold standard" imaging technique in IBD and is widely used to determine mucosal irregularities, indicating the presence of small bowel CD. UGI-SBFT can also detect

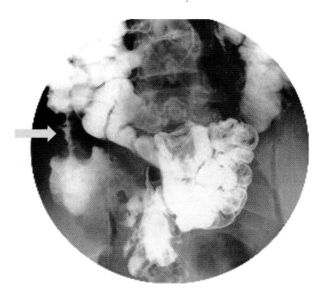

FIGURE 16–8 ■ Upper gastrointestinal series with small bowel follow-through showing apple core stricture of terminal ileum in Crohn's disease (yellow arrow).

strictures (Figure 16–8) and fistulas (Figure 16–9). It becomes even more sensitive if done by enteroclysis, in which contrast is injected directly into the jejunum through a nasojejunal tube. However, this technique requires increased fluoroscopy time and greater expertise, and is uncomfortable for the patient. Its use is usually therefore restricted to special situations in children.

Abdominal/pelvic CT scans have proven to be helpful in the evaluation of strictures in known disease

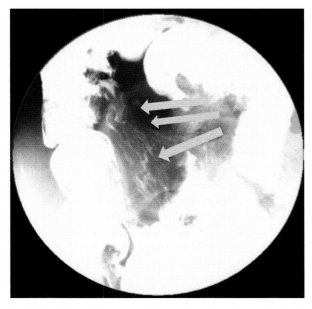

FIGURE 16–9 ■ Upper gastrointestinal series with small bowel follow-through showing intestine to intestine fistulous tract (yellow arrows).

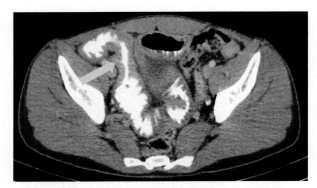

FIGURE 16–10 ■ CT scan showing stricture in Crohn's disease (yellow arrow).

(Figure 16–10), and especially to rule out an abscess or fistula that cannot be seen on UGI. Intravenous and oral contrast and in some instances rectal contrast should be used. The major disadvantage of CT scan is the large radiation exposure.

In recent years, *MRI* has overcome several obstacles that had prevented it from being widely used for imaging IBD in the past. Oral contrast has been optimized for bowel imaging, IV gadolinium has been added to protocols, and ultrafast sequences have increased MRI ability to give good soft tissue and 3D imaging. CT may be superior for large bowel imaging, but MRI can be superior to CT scan in evaluating small bowel disease. MRI is advantageous in patients with equivocal studies and is a crucial tool in distinguishing inflammation from fibrosis in patients with obstructive symptoms. In addition, MRI has become the imaging modality of choice for perianal disease. Most children with IBD receive multiple radiological exams throughout their life, increasing their lifetime radiation exposure, making MRI especially promising in the pediatric population because of the lack of ionizing radiation.[29]

Abdominal US has shown to be sensitive and specific in the detection of CD, especially when Doppler is used. However, this is highly dependent on the experience of the technician and the reading radiologist. It is recommended only in centers that have experience with this technique.[29]

White blood cell scan (scintigraphy) is highly indicative of IBD in the pediatric population. WBC scan can also help distinguish between CD and UC. In UC, the scan would not have uptake in the small bowel and uptake should be continuous, starting in the rectum. Any uptake in the small bowel would indicate CD and could have discontinuous uptake throughout the large and small bowels. It could also aid in deciding if luminal narrowing is due to fibrosis versus inflammation, since WBC scan should only show uptake in active inflammation. Limitations of the WBC scan are its inability to

identify strictures and fistulas and less sensitivity in evaluating proximal small bowel disease. Other drawbacks to scintigraphy include exposure to ionizing radiation (although less than CT), the long duration of the examination, and false negatives in early disease and patients on steroids.[31] *Positron emission tomography* (PET) scan has been shown to be as accurate as WBC scan in detecting an inflamed GI tract in children. However, the data are limited and PET scans are not widely available; therefore, they currently have minimal role in evaluating IBD in children.[31]

Video Capsule Endoscopy

One of the most promising additions in imaging has been *video wireless capsule endoscopy* (WCE). WCE allows small bowel visualization with no radiation. It has been shown to be well tolerated in the pediatric population. In most cases, it requires no sedation. In young children who are unable to swallow the capsule, endoscopy may be necessary to place the device in the small bowel; most older children can simply swallow it with water. The capsule is the size of a large multivitamin (1.1 × 2.6 cm or 1 × 0.5 in.) and contains a video chip, radio transmitter, and battery; video images are transmitted to a portable recording device via an abdominal antenna array. These are later downloaded to a computer and read by a gastroenterologist. Small bowel transit time is approximately 4 hours, and the single-use capsule is passed in the stool within 24–48 hours. The main risk of this procedure is retention of the capsule. Capsule retention requiring intervention has been reported in <1% of subjects. Nevertheless, WCE is contraindicated in patients with known or suspected stricture. WCE does have limitations. It can detect nonspecific lesions (that may or may not be IBD), lesions cannot be biopsied, and it cannot detect extraluminal abnormalities. However, this technology has made evaluation of the small bowel more sensitive.[32]

Endoscopy

The diagnosis of IBD is virtually impossible without endoscopic evaluation. *Endoscopy with biopsy* is the most sensitive and specific evaluation of colon/ileum. During initial work-up, endoscopy aids in diagnosing IBD, differentiating between UC and CD, and assessing extent and severity of disease. Macroscopic findings (Figures 16–11 and 16–12), depending on disease, can include patchy or continuous inflammation, ulcerations, nodularity, and strictures. After diagnosis, endoscopy is used to monitor response to therapy, to perform cancer surveillance, and to provide therapies such as stricture dilatation. Endoscopic work-up of IBD differs in adults and children. For example, pediatric gastroenterologists

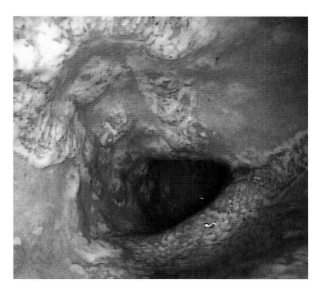

FIGURE 16–11 ■ Linear ulcerations in Crohn's disease.

are more likely to consider an exam without ileal intubation to be incomplete, and generally perform random biopsies from every examined part of the GI tract even in the absence of macroscopic disease. In addition, after several studies showed that performing an esophagogastroduodenoscopy (EGD or upper endoscopy) during the work-up for pediatric IBD resulted in higher rates of confirming a diagnosis, it is now considered standard practice to perform upper endoscopy as part of the diagnostic regimen.[33]

Anesthesia is one of the major concerns for parents when their child undergoes endoscopy. Anesthesia choices include: anxiolysis, moderate sedation, deep sedation, and general anesthesia. Pediatric practice has shifted from sedation toward general anesthesia for

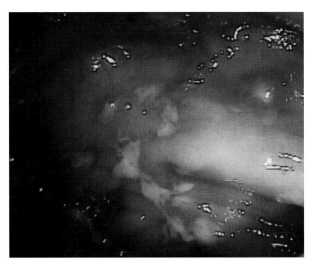

FIGURE 16–12 ■ Exudative ulcers in Crohn's disease.

most endoscopic procedures. In the past there was concern of increased risk of perforation with general anesthesia because patient discomfort is not recognized, but evidence for this concern is lacking. General anesthesia provides some advantages: a certified PALS provider is in charge of airway, the endoscopist can focus on the procedure, and the patient is cooperative and comfortable, all leading to a better overall examination.[33]

Histology

Biopsies taken during endoscopy aid in the diagnosis of IBD and the differentiation between UC and CD. Biopsies are usually taken from all areas examined, even in the absence of obvious lesions, because histological abnormalities can be present in biopsies of "normal" appearing tissue.

Certain histological findings are helpful in confirming an IBD diagnosis and distinguishing between UC and CD. *Noncaseating granulomas* are virtually pathognomonic for CD; however, 60% of biopsies will not show granulomas and the diagnosis must be made from other radiological, histological, or endoscopic findings.[34]

TREATMENT AND MANAGEMENT

Induction of remission and maintenance of remission are the main goals of treatment in IBD. However, since this is a chronic multisystem disease, other areas also have to be addressed. Optimal treatment consists of a multidisciplinary approach including medications, nutrition, psychological assessment, enrollment of primary care providers, and, if necessary, other specialists to help with complications and EIM. Physicians and others involved in the care of these patients should not consider disease *remission* as the only end point. *Long-term goals* should include *preventing relapses* (which include encouraging compliance), *optimizing growth and development*, improving *quality of life*, and *limiting complications*.

Medications

Medical therapy has evolved significantly over the last 15 years. Before 2000, the main therapy consisted of *corticosteroids* and *aminosalicylates*, with few other options. Today, there are many options in treating IBD. Use of medications that "spare corticosteroids" minimizes the many complications that were previously common with chronic use of glucocorticoids. Classes of drugs in current use include *aminosalicylates*, *immuno-modulators*, and *biologics*. As knowledge of the genetics of IBD and the pathways involved in the development of

Table 16–3.

Commonly Used Pharmacologic Therapies for Ulcerative Colitis

Treatment	Dose	Indication	Comments
Induction of remission			
Prednisone	1 mg/kg/day (40 mg maximum), and then taper	Moderate to severe disease	Rapid onset of action; many long-term side effects
Aminosalicylates		Mild to moderate disease	Minimally effective; generally well tolerated; requires multiple pills daily
Sulfasalazine	30–60 mg/kg/day		
Mesalamine	50–100 mg/kg/day		
Balsalazide, infliximab	5 mg/kg at 0, 2, and 6 weeks	Refractory disease, steroid dependency, fistulizing disease	Infusion reactions may occur; requires no daily medications; expensive
Maintenance of remission			
6-Mercaptopurine, azathioprine	1–1.5 mg/kg/day; 2–3 mg/kg/day	Moderate to severe disease	
Aminosalicylates		Mild to moderate disease	Minimally effective; generally well tolerated; requires multiple pills daily
Sulfasalazine	30–60 mg/kg/day		
Mesalamine	50–100 mg/kg/day		
Balsalazide, infliximab	5 mg/kg every 6–8 weeks	Refractory disease, steroid dependency, fistulizing disease	Infusion reactions may occur; requires no daily medications; expensive

IBD increases, it is anticipated that drugs that can specifically target those pathways will be developed, resulting in improved outcomes. Many treatment medications overlap between UC and CD but there are some clear indications that differ (Tables 16–3 and 16–4).

Steroids

Corticosteroids are still used for *induction of remission* in moderate to severe CD and UC. They induce rapid improvement of inflammation. No evidence suggests that they provide mucosal healing, and steroids should not be used as maintenance therapy. They are typically used in conjunction with a maintenance therapy to induce remission; the slower acting maintenance drug takes effect as the steroids are slowly weaned. IV *methylprednisolone* can be used in severe UC and CD to induce remission. Oral *prednisone* dosing is 1 mg/kg/day with a maximum of 40 mg/kg/day, since doses greater than this have not shown increased efficacy.[35] *Budesonide* is an oral steroid preparation that is released in the distal ileum and proximal colon. Because it undergoes rapid "first pass" metabolism in the liver, it has fewer systemic side effects than prednisone, but is not completely without them, and quick withdrawal can lead to adrenal insufficiency. Budesonide can be considered in patients with limited disease of the distal ileum and proximal colon. Rectal *steroid enemas* are available and can be used for proctitis and sigmoid disease without the systemic side effects.

Steroids have multiple side effects. Reversible short-term side effects include moon facies, acne, weight gain, hirsuitism, mood swings, and psychoses. Long-term side effects are the result of cumulative doses. They include growth retardation, osteopenia, permanent skin striae, and cataracts. For these reasons, in addition to the lack of efficacy in maintenance and healing of IBD and introduction of newer medications, they should be used only as short-term treatment, ideally <3 months.

Aminosalicylates

Aminosalicylates include a group of medications containing mesalamine (5-aminosalicylic acid, 5-ASA) as the active agent. Because of rapid absorption of naked 5-ASA by the proximal gut, the drug is delivered to the downstream bowel either linked to a carrier molecule or packaged in a matrix for controlled release. These agents have proven efficacy in induction and maintenance of remission in mild to moderate UC and are the first line of therapy in this disorder.[36,37] They also have some benefit in maintenance of remission in mild CD.[38] The delivery systems used for 5-ASA target specific parts of the bowel, so when choosing which aminosalicylate to use, knowing the disease distribution for that patient and the particular characteristics of each available drug is extremely

Table 16–4.

Commonly Used Pharmacologic Therapies for Crohn's Disease

Treatment	Dose	Indication	Comments
Induction of remission			
Prednisone	1 mg/kg/day (40 mg maximum), and then taper	Moderate to severe disease	Rapid onset of action; many long-term side effects
Budesonide	9 mg/day, and then taper	Ileocecal CD	Used for localized disease and prednisone intolerance
Infliximab	5 mg/kg at 0, 2, and 6 weeks	Refractory disease, steroid dependency, fistulizing disease	Infusion reactions may occur; requires no daily medications; expensive
Maintenance of remission			
6-Mercaptopurine, azathioprine	1–1.5 mg/kg/day; 2–3 mg/kg/day	Moderate to severe disease	Slow onset of action; well tolerated; adverse effects of myelosuppression; pancreatitis; and hepatitis
Methotrexate	15–25 mg/m^2 IM or oral every week	Moderate to severe disease	
Aminosalicylates		Mild to moderate disease	Minimally effective; generally well tolerated; requires multiple pills daily
Mesalamine Balsazide	50–100 mg/kg/day		
Infliximab	5 mg/kg every 6–8 weeks	Refractory disease, steroid dependency, fistulizing disease	Infusion reactions may occur; requires no daily medications; expensive

important. In general, these medications are well tolerated. The main side effects include headache and rash; rare but more serious side effects include hepatitis, pancreatitis, colitis, and decreased sperm count in males. Reactions to the carrier molecule can occur with some aminosalicylate drugs; allergy to the sulfapyradine component of *sulfasalazine* is the most frequent example.

6-Mercaptopurine and Azathioprine

Azathioprine and its metabolite, *6-mercaptopurine* (6-MP), are in the class of thiopurine immunomodulators. They have been used for steroid-refractory CD for decades and are also used in maintenance of remission in moderate to severe UC and CD.[39–41] These drugs are not used in the induction of remission because they have a very slow onset of action and may take 3–6 months to reach maximal effect. However, they are often started in conjunction with steroids in moderate to severe disease and, when used in this way, can decrease the duration of steroid use. These drugs have both idiosyncratic and dose-dependent side effects. Idiosyncratic side effects include pancreatitis, fevers, and myalgias. Dose-dependent side effects include myelosuppression, infections, and elevated liver enzymes. Patients must be monitored due to these side effects.

Additionally, it was discovered that patients have different genotypes for thiopurine methyl transferase activity (TPMT), the enzyme that metabolizes the drugs. Laboratory tests to determine genotypes or to measure TPMT activity directly are commercially available and can be done before starting therapy to help guide dosing.[42] Slow metabolizers are at higher risk for myelosuppression and require reduced doses of the medication. Although rare, there are patients who have no or very low TPMT activity. Using thiopurines for them is dangerous and is clearly contraindicated. 6-Thioguanine nucleotide levels can be monitored to optimize the dose or check compliance.

Methotrexate

Methotrexate is an immunomodulator that has been proven efficacious in inducing and maintaining remission in adult CD patients.[43] To date there have been no controlled trials of its use in pediatric CD, but reports from retrospective reviews and uncontrolled trials have shown good remission rates in patients that fail 6-MP or are intolerant to thiopurines.[44,45] Methotrexate is a teratogen and a powerful abortifacient, so pregnancy counseling should be given to all females of child-bearing age who are started on this treatment.

Biologic Therapies

Biologic therapies have dramatically changed the treatment and management of IBD over the last few years. One class of these drugs is the anti-tumor necrosis factor alpha (TNF-α) agents. TNF-α is a cytokine involved in systemic inflammation and can stimulate the acute-phase reaction. *Infliximab* blocks the action of TNF-α by preventing it from binding to its receptor in the cell. Infliximab, the first in this class to be approved in pediatric IBD, is a chimeric monoclonal IgG1antibody (part mouse and part human) that is given intravenously. This biologic agent is approved for adult patients with moderate to severe UC and CD[46,47] and pediatric patients with moderate to severe CD.[48] Infliximab is also effective in fistulizing and perianal CD.[49]

The most common side effects of infliximab include infusion reactions, infections, and abnormal ALT elevations. Infusion reactions are usually mild and respond to slower infusion rates and antihistamine therapy. This is not necessarily a contraindication for further infusions, but patients do need to be premedicated with diphenhydramine. The most commonly reported infections are upper respiratory tract infection and pharyngitis. Serious infections have not been seen more frequently. Infliximab can reactivate latent *Mycobacterium tuberculosis* and all patients should have a documented negative PPD before starting treatment.

Although an overall slightly increased risk of lymphoma has been reported in patients with IBD who have been exposed to biologic or immunomodulator therapy, a rare fatal form of lymphoma, "hepatosplenic T-cell lymphoma," has occurred in children and young adults with IBD exposed to immunomodulators while taking biologics. Infliximab has a black box warning regarding this rare lymphoma. At the time of this writing, approximately 18 cases of HTLC have been reported, all in individuals taking both 6-MP/AZA and infliximab. These cases reveal preponderance for young male patients, although the mechanism of this observation is unknown. For this reason, most pediatric patients do not receive concomitant therapy with these two classes of medications (there are some exceptions in severe disease).

Other anti-TNF agents have been approved for treatment of IBD in adults and are undergoing trials in pediatrics.[50,51] *Adalimumab* is a recombinant human IgG1 monoclonal antibody. Unlike infliximab, which has a significant murine-derived portion, adalimumab is primarily human and therefore is seldom the target of antibody formation. An additional advantage of adalimumab is that it is given as a subcutaneous injection instead of an intravenous infusion such as infliximab.[52] Most recently, a polyethylene glycol-linked, humanized anti-TNF-α antibody fragment, *certolizumab pegol*, has been introduced for treatment of adult IBD.[53,54] It is different from the other two anti-TNF drugs in that it does not induce apoptosis of T cells or monocytes, and does not fix complement. Whether this has clinical significance is still under investigation. It is also given as a subcutaneous injection and is not approved in pediatrics to date.

Other Biologics

Natalizumab, a humanized antibody directed against α4 integrin, is the first drug developed in the class of selective adhesion molecule inhibitors. α4 integrin is required for white blood cells to move into organs from blood vessels. Natalizumab's mechanism of action is believed to involve the inhibition of neutrophils from crossing blood vessel walls to reach the gastrointestinal tract. It is FDA-approved for both induction of remission and maintenance of remission for moderate to severe CD.[55,56] The drug was originally approved for treatment of multiple sclerosis, but was temporarily pulled from the market after progressive multifocal leukoencephalopathy (PML), an opportunistic infection caused by the Jacob–Creutzfeldt virus, developed in seven patients. It has been brought back, but has a black box warning stating that the drug has only been linked to PML when combined with other immune-modulating drugs. Therefore, natalizumab is contraindicated for use with other immunomodulators. In addition, prescribing information from the package insert recommends that people taking corticosteroids for the treatment of CD have their doses reduced before starting natalizumab treatment to reduce immunosuppressive effects. The risk of developing PML was later estimated to be 1 in 1000 (0.1%) over 18 months, though the longer term risks of PML are unknown. Due to the uncertain risk of PML, natalizumab is only available through a restricted distribution program and patients must enter into a registry for monitoring.

Other classes of biologics are under investigation. This is an exciting area of research and discovery but still leaves many questions unanswered. This is especially important for the pediatric population as long-term side effects and complications of new drugs are unknown. The FDA now requires post-marketing studies to be incorporated into drug trials.

Other Treatment Modalities

Antibiotics are used widely in the treatment of IBD, with *metronidazole* and *ciprofloxacin* being at the top of the list. However, their efficacy in treating intestinal inflammation has not been proven.[57] In the cases of perianal abscess or fistulae, they may have some benefit.[58]

Cyclosporine is indicated only in severe refractory UC as a rescue therapy. It has not been shown efficacious in CD.[59,60] Due to the serious side effects including renal and hepatoxicity and increased risk of opportunistic infections, the risks and benefits must be weighed and other options exhausted.

Thalidomide is given in severe refractory CD but no standardized controlled trials have been done to accurately measure its efficacy or outweigh the risks and benefits.[61] Given the well-known risk of severe birth defects and other side effects, the use of thalidomide is only given in severe cases of refractory disease.

Tacrolimus is used in patients with treatment-resistant UC and can help in reducing symptoms. However, no benefit for induction of remission has been proven.[62] Tacrolimus is a potent immunosuppressant; therefore, risks and benefits need to be weighed before a patient is started on this medication. Other side effects can include finger tremor, sleepiness, hot flush, headache, stomach discomfort, hypomagnesaemia, kidney and liver problems, seizures, hypertension, diabetes mellitus, hyperkalemia, itching, insomnia, confusion, loss of appetite, hyperglycemia, weakness, depression, cramps, neuropathy, and infections.

Probiotics have not been shown to add any benefit to conventional therapy in maintaining remission of UC or CD. However, many patients and parents may add this to conventional therapy and at this time there are not contraindications to this.[63,64]

Nutrition

Nutritional therapy consists of using formula (both elemental and nonelemental) as primary therapy to induce and maintain remission in CD, as a supplement to improve growth, or to replenish micronutrient deficiency. Primary therapy means that the majority of the patient's caloric needs are being given as formula, and that they are typically not taking other medications (steroid sparing). In most cases, the enteral nutrition is administered through nasogastric tube; however, with the advent of better tasting formulas, some patients can do this orally. The evidence to support the use of enteral nutrition as primary therapy is controversial and this therapy is not widely practiced in the United States. It is more widely used in Europe and Canada, with remission rates in CD reported at 50–80%.[65] Studies in pediatric patients have had varying results. *Supplemental* nutritional therapy, on the other hand, is commonly used for patients who cannot maintain weight on "normal" caloric intake and cannot consume the needed 100–150% of recommended daily allowances through a regular diet. Other nutritional modifications, such as low residue diets and lactose-free or other elimination diets, have not been sufficiently studied. To date, there is no evidence to suggest they should be recommended in the general IBD population.[66] However, a low-fiber diet is recommended in patients who have active colitis or narrowing/stricture of the small bowel.

Surgical Management

Medical management remains the first-line treatment in IBD. Indications for surgery are relatively similar between UC and CD; however, the approach and the outcomes differ. Indications for surgery include fulminant colitis, massive hemorrhage, perforation, stricture, abscess, fistula (in CD), toxic megacolon, failure of medical therapy, steroid dependency, and dysplasia. Pediatric patients also have other indications including growth failure and pubertal delay. It has been shown that children will have catch-up growth after surgery.[67,68]

When deciding to perform surgery for UC, the diagnosis should be confirmed to the highest degree possible because the approach, follow-up, and outcomes vary between UC and CD. In UC, total colectomy and ileoanal pull-through anal anastomosis (IPAA) is the current standard surgical procedure for UC.[68] This removes the colon and rectal mucosa. The distal ileum of folded over and stapled to create J-shaped reservoir or "pouch," pulled through the muscular rectal stump, and anastomosed to the anus. This technique avoids permanent ileostomy and preserves anorectal function. The surgery is done in one to three stages, with months in between (with a temporary ileostomy) depending on the patient, the disease, and the surgeon. Laparoscopic surgery is also becoming an option for some patients. Complications include pouchitis (inflammation of the J-pouch), small bowel obstruction, anastomotic leak, fecal incontinence, strictures, fistula, and dysplasia of anal transition zone.[69]

Many patients with CD will require surgery during their life, although the number is decreasing due to improved medical therapy. The aim of surgery differs from that in UC. In CD, the goal is to resect as little bowel as possible since CD will recur in majority of patients within 5 years of surgery. This is also the reason CD is a relative contraindication to IPAA. Postoperative recurrence prevention is an area of debate and varies between physicians and patients and families.[67]

PROGNOSIS AND OUTCOMES

IBD is a relapsing disease that has high morbidity but low mortality. Most children with IBD lead active normal lives, with no limitations except during flares. However, patients with IBD are at increased risk for some malignancies. In UC, the greatest risk is colonic dysplasia/cancer. The risk has been estimated to be up to 25% after 30 years of disease.[70] Risk factors for development of colorectal cancer in UC patients are long duration of disease, early onset, chronic inflammation, family history of colorectal cancer, and PSC. Patients with colonic CD share the same risk factors as UC patients. CD patients are known to have a slightly increased risk of lymphoma over their lifetime.

CONCLUSIONS

The diagnosis and management of IBD in children has changed dramatically over the last decade, mainly due to increased awareness, availability of newer diagnostic modalities such as MRI and video capsule endoscopy, and newer and powerful treatments such as biologics. Advances in IBD research are occurring at an ever-increasing rate and include many diverse disciplines such as therapeutics, genetics, microbiology, and immunology. There is great hope that combined innovative research and advances in drug discoveries will continue to improve the natural history of IBD and will improve the lives of those who suffer from this disorder.

REFERENCES

1. Kugathasan S, Amre D. Inflammatory bowel disease—environmental modification and genetic determinants. *Pediatr Clin North Am.* 2006;53:727–749.
2. Kugathasan S, Judd RH, Hoffmann RG, et al. Epidemiologic and clinical characteristics of children with newly diagnosed inflammatory bowel disease in Wisconsin: a statewide population-based study. *J Pediatr.* 2003;143:525–531.
3. Van Limbergen J, Russell RK, Drummond HE, et al. Definition of phenotypic characteristics of childhood-onset inflammatory bowel disease. *Gastroenterology.* 2008;135:1114–1122.
4. Loftus EV Jr. Clinical epidemiology of inflammatory bowel disease: incidence, prevalence, and environmental influences. *Gastroenterology.* 2004;126:1504–1517.
5. Bach JF. The effect of infections on susceptibility to autoimmune and allergic diseases. *N Engl J Med.* 2002;347:911–920.
6. Hugot JP, Chamaillard M, Zouali H, et al. Association of NOD2 leucine-rich repeat variants with susceptibility to Crohn's disease. *Nature.* 2001;411:599–603.
7. Ogura Y, Bonen DK, Inohara N, et al. A frameshift mutation in NOD2 associated with susceptibility to Crohn's disease. *Nature.* 2001;411:603–606.
8. The Wellcome Trust Case Control Consortium. Genome-wide association study of 14,000 cases of seven common diseases and 3,000 shared controls. *Nature.* 2007;447:661–678.
9. Abreu MT, Taylor KD, Lin YC, et al. Mutations in NOD2 are associated with fibrostenosing disease in patients with Crohn's disease. *Gastroenterology.* 2002;123:679–688.
10. Faubion A. Gut immunity and inflammatory bowel disease. In: Mamula P, ed. *Pediatric Inflammatory Bowel Disease.* New York City: Springer; 2008:15–29.
11. Bousvaros A, Antonioli DA, Colletti RB, et al. Differentiating ulcerative colitis from Crohn disease in children and young adults: report of a working group of the North American Society for Pediatric Gastroenterology, Hepatology, and Nutrition and the Crohn's and Colitis Foundation of America. *J Pediatr Gastroenterol Nutr.* 2007;44:653–674.
12. Fish D, Kugathasan S. Inflammatory bowel disease. *Adolesc Med Clin.* 2004;15:67–90, ix.
13. Baldassano RN, Piccoli DA. Inflammatory bowel disease in pediatric and adolescent patients. *Gastroenterol Clin North Am.* 1999;28:445–458.
14. Griffiths AM, Nguyen P, Smith C, MacMillan JH, Sherman PM. Growth and clinical course of children with Crohn's disease. *Gut.* 1993;34:939–943.
15. Kanof ME, Lake AM, Bayless TM. Decreased height velocity in children and adolescents before the diagnosis of Crohn's disease. *Gastroenterology.* 1988;95:1523–1527.
16. Sawczenko A, Sandhu BK. Presenting features of inflammatory bowel disease in Great Britain and Ireland. *Arch Dis Child.* 2003;88:995–1000.
17. Sawczenko A, Ballinger AB, Croft NM, Sanderson IR, Savage MO. Adult height in patients with early onset of Crohn's disease. *Gut.* 2003;52:454–455 [author reply 5].
18. Ballinger AB, Savage MO, Sanderson IR. Delayed puberty associated with inflammatory bowel disease. *Pediatr Res.* 2003;53:205–210.
19. Greenstein AJ, Janowitz HD, Sachar DB. The extra-intestinal complications of Crohn's disease and ulcerative colitis: a study of 700 patients. *Medicine (Baltimore).* 1976;55:401–412.
20. Danese S, Semeraro S, Papa A, et al. Extraintestinal manifestations in inflammatory bowel disease. *World J Gastroenterol.* 2005;11:7227–7236.
21. Hyams JS. Extraintestinal manifestations of inflammatory bowel disease in children. *J Pediatr Gastroenterol Nutr.* 1994;19:7–21.
22. Jose FA, Heyman MB. Extraintestinal manifestations of inflammatory bowel disease. *J Pediatr Gastroenterol Nutr.* 2008;46:124–133.
23. Bernstein CN. Osteoporosis and other complications of inflammatory bowel disease. *Curr Opin Gastroenterol.* 2002;18:428–434.
24. Sylvester FA. Pediatric inflammatory bowel disease. In: Mamula P, ed. *Pediatric Inflammatory Bowel Disease.* New York City: Springer; 2008:119–132.
25. Srirajaskanthan R, Winter M, Muller AF. Venous thrombosis in inflammatory bowel disease. *Eur J Gastroenterol Hepatol.* 2005;17:697–700.
26. Mack DR, Langton C, Markowitz J, et al. Laboratory values for children with newly diagnosed inflammatory bowel disease. *Pediatrics.* 2007;119:1113–1119.
27. Bossuyt X. Serologic markers in inflammatory bowel disease. *Clin Chem.* 2006;52:171–181.
28. Austin GL, Shaheen NJ, Sandler RS. Positive and negative predictive values: use of inflammatory bowel disease serologic markers. *Am J Gastroenterol.* 2006;101:413–416.
29. Mackalski BA, Bernstein CN. New diagnostic imaging tools for inflammatory bowel disease. *Gut.* 2006;55:733–741.
30. Horsthuis K, Bipat S, Bennink RJ, Stoker J. Inflammatory bowel disease diagnosed with US, MR, scintigraphy, and CT: meta-analysis of prospective studies. *Radiology.* 2008;247:64–79.
31. Nwomeh B. Radiologic evaluation of inflammatory bowel disease. In: Mamula P, ed. *Pediatric Inflammatory Bowel Disease.* New York City: Springer; 2008:193–210.
32. Girardin M. Video capsule endoscopy in pediatric inflammatory bowel disease. In: Mamula P, ed. *Pediatric Inflammatory Bowel Disease.* New York City: Springer; 2008:263–273.
33. Venkatesh K. Endoscopic modalities in pediatric inflammatory bowel disease. In: Mamula P, ed. *Pediatric Inflammatory Bowel Disease.* New York City: Springer; 2008:211–235.

34. De Matos V, Russo PA, Cohen AB, Mamula P, Baldassano RN, Piccoli DA. Frequency and clinical correlations of granulomas in children with Crohn disease. *J Pediatr Gastroenterol Nutr.* 2008;46:392–398.

35. Benchimol EI, Seow CH, Steinhart AH, Griffiths AM. Traditional corticosteroids for induction of remission in Crohn's disease. *Cochrane Database Syst Rev.* 2008:CD006792.

36. Sutherland L, Macdonald JK. Oral 5-aminosalicylic acid for maintenance of remission in ulcerative colitis. *Cochrane Database Syst Rev.* 2006:CD000544.

37. Sutherland L, Macdonald JK. Oral 5-aminosalicylic acid for induction of remission in ulcerative colitis. *Cochrane Database Syst Rev.* 2006:CD000543.

38. Akobeng AK, Gardener E. Oral 5-aminosalicylic acid for maintenance of medically-induced remission in Crohn's Disease. *Cochrane Database Syst Rev.* 2005:CD003715.

39. Markowitz J, Grancher K, Kohn N, Lesser M, Daum F. A multicenter trial of 6-mercaptopurine and prednisone in children with newly diagnosed Crohn's disease. *Gastroenterology.* 2000;119:895–902.

40. Markowitz J, Rosa J, Grancher K, Aiges H, Daum F. Long-term 6-mercaptopurine treatment in adolescents with Crohn's disease. *Gastroenterology.* 1990;99:1347–1351.

41. Verhave M, Winter HS, Grand RJ. Azathioprine in the treatment of children with inflammatory bowel disease. *J Pediatr.* 1990;117:809–814.

42. Dubinsky MC, Yang H, Hassard PV, et al. 6-MP metabolite profiles provide a biochemical explanation for 6-MP resistance in patients with inflammatory bowel disease. *Gastroenterology.* 2002;122:904–915.

43. Alfadhli AA, McDonald JW, Feagan BG. Methotrexate for induction of remission in refractory Crohn's disease. *Cochrane Database Syst Rev.* 2005:CD003459.

44. Turner D, Grossman AB, Rosh J, et al. Methotrexate following unsuccessful thiopurine therapy in pediatric Crohn's disease. *Am J Gastroenterol.* 2007;102:2804–2812 [quiz 3, 13].

45. Uhlen S, Belbouab R, Narebski K, et al. Efficacy of methotrexate in pediatric Crohn's disease: a French multicenter study. *Inflamm Bowel Dis.* 2006;12:1053–1057.

46. Hanauer SB, Feagan BG, Lichtenstein GR, et al. Maintenance infliximab for Crohn's disease: the ACCENT I randomised trial. *Lancet.* 2002;359:1541–1549.

47. Rutgeerts P, Sandborn WJ, Feagan BG, et al. Infliximab for induction and maintenance therapy for ulcerative colitis. *N Engl J Med.* 2005;353:2462–2476.

48. Hyams J, Crandall W, Kugathasan S, et al. Induction and maintenance infliximab therapy for the treatment of moderate-to-severe Crohn's disease in children. *Gastroenterology.* 2007;132:863–873 [quiz 1165–1166].

49. Sands BE, Anderson FH, Bernstein CN, et al. Infliximab maintenance therapy for fistulizing Crohn's disease. *N Engl J Med.* 2004;350:876–885.

50. Colombel JF, Sandborn WJ, Rutgeerts P, et al. Adalimumab for maintenance of clinical response and remission in patients with Crohn's disease: the CHARM trial. *Gastroenterology.* 2007;132:52–65.

51. Wyneski MJ, Green A, Kay M, Wyllie R, Mahajan L. Safety and efficacy of adalimumab in pediatric patients with Crohn disease. *J Pediatr Gastroenterol Nutr.* 2008;47:19–25.

52. Sandborn WJ, Hanauer SB, Rutgeerts P, et al. Adalimumab for maintenance treatment of Crohn's disease: results of the CLASSIC II trial. *Gut.* 2007;56:1232–1239.

53. Sandborn WJ, Feagan BG, Stoinov S, et al. Certolizumab pegol for the treatment of Crohn's disease. *N Engl J Med.* 2007;357:228–238.

54. Schreiber S, Khaliq-Kareemi M, Lawrance IC, et al. Maintenance therapy with certolizumab pegol for Crohn's disease. *N Engl J Med.* 2007;357:239–250.

55. Sandborn WJ, Colombel JF, Enns R, et al. Natalizumab induction and maintenance therapy for Crohn's disease. *N Engl J Med.* 2005;353:1912–1925.

56. Targan SR, Feagan BG, Fedorak RN, et al. Natalizumab for the treatment of active Crohn's disease: results of the ENCORE Trial. *Gastroenterology.* 2007;132:1672–1683.

57. Jacobstein D. Antibiotic therapy. In: Mamula P, ed. *Pediatric Inflammatory Bowel Disease.* New York City: Springer; 2008:329–336.

58. Brandt LJ, Bernstein LH, Boley SJ, Frank MS. Metronidazole therapy for perineal Crohn's disease: a follow-up study. *Gastroenterology.* 1982;83:383–387.

59. Shibolet O, Regushevskaya E, Brezis M, Soares-Weiser K. Cyclosporine A for induction of remission in severe ulcerative colitis. *Cochrane Database Syst Rev.* 2005:CD004277.

60. McDonald JW, Feagan BG, Jewell D, Brynskov J, Stange EF, Macdonald JK. Cyclosporine for induction of remission in Crohn's disease. *Cochrane Database Syst Rev.* 2005:CD000297.

61. Srinivasan R, Akobeng AK. Thalidomide and thalidomide analogues for induction of remission in Crohn's disease. *Cochrane Database Syst Rev.* 2009:CD007350.

62. Baumgart DC, Macdonald JK, Feagan B. Tacrolimus (FK506) for induction of remission in refractory ulcerative colitis. *Cochrane Database Syst Rev.* 2008:CD007216.

63. Mallon P, McKay D, Kirk S, Gardiner K. Probiotics for induction of remission in ulcerative colitis. *Cochrane Database Syst Rev.* 2007:CD005573.

64. Rolfe VE, Fortun PJ, Hawkey CJ, Bath-Hextall F. Probiotics for maintenance of remission in Crohn's disease. *Cochrane Database Syst Rev.* 2006:CD004826.

65. Akobeng AK, Thomas AG. Enteral nutrition for maintenance of remission in Crohn's disease. *Cochrane Database Syst Rev.* 2007:CD005984.

66. Kleinman RE, Baldassano RN, Caplan A, et al. Nutrition support for pediatric patients with inflammatory bowel disease: a clinical report of the North American Society for Pediatric Gastroenterology, Hepatology and Nutrition. *J Pediatr Gastroenterol Nutr.* 2004;39:15–27.

67. von Allmen D. Surgical management of Crohn's disease. In: Mamula P, ed. *Pediatric Inflammatory Bowel Disease.* New York City: Springer; 2008:455–468.

68. Mattei P. Surgical treatment of ulcerative colitis. In: Mamula P, ed. *Pediatric Inflammatory Bowel Disease.* New York City: Springer; 2008:469–483.

69. Shen B, Fazio VW, Remzi FH, Lashner BA. Clinical approach to diseases of ileal pouch-anal anastomosis. *Am J Gastroenterol.* 2005;100:2796–2807.

70. Eaden JA, Mayberry JF. Colorectal cancer complicating ulcerative colitis: a review. *Am J Gastroenterol.* 2000 Oct;95(10):2710–2719.

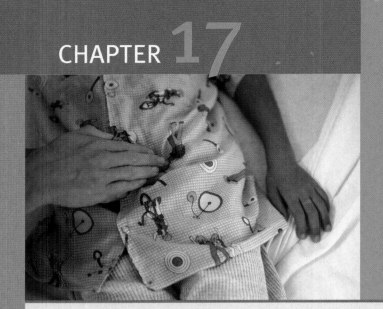

CHAPTER 17

Food Allergy and Intolerance

*Jonathan E. Markowitz
and Chris A. Liacouras*

DEFINITIONS AND EPIDEMIOLOGY

Food allergy is a common problem in the pediatric age group, one that has numerous manifestations and touches on many organ systems. As such, food allergy is often first seen and managed by the generalist such as the pediatrician or family practitioner. However, various aspects of food allergy may also necessitate the involvement of a subspecialist. For the purposes of this chapter, we will focus on the aspects of food allergy and intolerance that involve the gastrointestinal tract and may require the assistance of a gastroenterologist.

Immune-mediated food reactions are typical (IgE-mediated or type 1) food allergy as well as several types of food reactions that involve either mixed (IgE and non-IgE) or delayed (non-IgE) hypersensitivity. GI manifestations of type 1 food allergy include the oral allergy syndrome (OAS) and immediate hypersensitivity reactions. From this point forward, the term food allergy will refer to *immune-mediated* food reactions, with a particular emphasis on the gastrointestinal manifestations of each of these reactions.

Type I (IgE-mediated) immediate hypersensitivity reactions to foods are most common in young children, with 50% of these reactions occurring in the first year of life. The majority are reactions to cow's milk or to soy protein from infant formulas.[1] Other food allergies begin to predominate in older children, including egg, fish, peanut, and wheat. Together with milk and soy, these account for more than 90% of food allergy in children.[2]

There are several gastrointestinal illnesses that manifest as a result of mixed and non-IgE allergies. Some, such as gastroesophageal reflux (GER), infantile colic, constipation, and diarrhea, are multifactorial illnesses, in which food allergy may play a prominent role in a proportion of patients with refractory symptoms. Others, such as infantile allergic proctocolitis (AP), eosinophilic esophagitis (EoE), and in some cases eosinophilic gastroenteritis (EoG), are disorders where food allergy has been demonstrated as the main (if not only) causative factor.

PATHOGENESIS

The gastrointestinal tract plays a major role in the development of oral tolerance to foods. Through the process of endocytosis by the enterocyte, food antigens are generally degraded into non-antigenic proteins.[3,4] Although the gastrointestinal tract serves as an efficient barrier to ingested food antigens, this barrier may not be mature for the first few months of life.[5] As a result, ingested antigens may have an increased propensity for being presented intact to the immune system. These intact antigens have the potential for stimulating the immune system, and driving an inappropriate response directed at the gastrointestinal tract.

With IgE-mediated food allergy, the rapid onset of GI symptoms after food ingestion correlates highly with positive IgE–RAST or skin prick tests to the offending antigen, demonstrating that these reactions are related to typical type 1 hypersensitivity. On the other hand, in patients with OAS, symptoms relate to cross-reaction between similar epitopes on certain pollens and certain fruits and vegatables.[6]

EoE and gastroenteritis are thought to arise from the interaction of genetic and environmental factors. Of note, approximately 10% of individuals with one of these disorders have a family history in an immediate family member.[7] In addition, there is evidence for the role of allergy in the etiology of these conditions, including the observations that up to 75% of patients are atopic[8,9] and that an allergen-free diet can sometimes reverse disease activity.[8–10] Interestingly, only a minority of individuals with eosinophilic gastroenteropathies have food-induced anaphylaxis,[11] as evidence that these are not pure IgE-mediated food allergies.

CLINICAL PRESENTATION

IgE-mediated Food Allergies

Oral allergy syndrome

Oral allergy syndrome may begin in childhood or may be adult onset. It is manifested by a combination of oral itching, burning, swelling, and erythema, but rarely results in systemic symptoms.[6] Table 17–1 outlines the common foods and pollens that cause OAS.

Gastrointestinal hypersensitivity reaction

Immediate GI hypersensitivity usually occurs in the setting of a systemic allergic reaction such as anaphylaxis and typically involves a combination of nausea, abdominal pain, vomiting, and diarrhea. Onset may be anywhere from seconds to several hours after food ingestion. Resolution of gastrointestinal symptoms may also be rapid, and occasionally forceful vomiting induces complete resolution of symptoms after the stomach has been completely emptied of the inciting antigen.[12]

Mixed and Non-IgE-mediated Food Allergies

Infantile allergic proctocolitis (allergic colitis)

AP, also known as allergic colitis or milk–protein proctocolitis, has been recognized as one of the most

Table 17–1.

Foods that are Associated with the Oral Allergy Syndrome (OAS)

Pollen	Potential Cross-reactive Foods
Ragweed	Bananas, melons (watermelon, cantaloupe, honeydew) zucchini, cucumber, dandelions, chamomile tea
Birch	Apples, pears, peaches, apricots, cherries, plums, nectarines, prunes, kiwi, carrots, celery, potatoes, peppers, fennel, parsley, coriander, parsnips, hazelnuts, almonds, walnuts
Grass	Peaches, celery, melons, tomatoes, oranges
Mugwort	Celery, apple, kiwi, peanut, fennel, carrots, parsley, coriander, sunflower, peppers
Alder	Celery, pears, apples, almonds, cherries, hazelnuts, peaches, parsley
Latex	Bananas, avocado, kiwi, chestnut, papaya

common etiologies of rectal bleeding in infants.[13,14] This disorder is characterized by the onset of rectal bleeding, generally in children less than 2 months of age.

Diarrhea, rectal bleeding, and increased mucus production are the typical symptoms seen in patients who present with AP.[14,15] The typical infant with AP is well appearing with no constitutional symptoms. Rectal bleeding begins gradually, initially appearing as small flecks of blood. Usually, increased stool frequency occurs, accompanied by water loss or mucus streaks. The development of irritability or straining with stools is also common and can falsely lead to the initial diagnosis of anal fissuring. Atopic symptoms, such as eczema and reactive airway disease, may be associated. Continued exposure to the inciting antigen causes increased bleeding and may, on rare occasions, cause anemia and poor weight gain. Despite the progression of symptoms, the infants generally appear to be well. Other manifestations of gastrointestinal tract inflammation, such as vomiting, abdominal distention, or weight loss, almost never occur.

Eosinophilic esophagitis

EoE, also known as allergic esophagitis, has come to the forefront in individuals previously suspected as having severe, chronic gastroesophageal reflux disease (GERD). EoE is a disease of children and adults characterized by an isolated, severe eosinophilic infiltration of the esophagus manifested by GER-like symptoms, such as regurgitation, epigastric and chest pain, vomiting, heartburn, feeding difficulties, and dysphagia.[16] Classically, the presentation is that of GER, refractory to treatment with acid suppression therapy. Younger children tend to present with more non-specific symptoms such as abdominal pain and feeding refusal, while older children and adults often present with dysphagia and esophageal food impactions. Uncommon symptoms include growth failure, hematemesis, globus, and water brash (Table 17–2).

The clinical features of EoE may evolve over years. Symptoms such as abdominal pain and heartburn occur regularly; however, patients with vomiting or dysphagia may display these symptoms sporadically, complaining only once or twice a month. Although the use of acid-suppressing medication often improves the patient's symptoms, it does not eliminate the symptoms or change the abnormal esophageal histology. Approximately 50% of affected children also exhibit other allergic signs and symptoms, including bronchospasm, allergic rhinitis, and eczema. Frequently, there is a strong family history of food allergies or other allergic disorders.

Eosinophilic gastroenteritis

EoG is a general term that describes a constellation of symptoms attributable to the gastrointestinal tract, in combination with pathologic infiltration by eosinophils. This group includes eosinophilic gastritis, gastroenteritis, and enteritis. There are no strict diagnostic criteria

Table 17–2.

Comparison between Eosinophilic Esophagitis and Gastroesophageal Reflux

	Eosinophilic Esophagitis	Gastroesophageal Reflux
Symptoms	Nausea, vomiting, epigastric pain, dysphagia	Nausea, vomiting, epigastric pain, dysphagia
Endoscopic findings	Esophageal furrows, rings, white specks	Esophageal ulceration, erythema
Histologic findings	Usually 20 or more eosinophils/HPF	Usually 5 or less eosinophils/HPF
Esophageal strictures	Mid-esophagus if present	Distal esophagus if present
pH studies	Essentially normal, with some increased frequency of reflux episodes	Abnormal
Peripheral eosinophils	Usually increased	Usually normal
Serum IgE	Usually increased	Usually normal
Atopic history	Increased rates of atopic disease	Baseline rates of atopic disease
Family history	Increased family history of atopic disease	Baseline family rates of atopic disease
Response to acid blockade	Partially responsive symptoms; histologic findings unresponsive	Symptoms and histologic findings respond
Response to fundoplication	Symptoms and histologic findings persist	Symptoms and histologic findings respond
Response to corticosteroids	Symptoms and histologic findings respond	Symptoms and histologic findings persist
Response to elimination diet	Symptoms and histologic findings respond	Symptoms and histologic findings persist

for this disorder and it has been largely delineated by multiple case reports and series. A combination of gastrointestinal complaints with supportive histologic findings is sufficient to make the diagnosis. These conditions are grouped together under the term EoG for the discussion here, though it is likely that they are distinct entities in most patients.

The most common symptoms of EoG include colicky abdominal pain, bloating, diarrhea, weight loss, dysphagia, and vomiting.[17,18] In addition, up to 50% have a past or family history of atopy.[14] Features of severe disease include gastrointestinal bleeding, iron deficiency anemia, protein-losing enteropathy (hypoalbuminemia), and growth failure.[17] Approximately 75% of affected patients have an elevated blood eosinophilia.[19] Males are more commonly affected than females. Rarely, ascites can occur.[19,20]

In an infant, EoG may present in a manner similar to hypertrophic pyloric stenosis, with progressive vomiting, dehydration, electrolyte abnormalities, and thickening of the gastric outlet.[21,22] When an infant presents with this constellation of symptoms, in addition to atopic symptoms such as eczema and reactive airway disease, an elevated eosinophil count, or a strong family history of atopic disease, EoG should be considered in the differential diagnosis before surgical intervention if possible.

Uncommon presentations of EoG include acute abdomen (even mimicking acute appendicitis)[23] or colonic obstruction.[24] There have also been reports of serosal infiltration with eosinophils, with associated complaints of abdominal distention, eosinophilic ascites, and bowel perforation.[20,25–29]

Other Manifestations of Gastrointestinal Allergy in Infants and Children

Gastroesophageal reflux

GER is a common complaint among infants, children, and adults. Up to two-thirds of 4-month-old infants experience regurgitation on a daily basis,[30] with other complaints such as forceful vomiting, arching, irritability, and feeding refusal occurring to varying degrees. Furthermore, many infants and children may experience GER without the presence of any overt signs or symptoms. Most cases of GER are not attributable to a specific underlying cause; however, one of the leading identifiable causes of GER in this population is food allergy.[31,32]

Relatively recently, the association between GER and cow's milk allergy (CMA) was prospectively investigated.[32] In a 3-year prospective study, infants with symptoms compatible with GER underwent pH monitoring and endoscopy to confirm the presence of GER. Patients with a reflux index (percentage of time with acid reflux) greater than 5% and the presence of esophagitis were considered to have GER. The presence of CMA in these patients was assessed using skin prick tests, the presence of eosinophils in fecal mucus, nasal mucus, or peripheral blood, and by circulating levels of anti-beta-lactoglobulin IgG. Patients who had positive assays for CMA and GER were placed on a cow's milk restricted diet with a protein hydrolysate formula. After 3 months, a double-blind cow's milk challenge was performed to confirm the diagnosis of CMA.

This stringent method of diagnosing both GER and CMA revealed a surprisingly high prevalence (42%) of patients with GER who also had CMA. Further, this author group went on to show that 14 of 47 patients (30%) had GER that was attributable to the CMA itself, based on resolution of symptoms on restricted diet followed by return of symptoms when re-challenged.

Whether cow's milk or other food allergies are responsible for such a high proportion of GER in all populations remains to be seen; however, these results imply that refractory cases of GER warrant consideration of food allergy as a contributing factor.

Infantile colic

Infantile colic is a term that is generally used to describe acute self-limited episodes of irritability (presumably due to abdominal pain) that occur in otherwise healthy infants in the first several months of life.[33] Although labeling an infant as having "colic" implies there is no organic disease responsible, a subset of infants diagnosed with colic will have an underlying organic cause. Food allergies, and specifically CMA, have been highly implicated in the organic etiologies of infantile colic.

In a trial of 70 formula-fed infants, 50 (71%) had resolution of colic symptoms when cow's milk protein was removed from the diet, with 100% relapse rate after two successive reintroductions of the protein.[34] Similarly, in a double-blind crossover study, CMA was implicated in 24 of 27 infants with colic with significant reductions in daily crying when cow's milk protein was removed from the diet,[35] with worsening of symptoms when whey was reintroduced into the diet in a blinded fashion.

Traditionally, changing the infant's formula is a common way of dealing with colic; often several formula changes are made (e.g., from cow's milk based to soy based to hydrolyzed protein). It is often unclear, however, whether the formula change is responsible for the eventual resolution of symptoms, as colic by definition begins to resolve by 4–5 months of age.

Diarrhea

The presence of diarrhea in the context of food allergies can be multifactorial. As discussed in previous sections, EoG and AP may both lead to intestinal mucosal damage and subsequent diarrhea. However, food allergy may also result in diarrhea in the absence of mucosal damage or eosinophilic infiltration.

Gastrointestinal symptoms, in particular diarrhea, are commonly seen among children with atopic eczema[36,37]; avoidance of particular foods in these patients will alleviate the symptoms.[37] In patients with GI symptoms related to milk ingestion (confirmed by double-blind challenge), the instillation of milk into the intestinal lumen resulted in increased production of histamine and eosinophil cationic protein within 20 minutes.[38] Albumin concentration in the intestine also increased, suggesting increased gut permeability and leakage; none of these findings were seen in normal controls.

Animal models suggest that food allergy may also increase intestinal motility, which in turn may lead to diarrhea.[39] Increased intestinal mast cell counts have been seen in subjects with increased intestinal motility.[40] However, diarrhea in relation to food allergy is almost certainly a multifactorial event that may involve other processes such as secondary carbohydrate malabsorption or overingestion of non-absorbable sugars.

Constipation

Constipation is a common problem among infants and children, and although often short-lived or self-limited, a substantial proportion may have symptoms that persist for 6 months or more.[41] It has long been suggested that cow's milk plays a role in the development of chronic constipation,[42] and there is evidence that CMA is a causative factor. One of the most compelling studies involved a blinded crossover study of cow's milk restriction in children with chronic constipation.[43] In this trial, 65 children with chronic constipation (all of whom received cow's milk in their regular diet) were randomized to receive either cow's milk or soy milk for 15 days, followed by a washout period and reversal of the previous diet. Sixty-eight percent of the children had improvement in their constipation while taking soy milk, while none had improvement on cow's milk. Rechallenging the responders with cow's milk resulted in return of constipation. Evidence of CMA was based on higher frequencies of co-existent rhinitis, dermatitis, and bronchospasm in responders, as well as increased likelihood of elevated IgE to cow's milk antigens and inflammatory cells on rectal biopsy. A subsequent study revealed further evidence of the causative nature of CMA in constipation.[44]

DIFFERENTIAL DIAGNOSIS

The differential diagnosis of the various disorders outlined above depends on several factors including clinical presentation, associated symptoms, and timing with regard to food ingestion. See Figure 17–1. First and foremost, it is important to differentiate between food allergy and other types of food reaction.

Toxic reactions do not involve the immune system, but may present in a fashion similar to immune-mediated food reactions. For example, scombroid is a food-related illness following the ingestion of improperly stored fish. When certain fish are not properly refrigerated, bacterial production of biogenic amines, in particular histamine, can occur, leading to markedly increased levels.

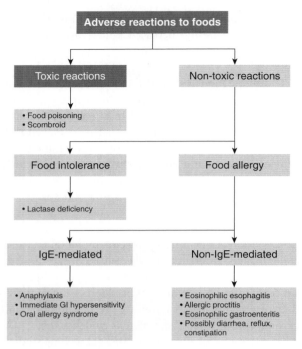

FIGURE 17–1 ■ Thought process to consider in the diagnosis of food allergy versus intolerance in children.

Ingestion leads to histamine-mediated reactions in the GI tract including flushing, nausea, vomiting, and diarrhea.

In addition to toxic reactions, other *non-immune-mediated food intolerances* may produce gastrointestinal symptoms. Lactose intolerance from congenital or acquired deficiency of the intestinal brush border enzyme lactase may lead to symptoms of abdominal pain, distention, gas, bloating, and diarrhea following the ingestion of lactose. Similar syndromes can be seen with the malabsorption of other carbohydrates such as sucrose, fructose, trehalose, and stachyose as well as sugar alcohols such as sorbitol. Celiac disease represents an immune-mediated food reaction, but is not considered to be an allergy.

Because many of the manifestations of GI allergy, such as GER, abdominal pain, vomiting, diarrhea, and rectal bleeding, are non-specific, other common causes of each of these must be considered within the differential diagnosis (Table 17–3). Additionally, EoE and gastroenteritis must be differentiated from other causes of tissue eosinophilia such as parasitic infection and inflammatory conditions such as Crohn's disease (Table 17–4).

Table 17–4.

Differential Diagnosis of Gastrointestinal Eosinophilia

Esophagus
Eosinophilic esophagitis
Gastroesophageal reflux
Food allergy

Stomach
Eosinophilic gastroenteritis
Menetrier's disease
Chronic granulomatous disease
Vasculitis
Oral gold therapy
Hyper-IgE syndrome
Idiopathic hypereosinophilic syndrome

Small intestine
Eosinophilic gastroenteritis
Inflammatory bowel disease (Crohn's disease)
Infectious (parasites)
Food allergy
Vasculitis
Oral gold therapy
Hyper-IgE syndrome
Idiopathic hypereosinophilic syndrome

Colon
Food allergy
Eosinophilic gastroenteritis
Inflammatory bowel disease (Crohn's or ulcerative colitis)
Infectious (parasites)
Vasculitis

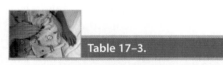

Table 17–3.

Differential Diagnosis of Eosinophilic Esophagitis

The differential diagnosis is broad prior to performing the diagnostic test for eosinophilic esophagitis. After endoscopy the differential decreases significantly

Differential diagnosis at presentation
■ Gastroesophageal reflux disease (GERD)
■ Eosinophilic esophagitis
■ Gastritis
■ Peptic ulcer disease
■ Esophageal dysmotility
■ Esophageal stricture
■ Infection, that is, *Helicobacter pylori*
■ Inflammatory bowel disease
■ Connective tissue disease

Differential diagnosis after biopsy-proven eosinophilia in the esophagus
■ Eosinophilic esophagitis
■ Eosinophilic gastroenteritis
■ GERD
■ Recurrent vomiting
■ Parasitic or fungal infections
■ Inflammatory bowel disease
■ Esophageal leiomyomatosis
■ Myeloproliferative disorder

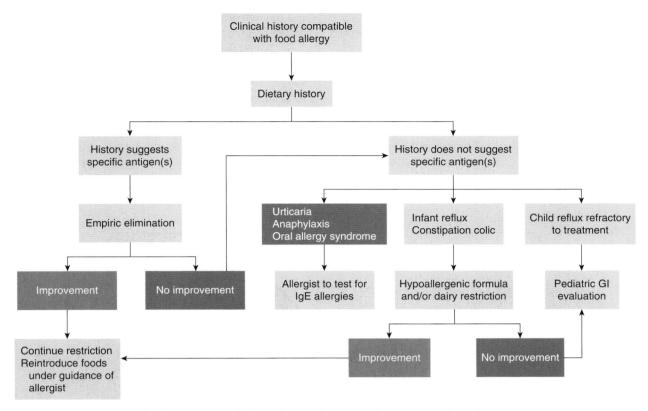

FIGURE 17–2 ■ Diagnostic algorithm to consider in the evaluation of patients with suspected food allergies.

DIAGNOSIS

See Figure 17–2 for an algorithm outlining diagnostic thought process.

IgE-mediated Food Allergies

Patients with a history of a significant reaction to one or more foods should be tested by skin prick against those foods and against a limited battery of common food allergens (milk, soy, egg, peanut, fish, and wheat). Skin testing has a sensitivity of 90–100% depending on the antigen, so patients with negative skin testing are very unlikely to have IgE-mediated disease and should be challenged openly with the food in question. The specificity of skin prick testing for food allergies ranges from 40% to 80%, which implies that the possibility of a false-positive skin test is not inconsequential.[45] Therefore, the use of skin testing in the evaluation of food allergy should be limited to cases where there is a high clinical suspicion of allergies as the etiology of symptoms, which increases the positive predictive value of the test.

Non-IgE-mediated hypersensitivity may still cause symptoms on challenge, but these may be delayed for hours or days. IgE–RAST testing for specific foods does not have greater positive or negative predictive

value than skin prick testing, and combining the two does not improve the diagnostic yield.[46] IgG-RAST testing for food allergies is commercially available; however, the results of IgG-RAST do not correlate with food allergies, and this type of test should not be used.[45]

In patients with suspected OAS, skin prick or RAST testing for the pollens associated with OAS should be done. A combination of supportive history and positive testing for specific IgE antibodies is adequate to make the diagnosis of OAS.

Non-IgE-mediated Food Allergy

Allergic proctocolitis

AP is primarily a clinical diagnosis, although several laboratory parameters and diagnostic procedures may be useful. Initial assessment should be directed at the overall health of the child. A toxic-appearing infant is not consistent with the diagnosis of AP and should prompt evaluation for other causes of gastrointestinal bleeding. A complete blood count is useful, as the majority of infants with AP have a normal or borderline low hemoglobin. An elevated serum eosinophil count may be present. Stool studies for bacterial pathogens, such as *Salmonella* and *Shigella*, should be performed in the setting of rectal bleeding. In particular, an assay for

Clostridium difficile toxins A and B should also be considered. While *C. difficile* may cause colitis, infants may be asymptomatically colonized with this organism.[47,48] A stool specimen may be analyzed for the presence of white blood cells, and specifically for eosinophils. The sensitivity of these tests is not well documented, and the absence of a positive finding on these tests does not exclude the diagnosis.[49] Eosinophils can also accumulate in the colon in other conditions such as pinworm and hookworm infections, drug reactions, vasculitis,

and inflammatory bowel disease, and it may be important to exclude these, especially in older children.

Although not always necessary, flexible sigmoidoscopy may be useful to demonstrate the presence of colitis. Visually, one may find erythema, friability, or frank ulceration of the colonic mucosa. Alternatively, the mucosa may appear normal, or show evidence of lymphoid hyperplasia.[50,51] Histologic findings typically include increased eosinophils in focal aggregates within the lamina propria, with generally preserved crypt architecture.

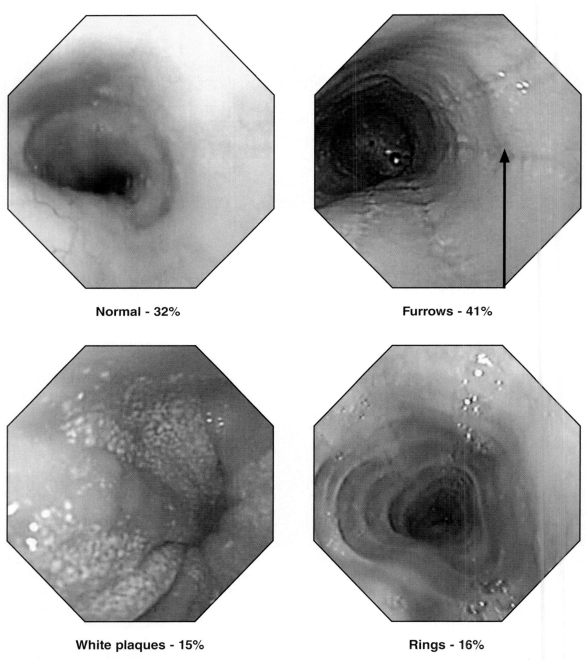

Normal - 32%

Furrows - 41%

White plaques - 15%

Rings - 16%

FIGURE 17–3 ■ Endoscopic findings in eosinophilic esophagitis.

Findings may be patchy, so that care should be taken to examine many levels of each specimen if necessary.[52,53]

Eosinophilic esophagitis

Children with chronic refractory symptoms of GERD or dysphagia should undergo evaluation for EoE. While laboratory and radiologic assessment is appropriate, patients with suspected EoE should undergo an upper endoscopy with biopsy. The diagnosis of EoE can only be confirmed endoscopically. Although there are several endoscopic findings that are suggestive of EoE (Figure 17–3), definitive diagnosis is made when an isolated histologic esophagitis with 20 or more eosinophils per microscopic high-powered field equivalent to 40× (HPF) is present in the appropriate clinical setting.[16] In the past, a 24-hour pH probe was required to demonstrate that the esophageal disease was not acid induced. Subsequently, convention became that EoE could be diagnosed on the basis of 20 eosinophils/HPF, regardless of pH probe results because individuals with reflux esophagitis typically show less than 5 eosinophils/HPF.[54] However, some recent reports have shown that occasionally acid reflux alone may result in significant esophageal eosinophilia.[55] Therefore, the current guidelines for diagnosis include that acid reflux be ruled out as a potential etiology by medical therapy with proton pump inhibitors prior to endoscopy (usually at least 4 weeks) or pH-metry that reveals minimal to no acid reflux[16] (Table 17–5).

Eosinophilic gastroenteritis

EoG should be considered in any patient with a history of chronic symptoms including vomiting, abdominal pain, diarrhea, anemia, hypoalbuminemia, or poor weight gain in combination with the presence of eosinophils in the gastrointestinal tract. Other causes of eosinophilic infiltration of the gastrointestinal tract include EoE and AP, as well as parasitic infection, inflammatory bowel disease, neoplasm, chronic granulomatous disease, collagen vascular disease, and the hypereosinophilic syndrome.[56–60]

A number of tests may aid in the diagnosis of EoG; however, no single test is pathognomonic and there are no standards for diagnosis. Eosinophils in the gastrointestinal tract must be documented before EoG can be truly entertained as a diagnosis. This is most readily done with biopsies of either the upper gastrointestinal tract through esophagogastroduodenoscopy or the lower tract through flexible sigmoidoscopy or colonoscopy. A history of atopy supports the diagnosis, but is not a necessary feature. Peripheral eosinophilia or an elevated IgE level occurs in approximately 70% of affected individuals.[61] Measures of absorptive activity such as the *D-xylose* absorption test and lactose hydrogen breath testing may reveal evidence of malabsorption, reflecting small intestinal damage. Radiographic contrast studies may demonstrate mucosal irregularities or edema, wall thickening, ulceration, or lumenal narrowing. A lacy mucosal pattern of the gastric antrum known as *areae gastricae* is a finding that may be present in patients with EoG.[62]

Evaluation of other causes of eosinophilia should be undertaken, including stool analysis for ova and parasites. Signs of intestinal obstruction warrant abdominal imaging. RAST testing, as well as skin testing for environmental antigens, is rarely useful. Skin testing using both traditional prick tests and patch tests may increase the sensitivity for identifying foods responsible for EoG by evaluating both IgE-mediated and T-cell-mediated sensitivities.[9]

Other GI manifestations of food allergy

The diagnosis of some of the non-specific GI manifestations of allergy, such as reflux, colic, constipation, and diarrhea requires a multifaceted approach. First, in order to implicate food allergy as an etiological factor in one of these disorders, one should first demonstrate that there is not another etiology or effective therapy. As an example, it would not be appropriate to attribute reflux in an infant to milk protein allergy without first giving a trial of an anti-secretory agent such as ranitidine. Likewise, it would not be appropriate to label diarrhea as food allergy related in the setting of rotavirus infection. Because these problems are considered mixed or non-IgE-mediated, skin prick testing or RAST testing is unlikely to aid in diagnosis. Therefore, empiric dietary elimination is often the first diagnostic test utilized. If empiric dietary elimination fails to result in clinical

Table 17–5.

Diagnostic Testing for Suspected Eosinophilic Disorders

Radiographic upper gastrointestinal series to the ligament of Treitz (anatomic causes)

Clinical history (including past medical and family history) and physical examination attempting to identify stigmata of allergic disease

Laboratory studies including complete blood count (differential); comprehensive chemistry panel; quantitative IgE level, sedimentation rate

Upper endoscopy with biopsy of esophagus (middle and distal); antrum and duodenum (with patient on proton pump inhibitor if reflux symptoms exist)

Colonoscopy if diarrhea or rectal bleeding present

Consider 24-hour pH probe (performed off acid blockade) or impedance monitoring to determine if acid reflux is the cause of problem improvement, further guidance may be provided by an allergist or gastroenterologist.

TREATMENT

As a general rule, the optimal treatment for food allergies is elimination of the appropriate food antigens from the diet. The practicality of this approach varies, however, based on several factors: reliability of the diagnosis, the accuracy of allergy testing, and the number of foods the patient is allergic to. In the patient with IgE-mediated immediate GI hypersensitivity, if IgE–RAST or skin prick tests are positive, the food should be avoided for at least 3 weeks; if symptoms improve, the elimination diet is continued. If there is no improvement, then open or single-blind challenges with the food are given to try to elicit a response. These challenges should be performed in a setting in which access to emergency treatment of allergic reactions is available and this is generally best handled by an allergist.

Positive challenges should lead to consultation with a dietitian to educate the patient and family concerning avoidance of the food and to ensure that adequate nutrition is maintained. Groups such as the Food Allergy and Anaphylaxis Network (FAAN) and the American Partnership for Eosinophilic Disorders (APFED) provide support and educational materials for families. Patients with a history of serious reactions to foods should be provided with an epinephrine kit for home use, proper instruction on how the device is used, and a MedicAlert bracelet.

In the case of OAS, elimination of cross-reacting foods can be performed based on skin prick or RAST testing. Because serious complications are unlikely, unblinded food challenge can be done to confirm which particular foods should continue to be eliminated. Histamine blockers such as diphenhydramine may be useful to manage symptoms. See Table 17–6 for treatment guidelines for GI manifestations of food allergy, including when to consult a specialist. While desensitization therapy (the administration of small amounts of a substance for which the patient is allergic in order to desensitize the patient to the allergen) is useful for patients who have IgE-mediated allergies or allergies to antibiotics, there have been no studies demonstrating its effectiveness in patients with EoE or other eosinophilic gastrointestinal disorders.

Eosinophilic Esophagitis

The identification and removal of allergic dietary antigens is the mainstay of treatment for EoE. While removal of the offending food(s) reverses the disease process in patients with EoE, in many cases the isolation of these foods is extremely difficult. Often, patients with EoE cannot correlate their gastrointestinal symptoms with the ingestion of a specific food. This occurs due to the delayed hypersensitivity response. Several reports have demonstrated that it may take several days for symptoms to recur on ingestion of antigens that cause EoE.[63,64] Even when a particular food causing EoE has been isolated, it may take days or weeks for the symptoms to resolve.[10] In addition, although one food may be identified, there may be several other foods (not identified) that could also be contributing.

While attempts should be made to identify and eliminate potential food allergens through a careful history and the use of allergy testing, it is often difficult to determine the responsible allergic foods. Currently, there are no specific diagnostic tests that can perfectly exclude those food antigens that cause EoE. Several methods of dietary restriction have been utilized for patients with EoE. Dietary restriction based on skin prick and atopy patch testing has been found useful in up to 75% of patients.[65] Alternatively, instead of using allergy testing, Kagalwalla et al. reported that the administration of a directed diet based on the removal of the most likely food allergens (dairy, soy, wheat, fish, nuts, and shellfish) was also effective in up to 75% of patients with EoE.[66]

Unfortunately, under the best of circumstances, directed dietary therapy is still unsuccessful in 25–50% of patients; in these cases, the administration of a strict diet, utilizing an amino acid-based formula, is a preferred option. As established previously, the use of an elemental diet rapidly improves both clinical symptoms and histology in patients with EoE.[10,64,67] Because of poor palatability, the elemental formula is most often provided by continuous nasogastric feeding. The diet may be supplemented with water, and at the discretion of the physician sometimes a fruit (e.g., apple and grape) or foods with pure sugar and no protein such as a pure fruit juice. Reversal of symptoms typically occurs within 10 days, with histologic improvement in 4 weeks. After the symptoms and esophagitis have resolved, specific foods can be reintroduced in an attempt to determine those foods responsible for the disease. Based on previous reports, foods can be introduced from those least likely to produce disease (vegetables and fruits) to those most likely to cause disease (milk, soy, and wheat). (REF) Typically several foods are reintroduced, one at a time, for a period of 4–8 weeks. The patient's symptoms are monitored and if symptoms occur the food(s) are eliminated. However, because the disease may cause intermittent symptoms, a repeat upper endoscopy with biopsy is almost always performed after each series of food trials. Unfortunately, up to 20% of patients have been found to be allergic to almost every food and remain on enteral

Table 17–6.

Treatment Guidelines for Food Allergies, Including When to Consult Specialists

Treatment algorithm: continue with stepwise progression if symptoms do not improve
Eosinophilic disorders

Allergic proctocolitis (AP)
Step 1. Remove milk/soy from diet (and from mother's diet if breastfeeding)
Step 2. Use hydrolysate formula
Step 3. Remove all intact food antigens from diet. Use amino acid-based formula
After resolution of AP (on above therapy), foods may be reintroduced at 1 year of age. Challenge should be performed in an office setting when the history of symptoms is mild and in a hospital setting if anaphylaxis is a possibility. If anaphylaxis is a possibility, pediatric allergist should be consulted

Eosinophilic gastroenteritis (EoG)
Step 1. Consult gastroenterologist to confirm eosinophilic disease
Step 2. Consult allergist for allergy testing (skin prick and skin patch)
Step 3a. If allergy testing yields positive result, eliminate foods from diet and monitor symptoms
Step 3b. If allergy testing yields negative result, consider strict elemental diet using amino acid-based formula
Step 4. Administer a trial of corticosteroids and cromolyn sodium
Step 5. Consider other immunosuppressive agents (6-MP, imuran)

Eosinophilic esophagitis (EoE)
Step 1. Consult gastroenterologist to perform endoscopy with biopsy on aggressive acid blockade (proton pump inhibitor)
Step 2. Consult allergist; remove suspected foods; repeat endoscopy with biopsy in 4–6 weeks
Step 3. Administer strict amino acid-based formula for 4 weeks followed by repeat endoscopy with biopsy
Non-eosinophilic disorders

Reflux, diarrhea, constipation, colic (when suspected to be related to allergy)
Step 1. Remove milk +/− soy from diet (and from mother's diet if breastfeeding)
Step 2a. For infants, consider hydrolysate formula
Step 2b. Remove all intact food antigens from diet. Use amino acid-based formula
Step 3. Re-challenge to confirm symptoms were due to allergy
If no resolution of symptoms on food elimination, consider other causes of symptoms

Oral allergy syndrome (OAS)
Step 1. Consult allergist for allergy testing to typical antigens (skin prick or RAST)
Step 2a. If allergy testing yields positive result, eliminate cross-reactive foods from diet and monitor symptoms
Step 2b. If allergy testing yields negative result, consider other causes
Step 3. Administer a trial of corticosteroids and cromolyn sodium
Step 4. Consider other immunosuppressive agents (6-MP, imuran)

Immediate GI hypersensitivity/anaphylaxis
Step 1. Consult allergist for allergy prick/RAST testing
Step 2a. Remove foods with positive reactions from diet. Obtain EpiPen training and MedicAlert bracelet
Step 2b. Consult with dietitian for further advice on allergen avoidance

feedings utilizing an amino acid-based formula for a prolonged period of time. Although the strict use of an amino acid-based formula may initially be difficult for patients (and parents) to accept, in general its benefits outweigh the risks of other treatments and the rapid improvement in symptoms proves reinforcement to families. While the use of other medications, such as corticosteroids, may temporarily improve the disease and its symptoms, on their discontinuation the disease recurs. In contrast, when foods that cause EoE are identified through a combination of allergy testing, endoscopy, elimination, and selective reintroduction,

the disease for the individual patient is in effect cured, and should not recur.

Treatment of EoE with aggressive acid blockade, including medical and surgical therapy, has not been proven effective. Several published reports have demonstrated the failure of H2 blocker and proton pump therapy in patients with EoE.[68–70] While acid blockade may improve clinical symptoms by improving acid reflux caused by inflamed esophageal mucosa, it does not reverse the esophageal histologic abnormality or the underlying disease process. Although some case reports suggested that fundoplication may be beneficial for patients with EoE, two pediatric studies demonstrate failure of fundoplication to result in symptomatic or histologic resolution of the disease process.[17,71] In the report by Liacouras, two patients underwent fundoplication for presumed acid reflux esophagitis unresponsive to medical therapy. However, post-surgical evaluation of both patients revealed ongoing clinical symptoms. Repeat EGD demonstrated persistent esophageal eosinophilia. Subsequently, both patients responded to oral corticosteroids with resolution of symptoms and histologic improvement.

Prior to 1997, reports suggested that systemic corticosteroids improved the symptoms of EoE in adults identified with a severe EoE.[72,73] In 1997, Liacouras et al. were the first to publish the use of oral corticosteroids in 20 children diagnosed with EoE.[69] These patients were treated with oral methylprednisolone (average dose 1.5 mg/kg/day; maximum dose 48 mg/kg/day) for 1 month. Symptoms were significantly improved in 19 of 20 patients by an average of 8 days. A repeat endoscopy with biopsy, 4 weeks after the initiation of therapy, demonstrated a significant reduction of esophageal eosinophils, from 34 to 1.5 eosinophils/HPF. However, on discontinuation of corticosteroids, 90% had recurrence of symptoms.

In 1998, Faubion et al. reported that swallowing a metered dose of corticosteroids dispensed into the mouth by an inhaler was also effective in treating the symptoms of EoE in children.[74] Four patients diagnosed with EoE manifested by epigastric pain, dysphagia, and severe esophageal eosinophilia unresponsive to aggressive acid blockade were given fluticasone, four puffs swallowed twice a day. Patients were instructed not to inhale, but to immediately swallow after dispensing the medication in the mouth to deliver the medication to the esophagus. Histologic improvement was not determined. Within 2 months, all four patients responded with an improvement in symptoms. Two patients required repeat use of inhalation therapy. Success with this therapy was recently confirmed.[70]

As an alternative, Konikoff et al. performed a randomized double-blind placebo-controlled trial utilizing swallowed fluticasone in patients with EoE.[75] The study revealed symptom improvement and decreased esophageal eosinophils in those who received study drug compared to those who received placebo. In addition to swallowed fluticasone, Aceves et al. reported an effective alternative by using budesonide mixed with a sucralose suspension.[76]

While this approach to therapy can improve EoE, to date there is no evidence that topical steroids result in histologic remission (as opposed to histologic improvement). Additionally, the side effects can include esophageal candidiasis and growth failure.[77,78] As with all therapies that do not involve removal of antigens,

symptoms often recur in patients on discontinuation of the therapy.[70]

Other forms of medical therapy that have been evaluated previously include the mast-cell-stabilizing agent cromolyn sodium and the leukotriene antagonist montelukast.[18,79–82] While each of these medications represents appealing options from a pathophysiologic standpoint, the available data do not support their use, based on either lack of clinical improvement or minimal to no histologic resolution.

The latest innovation in therapy includes the use of biologic agents directed at the cyotokine interleukin 5 (IL-5). IL-5 plays in important role in eosinophil recruitment, activation, and proliferation. In the past, two small studies demonstrated the effectiveness of anti IL-5 in improving both symptoms and esophageal histology.[83,84] Currently, in 2009, the two first large-scale pediatric trials utilizing an anti-IL-5 antibody are underway. The results to date are still pending. If effective, this therapy may represent an additional option to a subset of patients with EoE.

Eosinophilic Gastroenteritis

Just as the diagnosis of EoG can be difficult due to its overlap with other diseases, the optimal treatment remains a point of debate and confusion. Because food allergy is considered one of the potential contributors to cases of EoG, the elimination of pathogenic foods, as identified by any form of allergy testing, or by random removal of the most likely antigens, should be considered a first line treatment. Unfortunately, this approach results in improvement in a limited number of patients. In severe cases, or when other treatment options have failed, the administration of a strict diet, utilizing an elemental formula, has been shown to be successful with resolution of clinical symptoms and tissue eosinophilia.[85,86]

When the use of a restricted diet fails, corticosteroids are often employed due to their high likelihood of success in attaining remission.[18] However, when weaned, the duration of remission is variable and can be short-lived, leading to the need for repeated courses or continuous low doses of steroids. In addition, the chronic use of corticosteroids carries an increased likelihood of undesirable side effects, including cosmetic problems (cushingoid facies, hirsutism, and acne), decreased bone density, impaired growth, and personality changes. A response to these side effects has been to look for substitutes that may act as steroid-sparing agents, while still allowing for control of symptoms.

Orally administered cromolyn sodium has been used with some success,[18,87–89] and recent reports have detailed the efficacy of other oral anti-inflammatory medications. Montelukast, a selective leukotriene receptor antagonist used to treat asthma, has been reported to successfully treat two patients with EoG.[81,90] Treatment of EoG with inhibition of leukotriene D4, a potent chemotactic factor for eosinophils, relies on the theory that the inflammatory response in EoG is perpetuated by the presence of the eosinophils already present in the mucosa causing an interruption in the chemotactic cascade breaking the inflammatory cycle. Suplatast tosilate, another suppressor of cytokine production, has also been reported as a treatment for EoG.[91]

Given the possibilities for treatment of EoG, the combination of therapies incorporating the best chance of success with the smallest likelihood of side effects should be employed. As with any potential food reaction, elimination of food antigens (whether directed or empiric) is our preferred approach when successful. Incorporating non-steroid pharmacologic treatment would seem the next best option, and when other treatments fail, corticosteroids remain a reliable treatment for EoG, with attempts at limiting the total dose, or the number of treatment courses where possible. Due to the diffuse and inconsistent nature of symptoms in this disease, serial endoscopy with biopsy is a useful and important modality for monitoring disease progression.

Allergic Proctocolitis

In a well-appearing patient with a history consistent with AP, it is acceptable to make an empiric change in the protein source of the formula. Because of the high degree of cross-reactivity between milk and soy protein in sensitized individuals, a protein hydrolysate formula is often the best choice.[92] Resolution of symptoms begins almost immediately after the elimination of the problematic food. Although symptoms may linger for several days to weeks, continued improvement is the rule. If symptoms do not quickly improve or persist beyond 4–6 weeks, other antigens should be considered, as well as other potential causes of rectal bleeding. In breast-fed infants, dietary restriction of milk and soy-containing products for the mother may result in improvement; however, care should be taken to ensure that the mother maintains adequate protein and calcium intake from other sources.

AP in infancy is generally benign and withdrawing the milk protein trigger resolves the condition. Though gross blood in the stool usually disappears within 72 hours, occult blood loss may persist for longer.[93] The prognosis is excellent and the majority of patients are able to tolerate the culprit milk protein by 1–3 years of age. In older individuals, it is more difficult to identify the food triggers and therefore patients usually require medical management. Though there is a paucity of clinical data regarding therapy for this condition, it appears that glucocortociods and aminosalicylates are efficacious.[94] The prognosis for older onset AP is less favorable than the infant presentation and is typically chronic and relapsing.

Approach to the Potentially Allergic Infant with Non-specific GI Symptoms

Because GI complaints such as colic, reflux, diarrhea, and constipation are common in the infant population, the practitioner who cares for infants will commonly be faced with the issue of when to implicate food allergy. Further complicating the issue is that general allergic complaints such as atopic eczema and rhinitis are also quite common in this population. Optimally, the allergic contribution to any GI complaint would be investigated by allergists through diagnostic testing and double-blind food challenges. However, this is not practical for all patients who present to most practitioners with concerns of food allergy.

It is important for physicians to understand the pathophysiology, the clinical symptoms, diagnosis, and treatment of food allergies in children. Many parents believe that food allergy is the primary cause of many symptoms such as atopic dermatitis, respiratory disease, and lower gastrointestinal symptoms. In fact, many patients with these symptoms do not have primary food allergy. In contrast, many parents do not correlate food allergy with upper gastrointestinal symptoms (reflux-like). It is essential that physicians are well versed not only in the various ways that food allergens can cause gastrointestinal disease, but also with the limitation of diagnostic allergy testing. It is equally important that physicians allay the concerns of parents and prevent them from restricting foods from their children until appropriate testing is conducted and a diagnosis of food allergy is made.

Any infant with GI symptoms refractory to standard treatment may be manifesting signs of food allergy. Because CMA is implicated most commonly in this population, removal of this antigen from the diet is a reasonable approach. However, this change should be made in concert with appropriate investigations for other etiological factors (e.g., anatomic studies such as upper GI series in chronic reflux and stool cultures in chronic diarrhea). Soy formula may be substituted for cow's milk formula, with the understanding that there is a high cross-reactivity between cow's milk and soy protein in sensitized individuals. Protein hydrolysate formulas represent a good option, more likely to result in improvement in a truly allergic infant. Breastfeeding mothers may need to restrict their intake of milk and soy for several weeks before the antigens no longer appear in breast milk. The use of amino acid-based elemental formulas should be reserved for those who have failed hydrolyzed protein formulas, and preferably, in those who have some other objective positive findings of allergy. It should be remembered that the natural history of allergy in the infant is often self-limited, and thus improvement with dietary elimination does not independently confirm food allergy. Formally re-challenging the infant with the suspected food antigen is a better way to confirm that allergy existed and was responsible for the symptoms in question. Formal consultation with an allergist in this context is highly advisable.

SUMMARY AND CONCLUSIONS

Food allergies are common in infants and children. Gastrointestinal problems are common in infants and children. With this in mind, it should be expected that those who care for infants in children will encounter both of these conditions numerous times, and that in a proportion of these cases the two problems will be related.

Because the GI manifestations of food allergy are variable in terms of symptoms and severity, there is no single treatment that will be effective in all cases. However, a common approach that involves attempts at identifying causative food antigens, followed by directed elimination, should provide opportunity for improvement in many children. When this approach fails, a combination of empiric elimination and medical therapy will benefit another proportion of patients. It is also important to remember that because many of the symptoms of GI allergy occur in other diseases, when the usual treatments for allergy fail, other causes of the symptoms should be investigated. A pediatric-trained allergist and gastroenterologist can be invaluable resources for more difficult cases.

REFERENCES

1. Sampson HA. Differential diagnosis in adverse reactions to foods. *J Allergy Clin Immunol.* 1986;78:212–219.
2. Bock SA, Atkins FM. Patterns of food hypersensitivity during sixteen years of double-blind, placebo-controlled food challenges. *J Pediatr.* 1990;117:561–567.
3. Heyman M, Grasset E, Ducroc R, et al. Antigen absorption by the jejunal epithelium of children with cow's milk allergy. *Pediatr Res.* 1988;24:197–202.
4. Husby S, Host A, Teisner B, et al. Infants and children with cow milk allergy/intolerance. Investigation of the uptake of cow milk protein and activation of the complement system. *Allergy.* 1990;45:547–551.
5. Kerner JA Jr. Formula allergy and intolerance. *Gastroenterol Clin North Am.* 1995;24:1–25.
6. Høst A, Halken S. Approach to feeding problems in the infant and young child. In: Leung DYM, Sampson HA, Geha RS, Szefler SJ, eds. *Pediatric Allergy: Principles and Practice.* St. Louis, MO: Mosby; 2003:488–494.
7. Guajardo JR, Plotnick LM, Fende JM, et al. Eosinophil-associated gastrointestinal disorders: a world-wide-web based registry. *J Pediatr.* 2002;141:576–581.
8. Walsh SV, Antonioli DA, Goldman H, et al. Allergic esophagitis in children: a clinicopathological entity. *Am J Surg Pathol.* 1999;23:390–396.
9. Spergel JM, Beausoleil JL, Mascarenhas M, et al. The use of skin prick tests and patch tests to identify causative foods in eosinophilic esophagitis. *J Allergy Clin Immunol.* 2002;109:363–368.
10. Markowitz JE, Spergel JM, Ruchelli E, et al. Elemental diet is an effective treatment for eosinophilic esophagitis in children and adolescents. *Am J Gastroenterol.* 2003;98:777–782.
11. Sampson HA. Food allergy. Part 2: diagnosis and management. *J Allergy Clin Immunol.* 1999;103:981–989.
12. Bock SA, Sampson HA. Evaluation of food allergy. In: Leung DYM, Sampson HA, Geha RS, Szefler SJ, eds. *Pediatric Allergy: Principles and Practice.* St. Louis, MO: Mosby; 2003:478–487.
13. Jenkins HR, Pincott JR, Soothill JF, et al. Food allergy: the major cause of infantile colitis. *Arch Dis Child.* 1984;59:326–329.
14. Goldman H, Proujansky R. Allergic proctitis and gastroenteritis in children. Clinical and mucosal biopsy features in 53 cases. *Am J Surg Pathol.* 1986;10:75–86.
15. Katz AJ, Twarog FJ, Zeiger RS, et al. Milk-sensitive and eosinophilic gastroenteropathy: similar clinical features with contrasting mechanisms and clinical course. *J Allergy Clin Immunol.* 1984;74:72–78.
16. Furuta GT, Liacouras CA, Collins MH, et al. Eosinophilic esophagitis in children and adults: a systematic review and consensus recommendations for diagnosis and treatment. *Gastroenterology.* 2007;133:1342–1363.
17. Kelly KJ. Eosinophilic gastroenteritis. *J Pediatr Gastroenterol Nutr.* 2000;30:S28–S35.
18. Whitington PF, Whitington GL. Eosinophilic gastroenteropathy in childhood. *J Pediatr Gastroenterol Nutr.* 1988;7:379–385.
19. Talley NJ, Shorter RG, Phillips SF, et al. Eosinophilic gastroenteritis: a clinicopathological study of patients with disease of the mucosa, muscle layer, and subserosal tissues. *Gut.* 1990;31:54–58.
20. Santos J, Junquera F, de Torres I, et al. Eosinophilic gastroenteritis presenting as ascites and splenomegaly. *Eur J Gastroenterol Hepatol.* 1995;7:675–678.
21. Aquino A, Domini M, Rossi C, et al. Pyloric stenosis due to eosinophilic gastroenteritis: presentation of two cases in mono-ovular twins. *Eur J Pediatr.* 1999;158:172–173.
22. Khan S, Orenstein SR. Eosinophilic gastroenteritis masquerading as pyloric stenosis. *Clin Pediatr (Phila).* 2000;39:55–57.
23. Redondo-Cerezo E, Cabello MJ, Gonzalez Y, et al. Eosinophilic gastroenteritis: our recent experience: one-year experience of atypical onset of an uncommon disease. *Scand J Gastroenterol.* 2001;36:1358–1360.
24. Shweiki E, West JC, Klena JW, et al. Eosinophilic gastroenteritis presenting as an obstructing cecal mass—a case report and review of the literature. *Am J Gastroenterol.* 1999;94:3644–3645.
25. Huang FC, Ko SF, Huang SC, et al. Eosinophilic gastroenteritis with perforation mimicking intussusception. *J Pediatr Gastroenterol Nutr.* 2001;33:613–615.

26. Deslandres C, Russo P, Gould P, et al. Perforated duodenal ulcer in a pediatric patient with eosinophilic gastroenteritis. *Can J Gastroenterol.* 1997;11:208–212.

27. Wang CS, Hsueh S, Shih LY, et al. Repeated bowel resections for eosinophilic gastroenteritis with obstruction and perforation. Case report. *Acta Chir Scand.* 1990;156: 333–336.

28. Hoefer RA, Ziegler MM, Koop CE, et al. Surgical manifestations of eosinophilic gastroenteritis in the pediatric patient. *J Pediatr Surg.* 1977;12:955–962.

29. Lerza P. A further case of eosinophilic gastroenteritis with ascites. *Eur J Gastroenterol Hepatol.* 1996;8:407.

30. Nelson SP, Chen EH, Syniar GM, et al. Prevalence of symptoms of gastroesophageal reflux during infancy. A pediatric practice-based survey. Pediatric Practice Research Group. *Arch Pediatr Adolesc Med.* 1997;151: 569–572.

31. Iacono G, Carroccio A, Cavataio F, et al. Gastroesophageal reflux and cow's milk allergy in infants: a prospective study. *J Allergy Clin Immunol.* 1996;97:822–827.

32. Cavataio F, Carroccio A, Iacono G. Milk-induced reflux in infants less than one year of age. *J Pediatr Gastroenterol Nutr.* 2000;30(suppl):S36–S44.

33. Wessel MA, Cobb JC, Jackson EB, et al. Paroxysmal fussing in infancy, sometimes called colic. *Pediatrics.* 1954;14:421–435.

34. Iacono G, Carroccio A, Montalto G, et al. Severe infantile colic and food intolerance: a long-term prospective study. *J Pediatr Gastroenterol Nutr.* 1991;12:332–335.

35. Lothe L, Lindberg T. Cow's milk whey protein elicits symptoms of infantile colic in colicky formula-fed infants: a double-blind crossover study. *Pediatrics.* 1989;83:262–266.

36. Ruuska T. Occurrence of acute diarrhea in atopic and nonatopic infants: the role of prolonged breast-feeding. *J Pediatr Gastroenterol Nutr.* 1992;14:27–33.

37. Caffarelli C, Cavagni G, Deriu FM, et al. Gastrointestinal symptoms in atopic eczema. *Arch Dis Child.* 1998;78: 230–234.

38. Bengtsson U, Knutson TW, Knutson L, et al. Eosinophil cationic protein and histamine after intestinal challenge in patients with cow's milk intolerance. *J Allergy Clin Immunol.* 1997;100:216–221.

39. Scott RB, Tan DT. Mediation of altered motility in food protein induced intestinal anaphylaxis in Hooded–Lister rat. *Can J Physiol Pharmacol.* 1996;74:320–330.

40. Gwee KA, Leong YL, Graham C, et al. The role of psychological and biological factors in postinfective gut dysfunction. *Gut.* 1999;44:400–406.

41. Loening-Baucke V. Constipation in children. *N Engl J Med.* 1998;339:1155–1156.

42. Clein NW. Cow's milk allergy in infants. *Pediatr Clin North Am.* 1954;25:949–962.

43. Iacono G, Cavataio F, Montalto G, et al. Intolerance of cow's milk and chronic constipation in children. *N Engl J Med.* 1998;339:1100–1104.

44. Daher S, Tahan S, Sole D, et al. Cow's milk protein intolerance and chronic constipation in children. *Pediatr Allergy Immunol.* 2001;12:339–342.

45. Bernstein IL, Li JT, Bernstein DI, et al. Allergy diagnostic testing: an updated practice parameter. *Ann Allergy Asthma Immunol.* 2008;100:S1–S148.

46. Sampson HA, Albergo R. Comparison of results of skin tests, RAST, and double-blind, placebo-controlled food challenges in children with atopic dermatitis. *J Allergy Clin Immunol.* 1984;74:26–33.

47. Donta ST, Myers MG. *Clostridium difficile* toxin in asymptomatic neonates. *J Pediatr.* 1982;100:431–434.

48. Cooperstock MS, Steffen E, Yolken R, et al. *Clostridium difficile* in normal infants and sudden infant death syndrome: an association with infant formula feeding. *Pediatrics.* 1982;70:91–95.

49. Hirano K, Shimojo N, Katsuki T, et al. Eosinophils in stool smear in normal and milk-allergic infants. *Arerugi.* 1997;46:594–601.

50. Anveden-Hertzberg L, Finkel Y, Sandstedt B, et al. Proctocolitis in exclusively breast-fed infants. *Eur J Pediatr.* 1996;155:464–467.

51. Odze RD, Bines J, Leichtner AM, et al. Allergic proctocolitis in infants: a prospective clinicopathologic biopsy study. *Hum Pathol.* 1993;24:668–674.

52. Machida HM, Catto Smith AG, Gall DG, et al. Allergic colitis in infancy: clinical and pathologic aspects. *J Pediatr Gastroenterol Nutr.* 1994;19:22–26.

53. Goldman H. Allergic disorders. In: Ming S-C, Goldman H, eds. *Pathology of the Gastrointestinal Tract.* Philadelphia: WB Saunders; 1992:171–187.

54. Winter HS, Madara JL, Stafford RJ, et al. Intraepithelial eosinophils: a new diagnostic criterion for reflux esophagitis. *Gastroenterology.* 1982;83:818–823.

55. Ngo P, Furuta GT, Antonioli DA, et al. Eosinophils in the esophagus—peptic or allergic eosinophilic esophagitis? Case series of three patients with esophageal eosinophilia. *Am J Gastroenterol.* 2006;101:1666–1670.

56. DeSchryver-Kecskemeti K, Clouse RE. A previously unrecognized subgroup of "eosinophilic gastroenteritis". Association with connective tissue diseases. *Am J Surg Pathol.* 1984;8:171–180.

57. Dubucquoi S, Janin A, Klein O, et al. Activated eosinophils and interleukin 5 expression in early recurrence of Crohn's disease. *Gut.* 1995;37:242–246.

58. Levy AM, Yamazaki K, Van Keulen VP, et al. Increased eosinophil infiltration and degranulation in colonic tissue from patients with collagenous colitis. *Am J Gastroenterol.* 2001;96:1522–1528.

59. Griscom NT, Kirkpatrick JA Jr, Girdany BR, et al. Gastric antral narrowing in chronic granulomatous disease of childhood. *Pediatrics.* 1974;54:456–460.

60. Harris BH, Boles ET Jr. Intestinal lesions in chronic granulomatous disease of childhood. *J Pediatr Surg.* 1973;8:955–956.

61. Caldwell JH, Tennenbaum JI, Bronstein HA. Serum IgE in eosinophilic gastroenteritis. Response to intestinal challenge in two cases. *N Engl J Med.* 1975;292:1388–1390.

62. Teele RL, Katz AJ, Goldman H, et al. Radiographic features of eosinophilic gastroenteritis (allergic gastroenteropathy) of childhood. *AJR Am J Roentgenol.* 1979;132:575–580.

63. Liacouras CA, Markowitz JE. Eosinophilic esophagitis: a subset of eosinophilic gastroenteritis. *Curr Gastroenterol Rep.* 1999;1:253–258.

64. Kelly KJ, Lazenby AJ, Rowe PC, et al. Eosinophilic esophagitis attributed to gastroesophageal reflux: improvement with an amino acid-based formula. *Gastroenterology.* 1995;109:1503–1512.

65. Spergel JM, Brown-Whitehorn T, Beausoleil JL, et al. Predictive values for skin prick test and atopy patch test for eosinophilic esophagitis. *J Allergy Clin Immunol.* 2007;119:509–511.

66. Kagalwalla AF, Sentongo TA, Ritz S, et al. Effect of six-food elimination diet on clinical and histologic outcomes in eosinophilic esophagitis. *Clin Gastroenterol Hepatol.* 2006;4:1097–1102.

67. Liacouras CA, Spergel JM, Ruchelli E, et al. Eosinophilic esophagitis: a 10-year experience in 381 children. *Clin Gastroenterol Hepatol.* 2005;3:1198–1206.

68. Ruchelli E, Wenner W, Voytek T, et al. Severity of esophageal eosinophilia predicts response to conventional gastroesophageal reflux therapy. *Pediatr Dev Pathol.* 1999;2:15–18.

69. Liacouras CA, Wenner WJ, Brown K, et al. Primary eosinophilic esophagitis in children: successful treatment with oral corticosteroids. *J Pediatr Gastroenterol Nutr.* 1998;26:380–385.

70. Teitelbaum JE, Fox VL, Twarog FJ, et al. Eosinophilic esophagitis in children: immunopathological analysis and response to fluticasone propionate. *Gastroenterology.* 2002;122:1216–1225.

71. Liacouras CA. Failed Nissen fundoplication in two patients who had persistent vomiting and eosinophilic esophagitis. *J Pediatr Surg.* 1997;32:1504–1506.

72. Vitellas KM, Bennett WF, Bova JG, et al. Idiopathic eosinophilic esophagitis. *Radiology.* 1993;186:789–793.

73. Lee RG. Marked eosinophilia in esophageal mucosal biopsies. *Am J Surg Pathol.* 1985;9:475–479.

74. Faubion WA Jr, Perrault J, Burgart LJ, et al. Treatment of eosinophilic esophagitis with inhaled corticosteroids. *J Pediatr Gastroenterol Nutr.* 1998;27:90–93.

75. Konikoff MR, Noel RJ, Blanchard C, et al. A randomized, double-blind, placebo-controlled trial of fluticasone propionate for pediatric eosinophilic esophagitis. *Gastroenterology.* 2006;131:1381–1391.

76. Aceves SS, Bastian JF, Newbury RO, et al. Oral viscous budesonide: a potential new therapy for eosinophilic esophagitis in children. *Am J Gastroenterol.* 2007;102:2271–2279 [quiz 80].

77. Simon MR, Houser WL, Smith KA, et al. Esophageal candidiasis as a complication of inhaled corticosteroids. *Ann Allergy Asthma Immunol.* 1997;79:333–338.

78. Sharek PJ, Bergman DA. The effect of inhaled steroids on the linear growth of children with asthma: a meta-analysis. *Pediatrics.* 2000;106:E8.

79. Dahl R. Disodium cromoglycate and food allergy. The effect of oral and inhaled disodium cromoglycate in a food allergic patient. *Allergy.* 1978;33:120–124.

80. Businco L, Cantani A. Food allergy in children: diagnosis and treatment with sodium cromoglycate. *Allergol Immunopathol (Madr).* 1990;18:339–348.

81. Schwartz DA, Pardi DS, Murray JA. Use of montelukast as steroid-sparing agent for recurrent eosinophilic gastroenteritis. *Dig Dis Sci.* 2001;46:1787–1790.

82. Attwood SE, Lewis CJ, Bronder CS, et al. Eosinophilic oesophagitis: a novel treatment using montelukast. *Gut.* 2003;52:181–185.

83. Garrett JK, Jameson SC, Thomson B, et al. Anti-interleukin-5 (mepolizumab) therapy for hypereosinophilic syndromes. *J Allergy Clin Immunol.* 2004;113:115–119.

84. Stein ML, Collins MH, Villanueva JM, et al. Anti-IL-5 (mepolizumab) therapy for eosinophilic esophagitis. *J Allergy Clin Immunol.* 2006;118:1312–1319.

85. Vandenplas Y, Quenon M, Renders F, et al. Milk-sensitive eosinophilic gastroenteritis in a 10-day-old boy. *Eur J Pediatr.* 1990;149:244–245.

86. Justinich C, Katz A, Gurbindo C, et al. Elemental diet improves steroid-dependent eosinophilic gastroenteritis and reverses growth failure. *J Pediatr Gastroenterol Nutr.* 1996;23:81–85.

87. Van Dellen RG, Lewis JC. Oral administration of cromolyn in a patient with protein-losing enteropathy, food allergy, and eosinophilic gastroenteritis. *Mayo Clin Proc.* 1994;69:441–444.

88. Moots RJ, Prouse P, Gumpel JM. Near fatal eosinophilic gastroenteritis responding to oral sodium chromoglycate. *Gut.* 1988;29:1282–1285.

89. Di Gioacchino M, Pizzicannella G, Fini N, et al. Sodium cromoglycate in the treatment of eosinophilic gastroenteritis. *Allergy.* 1990;45:161–166.

90. Neustrom MR, Friesen C. Treatment of eosinophilic gastroenteritis with montelukast. *J Allergy Clin Immunol.* 1999;104:506.

91. Shirai T, Hashimoto D, Suzuki K, et al. Successful treatment of eosinophilic gastroenteritis with suplatast tosilate. *J Allergy Clin Immunol.* 2001;107:924–925.

92. Juvonen P, Mansson M, Jakobsson I. Does early diet have an effect on subsequent macromolecular absorption and serum IgE? *J Pediatr Gastroenterol Nutr.* 1994;18:344–349.

93. Hill SM, Milla PJ. Colitis caused by food allergy in infants. *Arch Dis Child.* 1990;65:132–133.

94. Rothenberg ME. Eosinophilic gastrointestinal disorders (EGID). *J Allergy Clin Immunol.* 2004;113:11–28 [quiz 9].

CHAPTER 18

Celiac Disease

Edward Hoffenberg
and Thomas Flass

DEFINITIONS AND EPIDEMIOLOGY

Celiac disease (CD) is "a permanent sensitivity to gluten in wheat and related proteins found in barley and rye, occurring in genetically susceptible individuals, and manifesting as an immune mediated enteropathy as defined by characteristic changes seen on intestinal histology."[1] A *conservative definition* requires the following:

- typical signs or symptoms;
- presence of CD-associated antibodies;
- a small intestinal biopsy showing villous atrophy;
- resolution of clinical manifestations with a gluten-free diet (GFD), including complete healing of the intestinal mucosa;
- reduction or disappearance of the CD-associated antibodies on a GFD.

In practice, it is questionable whether it is necessary to meet all aspects of this definition. Controversy continues about whether a small bowel biopsy is required to diagnose CD. Because of numerous reports of CD-associated seropositive individuals with no signs or symptoms of CD, guidelines continue to require a biopsy to confirm the diagnosis and need for treatment.

Different terms have been applied to common clinical situations:

- *Classic CD* refers to a presentation with typical clinical features such as diarrhea, abdominal pain, failure to thrive, or abdominal distention.
- *Atypical CD* describes a non-traditional presentation, primarily with extraintestinal manifestations, such as arthritis or iron deficiency anemia. In older children and adults, the atypical presentation may be more common than the "classic" presentation.
- *Silent CD* describes the situation of an individual without signs or symptoms of CD, but who has small bowel biopsy evidence of CD; usually these patients have an associated condition or a family history of CD, and are identified on screening as having CD-associated antibodies.
- *Latent CD* applies to individuals without signs or symptoms of CD, but who have some risk for future development of CD, such as expression of CD-related antibodies or DQ2 or DQ8 permissive genes, family history of CD, or having an associated condition. These individuals do not have small bowel biopsy changes, but may have CD-associated antibodies.
- *Refractory CD* describes an individual with defined CD who continues to have signs or symptoms of active CD despite pursuing a GFD. In this situation, considerations include considered exposure to gluten, enteropathy-associated T-cell lymphoma (EATL), or possibly another condition such as allergy or inflammatory bowel disease.

Incidence and Prevalence

The prevalence in the United States and Europe is roughly 3–13 cases per 1000 individuals (1:300 to 1:80).[1] There is a female predominance with a ratio of roughly 2:1.[2] These estimates indicate that there are approximately 3 million people with CD in the United States alone, and a roughly equal number in Europe, of which 90% are undiagnosed (Table 18–1). Recent screening studies suggest that in developing countries in Africa, parts of Asia, and South America, the frequency is similar to that of the U.S. and European countries.[3] To date, there are very little data exploring

Table 18–1.

Worldwide Disease Prevalence Based on Screening Data	
Argentina	1:167
Australia	1:251
Brazil	1:66 to 1:119
Egypt	1:187
Finland	1:99 to 1:67
India	1:310
Iran	1:166 to 1:104
Israel	1:157
Italy	1:106
Netherlands	1:198
Russia	1:133
Spain	1:118
Sweden	1:77
Tunisia	1:157
Turkey	1:115
United Kingdom	1:100
United States	1:105

Table 18–2.

Conditions Associated with Increased Risk for CD in Children and Adults[1,4,11]	
Condition	Prevalence of CD (%)
Type 1 diabetes	8–16
Down syndrome	3–15
Turner syndrome	4–8
Williams syndrome	10
IgA deficiency	2–8
Autoimmune thyroiditis	8
First-degree relatives with CD	5–18
Second-degree relatives	3
Dermatitis herpetiformis	80–100
Short stature/delayed puberty	
Dental enamel defects	
Adults specifically:	
■ Irritable bowel syndrome	
■ Persistent aphthous stomatitis	
■ Peripheral neuropathy	
■ Unexplained cerebellar ataxia	
■ Elevated transaminases	
■ Unexplained iron deficiency anemia	
■ Decreased bone mineral density	
■ Infertility	

the rates of CD in China, Japan, and Southeast Asian countries, and these populations are thought to be at lower genetic risk for CD. A number of conditions are associated with an increased risk of CD in children and adults (Table 18–2).

Genetic Considerations

Specific HLA types are permissive for development of CD. HLA molecules bind peptide antigens and present them to CD4$^+$ helper T cells. An estimated 95% of CD patients express the HLA-DQ2 gene and the remainder express DQ8.[5] HLA II molecules are made up of dimers, expressing one alpha and one beta chain. The vast majority of CD patients express the HLA II subtype DQ2 coded by alleles DQA1*0501 and DQB*0201, or DQ8 coded by alleles DRB*04-DQA1*03-DQB1*0302. The DQ2 dimer contains specific pockets that bind deamidated gluten peptides and present them to CD4$^+$ lymphocytes. Expressing two copies of HLA-DQ2 (homozygous state) increases the risk for developing CD, and an estimated 25% of CD patients are DQ2 homozygous. The genes coding for HLA II are located on chromosome 6p21, termed the CELIAC1 locus.

However, other genetic factors are important, and the absolute necessity of DQ2/DQ8 for development of CD has been questioned, as apparent cases of CD occur in individuals who do not express DQ2 or DQ8.[2,4] The DQ2 gene is expressed by approximately 30% of Caucasians, but only 3% of these develop CD.

Having a first-degree relative with CD increases the risk of CD to between 5% and 18%.[4] There is an estimated 70–86% concordance in monozygotic twins with CD, but only 30–40% with HLA-matched twins, and less than 20% concordance in dizygotic twins and first-degree relatives.[6] Expression of DQ2 or DQ8 only accounts for approximately 36–53% of the disease risk. Therefore, other genetic and environmental factors are important.[7,8] Gene linkage analysis and genetic-associated studies, including genome-wide association studies, have identified a number of other loci of possible importance in CD[5,9] (Tables 18–3 and 18–4).

Table 18–3.

Genetic Linkage Studies[5,9]		
Locus	Gene Region	Function
CELIAC1	6p21	HLA II coding region
CELIAC2	5q31–5q33	Cytokine gene cluster
CELIAC3	2q33	T-cell regulatory genes
CELIAC4	19p13.1	MYO9B—unconventional myosin molecule

Table 18–4.

Genetic Association Studies[5,43–45]

Gene Region	Function/Association
1q31	Contains RGS1, regulator of G protein signaling molecule. Involved in B-cell activation/proliferation; found in intestinal intraepithelial lymphocytes
2q11–2q12	2 genes coding for receptor for IL-18 that stimulates T-cell synthesis of IFN-gamma
3p21	Large cluster of chemokine receptor genes CCR1, CCR2, CCR3, CCR5, CCRL2, and XCR1
3q25–3q26	Immediately 5′ of IL-12 gene. IL-12 induces Th1 IFN-gamma secretion
3q28	Associated with LPP gene of unclear significance
4q27	Strongest current association with CD outside HLA locus. Cluster of 8 associated single nucleotide polymorphisms; 2 contain genes for IL2 and IL21, involved in T-cell activation. Associated with type 1 diabetes and rheumatoid arthritis
6q25	Contains TAGAP gene (T-cell activation GTPase-activating protein) expressed in activated T cells
12q24	Contains LNK and ATXN2—strongly expressed in monocytes, dendritic cells, and small intestine

Pathogenesis

The exact mechanism by which ingestion of gluten proteins by genetically susceptible individuals leads to immune-mediated intestinal injury remains unclear (Figure 18–1). An inciting event such as a viral infection, plus additional genetic factors, may be important to development of CD. Both innate and adaptive immunity are thought to be involved.

Gluten proteins are found in wheat and related grains, and can be divided into gliadin and glutenin components. Hordeins in barley and secalins in rye are equivalent proteins that promote the CD process. The oat avedin protein is more distantly related to *Triticeae*

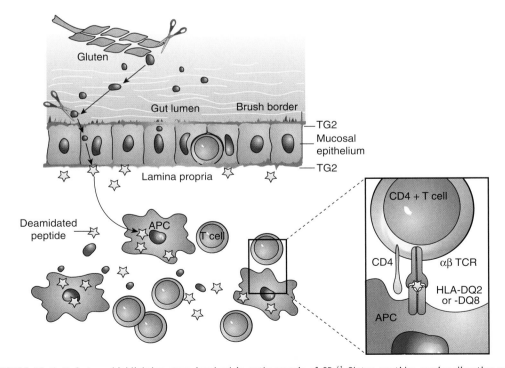

FIGURE 18–1 ■ Cartoon highlighting steps involved in pathogenesis of CD.[41] Gluten peptides survive digestion and cross the mucosal epithelium, where deamidation by tissue transglutaminase (TG2) occurs. HLA-DQ2 or -DQ8 molecules on antigen-presenting cells present these peptides in the intestinal lamina propria where they are recognized by specific CD4[+] T cells Adapted by permission from Ref.[41] (Macmillan Publishers Ltd).

glutens, and seems to be non-immunogenic for most CD patients.[10]

Several properties of gluten may be important in stimulating the immune response of CD:

- Gliadin stimulation of IL-15 secretion through a non-HLA-binding mechanism.
- Gliadin induction of zonulin expression in small intestinal epithelium, with subsequent increase in intestinal permeability, CD4$^+$T-cell antigen exposure, and alteration in cell morphology.
- The high proline (15%) and glutamine (35%) content confers important chemical properties to gluten. First, gluten peptides resist human acid and peptic digestion, and reach the intestinal mucosa in antigenic segments. Second, constitutively expressed tissue transglutaminase (TTG) in the small intestine alters gliadin peptides by deamidating specific glutamine residues to the negatively charged glutamate. Individuals with CD express antibodies to both TTG and deamidated gliadin peptides; these antibodies are specific serologic markers for CD. Deamidated gliadin peptides show enhanced binding to specific pockets in the DQ2 molecule, resulting in enhanced presentation to CD4$^+$T cells by local antigen-presenting cells (APCs).

Both activated APCs and CD4$^+$ T cells secrete increased amounts of inflammatory cytokines such as IFN-gamma and IL-15, causing local recruitment of fibroblasts and clonal expansion of cytotoxic intraepithelial lymphocytes (IELs). The increased numbers of IELs and the subsequent mucosal damage are the classic changes seen on intestinal biopsy of CD patients.

CLINICAL PRESENTATION

Well-recognized clinical presentations of pediatric CD include: failure to thrive, chronic diarrhea, distended abdomen, irritability, constipation, and growth or pubertal delay (Table 18–5).[1,11] Extraintestinal manifestations such as arthritis, iron deficiency anemia, dental enamel defects, and dermatitis herpetiformis (DH) are also common. Asymptomatic children may be identified on screening because of increased risk due to having an associated condition or a family history of CD or diabetes (Table 18–2). Recently, a variety of presentations have been imputed to be related to undiagnosed CD in adults (Table 18–2). These include neuropsychiatric presentations such as ataxia and epilepsy, as well as infertility. Because the signs and symptoms may be mild, vague, and non-specific, delays in diagnosis are common.[11–13]

"Celiac crisis" is a rare medical emergency characterized by explosive, watery diarrhea and dehydration/electrolyte imbalances, marked abdominal distension, hypotension, and lethargy. It is typically seen in toddlers and responds to corticosteroids within a few days.

Clinical Course/Progression of Disease

With institution of a GFD, symptoms often improve by the second week, but may take months to completely resolve. Normalization of the intestinal histology may take 6–12 months. Lactose intolerance tends to resolve within a few weeks. Treatment of nutritional deficiencies, such as iron deficiency, is generally not needed over long term. Adults tend to improve more slowly.

For those with silent or latent CD, continued exposure to gluten leads to eventual clinical manifestations in

Table 18–5.

Manifestations of CD[1,11]

Classic CD	Extraintestinal	Neuropsychiatric Symptoms
Failure to thrive*	Dermatitis herpetiformis*	Ataxia†
Diarrhea*	Dental enamel defects*	Epilepsy +/− cerebral calcifications†
Abdominal distension*	Anemia*	Migraines†
Vomiting*	Aphthous stomatitis*	Depression†
Abdominal pain*	Arthritis/arthralgias†	Fatigue/malaise†
Constipation*	Abnormal liver function tests*	Anxiety†
	Pubertal delay/short stature*	Peripheral neuropathy†
	Osteoporosis/osteopenia*	
	Infertility†	
	Recurrent fetal loss†	

*Strong evidence for association.
†Less strong.

at least some individuals.[14] Data from the adult literature also show a mortality risk significantly above the standard mortality rate (SMR) by a factor of two- to three-fold for patients not adhering to a GFD, not responding to the GFD, or with lengthy delay in diagnosis.[15] There is reasonable evidence that early compliance with a GFD reduces the risk of mortality to close to baseline.[16]

Malignancy

The two- to three-fold increase in all-cause mortality in CD adult patients, as compared to controls, is mostly due to gastrointestinal malignancies such as EATL, non-Hodgkin lymphoma (NHL), and small bowel adenocarcinoma. CD is associated with an increased relative risk 2.1–6.6 times above baseline for NHL and a 30-fold increased risk for small bowel adenocarcinoma.[16]

Dermatitis Herpetiformis

DH is the most common skin lesion associated with CD, occurring in up to 24% of adult patients with CD, but is rare in children. Classic DH is a chronic, pruritic, papular/vesicular rash symmetrically located on the extensor surfaces of the elbows, knees, buttocks, back, and sacrum, and occasionally is seen on the face, neck, and trunk. Biopsy of skin lesions shows microabscesses with neutrophils and eosinophils in the dermal papillae. Immunofluorescence of adjacent skin shows IgA deposits in the papillary dermis directed toward an unknown antigen, but theorized to possibly be epidermal transglutaminase. Markers of CD are often elevated in DH, with positive TTG IgA, endomyseal antibody assay (EMA), and anti-gliadin antibody assays (AGA). The vast majority of DH patients will have villous flattening or increased IELs, even in the absence of overt gastrointestinal symptoms. Most, 85–90%, are HLA B8 positive, and there is a strong association with HLA DW3, and DRW3. A gluten-containing diet is necessary to manifest the lesions of DH, and symptoms often resolve with GFD. Dapsone is often used as a suppressive medication.[1,17,18]

Skeletal Manifestations

There is strong evidence supporting the increased risk for osteopenia and osteoporosis in untreated CD. Bone mineral density, area, and content may be reduced but assessment should adjust for growth and pubertal delay. In children, bone density normalizes within 1–2 years of treatment with GFD.[19]

Association with Other Autoimmune Diseases

The most commonly seen concurrent autoimmune diseases are type 1 diabetes and Hashimoto thyroiditis. Less common are associations with juvenile arthritis, alopecia areata, vitiligo, hepatitis and cholangitis, Sjogren's syndrome, Addison's disease, peripheral neuropathy, psoriasis, and autoimmune cardiomyopathy.

DIFFERENTIAL DIAGNOSIS

Because of its many and varied clinical features, CD can be a great imitator of other disorders, and it can also be silent. The differential diagnosis depends on the way it manifests as well as the age of the patient (Table 18–6). The presentation of diarrhea, abdominal distention, irritability, and vomiting may mimic gastroesophageal reflux, milk or soy protein allergy, *Giardia* infection, malrotation, lymphangiectasia, and iron deficiency anemia in toddlers. The same presentation in school age children and adolescents should lead to considerations

Table 18–6.

Differential Diagnosis

Toddler	School Age and Adolescent	Flattened Mucosa (Villous Atrophy)
Gastroesophageal reflux	Irritable bowel syndrome	Malnutrition
Milk or soy protein allergy	Functional abdominal pain	Infectious enteropathy: *Giardia*
Giardia	Post-infectious chronic diarrhea	Tropical sprue
Lymphangiectasia	Small bowel bacterial overgrowth	IgA/immunodeficiency
Malrotation	Immunodeficiency (IgA deficiency, HIV, other)	Allergic enteropathy: cow/soy milk
Iron deficiency anemia	IBD (Crohn's disease)	Autoimmune enteropathy
Chronic constipation/ Hirschsprung's	Growth hormone deficiency	Zollinger–Ellison syndrome
	Fibromyalgia	
	Acid peptic disease, ulcer	

of irritable bowel syndrome, inflammatory bowel disease, lactose intolerance, ulcer, post-infectious diarrhea/bacterial overgrowth, as well as parasite infection, and immunodeficiency such as IgA deficiency or HIV. Of note, lactose intolerance may be a consequence of the intestinal injury of CD and often resolves with therapy.

The histological hallmark of CD is the small bowel biopsy showing increased numbers of IELs and villous atrophy. The differential diagnosis for this histological finding includes HIV and immunodeficiency, allergy, *Giardia* infection, viral gastroenteritis, autoimmune enteropathy, Zollinger–Ellison syndrome, tropical sprue, and malnutrition (Table 18–6).

DIAGNOSIS

The criteria for diagnosis of CD have been recently updated separately by the North American Society for Pediatric Gastroenterology, Hepatology and Nutrition (NASPGHAN),[1] the Federation of International Societies of Pediatric Gastroenterology Hepatology and Nutrition,[20] the National Institutes of Health (NIH),[11] and the American Gastroenterological Society (AGA).[21,15] Unfortunately, these guidelines are not uniform. In general, the diagnostic algorithm depends on whether the presentation includes clinical signs or symptoms (Figure 18–2), or whether identified because of associated conditions or risks (Figure 18–3).

The current NASPGHAN and FISPGHAN recommendations are to use TTG antibody assays or EMA as the single screening test. These tests have sensitivity and specificity above 0.95. The role of new serologic tests such as the deamidated gliadin peptide antibody test is not yet clear. There is no benefit to a celiac "panel" of multiple antibody tests. Because of the rare case of CD in a patient with IgA deficiency, and to increase the confidence in a negative result, quantitative IgA levels may be obtained, or IgA plus IgG-based TTG tests ordered. AGA are no longer recommended for any patient suspected to be at risk for CD as it has a low specificity and high false-positive rate.

A positive serologic screening test should be followed by a small bowel biopsy showing villous atrophy in order to confirm the diagnosis of CD, and to exclude other causes for the symptoms. The presence of increased IELs alone, the Marsh 1 lesion, is commonly seen in other conditions and experts do not consider it enough for diagnosis of CD. Multiple biopsies (four to six) should be taken from the second portion and distal duodenum. Villous atrophy with increase in IELs is the characteristic finding (Figure 18–4), but is not specific for CD (see Table 18–6). Finally, a complete resolution of symptoms within weeks of following a GFD clinches the diagnosis in the child with a clinical presentation of CD.

Value of DQ2/DQ8 Testing

Virtually all patients with CD will test positive for DQ2 or DQ 8. However, 30–40% of Caucasians will express DQ2 or DQ8, and fewer than 5% will ever develop CD. Therefore, the value of HLA haplotype testing is in its

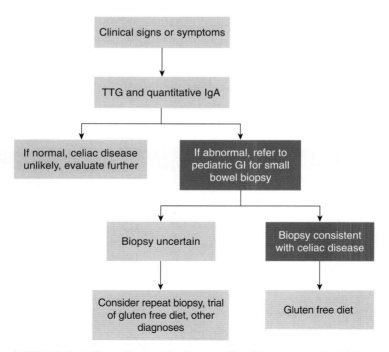

FIGURE 18–2 ■ Diagnostic algorithm for evaluation of the symptomatic child.

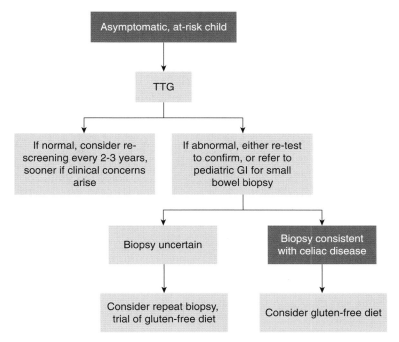

FIGURE 18-3 ■ Diagnostic algorithm for evaluation of the asymptomatic child with a risk.

high negative predictive value. Situations to consider DQ2/8 testing include those individuals with an unclear diagnosis and those with a risk factor but negative initial screening. In this situation, if testing is negative for DQ2 or DQ8, CD is unlikely.

Current recommendations for biopsy-positive individuals are to recheck TTG 6 months after initiating GFD to measure compliance and response, as serology should normalize during this time with good compliance. For the asymptomatic patient, TTG should be rechecked at intervals of 1 year or longer. Gluten challenge and repeat biopsy are no longer recommended if patient improves on GFD. If the patient has been on a GFD after serologic testing but prior to biopsy, or if the patient is receiving corticosteroids or immunosuppressants, biopsy results may not reflect true level of disease. In this situation, a gluten

"load" of 2–4 weeks of a gluten-containing diet usually is sufficient to produce typical CD changes on biopsy.

CONTROVERSIES

Stool Testing

Fecal tests for CD-associated antibodies are commercially available but have not been well validated in adults and have not been studied in children.

Rapid In-office Assays

Rapid whole blood assays for TTG are also being commercialized, with as yet limited data on use in clinical practice.

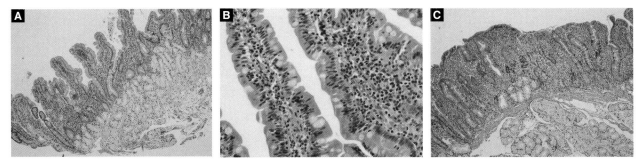

FIGURE 18-4 ■ Small bowel biopsy features of CD, hematoxylin and eosin stain. Panel A shows normal small bowel biopsy with tall slender villi, 10x magnification (Marsh score 0) Panel B shows tall villi with increased numbers of intra-epithelial lymphocytes, 40x magnification (Marsh score 1) Panel C shows total villous atrophy typical of celiac disease, 10x magnification (Marsh score 3).

Non-celiac Gluten Sensitivity

"Gluten sensitivity," "gluten intolerance," and "gluten syndrome" are terms used by a growing number of alternative and complementary care practitioners to describe a condition in which patients report myriad intestinal or extraintestinal manifestations that are attributed to ingestion of gluten proteins but do not meet diagnostic criteria for CD. These patients generally report neuropsychiatric, dermatologic, rheumatologic, and non-celiac gastrointestinal complaints such as headache, sinusitis or rhinorrhea, concentration and learning problems, fatigue, fibromyalgia, and malaise. This entity is becoming more popular with the lay public, with estimates that 10% of the population may be affected. The theory is that ingested gluten induces immunologic response affecting the body without intestinal involvement, and without development of TTG or deamidated gliadin peptide antibodies. The presence of higher titer anti-gliadin antibodies is viewed as consistent with this entity.

TREATMENT

The only known treatment for CD currently is strict lifelong adherence to a GFD. With the seeming omnipresence of gluten-containing foods in the food supply, this requires considerable education, effort, and discipline. There exist both overt and occult sources of gluten in the diet, and failure of the CD patient to improve clinically is often the result of these hidden sources. A list of common gluten-free ingredients, foods to question, and common sources of gluten exposure is shown in Table 18–7. More comprehensive and updated information is provided by the multiple CD or gluten intolerance organizations, listed in Table 18–8.

Consideration should be given to identifying and treating specific nutritional deficiencies associated with CD. In most pediatric patients, these deficiencies resolve with GFD and supplementation is usually only short term. Testing should be considered for: iron deficiency anemia (iron studies including TIBC, ferritin, and transferrin), B_{12}, folate, and zinc as well as vitamin D and calcium. Deficiency of vitamins A, E, and K and phosphorus is rare.

How Much Gluten is Safe?

Based on a double-blind, placebo-controlled study, patients with CD should ingest less than 50 mg of gluten per day in order to remain symptom-free.[22] The Food Allergen Labeling and Consumer Protection Act

Table 18–7.

Food and Ingredient List for the Gluten-free Diet

Food Item	Foods/Ingredients Allowed	Foods/Ingredients to Question	Foods/Ingredients Not Allowed
Grains and flours	Amaranth, arrowroot, bean flour (lentil, romano, garbanzo, etc.), buckwheat, carob flour, chickpea flour, corn flour, corn meal, cornstarch, job's tears, kasha (roasted buckwheat), kudzu root starch, maize, maize waxy, masa flour, harina, millet, Montina Flour (Indian ricegrass), nut flour (almond, chestnut, etc.), pea flour (chickpea, besan, cowpea, etc.), potato flour, potato starch, quinoa, ragi, rape, rice flour (white, brown, sweet, bran), sago flour, soba flour, sorghum, soy flour, tapioca flour, taro root, teff flour, yam flour	Safe flours in bulk bins in stores	Barley (malt, pearl, grass, etc.), bleached flour, bran, bread flour, brown flour, farina, graham, fu (dried wheat gluten), gluten flour, graham flour, granary flour
		Groats can be from either safe or unsafe grains	Groats (arley, heat), alt, matzo semolina, ats, ye, emolina, pelt, heat (emolina, prouted, urum, tarch, bulgar, Kamut, rass, etc.), hole-eal lour Wheat germ
Cereals	Hot and cold cereals made from the allowed grains, cream of rice, cream of buckwheat, grits corn, hominy grits	Commercial cereals made in a non-dedicated facility	Hot and cold cereals containing a grain not allowed Cereals made with malt or malt extract

Table 18–7. (Continued)

Food and Ingredient List for the Gluten-free Diet

Food Item	Foods/Ingredients Allowed	Foods/Ingredients to Question	Foods/Ingredients Not Allowed
Pastas, potatoes, and other starches	Pastas made from allowed grains, rice including white brown and wild, corn tacos and corn tortillas, potatoes, saifun (bean threads), rice noodles	Commercial rice and pasta mixes, French fries, fried restaurant foods (gluten-contaminated grease), polenta	All pastas made from grains not allowed, couscous, tabbouleh, soba noodles
Fruits and fruit products	Fresh fruit, pure fruit juices	Thickened or prepared fruits and pie fillings, dried fruit mixes, jelly and jam	
Beverages	Tea (black, green, and white), coffee (plain), pure fruit juices, cider	Soy and rice beverages, instant tea and coffee, flavored tea and coffee, hot cocoa, hot chocolate, soda, sports drinks, nutritional supplements	Malted beverages, ground coffee with added grains
Vinegar	Vinegars (apple cider, rice, wine, and balsamic)	Flavored vinegars	Malt vinegar
Condiments	Salt, pepper (black, white, and red), pure herbs, pure spices, pure flavoring extracts, wheat-free soy sauce, cream of tartar, pickles, honey	Ground spices, seasoning and spice mixes, gravy cubes and mixes, bouillon cubes and powder, ketchup, mustard, mustard powder, Worcestershire sauce, salad dressings, soy sauce, teriyaki sauce, relish	Most soy sauces contain wheat
Miscellaneous	Seaweed (algin, algae, alginate), alfalfa, aspic	Yeast, yeast flakes, bicarbonate of soda, baking soda, baking powder, powdered sugar, molasses, rice paper, confectioner sugar	Communion wafers, brewer's yeast
Non-food		Lotions, creams, cosmetics, lip gloss, lip balm, sunscreen, toothpaste, mouthwash, products used in dental offices, medications: prescription and over the counter (many contain gluten), laxatives, vitamins, stamps, envelopes, and gummed labels, Play Doh, paper mache	

(FALCPA), which took effect on January 1, 2006, requires food labels to clearly identify eight common food allergens: wheat, eggs, fish, milk, peanuts, shellfish, soybeans, and tree nuts. This law does not, however, address the use of barley (malt), rye, or oats. FALCPA also requires the U.S. Food and Drug Administration to develop rules for the use of the term "gluten-free" on product labels. The final ruling is still pending, although the FDA proposal is available from the federal register at http://www.cfsan.fda.gov/%7Elrd/fr070123.html. The parameter for a naturally gluten-free product is 20 ppm per serving, and for a food rendered gluten-free is 200 ppm.

NEW THERAPIES UNDER INVESTIGATION

While the only current treatment for CD is lifelong adherence to a GFD, several alternative treatments are currently being investigated as possible adjunctive therapies.

Bacterial Prolyl-endopeptidases

One of the properties of gluten that makes it immunogenic is the ability to reach the lamina propria in large, antigenically intact peptide fragments. This is due to lack of native peptidases capable of cleavage of peptide

Table 18–8.

Celiac Disease and Gluten Sensitivity Resources

www.celiac.com: celiac and gluten-free information
www.celiac.org: Celiac Disease Foundation
www.gluten.net: Gluten Intolerance Group of North America
www.celiac.nih.gov: Celiac Disease Awareness Campaign
www.celiaccentral.org: National Foundation for Celiac
    Awareness
www.celiachealth.org: Children's Digestive Health and
    Nutrition Foundation
www.americanceliac.org: American Celiac Disease Alliance
www.eatright.org: American Dietetic Association
www.csaceliacs.org: Celiac Sprue Association
www.cdhnf.org: Children's Digestive Health and Nutrition
    Foundation

bonds of proline residues. Currently being investigated is the use of exogenous bacterial derived prolyl-endopeptidases to cleave these peptides into smaller, less immunogenic fragments prior to reaching the lamina propria. There are published data on in vitro and in vivo animal models, and ex vivo human T cells, with promising results. Controlled studies in CD patients using these enzymes are yet to be published.[23–29]

Inhibition of Intestinal tTG

Early work is underway at developing a site-specific inhibitor of intestinal tTG, to prevent the local deamidation and binding enhancement of gluten peptides. There are potential side effects with such an inhibitor, such as impaired wound healing and perturbation of the extracellular matrix.[30,31]

DQ2/DQ8-binding Peptides

Theoretically, a compound can be formulated that will occupy the binding groove on HLA-DQ2 or -DQ8 and prevent gluten peptide antigen presentation. This would effectively block the immunogenic reaction. To our knowledge, no such compound has yet been formulated.[30]

T-cell Silencing

Another theoretic therapy would be to stimulate apoptosis in gluten-specific T cells, or induce tolerance in these T cells by targeting tolerogenic dendritic cells. These therapies again are still in theoretic stages.[30]

Cytokine Therapy

Several trials of anti-inflammatory cytokine therapy are underway for other chronic diseases such as RA and IBD. IL-15 antagonists have been developed by several pharmaceutical companies for treatment of RA, but have therapeutic potential for CD as well. IFN-γ antagonists have been developed and are in phase II testing for reduction of inflammation in IBD, but are being recognized for potential in CD treatment as well. IL-10 has been tested in both refractory CD and IBD for its potential ability to shift away from TH1 immune reaction. Unfortunately, neither trial has so far showed any success.[30,32–34]

Genetically Modified Wheat

Work is currently underway to evaluate the feasibility of engineering and cultivating a modified, gluten-free strain of wheat that would lack immunogenic peptides. Barriers to this would include cost, palatability, and industrial quality of the flour derived from such a strain. This project is in its early stages, and would not be available to the mass market for many years, if ever.

Other Possibilities

Monoclonal antibodies to the adhesion molecule integrin a4 are currently being used for multiple sclerosis and are also in phase II trials for IBD. These compounds may have potential for CD by prevention of T-cell migration into the lamina propria. Zonulin antagonists are being looked at for prevention of gluten-induced intestinal hyper-permeability. The concept of using NGK2D antagonists to prevent the phenotypic conversion of CD4 T cells to cytotoxic T cells in the intestinal epithelium has also been raised.[30]

PREVENTION

With a more thorough understanding of the pathogenesis of CD, more emphasis may start being placed on the prevention of development rather than treatment.

In a recent meta-analysis of breastfeeding practices and effect on CD, the authors concluded that duration of breastfeeding and breastfeeding during introduction of grains reduced future risk of CD development.[35,36] This is not uniformly accepted, however, and some investigators feel that breastfeeding may delay or mask, but not prevent the development of CD.[37] The mechanism is speculative, but involvement of probiotic bacteria is thought to be important for development of tolerance to food proteins and maintenance of intact intestinal epithelial barrier in infancy. It is also speculated that probiotic therapy in at-risk individuals may help to promote tolerance and prevent CD.

Timing of introduction of gluten and quantity of gluten in the diet are other controversial topics in prevention of CD. Early (prior to 3 months of age) and late (after 7 months) introduction of gluten were associated with increased risk of CD in one prospective study.[37] Several recent papers documented a four-fold rise in incidence of CD in Sweden in children less than 2 years old, after a significant increase in gluten intake in this population. A later decrease in gluten consumption corresponded to a drop in CD.[38]

Prevention of infectious triggers such as rotavirus and the subsequent effect on CD risk is another area currently being researched. If the increased permeability and inflammation corresponding with infection can be avoided in at-risk individuals, perhaps breakdown of tolerance will not occur.[36,39,40]

REFERENCES

1. Hill ID, Dirks MH, Liptak GS, et al. Guideline for the diagnosis and treatment of celiac disease in children: recommendations of the North American Society for Pediatric Gastroenterology, Hepatology and Nutrition. *J Pediatr Gastroenterol Nutr.* 2005;40:1–19.
2. Megiorni F, Mora B, Bonamico M, et al. HLA-DQ and susceptibility to celiac disease: evidence for gender differences and parent-of-origin effects. *Am J Gastroenterol.* 2008;103:997–1003.
3. Cataldo F, Montalto G. Celiac disease in the developing countries: a new and challenging public health problem. *World J Gastroenterol.* 2007;13:2153–2159.
4. Bonamico M, Ferri M, Mariani P, et al. Serologic and genetic markers of celiac disease: a sequential study in the screening of first degree relatives. *J Pediatr Gastroenterol Nutr.* 2006;42:150–154.
5. Wolters VM, Wijmenga C. Genetic background of celiac disease and its clinical implications. *Am J Gastroenterol.* 2008;103:190–195.
6. Nistico L, Fagnani C, Coto I, et al. Concordance, disease progression, and heritability of coeliac disease in Italian twins. *Gut.* 2006;55:803–808.
7. Kagnoff MF. Celiac disease: pathogenesis of a model immunogenetic disease. *J Clin Invest.* 2007;117:41–49.
8. Sollid LM. Hunting for celiac disease genes. *Gastroenterology.* 2008;134:869–871.
9. Catassi C, Fasano A. Celiac disease. *Curr Opin Gastroenterol.* 2008;24:687–691.
10. Kemppainen T, Janatuinen E, Holm K, et al. No observed local immunological response at cell level after five years of oats in adult coeliac disease. *Scand J Gastroenterol.* 2007;42:54–59.
11. National Institutes of Health Consensus Development Conference Statement on Celiac Disease, June 28–30, 2004. *Gastroenterology.* 2005;128:S1–S9.
12. NIH Consensus Development Conference on Celiac Disease. *NIH Consens State Sci Statements.* 2004;21:1–23.
13. Fasano A. Clinical presentation of celiac disease in the pediatric population. *Gastroenterology.* 2005;128: S68–S73.
14. Troncone R, Auricchio R, Granata V. Issues related to gluten-free diet in coeliac disease. *Curr Opin Clin Nutr Metab Care.* 2008;11:329–333.
15. Rostom A, Murray JA, Kagnoff MF. American Gastroenterological Association (AGA) Institute technical review on the diagnosis and management of celiac disease. *Gastroenterology.* 2006;131:1981–2002.
16. Halfdanarson TR, Litzow MR, Murray JA. Hematologic manifestations of celiac disease. *Blood.* 2007;109:412–421.
17. Collin P, Reunala T. Recognition and management of the cutaneous manifestations of celiac disease: a guide for dermatologists. *Am J Clin Dermatol.* 2003;4:13–20.
18. Zone JJ. Skin manifestations of celiac disease. *Gastroenterology.* 2005;128:S87–S91.
19. Zanchi C, Di Leo G, Ronfani L, Martelossi S, Not T, Ventura A. Bone metabolism in celiac disease. *J Pediatr.* 2008;153:262–265.
20. Fasano A, Araya M, Bhatnagar S, et al. Federation of International Societies of Pediatric Gastroenterology, Hepatology, and Nutrition consensus report on celiac disease. *J Pediatr Gastroenterol Nutr.* 2008;47:214–219.
21. AGA Institute medical position statement on the diagnosis and management of celiac disease. *Gastroenterology.* 2006;131:1977–1980.
22. Catassi C, Fabiani E, Iacono G, et al. A prospective, double-blind, placebo-controlled trial to establish a safe gluten threshold for patients with celiac disease. *Am J Clin Nutr.* 2007;85:160–166.
23. Cerf-Bensussan N, Matysiak-Budnik T, Cellier C, Heyman M. Oral proteases: a new approach to managing coeliac disease. *Gut.* 2007;56:157–160.
24. Matysiak-Budnik T, Candalh C, Cellier C, et al. Limited efficiency of prolyl-endopeptidase in the detoxification of gliadin peptides in celiac disease. *Gastroenterology.* 2005;129:786–796.
25. Gass J, Bethune MT, Siegel M, Spencer A, Khosla C. Combination enzyme therapy for gastric digestion of dietary gluten in patients with celiac sprue. *Gastroenterology.* 2007;133:472–480.
26. Mitea C, Havenaar R, Drijfhout JW, Edens L, Dekking L, Koning F. Efficient degradation of gluten by a prolyl endoprotease in a gastrointestinal model: implications for coeliac disease. *Gut.* 2008;57:25–32.
27. Stepniak D, Spaenij-Dekking L, Mitea C, et al. Highly efficient gluten degradation with a newly identified prolyl endoprotease: implications for celiac disease. *Am J Physiol Gastrointest Liver Physiol.* 2006;291:G621–G629.
28. Marti T, Molberg O, Li Q, Gray GM, Khosla C, Sollid LM. Prolyl endopeptidase-mediated destruction of T cell epitopes in whole gluten: chemical and immunological characterization. *J Pharmacol Exp Ther.* 2005;312:19–26.
29. Shan L, Marti T, Sollid LM, Gray GM, Khosla C. Comparative biochemical analysis of three bacterial prolyl endopeptidases: implications for coeliac sprue. *Biochem J.* 2004;383:311–318.
30. Sollid LM, Khosla C. Future therapeutic options for celiac disease. *Nat Clin Pract Gastroenterol Hepatol.* 2005;2: 140–147.

31. Schuppan D, Dieterich W. A molecular warhead and its target: tissue transglutaminase and celiac sprue. *Chem Biol*. 2003;10:199–201.

32. Gianfrani C, Auricchio S, Troncone R. Possible drug targets for celiac disease. *Expert Opin Ther Targets*. 2006;10:601–611.

33. Di Sabatino A, Ciccocioppo R, Cupelli F, et al. Epithelium derived interleukin 15 regulates intraepithelial lymphocyte Th1 cytokine production, cytotoxicity, and survival in coeliac disease. *Gut*. 2006;55:469–477.

34. Salvati VM, Mazzarella G, Gianfrani C, et al. Recombinant human interleukin 10 suppresses gliadin dependent T cell activation in ex vivo cultured coeliac intestinal mucosa. *Gut*. 2005;54:46–53.

35. Akobeng AK, Heller RF. Assessing the population impact of low rates of breast feeding on asthma, coeliac disease and obesity: the use of a new statistical method. *Arch Dis Child*. 2007;92:483–485.

36. Troncone R, Auricchio S. Rotavirus and celiac disease: clues to the pathogenesis and perspectives on prevention. *J Pediatr Gastroenterol Nutr*. 2007;44:527–528.

37. Norris JM, Barriga K, Hoffenberg EJ, et al. Risk of celiac disease autoimmunity and timing of gluten introduction in the diet of infants at increased risk of disease. *JAMA*. 2005;293:2343–2351.

38. Ivarsson A. The Swedish epidemic of coeliac disease explored using an epidemiological approach—some lessons to be learnt. *Best Pract Res Clin Gastroenterol*. 2005;19:425–440.

39. Pavone P, Nicolini E, Taibi R, Ruggieri M. Rotavirus and celiac disease. *Am J Gastroenterol*. 2007;102:1831.

40. Stene LC, Honeyman MC, Hoffenberg EJ, et al. Rotavirus infection frequency and risk of celiac disease autoimmunity in early childhood: a longitudinal study. *Am J Gastroenterol*. 2006;101:2333–2340.

41. Sollid LM. Coeliac disease: dissecting a complex inflammatory disorder. *Nat Rev Immunol*. 2002;2:647–655.

42. Hoffenberg EJ, Bao F, Eisenbarth GS, et al. Transglutaminase antibodies in children with a genetic risk for celiac disease. *J Pediatr*. 2000;137:356–360.

43. Dubois PC, van Heel DA. Translational mini-review series on the immunogenetics of gut disease: immunogenetics of coeliac disease. *Clin Exp Immunol*. 2008;153:162–173.

44. Hunt KA, Zhernakova A, Turner G, et al. Newly identified genetic risk variants for celiac disease related to the immune response. *Nat Genet*. 2008;40:395–402.

45. Smyth DJ, Plagnol V, Walker NM, et al. Shared and distinct genetic variants in type 1 diabetes and celiac disease. *N Engl J Med*. 2008;359:2767–2777.

CHAPTER 19

Disorders of Gastrointestinal Motility

Hayat Mousa

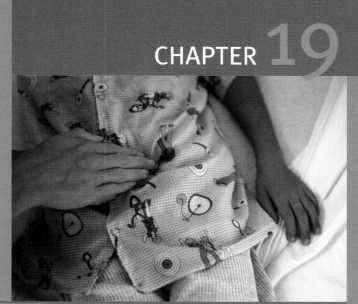

INTRODUCTION

Gastrointestinal (GI) motility disorders (GMDs) are represented by a spectrum of conditions that range from benign prevalent disorders (gastroesophageal reflux (GER) and childhood constipation) to more rare and severe entities (chronic intestinal pseudo-obstruction (CIP) and Hirschsprung's disease). Altered GI motility adds considerable co-morbidity to structural anomalies such as intestinal atresia, stenosis, or gastroschisis. Pediatric GMDs are classified according to the results of GI motility testing. It is likely that with advanced methods of studying the brain–gut axis, classification of these disorders will eventually be based on pathophysiology. Within the pediatric population, GMDs are also known to be either congenital or acquired, depending on the presence or absence of symptoms at birth.[1,2] Congenital disorders usually cause symptoms within the first 2 months of life and can be sporadic or familial. Acquired motility disorders present later in life and can be secondary to a variety of insults including infections and adverse reactions to medications.[3] Within the pediatric population, GMDs account for up to 15% of all intestinal failures.

Based on histopathology and patterns of motility abnormalities, traditionally the causes of GMDs are also classified as visceral neuropathy or visceral myopathy.[3] Neuropathic disorders are more common, but myopathies are usually associated with more severe symptoms.[2,3] The role of genetic mutations in visceral neuropathies or myopathies has not yet been thoroughly elucidated.

Other possible causes of motility disorders include intrauterine ischemic insults, exposure to amniotic fluid,[4] delayed maturation of either the enteric nervous system or the interstitial cells of Cajal,[5] and disorder of the mitochondrial electron transport chain enzymes.[6] Inflammation within the myenteric ganglia may cause severe progressive neuropathic CIP in conjunction with autoimmune disease and circulating antienteric neuronal antibodies.[7] Mitochondrial myopathies are known to be associated with a variety of clinical syndromes including CIP.[8] Patients with mitochondrial neurogastrointestinal encephalomyopathy (MNGIE) have GI dysmotility, peripheral neuropathy, and ophthalmoparesis, and muscle biopsy shows histological features of mitochondrial myopathy.[1,9,10]

While treatment of motility disorders has improved significantly over the last two decades, treatment options remain relatively limited. Motility disorders produce nutritional and electrolyte deficiencies, chronic and recurrent vomiting, fecal incontinence, chronic and recurrent pain or discomfort, reduced independence in daily life, and reduced mobility. A wide range of clinical skills is often required to optimally treat these patients. Centers specializing in this care generally establish a multidisciplinary team approach. As part of the treatment, psychological and social support efforts are extremely necessary to achieve optimal outcomes.

Given the number of pediatric GMDs and the space limitations of this chapter, only the following six motility disorders will be reviewed:

- esophageal achalasia (EA);
- motility disorders following repair of congenital intestinal atresias;
- motility disorders associated with gastroschisis;
- CIP;
- motility disorders following intestinal transplantation;
- Hirschsprung's disease.

ESOPHAGEAL ACHALASIA

Definition and Epidemiology

EA is a primary esophageal motility disorder characterized by impaired relaxation of the lower esophageal sphincter (LES) in response to swallowing and by a lack of effective peristalsis. EA rarely occurs in adolescents and is seen even less frequently in younger children.[11]

Pathogenesis

EA occurs so rarely that little is known about related etiologies and pathogenesis. A study by Gockel et al. showed that a majority of patients with EA had a significantly reduced number of intramural ganglion cells in addition to severe fibrosis of the smooth muscle and myopathic changes of smooth muscle cells.[12] The disorder in young children is associated with trisomy 21, the

Table 19–1.

Signs and Symptoms of Common Intestinal Motility Disorders, Given in Order of Frequency

Motility Disorder	Signs and Symptoms
Esophageal achalasia	Dysphagia for liquids and solids Regurgitation (also during the night) Difficulty burping Chest pain Slow eating (as reported by family) Neck and back stretching movements after eating
Following repair of congenital intestinal atresia	Abdominal pain and distention Constipation or diarrhea Vomiting TPN-feeding intolerance
Associated with gastroschisis	Vomiting Bloating Abdominal pain Chronic diarrhea Significant feeding problems including TPN-feeding intolerance
Chronic intestinal pseudo-obstruction	Abdominal distension, pain Constipation Nausea, vomiting **Late manifestations include** ▪ Abdominal bloating ▪ Constipation ▪ Bilious vomiting (initially, normal intestinal transit) **Due to complications** ▪ Diarrhea from bacterial overgrowth ▪ Urinary voiding disorders (due to nerve, muscle involvement)
Following intestinal transplantation	Increased stoma output Fever Abdominal pain, distension Ileus
Hirschsprung's disease	Abdominal pain, discomfort Constipation Chronic diarrhea (with associated enterocolitis) Vomiting **Associated with enterocolitis (HAEC)** ▪ Explosive, foul-smelling diarrhea ▪ Fever ▪ Vomiting ▪ Abdominal pain, distension **Severe cases** ▪ Rectal bleeding ▪ Shock

Abbreviations: TPN = total parenteral nutrition; HAEC = Hirschsprung's-associated enterocolitis.

triple A (achalasia–addisonian–alacrima) syndrome, and familial dysautomonia.[13,14]

Clinical Presentation

The signs and symptoms of EA progress slowly (Table 19–1), and the disorder may remain undiagnosed for several years. Vomiting and difficulty swallowing solids and liquids are the primary clinical features, and some children may experience resultant weight loss. Parents may complain that their child burps frequently or regurgitates during the night. Heartburn is also a common complaint.[12]

Differential Diagnosis

Both malignant (gastric carcinoma) and nonmalignant disorders (esophageal stricture, esophagitis, and

"GER") may cause pseudo-achalasia (Table 19–2). A patient who has had symptoms for <6 months, has lost weight during that time, or had a difficult endoscopy most likely has a malignancy. Esophageal manometry may not distinguish between achalasia and pseudo-achalasia, and computerized tomography and repeated biopsies may be needed to make this differentiation.[15]

Diagnosis

Several diagnostic tests are used to differentiate EA (Table 19–3). Typically, an EA esophagram will show a dilated esophagus with retained contrast and a smooth tapering of the distal esophagus ("bird beak" appearance), as seen in Figure 19–1A. Disease onset is gradual, however, and a normal contrast esophagram does not rule out early stage disease. Esophageal manometry showing poor relaxation of the LES and aperistalsis of

Table 19–2.

Etiologies of Common Intestinal Motility Disorders, Given in Order of Severity

Motility Disorder	Common Conditions	Rare Conditions
Esophageal achalasia	Esophageal stricture	Amyloidosis
	Idiopathic CIP	Chagas disease (esophageal infection)
	Secondary or pseudo-achalasia	Fabry disease
	Malignancy (gastric, lung, esophagus)	
	GER	
Following repair of congenital intestinal atresias	Short bowel syndrome	Volvulus
	Malabsorption syndromes	Anomalies of annular pancreas and biliary tracts
	Prolonged adynamic ileus	Leakage of intestinal contents
	Severely impaired intestinal motility	
Associated with gastroschisis	Abdominal wall defects	Prolapse of intestine, viscera
	Atresia	Intestinal atresia
	"Apple-peel" jejunoileal lesion	Ischemia or midgut infarction
	Oligohydramnios	Short bowel syndrome
	Malrotation	Meckel's diverticulum
		Gallbladder atresia
Chronic intestinal pseudo-obstruction	Toxic megacolon	Trauma (fractures)
	Mechanical obstruction	Obstetrical, abdominal, orthopedic surgery
	Slow transit constipation	Neurologic conditions
	Crohn's disease	
Following intestinal transplantation	Impaired absorption	Hepatic artery thrombosis
	Spontaneous small bowel perforation	Biliary anastomotic leak
	Abdominal compartment syndrome	
	Duodenal stump leak	
	Intestinal anastomotic leak	
Hirschsprung's disease	Enterocolitis	Volvulus
	Idiopathic constipation	
	Distal intestinal obstruction	
	Toxic megacolon	
	Anorectal malformations	

Abbreviations: CIP = chronic intestinal pseudo-obstruction; GER = gastroesophageal reflux.

Table 19–3.

Required Diagnostic Tests of Common Motility Disorders

Motility Disorder	Diagnostic Tests	When to Order Diagnostic Tests
Esophageal achalasia	Barium esophagram	Primary screening test
	Esophageal manometry	Required for confirmation
	Endoscopy	To exclude malignancies
	Endoscopic ultrasound or CT scan	To characterize tumors
Following repair of congenital intestinal atresias	CBC and differential	Early screening tests
	Serum electrolytes	To determine obstruction
	BUN and creatinine	
	Blood culture (if suspected sepsis)	
	Abdominal X-rays	
Associated with gastroschisis	Serial ultrasound	Prenatal testing
	Fetal karyotype	
	Antepartum fetal surveillance	
Chronic intestinal pseudo-obstruction	Abdominal and upper GI	All necessary to confirm diagnosis
	Nutritional assessment (serum electrolytes and albumin)	If no underlying disease, determine underlying neurologic disorder
	Scintigraphy (gastric and small bowel transit test)	
	Manometry	
	Autonomic testing	
	Possible tests	
	■ Intestinal biopsy	
	■ Small bowel aspirate	
Following intestinal transplantation	D-Xylose absorption test	Early study
	Fecal fat determination	Early study
	Endoscopy, biopsy	For mucosal changes
	Magnification endoscopy	
	Bacterial/fungal studies	
Hirschsprung's disease	Contrast enema	All necessary to confirm diagnosis
	Digital rectal exam	
	Detailed anal exam	
	Colonic manometry	

Abbreviations: CT = computerized tomography; CBC = complete blood count; BUN = blood urea nitrogen.

the esophageal body establishes the diagnosis (Figure 19–1B). The LES may also be hypertensive. Endoscopy may demonstrate a distended esophagus, retaining food without any difficulty advancing the scope to the stomach. But scope passage in the distal esophagus is difficult if there is stricture or mass occluding lesion in distal esophagus.[15]

Referral to a specialist should be made at the early onset of symptoms, especially for children with a history of:

■ Down syndrome because of the increased incidence of achalasia and esophageal motility;
■ adrenal insufficiency (association with triple A syndrome);
■ persistent dysphagia;
■ weight loss (Table 19–4).

Treatment

Although the triggering events of primary achalasia remain undetermined, motility abnormality results from a reduction in the number of inhibitory neurons in the esophageal myenteric plexus.[12] Directing treatment of the underlying abnormality would require restoring the damaged neurons of this plexus. As these treatments are not yet available, current treatment is directed at relieving the distal esophageal obstruction in order to allow the passage of food into the stomach by gravity (Table 19–5).

Pneumatic balloon dilation

Dilation in EA, which is meant to rupture the muscle fibers of the LES, carries a significant risk (2–15%) of perforation.[16] While some practitioners report good

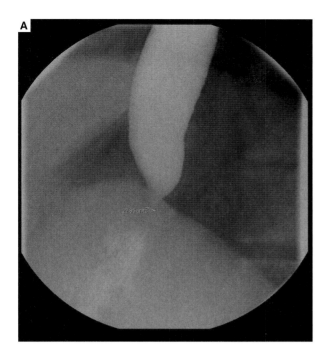

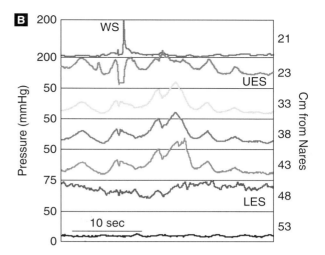

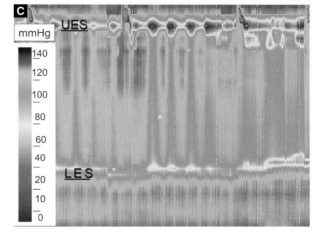

FIGURE 19–1 ■ Achalasia. (A) Contrast esophagram demonstrates typical findings in achalasia: gradual narrowing of the distal esophagus to obstruction at the lower esophageal sphincter. Body of the esophagus is dilated, with retention of contrast, an abnormal contraction pattern, and loss of coordinated peristalsis in the body of the esophagus. (B) Solid state esophageal motility shows a lack of distal progression of contraction waves in the body of the esophagus after a water swallow (WS) and a failure of the lower esophageal sphincter (LES) to relax in response to WS. (C) High-resolution esophageal motility shows no relaxation of the LES.

Table 19–4.

Specialist Referral for Common Motility Disorders

Motility Disorder	Specialist Referral
Esophageal achalasia	Persistent dysphagia with weight loss
	Delayed esophageal emptying on barium swallow
	Early onset of symptoms
	History of Down syndrome, adrenal insufficiency
Following repair of congenital intestinal atresia	Bilious emesis, abdominal distension, poor weight gain
Associated with gastroschisis	Vomiting, poor oral intake, poor growth, abdominal distension
Chronic intestinal pseudo-obstruction	Abdominal distension that limits activities
	Poor growth with dependency on TPN
	Fecal impaction refractory to medical therapy
Following intestinal transplantation	Diarrhea, poor weight gain, abdominal distension, lymphadenopathy, skin rash
Hirschsprung's disease	Fecal incontinence, abdominal distension, straining with stooling, fecal impaction refractory to medical therapy

Abbreviations: TPN = total parenteral nutrition.

Table 19–5.

Surgical, Nutritional, and Pharmacologic Approaches to Treating Common Intestinal Motility Disorders

Motility Disorder	Surgical Approach (Medical Support)	Nutritional Approach	Pharmacologic Approach Medication
Esophageal achalasia	Pneumatic balloon dilation LES myotomy Antireflux procedure		Botulinum toxin Calcium channel blockers Nitrates Phosphodiesterase Inhibitors Nifedipine
Following repair of congenital intestinal atresias	Revision of internal repair	Probiotics	Antimicrobial agents
		Oral feeding, if tolerated Continuous G-tube/J-tube feedings TPN for few weeks	Prokinetics Erythromycin Amoxicillin
Associated with gastroschisis	Surgical closure	Probiotics	Motility agents Bethanecol Antibiotics
Chronic intestinal pseudo-obstruction	Possible	Continuous G-tube/J-tube feedings	
	Ileostomy intestinal transplantation Surgical bypass Gastric/intestinal pacemakers (antegrade enemas)	TPN	
Following intestinal transplantation		Regular screening, monitoring	Anti-rejection medications
			Steroids Antibiotics Anticholinergics
Hirschsprung's disease	Surgical resection	Fiber therapy Structured meals	Anticholinergics

Abbreviations: LES = lower esophageal sphincter; G-tube = gastrostomy tube; J-tube = jejunostomy tube; TPN = total parenteral nutrition.

long-term results, it is difficult to balance the desire to disrupt the circular muscle fibers of the LES with the desire to avoid esophageal perforation, particularly in young small patients. In adults, a graded dilation for 60 seconds using a 30–35-mm balloon to efface the waist created by the LES is generally recommended. Repeated dilations may be needed to maintain symptomatic improvement. Given the need for long-term results in children and the data from some recent studies demonstrating better outcomes with surgical myotomy,[17] dilation is not a primary recommendation in children.

Surgical LES myotomy

Surgical myotomy relieves the LES obstruction by longitudinal transection of the sphincter. Laparoscopic Heller myotomy is comparable in result to the open procedure and has greatly reduced perioperative morbidity. An antireflux procedure, usually a partial-circumference fundoplication wrap using the Toupet technique, reduces GER symptoms and results in less postoperative dysphagia than full-circumference wrap

procedures. Even with this procedure, a significant proportion of patients will experience reflux symptoms and require proton pump inhibitor therapy.

In a large study of adults, Ortiz et al. found that at 1 year, ~97% of patients reported good to excellent results. However, with >15 year follow-up, they found a gradual reduction in the percentage of patients having satisfactory results; at ≥15 years post-procedure, only 75% of patients reported good to excellent results. This reduction in outcome success was primarily due to increased symptoms related to GER. Endoscopic peptic esophagitis developed in 11% of patients, although half of these patients were asymptomatic.[18] These results underline the importance of life-long follow-up in patients with achalasia.

The incidence of long-term complications after laparoscopic myotomy for EA in children is unknown, but persistent dysphagia is reported. Possible causes include incomplete myotomy, esophageal dysmotility, and relative obstruction from a fundoplication or post-surgical fibrosis in the distal esophagus. Evaluation should include a barium esophagram to exclude the presence of anatomic obstruction and to evaluate the emptying of the esophagus. If abnormal esophageal emptying is identified, esophageal manometry should be done to evaluate the effectiveness of the myotomy. Post-surgical LES pressures of <10 mm Hg predict a good long-term clinical response. In patients with persistent dysphagia and persistently elevated LES pressures after laparoscopic myotomy (with or without fundoplication), pneumatic dilations of the distal esophagus are considered, followed by repeat surgical intervention only if this fails. Persistent dysphagia after myotomy is reported. No randomized trials have shown that the performance of intraoperative esophageal manometry improves the outcome of surgical repair of achalasia (Heller myotomy). Algorithm for the management of post-surgical dysphagia is outlined in Figure 19–2.[19]

Pharmacologic approach

Currently available pharmacologic agents are of very limited usefulness in the treatment of EA, and are used only in patients unwilling or unable to undergo other procedures such as surgical myotomy. Agents that are sometimes used include calcium channel blockers, nitrites, and phosphodiesterase inhibitors (Table 19–5). Two small double-blind, placebo-controlled trials of nifedipine in adults with EA demonstrated modest improvements in esophageal manometry, with either no improvement in clinical symptoms or modest improvements in symptoms.[20]

Injecting botulinum toxin A into the LES blocks the release of the excitatory neurotransmitter, acetylcholine, from visceral motor efferent nerve terminals. This reduces the pressure in the LES and allows esophageal emptying. Botulinum toxin injection is a relatively low-risk procedure compared to dilations and surgical interventions and can be repeated in responding patients if the effect wears off.[21] Response to injections may last 6–12 months in responding patients. Patients who do not respond to the initial injections are unlikely to benefit from repeated injections.

MOTILITY DISORDERS FOLLOWING REPAIR OF CONGENITAL INTESTINAL ATRESIAS

Definition and Epidemiology

Congenital intestinal atresia, a narrowing or absence of a section of the intestine, is surgically corrected soon after birth. The likelihood of long-term complications following surgery depends on the associated anomalies (cardiac, genitourinary, and intestinal) and the remaining intestinal length. Despite high morbidity prior to surgery, survival rates are high. However, some children contend with long-term GI complications such as GER and malabsorption.[22]

Pathogenesis

Intestinal atresias are caused by an interruption of the normal development of the GI tract. The mechanism varies depending on the number and location of bowel segments affected. Following surgical repair, the prognosis depends on the length and function of the remaining bowel. Patients with atresias and gastroschisis may be at a high risk for short bowel syndrome. Other dysmotilities include anastomotic dysfunction, GER, malabsorption syndromes, stricture, adhesions, and obstruction.[23]

Clinical Presentation

Most infants with intestinal atresia have surgical repair within the first few days of life. Surgery is often delayed in infants with partial obstruction and delayed symptoms. Motility disorders immediately following surgery

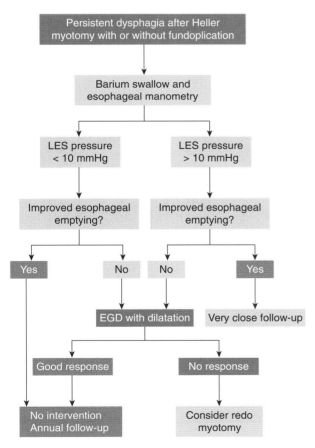

FIGURE 19–2 ■ Algorithm for the management of post-surgical dysphagia.

may result from anastomotic obstruction or leakage and prolonged adynamic ileus (Table 19–1). Adhesive bowel obstruction, GER, and late duodenal dysmotility are considered late complications.

Infants with duodenal atresia may present with stenosis, while colonic atresia is rarely associated with other abnormalities, such as gastroschisis and Hirschsprung's disease. Other intraoperative findings include volvulus, malrotation, and meconium peritonitis.[23]

Differential Diagnosis

Motility disorders following surgery for atresias often mimic short bowel syndrome, a major cause of morbidity and mortality (Table 19–2). This is especially true for infants with duodenal atresia and Down syndrome or for those with concurring severe atresias and gastroschisis. Despite having adequate intestinal length following surgery, some infants may have prolonged adynamic ileus and severely impaired intestinal motility.[24]

Diagnosis

Rarely following surgical correction, a patient experiences intestinal anastomotic leak and requires surgical reintervention. Blood cultures are run to check for sepsis (Table 19–3). After surgery, all children require regular follow-up to ensure adequate growth and development and to monitor nutritional deficiencies due to loss of intestine. Disinterest in feedings is one of the first signs of a mobility disorder. If partial obstruction is suspected, an upper GI contrast X-ray may demonstrate a stenosis of the small bowel, while a barium enema and X-ray will help rule out anomalies of rotation and fixation (Figure 19–3).[25] A specialist is required if symptoms, such as bilious emesis, abdominal distension, and poor weight gain, persist (Table 19–4).

Treatment

Manometry

Takahashi et al. performed antroduodenal manometry on patients after resection of an atretic duodenal segment. They reported low-amplitude contractions in the dilated segment. Several investigators had documented the existence of segmental intestinal muscular and neural[25,42] defects in dilated segments. Khen et al. identified evidence of delayed maturation of the myenteric plexus distal to the atretic segment and suggested that the fetal intestinal obstruction impairs development of the enteric nervous system.[26] Because the dilated segment has generally been identified as the main actor in the dysmotility and because patients often have multiple

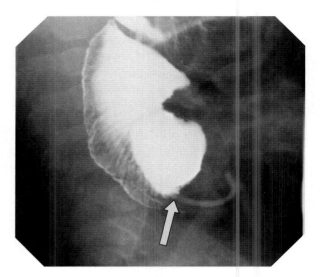

FIGURE 19–3 ■ Upper GI in a patient with duodenal atresia after surgical repair. Abrupt caliber change noted at the junction of the descending and transverse portions of the duodenum; findings are consistent with high-grade but partial duodenal obstruction (closed arrow).

atretic segments, physicians caring for these patients struggle with the risks of leaving in a dilated segment as seen in Figure 19–3, versus the risk of leaving the patient with insufficient gut for nutrient absorption (Figure 19–4). Some have advocated tapering procedures for the dilated segment to balance these risks, while others feel that this is leaving a dysmotile segment

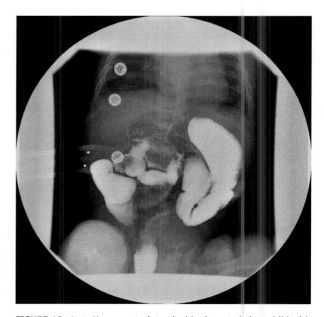

FIGURE 19–4 ■ Upper gastrointestinal barium study in a child with gastroschisis: short gut and prominent small bowel loops with very rapid transit time.

in place and argue for resection. Decisions to taper versus resect are individualized and based on the enteral feeding tolerance and the length of involved intestine (Table 19–5).[25,26]

Nutritional support and pharmacologic approach

Treatments of motility disorders following surgery include probiotics to attempt to prevent bacterial overgrowth and antimicrobial agents (most commonly metronidazole or sulfamethoxazole with trimethoprim) to reduce microbial overgrowth. When oral feedings are not tolerated or unable to support growth, continuous feeding into the stomach may be tolerated. If proximal motility is severely affected, it may be necessary to give jejunal feeds with continuous gastric decompression through a gastrostomy tube. Prokinetic agents, particularly erythromycin, may improve gastric emptying. Amoxicillin with clavulanic acid improves small bowel motility and can facilitate jejunal feedings in severely affected patients. Nutritional support is critical, and parenteral nutrition is frequently needed for a few months.

MOTILITY DISORDERS ASSOCIATED WITH GASTROSCHISIS

Definition and Epidemiology

Gastroschisis is a full-thickness congenital abdominal wall defect that includes para-umbilical herniation of bowel, and may create intestinal atresia. The disorder is rare, occurring in 2.6 infants per 10,000 live births. In a 17-year study by Vu et al. in California, the birth prevalence of gastroschisis increased 3.2-fold, in part due to young nulliparous mothers.[27]

Pathogenesis

The specific nature of motility problems associated with gastroschisis is not well defined. GER disease (GERD) is reported in about half of patients with gastoschisis, and enteral feeding tolerance is delayed.[28,29] Using esophageal manometry, Jadcherla et al. found a failure of pharyngoesophageal peristalsis and adaptive peristaltic reflexes in infants after gastroschisis repair compared to healthy infants. They also found impaired responses in the upper and LES.[28] Gastroschisis is strongly associated with very low maternal age and low maternal body mass index.[30]

Clinical Presentation

Gastroschisis is strongly associated with a high maternal serum alpha fetoprotein (MSAFFP) level in the second

trimester of pregnancy. An ultrasound at this time may detect anatomic abnormalities such as a cauliflower-like, eviscerated bowel. Infants with this disorder generally have significant feeding problems despite surgical repair. These problems are compounded by associated intestinal atresia, ischemia, and resections (Table 19–1).[28,29]

Differential Diagnosis

Gastroschisis may cause prolapse of the intestine and viscera, compounding what appears to be an abdominal wall defect. Up to 25% of infants with gastroschisis have associated GI anomalies including atresia, stenosis, and malrotation, most likely caused by herniation of the bowel (Table 19–2).[31,32] Up to 20% of affected infants may have a severe combination of gastroschisis/atresia/dysmotility. Despite adequate bowel length without obstruction, these children often have severe clinical symptoms of dysmotility.[27]

Diagnosis

Fetuses with gastroschisis are at risk for poor growth development and amniotic fluid abnormalities. Ultrasound examination at 2–4-week intervals enables careful monitoring of the fetus and fetal environment in addition to observing the intestine for complications such as dilatation, thickening, or edema (Table 19–3). If problems are detected, careful fetal monitoring may reduce complications.[33,34] Because gene polymorphisms may play a role in this disorder, fetal karyotyping is recommended.[35] Table 19–4 lists signs and symptoms that would require a specialist referral.

Treatment

Treatment of gastroschisis first should concentrate on adequate nutrient support. Continuous drip feeds are infused into the jejunum by nasojejunal or gastrojejunal feeding tubes. (Table 19–5). Parenteral nutrition is often needed, at least temporarily. Motility agents may be helpful; however, there are little objective data to support their use. Bethanecol can be used to improve esophageal motor function. A multicenter, randomized, double-blind, placebo-controlled trial of enteral erythromycin in infants after repair of uncomplicated gastroschisis failed to show efficacy in reducing the time to full enteral feedings.[36] Antibiotics and probiotics can treat and prevent *bacterial overgrowth* in dilated intestinal segments—a problem that not only interferes with nutrient absorption and enteral feeding tolerance, but can also lead to D-lactic acidosis.[37]

CHRONIC INTESTINAL PSEUDO-OBSTRUCTION

Definition and Epidemiology

CIP is a failure of the intestinal pump due to alteration of the enteric nervous system. The signs and symptoms suggest a bowel obstruction despite evidence to the contrary. Recent etiology studies are lacking, although past studies suggest that 100 infants are born with CIP each year in the United States. The sex ratio shows that more boys than girls are affected.[38]

Pathogenesis

The precise mechanism of CIP is unknown. The disorder may be caused by an impairment of the autonomic nervous system, although there is little evidence to support this theory. The resulting atonic and dilated bowel segment leads to symptoms similar to an obstruction. The disorder may be familial or sporadic, and congenital CIP may result from underlying neuropathic or myopathic pathologies.[39,40] CIP affects both children and adults alike, although the disorder in children is most often congenital (Table 19–6).

Clinical Presentation

Children with CIP may present with overlapping phenotypic features of mitochondrial myopathy, encephalopathy, lactic acidosis, and stroke-like episodes (MELAS) and mitochondrial neurogastrointestinal encephalopathy syndrome (MNGIE) or with different mitochondrial deficiencies (Table 19–1). At present, success of medical treatment in pseudo-obstruction remains limited, and most children with the most severe forms of the disease require parenteral nutrition. CIP is charac-

terized by chronic or repetitive episodes of bowel obstruction in the absence of a lumen-occluding lesion. The disorder often results in intestinal failure and requires life-long medical care.

Differential Diagnosis

Children who have undergone serious medical or surgical conditions or trauma are most likely to develop an autonomic imbalance, resulting in colonic atony and pseudo-obstruction. Colonic ischemia or perforation may follow if an accurate diagnosis is not readily made. Toxic megacolon and mechanical obstruction must be ruled out first, before an accurate CIP diagnosis can be made (Table 19–3).[39]

Diagnosis

Patients with suspected CIP are evaluated based on the presenting symptoms. Imaging studies should be done to rule out mechanical obstruction as suggested in the algorithm in Figure 19–5. On excluding mechanical obstruction, manometric studies should be done to evaluate the severity and map CIP. Manometry will define the pattern of CIP whether myopathic or neuropathic (Figure 19–6B). Abdominal radiographs and an upper GI series will rule out mechanical obstruction and reveal the dilated part(s) if any, as seen in Figure 19–6A. Patients should be monitored for hypokalemia, hypocalcemia, and hypomagnesemia. Serum electrolytes help to assess nutritional status.

Scintigraphy, taken 20 hours apart, evaluates transit through the colon.[41,42] Tests may also be run to rule out neuropathic dysmotility, especially in patients with previous evidence of a given neurologic disorder.[43,44] Abdominal distension-limiting activities, poor growth, or fecal impaction indicate the need for a specialist (Table 19–4).

Treatment

An algorithm of the treatment options for patients with CIP is present in Figure 19–7 and detailed below.

Nutritional support

While total parenteral nutrition (TPN) has extended the lives of infants and children with CIP,[45] complications related to parenteral feeding, including central venous catheter-associated sepsis, cholestasis, central venous thrombosis, and end-stage liver disease, are major contributing factors to CIP mortality and morbidity. However, pediatric patients with CIP may survive to be young adults with partial or full dependency on parenteral nutrition and its systemic complications.

Table 19–6.

General Differences Between Children and Adults with Chronic Intestinal Pseudo-obstruction

Children	Adults
Most primary	Most secondary
Mostly congenital	Mostly acquired
Neuropathy secondary to maturational arrest of plexus	Neuropathy secondary to plexus degeneration
TPN common	TPN rare
Motility predicts response to treatment	Autonomic testing predicts response to treatment
Death due to complications of CIP	Death due to primary disease

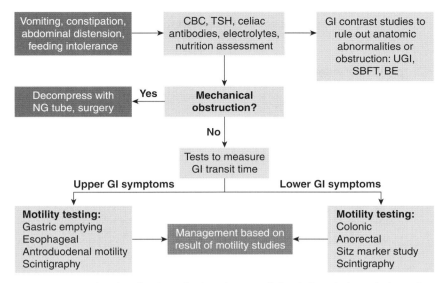

FIGURE 19–5 ■ Flowsheet for the evaluation of suspected chronic intestinal pseudoobstruction.

The management goals of CIP are to restore proper nutrition and fluid balance, relieve symptoms, improve intestinal motility, and treat complications (Table 19–5). When medical management is unsuccessful, decompressing the bowel through a gastrostomy or jejunostomy tube is reported to be the most beneficial intervention for patients with pseudo-obstruction. Gastrostomies and jejunostomies are also used for drip feeding prior to committing to parenteral nutrition. Every patient with pseudo-obstruction should have a trial of jejunal feeding and receive an ileostomy before considering TPN or intestinal transplantation. When constipation is the predominant symptom, use of antegrade enemas through a cecostomy or an appendicostomy may also be beneficial.

Surgical approach

Surgical bypass of diseased segments and loop enterostomies have been shown to benefit carefully selected patients (Table 19–5). The best results occur in rare situations where the disease is limited to an isolated segment of the bowel. Surgical implantation of gastric and intestinal pacemakers aimed at improving motility

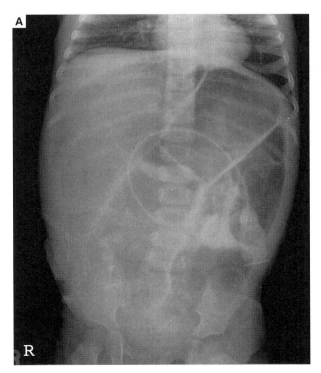

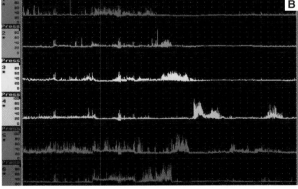

FIGURE 19–6 ■ Chronic intestinal pseudo-obstruction. Plain abdominal X-ray films in a 3-year-old girl with CIP after placement of ileostomy show (A) extremely dilated intestinal loops with gaseous detention and (B) Small bowel manometry showing antegrade retrograde MMC with disorganized migrating motor complex of normal amplitude.

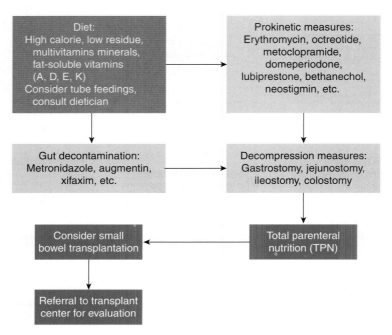

FIGURE 19–7 ■ Flowsheet showing treatment options for chronic intestinal pseudo-obstruction.

constitutes a promising investigational approach in patients with severe motility disorders. Use of the gastric pacemaker has been associated with significant improvement in nausea and vomiting,[46] although, as with gastroparesis, the pacemaker does not improve gastric emptying. Small bowel pacing, still in its infancy, is more challenging due to the length and complex function of the organ to be stimulated.

Total colectomy and ileorectal anastomosis may be considered for patients who have primarily colonic involvement, with clear clinical improvement after ileostomy placement, and who tolerate enteral feeding without exacerbation of CIP symptoms for >2 years. Two-thirds of such patients remain off parenteral nutrition for long periods of time, if not definitively necessary.

Children with GMDs are considered candidates for small bowel transplantation if they are dependent on TPN and have recurrent episodes of sepsis, limited intravenous access, or impending liver failure.

MOTILITY DISORDERS FOLLOWING INTESTINAL TRANSPLANTATION

Definition and Epidemiology

Intestinal transplantation is now considered the standard of care for children with intestinal failure who can no longer tolerate TPN. While survival rates have improved considerably, transplant rejection and surgical complications may occur. According to the Intestinal Transplant Registry, 141 transplants were performed in the United States in 2006, approximately 52% on children aged <1–18 years.[47]

Pathogenesis

Although success of intestinal transplantation has improved since the introduction of immunosuppressive agents, a variety of complications can occur. Despite therapies, the incidence of rejection is high, leading to abdominal pain, distension, impaired absorption, sepsis, and ileus. Graft versus host disease (GVHD) may result in diarrhea and GI ulcerations.[48]

Clinical Presentation

Technical complications to surgery include bleeding, hepatic artery thrombosis, biliary anastomotic leaks, and intra-abdominal or catheter-related sepsis (Table 19–1). Epstein–Barr virus infection or reactivation may result in lymphoproliferative disease.[49]

Following transplantation, patients with dysmotility may have poor intake and lack of appetite, thereby necessitating enteral feeding for many months. Switching from enteral feedings to oral feedings may cause symptoms of achalasia; if so, this disorder was most likely present prior to transplantation. Other transplant-related motility disorders include dumping syndrome, delayed gastric emptying, and recurrent gastric bezoars (accumulation of ingested materials).

Differential Diagnosis

Intestinal transplantation is associated with a high percentage of morbidity and mortality. Motility disturbances, bleeding, thrombosis, and bacterial infections must be watched for as possible signs of graft rejection, and should trigger immediate investigation and intervention (Table 19–2).

Diagnosis

In addition to observing the patient's tolerance of TPN and oral feedings, D-xylose absorption and fecal fat tests are used for early monitoring of intestinal function (Table 19–3). Endoscopy and biopsy determine whether there are activated lymphocytes, crypt injury, inflammation, and increased crypt cell apoptosis and indicate the grade of transplantation rejection. Magnification endoscopy is used to reveal early mucosal changes that may not be visible with standard endoscopy.[50] A specialist should be called if the patient develops symptoms such as diarrhea and poor weight gain (Table 19–4).

Treatment

Transplantation is the only viable option for patients with intractable GMDs who cannot tolerate TPN. Pseudo-obstruction disorders comprised 9% and other motility disorders 2% of the International Intestinal Transplant Registry (children and adults) as of May 2003. In recent years, outcome of small bowel transplantation has improved due to enhanced surgical technique, improved immunosuppressive regimens, and better perioperative care (Table 19–5). Small bowel transplantation should eventually evolve from being a "rescue" procedure to becoming a true therapeutic option.

Pretransplant evaluation in patients with motility disorders should include the evaluation of gastric, intestinal, and colonic functions. Multivisceral transplantation should be done instead of isolated intestinal transplantation whenever the gastric motility is abnormal. After receiving immunosuppressive medications, repeated episodes of urosepsis may occur in patients with bladder dysfunction. Chronic visceral pain may also create a co-morbid condition due to dependency on narcotics.

Studies on dogs undergoing intestinal autotransplantation revealed no extrinsic or reinnervation of the allografted bowel until 12 months postoperatively.[51] All extrinsic reinnervation occurred along the vascular anastomosis; none crossed the intestinal anastomosis. Antroduodenal motility studies performed on patients from 3 to 23 months after they received small bowel transplants found the following: (1) generation of migrating motor complex (MMC) by allograft bowel; (2) dissociation of MMCs across duodenojejunal anastomosis; (3) absence of motility pattern change from interdigestive to the feed pattern after meals; (4) propagation of giant waves from native bowel to allograft; (5) normal feed pattern only with patients who had undergone multivisceral transplantation, including stomach and duodenum; and (6) no MMCs in patients who suffered from exfoliative rejection.[52] It therefore appears that extrinsic innervation of allograft small bowel is not necessary for generation of MMC, and rejection adversely affects motility (Figure 19–8).

Cellular rejection

Acute cellular rejection in the GI tract is a regional process. It can be confined to one anatomic lesion, or it can be spotty in its distribution. The ileum and duodenum appear to be the most commonly involved areas. Acute cellular rejection is divided in three grades: mild (I), moderate (II), and severe (III). Watanabe et al. found that the degree of neuronal loss is closely correlated with the grade of rejection, with 0% loss in mild rejection, 19.3% loss in moderate rejection, and 61% neuronal loss in severe rejection.[53]

In classic chronic rejection, ischemic changes result in focal stricturing and patchy villous atrophy, with patchy intimal fibrosis of submucosal arteries. The obstruction progressively worsens; although initially it may transiently improve with steroids, recurrence usually occurs. Sclerosing peritonitis post-transplantation may also cause vascular changes; frozen bowel with inflammation involves the serosal surface of bowel and peritoneum. Management of post-transplantation dysmotility as a result of either acute or chronic rejection includes regular screening, monitoring, and management of post-transplant signs of dysmotility (Table 19–5). As a screening tool, we follow serum citrulline levels: levels >13 mg/kg have a negative predictive value for moderate or severe rejection of 96% and 99%, respectively. We also follow fecal calprotectin: levels >92 mg/kg detect rejection with a sensitivity of 83% and specificity of 77%.

Pharmacologic approach

Loperamide, clonidine, and octreotide are recommended for hypersecretion; erythromycin or metoclopramide for slow and obstructive symptoms; and alternating metronidazole with amoxicillin–clavulanate for bacterial overgrowth manifestations. After exfoliative rejection, patients may benefit from continuous enteral feedings and elemental feedings. When TPN dependence overtakes the patient, we list patients for retransplant.

A   NATIVE BOWEL

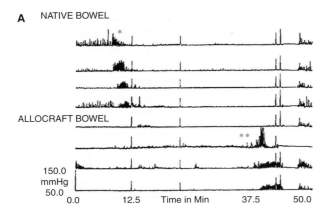

ALLOCRAFT BOWEL

B   NATIVE BOWEL

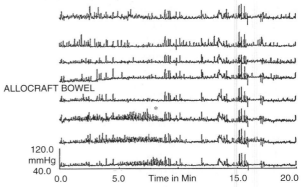

ALLOCRAFT BOWEL

C

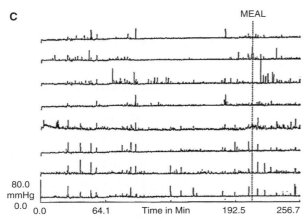

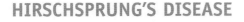

FIGURE 19–8 ■ Small intestinal motility following transplantation. (A) Antroduodenal motility study after small bowel transplantation showing MMC phase III (**) of allograft bowel dissociated in time from native bowel phase III (*). (B) Motility study showing the persistence of phase III after meal (*). (C) Motility study showing long period of motor quiescence after ingestion of meal in a child who had experienced severe acute cellular rejection.

HIRSCHSPRUNG'S DISEASE

Definition and Epidemiology

Hirschsprung's disease is a motor disorder of the colon, whereby the affected segment of the colon fails to relax and causes a functional obstruction. This disease may affect a short segment or the entire colon. According to the American Pediatric Surgical Association, Hirschsprung's disease affects 1 in 4400–7000 live births. As diagnosis and treatments have improved, the resultant mortality rate has dropped from 70% in 1954 to 1% in 2000.[54]

Pathogenesis

Hirschsprung's disease is a multigenic disorder with a complex inheritance. It is noted by the congenital absence of the myenteric and submucosal plexuses for a variable length of distal intestine. The lack of enteric neurons leads to tonic contraction of the aganglionic segment of gut and functional obstruction. Enteric nervous system progenitors colonize the developing gut in a cranial to caudal direction. The disease occurs when these progenitors fail to colonize a distal segment.[17]

Hirschsprung's disease is often associated with other congenital anomalies. It can be familial or sporadic and is generally categorized by the length of involved intestine, with ~75% of cases involving the colon distal to the splenic flexure (short-segment disease), ~20% of cases involving the colon distal to the ileo-cecal junction, and 5% of cases involving the entire colon and rarely involving the small intestine as well.[55]

Clinical Presentation

Typically, Hirschsprung's disease presents as constipation in neonates (Table 19–1). During the first 48 hours of life, 60–90% of children with Hirschsprung's disease fail to pass meconium. Failure to thrive is common. Occasionally the disease is not recognized until the child is older; however, a history of defecation difficulties (chronic constipation) in the neonatal period can almost always be elicited. Patients will also experience signs of intestinal obstruction.[56] Hirschsprung's-associated enterocolitis (HAEC) is a severe and lethal form of the disorder, usually producing explosive, foul-smelling diarrhea, fever, and possibly rectal bleeding and shock. Mild cases of HAEC, however, may be misdiagnosed as gastroenteritis.

Differential Diagnosis

If an accurate diagnosis of Hirschsprung's disease is not made in early infancy, the disorder may present later as enterocolitis or chronic idiopathic constipation (Table 19–2). Both of these conditions, in addition to fecal incontinence or toxic megacolon, are also long-term complications of Hirschsprung's.[57,58]

Diagnosis

Patients with defecation disorders >3 months after resection should generally have a contrast enema, a digital rectal examination, and a detailed exam of the anal canal (Table 19–3; Figure 19–9). Episodes of diarrhea, particularly with feces containing gross or occult blood, should be further evaluated with rectal and colonic biopsies (Table 19–4).

Patients with obstructive symptoms, but without a mechanical lesion on contrast study, should undergo a rectal suction biopsy (RSB) to evaluate the myenteric plexus. RSB is the most accurate test for diagnosing Hirschsprung's, with sensitivity and specificity rates of 93% and 100%, respectively. These numbers are not significantly different from the RSB rates noted with anorectal motility (83% and 93%, respectively). RSB also has the lowest rate of inconclusive test results and provides a histological diagnosis. Figure 19–1 outlines the diagnostic thought process for GMDs.

Distal propagation of high-amplitude propagating contractions

Colonic motility testing is useful for patients in whom the physical exam, contrast study, and biopsy are unrevealing. Colonic manometry can identify high-amplitude propagating contractions (HAPCs) and determine the appropriateness of the internal anal sphincter pressures. The healthy colon produces HAPCs that originate in the proximal colon and sweep distally to the rectosigmoid junction. These contractions are triggered by eating (gastrocolic reflex), are more frequent in children than adults, and do not occur during sleep. Normally, only 14% of HAPCs are propagated to the rectum. When the rectum has been resected, the contractions may move colon content to the anal verge, where pressures within the neorectum exceed the anal sphincter pressure, thereby leading to fecal incontinence. The patient's efforts to avoid incontinence may produce abdominal pain or discomfort. Following resection, some patients may experience more frequent day- and night-time contractions.

Hypomotility

Rarely, colonic manometry will demonstrate weak or ineffective HAPCs in all or part of the ganglion-containing colon of patients with Hirschsprung's. These patients benefit from diversion of the fecal stream and resection of the abnormal segment if the motility abnormality is persistent.

Treatment

Surgical resection

Until methods to repair the enteric nervous system are developed, the first stage of treatment for Hirschsprung's disease is surgical resection of the aganglionic segment (Table 19–5).[59] Unfortunately, a majority of patients will continue to have disordered defecation after this resection and will require careful evaluation. The post-resection defecation disorders are generally categorized as those primarily presenting with fecal incontinence or constipation. Rarely, Hirschsprung's disease is associated with intestinal neuronal dysplasia and CIP.

Incontinence can be the result of abnormal sphincter function or sensation, overflow incontinence from chronic constipation, or the propagation of high-amplitude colonic contractions (HAPCs) through the neorectum to the anal sphincter. Abnormal sphincter function or sensation is generally secondary to damage to the anal canal during the resection procedure. Post-resection enterocolitis may also present with incontinence, though this is usually also associated with diarrhea and abdominal pain. Chronic constipation can be the result of mechanical obstruction, persistent or acquired aganglionosis, absence of HAPCs in the colon, a hypertensive internal anal sphincter, or functional constipation.

Patients experiencing increased contractions may find some relief with fiber therapy, institution of structured meals, and avoidance of between-meal oral intake. Anticholinergic medications can also be very helpful and likely work by reducing the force and frequency of the propagating contractions as well as increasing internal anal sphincter pressures.[60] We usually start with loperamide but have also found amitriptyline and occasionally clonidine to be very useful.

LONG-TERM OUTCOMES

Despite ongoing improvements in nutrition, medical, and surgical therapies, children with severe motility disorders, such as CIP, continue to be plagued by significant morbidity and mortality.[2] Many of these patients receive long-term TPN, resulting in liver disease and sepsis, the most common causes of death.[2] A study of 85 children with congenital CIP by Mousa et al.[1] found a 25% mortality rate at a medium follow-up time of 2 years. Poor prognostic factors include midgut malrotation, short small intestine, urinary system involvement, and myopathy.[61]

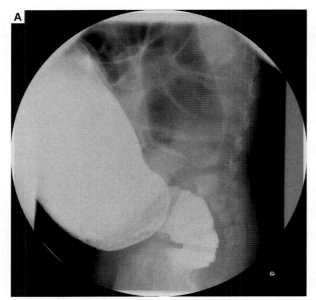

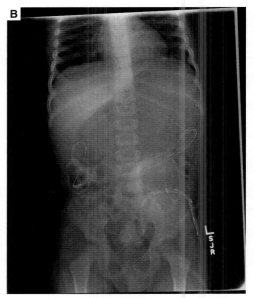

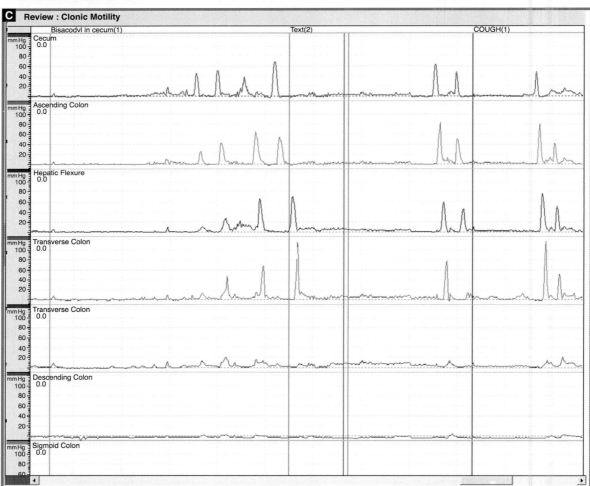

FIGURE 19–9 ■ Hirschsprung's disease. (A) Barium enema prior to pull-through procedure. (B) Placement of colonic motility catheter via colostomy after failed pull-through procedure. (C) Colonic motility study with clear abnormal motility in the distal colon.

While long-term outcomes for children with motility disorders, including their families, are still unclear, overall survival and quality of life are improving due to earlier recognition and aggressive nutritional and medical management.[2] Further studies are needed to define the long-term outcomes of patients with motility disorders.[9]

CONCLUSIONS

In summary, motility disorders represent a spectrum of diseases. Manometric evaluation is valuable in the clinical management of affected children. Classification of GMDs is better understood and managed based on the presenting symptoms and the anatomic involvement. Initial accurate diagnosis and resultant treatment leads to improved quality of life.

REFERENCES

1. Mousa H, Hyman PE, Cocjin J, et al. Long-term outcome of congenital intestinal pseudoobstruction. *Dig Dis Sci.* 2002;47:2298–2305.
2. Connor FL, Di Lorenzo C. Chronic intestinal pseudo-obstruction: assessment and management. *Gastroenterology.* 2006;130:S29–S36.
3. Guze CD, Hyman PE, Payne VJ. Family studies of infantile visceral myopathy: a congenital myopathic pseudo-obstruction syndrome. *Am J Med Genet.* 1999;82:114–122.
4. Srinathan SK, Langer JC, Blennerhassett MG, et al. Etiology of intestinal damage in gastroschisis. III: morphometric analysis of the smooth muscle and submucosa. *J Pediatr Surg.* 1995;25:1122–1126.
5. Simmons M, Georgeson KE. The effect of gestational age at birth on morbidity in patients with gastroschisis. *J Pediatr Surg.* 1996;31:1060–1062.
6. Chitkara D, Nurko S, Shoffner J, et al. Abnormalities in gastrointestinal motility are associated with diseases of oxidative phosphorylation in children. *Am J Gastroenterol.* 2003;98:871–877.
7. Schappi MG, Smith VV, Milla PJ, et al. Eosinophilic myenteric ganglionitis is associated with functional intestinal obstruction. *Gut.* 2003;52:752–755.
8. Hirano M, Silvestri G, Blake DM, et al. Mitochondrial neurogastrointestinal encephalomyopathy (MNGIE)—clinical, biochemical, and genetic features of an autosomal recessive mitochondrial disorder. *Neurology* 1994;44:721–727.
9. Schwankovsky L, Mousa H, Rowhani, A, et al. Quality of life outcomes in congenital chronic intestinal pseudo-obstruction. *Dig Dis Sci.* 2002:47:1965–1968.
10. Rudolph CD, Hyman PE, Altschuler SM, et al. Diagnosis and treatment of chronic intestinal pseudo-obstruction in children: report of consensus workshop. *J Pediatr Gastroenterol Nutr.* 1997;24:102–112.
11. Bohl J, Gockel I, Sultanov F, Eckardt V, Junginger T. Childhood achalasia: a separate entity? *Z Gastroenterol.* 2007;45:1273–1280.
12. Gockel I, Bohl JR, Doostkam S, Eckardt VF, Junginger T. Spectrum of histopathologic findings in patients with achalasia reflects different etiologies. *J Gastroenterol Hepatol.* 2006;21:727–733.
13. Brooks BP, Kleta R, Stuart C, et al. Genotypic heterogeneity and clinical phenotype in triple A syndrome: a review of the NIH experience 2000–2005. *Clin Genet.* 2005;68:215–221.
14. Wallace RA. Clinical audit of gastrointestinal conditions occurring among adults with Down syndrome attending a specialist clinic. *J Intellect Dev Disabil.* 2007;32:45–50.
15. Pohl D, Tutuian R. Achalasia: an overview of diagnosis and treatment. *J Gastrointest Liver Dis.* 2007;16:297–303.
16. Lamb PJ, Griffin SM. Achalasia of the cardia: dilatation or division? The case for balloon dilatation. *Ann R Coll Surg Engl.* 2006;88:9–11.
17. Wang L, Li YM, Li L. Meta-analysis of randomized and controlled treatment trials for achalasia. *Dig Dis Sci.* 2009 Nov;54(11):2303–2311
18. Ortiz A, de Haro LF, Parrilla P, et al. Very long-term objective evaluation of Heller myotomy plus posterior partial fundoplication in patients with achalasia of the cardia. *Ann Surg.* 2008;247:258–264.
19. Pensabene L, Nurko S. Approach to the child who has persistent dysphagia after surgical treatment for esophageal achalasia. *J Pediatr Gastroenterol Nutr.* 2008;47:92–97.
20. Triadafilopoulos G, Aaronson M, Sackel S, Burakoff R. Medical treatment of esophageal achalasia. Double-blind crossover study with oral nifedipine, verapamil, and placebo. *Dig Dis Sci.* 1991;36:260–267.
21. Annese V, Bassotti G, Coccia G, et al. A multicentre randomised study of intrasphincteric botulinum toxin in patients with oesophageal achalasia. GISMAD Achalasia Study Group. *Gut.* 2000;46:597–600.
22. Vecchia LD, Grosfeld J, West K, Rescorla F, Scherer L, Engum S. Intestinal atresia and stenosis: a 25-year experience with 277 cases. *Arch Surg.* 1998;133:490–496.
23. Phillips J, Raval M, Redden C, Weiner T. Gastroschisis, atresia, dysmotility: surgical treatment strategies for a distinct clinical entity. *J Pediatr Surg.* 2008;43: 2208–2212.
24. Werler M, Sheehan J, Mitchell A. Association of vasoconstrictive exposures with risks of gastroschisis and small intestinal atresia. *Epidemiology.* 2003;14:349.
25. Ozguner IF, Savas C, Ozguner M, Candir O. Intestinal atresia with segmental musculature and neural defect. *J Pediatr Surg.* 2005;40:1232–1237.
26. Khen N, Jaubert F, Sauvat F, et al. Fetal intestinal obstruction induces alteration of enteric nervous system development in human intestinal atresia. *Pediatr Res.* 2004;56:975–980.
27. Vu L, Nobuhara K, Laurent C, Shaw G. Increasing prevalence of gastroschisis: population-based study in California. *J Pediatr.* 2008;152:807–811.
28. Jadcherla SR, Gupta A, Stoner E, Fernandez S, Caniano D, Rudolph CD. Neuromotor markers of esophageal motility in feeding intolerant infants with gastroschisis. *J Pediatr Gastroenterol Nutr.* 2008;47:158–164.
29. Lund CH, Bauer K, Berrios M. Gastroschisis: incidence, complications, and clinical management in the neonatal intensive care unit. *J Perinat Neonatal Nurs.* 2007;21:63–68.
30. Siega-Riz A, Herring A, Olshan A, Smith J, Moore C. The joint effects of maternal prepregnancy body mass index and age on the risk of gastroschisis. *Paediatr Perinat Epidemiol.* 2009;23:51–57.

31. Abdullah F, Arnold M, Nabasweesi R, et al. Gastroschisis in the United States 1988–2003: analysis and risk categorization of 4344 patients. *J Perinatol.* 2007;27:50.

32. Houben C, Davenport M, Ade-Ajayi N, Flack N, Patel S. Closing gastroschisis: diagnosis, management, and outcomes. *J Pediatr Surg.* 2009;44:343–347.

33. Santiago-Munoz P, McIntire D, Barber R, Megison S, Twickler D, Dashe J. Outcomes of pregnancies with fetal gastroschisis. *Obstet Gynecol.* 2007;110:663.

34. Netta D, Wilson R, Visintainer P, et al. Gastroschisis: growth patterns and a proposed prenatal surveillance protocol. *Fetal Diagn Ther.* 2007;22:352.

35. Torfs C, Christianson R, Iovannisci D, Shaw G, Lammer E. Selected gene polymorphisms and their interaction with maternal smoking, as risk factors for gastroschisis. *Birth Defects Res A Clin Mol Teratol.* 2006;76:723.

36. Curry JI, Lander AD, Stringer MD. A multicenter, randomized, double-blind, placebo-controlled trial of the prokinetic agent erythromycin in the postoperative recovery of infants with gastroschisis. *J Pediatr Surg.* 2004;39:565–569.

37. Uchida H, Yamamoto H, Kisaki Y, Fujino J, Ishimaru Y, Ikeda H. D-Lactic acidosis in short-bowel syndrome managed with antibiotics and probiotics. *J Pediatr Surg.* 2004;39:634–636.

38. Di Lorenzo C. Pseudo-obstruction: current approaches. *Gastroenterology.* 1999;116:980–987.

39. Saunders M. Acute colonic pseudoobstruction. *Curr Gastroenterol Rep.* 2004;6:410–416.

40. Giorgio RD, Knowles C. Acute colonic pseudo-obstruction. *Br J Surg.* 2009;96:229–239.

41. Faxel A, Verne G. New solutions to an old problem: acute colonic pseudo-obstruction. *J Clin Gastroenterol.* 2005;39:17–20.

42. Camilleri M, Zinsmeister A, Greydanus M, Brown M, Proano M. Towards a costly but accurate test of gastric emptying and small bowel transit. *Dig Dis Sci.* 1991;36:609.

43. Camilleri M. Study of human gastroduodenojejunal motility: applied physiology in clinical practice. *Dig Dis Sci.* 1993;38:785.

44. Camilleri M. Disorders of gastrointestinal motility in neurologic diseases. *Mayo Clin Proc.* 1990;65:825.

45. Connor FL, Di Lorenzo C. Chronic intestinal pseudo-obstruction: assessment and management. *Gastroenterology.* 2006;130:S29–S36.

46. Forster J, Sarosiek I, Delcore R, Lin Z, Raju GS, McCallum RW. Gastric pacing is a new surgical treatment for gastroparesis. *Am J Surg.* 2001;182:676–681.

47. The Intestinal Transplant Registry. www.intestinaltransplant.org, accessed May 8, 2009.

48. Mazariegos G, Abu-Elmagd K, Jaffe R, et al. Graft versus host disease in intestinal transplantation. *Am J Transplant.* 2004;4:1459–1465.

49. Haghighi K, Sharif K, Mirza D, Mayer A, de Ville de Goyet J. Surgical complications of intestinal transplantation. In: *World Transplant Congress*, Boston, MA. *Am J Transplant.* 2006:216.

50. Kato T, Gaynor J, Nishida S, et al. Zoom endoscopic monitoring of small bowel allograft rejection. *Surg Endosc.* 2006;20:773.

51. Sugitani A, Reynolds JC, Tsuboi M, Todo S. Extrinsic intestinal reinnervation after canine small bowel autotransplantation. *Surgery.* 1998;123:25–35.

52. Mousa H, Bueno J, Griffiths J, et al. Intestinal motility after small bowel transplantation. *Transplant Proc.* 1998;30:2535–2536.

53. Watanabe T, Hoshino K, Tanabe M, et al. Correlation of motility and neuronal integrity with a focus on the grade of intestinal allograft rejection. *Am J Transplant.* 2008;8:529–536.

54. The American Pediatric Surgical Association. *Hirschsprung's Disease*; 2009 [accessed at http://www.eapsa.org/parents/resources/hirschsprungs.cfm].

55. Imseis E, Gariepy CE. Hirschsprung disease. In: Kleinman R, Goulet O, Miele-Vergani G, Sanderson I, Sherman P, Shneider B, eds. *Pediatric Gastrointestinal Disease: Pathophysiology, Diagnosis, and Management.* 5th ed. Hamilton, Ontario: B.C. Decker Inc.; 2008:683–691.

56. Singh SJ, Croaker GD, Manglick P, et al. Hirschsprung's disease: the Australian Paediatric Surveillance Unit's experience. *Pediatr Surg Int.* 2003;19:247–250.

57. Dasgupta R, Langer J. Evaluation and management of persistent problems after surgery for Hirschsprung disease in a child. *J Pediatr Gastroenterol.* 2008;46:13.

58. Martucciello G. Hirschsprung's disease, one of the most difficult diagnoses in pediatric surgery: a review of the problems from clinical practice to the bench. *Eur J Pediatr Surg.* 2008;18:140–149.

59. Haricharan RN, Georgeson KE. Hirschsprung disease. *Semin Pediatr Surg.* 2008;17:266–275.

60. Sun WM, Read NW, Verlinden M. Effects of loperamide oxide on gastrointestinal transit time and anorectal function in patients with chronic diarrhoea and faecal incontinence. *Scand J Gastroenterol.* 1997;32:34–38.

61. Heneyke S, Smith W, Spitz L, et al. Chronic intestinal pseudoobstruction: treatment and long term follow up of 44 patients. *Arch Dis Child.* 1999; 81:21–27.

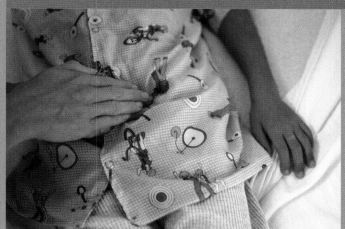

CHAPTER 20

Short Bowel Syndrome

Riad M. Rahhal

DEFINITIONS AND EPIDEMIOLOGY

Short bowel syndrome (SBS) is a disorder of malabsorption resulting from significant small bowel loss secondary to congenital disease or surgical resection. The incidence of SBS is estimated at 1200 per 100,000 live births.[1] SBS is the most common cause of *intestinal failure*. This is defined as a significant reduction in functional small bowel mass, leading to inadequate digestion and absorption, with subsequent growth failure. Other less common causes of intestinal failure include structural enterocyte defects and severe disorders of intestinal motility.[2]

At birth, the estimated small bowel length is approximately 250 cm for term or near-term infants and approximately 100–120 cm for premature infants <30 weeks gestation. Small bowel length is thought to double in the last trimester of pregnancy. Different systems have been used to describe SBS including those based on etiology, age, and anatomical considerations. In the context of surgical resection, the remaining small bowel length is often used to categorize disease severity. In a short resection, >100–150 cm of small bowel remains, compared to 40–100 cm with a large resection and <40 cm remaining after a massive resection.[2]

The small bowel has considerable adaptive capacity to compensate for intestinal loss. *Intestinal adaptation* is defined as a growth process of the remaining small bowel, through morphological and functional changes, leading to improved absorption. This process starts shortly after bowel loss but often continues for months to years. Depending on the segment and length of the lost small bowel, patients with SBS are frequently dependent on parenteral nutrition for prolonged periods of time, sometimes indefinitely. The use of parenteral nutrition has significantly improved the life expectancy

of children with SBS. On the other hand, long-term parenteral nutrition can be associated with a variety of complications, some of which can have grave consequences. Patients with SBS who fail medical therapy or develop complications may require surgical interventions, including transplantation. Because of the relatively high mortality, SBS is considered among the most lethal disorders in young children.[3]

PATHOGENESIS

The small bowel is a vital organ involved in digestion, absorption, and fluid balance. The small bowel is divided into three anatomical segments (Figure 20–1). The first is the *duodenum*, which extends from the pylorus to the duodenojejunal junction, defined by the ligament of Treitz. The proximal half of the remaining small intestine is composed of *jejunum* and the distal portion is *ileum*. Some absorption takes place in the duodenum,

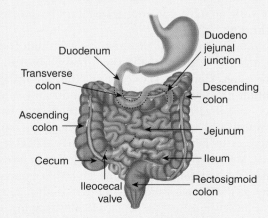

FIGURE 20–1 ■ Normal gastrointestinal anatomy.

including that of iron. The main function of the duodenum is to neutralize acidic gastric contents and mix them with intestinal, pancreatic, and hepatic digestive secretions. Absorption mostly takes place in the jejunum and ileum. The jejunum has an abundant surface area enhanced by folds and numerous tall villi. The luminal surface of enterocytes, or intestinal epithelial cells, is in turn covered with finger-like projections termed *microvilli*, which are collectively referred to as the *brush border*. Villi become shorter and less abundant in the ileum, which therefore has less absorptive surface area than the jejunum. The center of each villus is occupied by a capillary network that absorbs nutrients which are eventually transported to the liver by the portal venous system. The terminal ileum has a high concentration of lymphoid tissue that assists in immune regulation. The terminal ileum also has site-specific receptors for absorption of bile acids and vitamin B_{12}. The ileocecal valve, separating the ileum from the proximal colon, slows the movement of fluid into the cecum and limits bacterial migration from the colon into the small bowel.[4]

During embryonal development, the small intestine arises from the midgut, which extends from the mid-duodenum to the distal transverse colon. The duodenum has an extensive blood supply derived from the celiac axis and the superior mesenteric artery. This dual blood supply helps avoid ischemia if the supply from one of the major vessels becomes compromised. The remainder of the midgut, extending from the jejunum to the proximal two-thirds of the transverse colon, depends on blood supply from branches of the superior mesenteric artery. Therefore, extensive bowel loss can result from compromise of the superior mesenteric arterial blood flow. The midgut drains through the superior mesenteric vein, which joins the splenic vein in forming the portal vein.[4] About 70–80% of blood entering the liver is venous blood from the portal vein, and the remainder is arterial blood supplied by the hepatic artery. This is important as small bowel disease can have a significant negative impact on the liver with possible bacterial translocation and liver dysfunction.

Major physiologic disturbances can result from loss of large sections of the small bowel absorptive surface area. Consequences especially include malabsorption of fluid, electrolytes, macronutrients (proteins, carbohydrates, and fats), and micronutrients (vitamins and trace elements). In general, jejunal resections are better tolerated than is loss of ileal segments. When a significant portion of jejunum is lost, intestinal adaptation of the ileum can compensate for many of the jejunal functions. Certain jejunal functions, however, cannot be replaced, including loss of enteric hormone production (such as cholecystokinin

and motilin) that affects intestinal motility and digestion. Loss of jejunum is often accompanied by decreasing biliary and pancreatic secretions and increased gastrin levels, leading to gastric hypersecretion. Major ileal resections can reduce absorption of fluid, electrolytes, bile acids, and vitamin B_{12}. These functions cannot be taken over by the remaining jejunum. Bile acids, excreted into the duodenum by the liver, are required for the absorption of long-chain fatty acids and fat-soluble vitamins in the ileum. Loss of bile acids may therefore contribute to diarrhea by worsening fat malabsorption. Vitamin B_{12} binds to intrinsic factor, which is produced in the stomach, and the complex is subsequently absorbed in the terminal ileum. Bile acid and vitamin B_{12} absorption cannot be replaced by the jejunum. The ileocecal valve plays an important role in slowing intestinal transit to allow more time for absorption. The absence of the ileocecal valve, in addition to reducing transit time, can also lead to small bowel bacterial overgrowth (SBBO) from colonization by colonic bacteria. SBBO can result in mucosal injury and worsening diarrhea.[5] The colon, if present, can play an important role in absorbing water, sodium, and short-chain fatty acids in SBS patients. A summary of possible consequences of loss of specific intestinal segments is presented in Table 20–1.

In children, the causes of SBS are variable and can be classified by the age at the time of intestinal loss (Table 20–2).[3,5,6] The outcome will depend on the length and functionality of the remaining small bowel. Other contributing factors include the presence or absence of the ileocecal valve and colon, and associated complications, especially liver disease.

Table 20–1.

Possible Consequences of Specific Intestinal Resections

- Loss of duodenum
    - Iron malabsorption
- Loss of jejunum
    - Calcium malabsorption
    - Folate malabsorption
    - Fat-soluble vitamin malabsorption
    - Gastric hypersecretion
- Loss of ileum
    - Bile acid malabsorption
    - Vitamin B_{12} malabsorption
- Loss of the ileocecal valve
    - Small bowel bacterial overgrowth
    - Increased fluid and electrolyte losses

Table 20–2.

Causes of Short Bowel Syndrome in Children

- Prenatal/neonatal period
  - Intestinal atresia
  - Midgut or segmental volvulus
  - Gastroschisis
  - Omphalocele
  - Necrotizing enterocolitis
  - Extensive Hirschsprung's following resection
- Postnatal period
  - Midgut volvulus
  - Mesenteric infarction
  - Trauma
  - Crohn's disease requiring resection
  - Radiation enteritis
  - Intestinal tumor

CLINICAL PRESENTATION

History

A thorough review of the past medical and surgical history is essential. Children with SBS often have an obvious event or events that lead to bowel loss. Frequently noted causes include a major congenital anomaly such as gastroschisis or intestinal atresia, or the occurrence of an abdominal catastrophe such as midgut volvulus or extensive bowel resection after necrotizing enterocolitis (Table 20–2). Occasionally, patients may undergo large or multiple intestinal resections from Crohn's disease or extensive Hirschsprung's disease. Inquiring about the underlying etiology of SBS is important, because it can shed light on the portion of small bowel affected and the functionality of the remaining bowel. Other important historical aspects include the remaining length and segment of small bowel, the presence of an ileocecal valve and colon, and the continuity of the remaining bowel (versus presence of ostomies). These can be based on a thorough review of the surgical records and direct discussions with the surgical service.

It is critical to perform a thorough nutritional assessment. History of previous and current nutritional intake and tolerance should be obtained. Patients with SBS are typically on total or near-total parenteral nutrition through a central venous line. Most are receiving little to no enteral nutrition shortly after the event that leads to bowel loss. For parenteral nutrition, the amount of intravenous dextrose, amino acids, and lipids as well as the electrolyte, multivitamin, and trace element solutions should be determined. For enteral nutrition, the type (breast milk versus formula), caloric density, total volume, and mode (continuous versus bolus, oral versus tube feeding) of feedings should be known. Caloric intake should be assessed separately for parenteral and enteral nutrition. The aim of therapy is to gradually increase the caloric intake from enteral nutrition and decrease that from the parenteral route while maintaining appropriate growth and development.

Previous and current central line access should be reviewed. Any previous history of central line thrombosis or infection should be obtained, including causative organisms and related clinical complications. Frequent line infections requiring line changes can raise concern about line care quality, intestinal bacterial translocation, worsening-associated liver disease, and limited long-term vascular access. This complication can lead to adjustments in central line care and the feeding regimen, as well as earlier consideration for other surgical interventions, including transplantation.

The clinical symptoms associated with SBS can vary but often include diarrhea, weight loss or poor growth, fatigue, and lethargy. These symptoms arise from underlying dehydration, electrolyte abnormalities, and calorie and nutrient deficiencies. Stool output will be higher in children with SBS because of limited absorptive surface even with only partial enteral feeding. Worsening diarrhea can imply reaching or going beyond the maximum absorptive capacity of the remaining bowel. Diarrhea can also be seen with SBBO, which is common among SBS patients. A history of recurrent abdominal distention, foul-smelling stools, and flatulence should alert the managing physician to possible SBBO, especially when the ileocecal valve has been resected, allowing retrograde contamination of the small intestine with colonic contents. Weight loss or poor growth suggests inadequate caloric intake, and should lead to adjustments in the nutritional management. Certain vitamin and other micronutrient deficiencies can lead to specific symptoms that should be recognized and treated promptly (see Table 8–6).

Liver disease can affect 40–60% of infants receiving prolonged parenteral nutrition. The presence of liver disease, especially cholestasis, significantly worsens the outcome of children with SBS.[7] The history should therefore include an assessment for possible liver disease and related complications including portal hypertension, history of gastrointestinal bleeding, and signs of fat malabsorption.

PHYSICAL EXAMINATION

Accurate weight and height measurements are needed. The presence of temporal wasting, loss of muscle mass and subcutaneous fat, poor dentition, and peripheral edema suggest severe protein and energy malnutrition.

Other general features of malnutrition include dry skin, prominent nail ridges, and blunted lingual papillae.

Patients can have physical findings and symptoms related to specific micronutrient deficiencies. *Essential fatty acid deficiency* (linoleic acid and linolenic acid) may occur, manifesting as growth retardation, dermatitis, and alopecia. Patients with SBS and cholestasis should be closely monitored clinically and biochemically for fat-soluble vitamin deficiency (A, D, E, and K). *Vitamin A deficiency* is associated with significant ocular impairment. Vitamin A absorption and metabolism can also be impaired by underlying zinc deficiency. Signs of zinc deficiency include poor growth and wound healing, diarrhea, alopecia, and angular stomatitis. Manifestations of *vitamin E deficiency* can include ocular palsy, wide-based gait, and decreased deep tendon reflexes. The presence of ecchymoses, purpura, or bleeding diatheses should raise concern about vitamin K deficiency. *Vitamin D deficiency* is associated with rickets and osteomalacia. Biochemically, vitamin D-deficient patients can have hypocalcemia, hypophosphatemia, and elevated alkaline phosphatase levels.

Patients with significant resections of the distal ileum are at high risk of developing *vitamin B_{12} deficiency*. Deficiency in vitamin B_{12} (cobalamin) can result in megaloblastic anemia and demyelination. *Folic acid deficiency* can lead to megaloblastic anemia, neutropenia, and impaired growth. Iron deficiency can present with pallor, fatigue, spooned nails, and glossitis. In general, micronutrient deficiencies are uncommon occurrences with parenteral nutrition and are more likely to develop once parenteral nutrition is discontinued, as intestinal absorption may be suboptimal.

Physical signs of associated liver disease can include jaundice, scleral icterus, excoriations secondary to pruritis, splenomegaly, ascites, and poor growth. Abdominal distention and tympany may suggest SBBO from colonic bacterial translocation into the small bowel or from intestinal strictures following surgery.

DIFFERENTIAL DIAGNOSIS

Because children with SBS usually have a specific event leading to bowel loss or resection, the diagnosis is rarely confused with other conditions. However, some patients may have a long history of multiple enterectomies leading eventually to SBS, such as patients with small bowel Crohn's disease. Common symptoms in SBS patients, such as diarrhea and lack of growth, can be exacerbated by other factors, including gastrointestinal and extraintestinal infections, SBBO, intestinal strictures, loss of bowel function (despite reasonable remaining bowel length), dysmotility, and Munchausen by proxy. These possibilities should be investigated and addressed appropriately.

DIAGNOSIS

The diagnosis of SBS can be confirmed based on the surgical records that indicate the scope of bowel resection and the length of the remaining small bowel. Upper GI and small bowel contrast imaging can assist in determining the extent of the remaining bowel. Occasionally endoscopic evaluation with esophagogastroduodenoscopy and colonoscopy may help define the anatomy of the remaining bowel. The serum level of citrulline, an amino acid mainly produced by enterocytes, has been used as a quantitative biomarker to assess the remaining functional absorptive capacity. Reduced plasma citrulline levels are suggestive of intestinal failure.[8] A level ≥19 mmol/L has been postulated to predict achieving enteral autonomy in children with SBS.[9] Clinically, failure to tolerate enteral nutrition, with diarrhea and growth retardation despite having near-normal bowel length, may indicate dysfunction of the present bowel with intestinal failure.

Associated liver disease should be suspected based on biochemical tests including bilirubin and transaminase levels. Cholestasis is defined as a conjugated bilirubin level that is ≥20% of the total bilirubin. Many studies have used a conjugated bilirubin level of >2 mg/dL to report on parenteral nutrition-associated cholestasis. Hepatic synthetic function can be evaluated by serum albumin and prothrombin time, although these tests can be affected by the overall nutritional status. The gold standard for diagnosing liver disease is by liver biopsy. Histologic liver abnormalities can vary and include canalicular and intralobular cholestasis, steatosis, periportal inflammation, bile duct proliferation, portal fibrosis, and cirrhosis.

TREATMENT

Immediately after bowel loss, total parenteral nutrition is required until bowel function returns. The main challenge shortly after bowel resection is maintaining proper fluid balance. Once significant fluid and electrolyte losses are reduced, enteral feedings should be initiated. Depending on the severity, full enteral nutrition may be achieved within weeks to months. However, in some cases it is never achieved. It is important that every patient be given as much enteral nutrition as possible to facilitate the process of intestinal adaptation that leads to bowel growth and increased nutrient absorption, and diminishes the potentially hepatotoxic effects of parenteral nutrition.

Treatment of children with SBS involves a multidisciplinary approach engaging the pediatrician or family physician and an experienced center with pediatric gastroenterologists, nutritionists, speech and behavioral therapists, pediatric surgeons, and care coordinators. Insuring psychosocial support for the child and the family is essential. Proper education of the family about the management and expectations during the different phases of care should be provided.

Venous Nutrition

Parenteral nutrition is the mainstay of treatment for SBS. Its components include carbohydrate, protein, lipids, electrolytes, vitamins, and trace minerals. Parenteral nutrition should be individualized based on the child's caloric needs, nutritional status, and laboratory testing. The assistance of a dietitian and pharmacist can be vital in the management of parenteral nutrition. Estimated energy requirements by age are provided in Table 8–4. Most children may have been already on parenteral nutrition prior to the resection. Table 20–3 provides formulas to assist with calculations for components of parenteral nutrition. For patients who have not been started on parenteral nutrition, the following section may provide some guidelines.

The carbohydrate component is supplied as dextrose. Most infants will be euglycemic on an initial glucose infusion rate (GIR) of 5–8 mg/kg/minute that can be gradually increased to about 14 mg/kg/minute. A GIR of 12–14 mg/kg/minute is usually well tolerated in older children. Infusion rates in excess of 20 mg/kg/minute can promote fatty liver infiltration and should be avoided. A dextrose 12.5% solution should not be exceeded when using a peripheral intravenous line. With central lines, dextrose solutions as high as 25% can be gradually attained. Advancement in dextrose concentration by 2.5% increments per day in infants and 5% increments per day in older children is generally well tolerated. Monitoring serum glucose levels

with changing dextrose concentrations and/or infusion rates is important to identify and address significant fluctuations.

In the young infant, amino acid content can be started at 0.5–1 g/kg/day and then increased by increments of 0.5 g/kg/day to a target of 2.5–3 g/kg/day. In older children, amino acid content can be provided directly at the intended goal.

Intravenous lipids have the highest caloric density in parenteral nutrition and are important to avoid essential fatty acid deficiency when enteral intake is very limited. In infants, intravenous lipids can be started at 0.5 g/kg/day using a 20% solution and then increased by increments of 0.5 g/kg/day to a maximum of 3 g/kg/day. In older children, initial infusions at 1 g/kg/day can be used with target goals depending on age. Typically no more than 30–40% of total daily calories should come from lipids. Serum triglycerides should be monitored to insure lipid clearance from the circulation. Serum triglyceride levels are best checked 4 hours after the start of the fat infusion. Reductions in intravenous lipid delivery should be considered if serum triglyceride levels approach 250 mg/dL. Providing intravenous lipids over 20 hours/day has also been suggested to facilitate lipid clearance.

A pediatric formulation of trace elements should be provided in parenteral nutrition that includes zinc, copper, manganese, chromium, and selenium. Levels of these trace elements should be monitored. In the setting of established cholestasis, increased serum copper and manganese levels should be addressed as they are primarily liver excreted and may worsen liver disease. This should include a reduction in the copper content and an elimination of manganese from parenteral nutrition.[10] If removed or reduced, serum copper levels should still be followed to avoid copper deficiency that can lead to neutropenia and hypochromic anemia.[11] Monitoring for zinc deficiency is important; however, the optimal test remains unknown. Serum zinc only measures albumin-bound zinc and may not accurately assess total-body stores. In the setting of a low or low-normal serum zinc level and a low alkaline phosphatase level, zinc deficiency should be seriously considered and supplementation, either parenteral or enteral, should be started.[10]

Complications related to the use and changes in parenteral nutrition should be monitored including hypo-or hyperglycemia, electrolyte abnormalities, refeeding syndrome, and liver disease. Central line complications can be associated with significant morbidity and mortality and include infections, phlebitis, thrombosis, pulmonary embolism, and line occlusion. Suspected line infections should be treated aggressively with intravenous antibiotics until blood culture results with organism susceptibilities are available. The onset of fever, worsening cholestasis, hyperglycemia, acidosis,

Table 20–3.

Calculations for Parenteral Nutrition Components

Macronutrient content

GIR (mg/kg/minute) = [(% dextrose solution) × (total volume, mL)]/[(weight, kg) × 144]

Intravenous protein intake (g/kg/day) = [(% amino acid solution) × (total volume, mL)]/[100 × (weight, kg)]

Intravenous lipid intake (g/kg/day) = [(% lipid solution) × (total volume, mL)]/[100 × (weight, kg)]

Caloric intake

Calories from non-lipid components: [(3.4 × % dextrose solution) + (4 × % amino acid solution)]/100

Calories from lipid component: 2 kcal/mL for 20% lipid solution thrombocytopenia, and feeding intolerance should raise suspicion for a possible central line infection. Central lines should be handled with an aseptic technique to avoid infection. Lines impregnated with antibiotics or silver, or the use of antibiotic or ethanol locks, have been proposed to reduce bacterial colonization or treat persistent line infections.[12,13] As enteral nutrition is advanced, parenteral nutrition should be weaned with the ultimate goal of total discontinuation and central line removal.

Enteral Nutrition

Enteral nutrition should be initiated as soon as possible to start the process of intestinal adaptation, to stimulate gastrointestinal secretions and enhance production of trophic hormones. When enteral feeds are started, cycling parenteral nutrition over 12–20 hours may help alleviate liver dysfunction and allow more freedom for the child and family. The initiation and advancement of enteral nutrition by itself plays a pivotal role in reducing the frequency of associated liver disease.

There is no consensus on the optimal type or mode of enteral nutrition. Lactose-free formulas are usually preferred to avoid consequences of lactose malabsorption. Many centers utilize hydrolyzed or amino acid-based formulas to enhance intestinal absorption and address concerns about antigenic load related to gut inflammation and disruption in the mucosal barrier.[14] On the other hand, other centers use breast milk or polymeric formulas. Breast milk can provide trophic factors that promote intestinal growth. Use of polymeric formulas may enhance intestinal adaptation more than elemental formulas. Medium-chain triglyceride (MCT)-rich formulas or supplements are commonly used in the setting of cholestasis to enhance fat absorption and improve growth. MCTs can be better absorbed because they are not dependent on bile flow. It is important to note that MCTs do not provide essential fatty acids, so prolonged use of exclusive MCT formulas may lead to essential fatty acid deficiency.

Continuous tube feeds (nasogastric or gastrostomy) are often utilized initially. This allows for continuous saturation of the intestinal transporters to enhance absorption.[15] Subsequently, feeds can be adjusted to allow frequent small-volume boluses (orally or by feeding tube) during the day with continuous tube feeds at night. In general, enteral feeds are started using a non-concentrated formula given at a low rate. The caloric density and formula volume can be gradually advanced depending on feeding tolerance and stool output. Many children with SBS may have feeding difficulties with oral aversion and would benefit from early consultation with a behavioral feeding specialist. Even if a continuous feeding regimen is chosen, an oral stimulation program should be instituted early. Trails with age-appropriate solid food orally should not be withheld. Beverages rich in simple carbohydrates (such as juices) should be limited and preferably eliminated to avoid osmotic diarrhea.[16]

As enteral feeds are being advanced, children with SBS should be monitored for increasing stool output, dehydration, electrolyte abnormalities, and perineal dermatitis. Although there is no consensus on the acceptable upper limit of stool output, many centers use 40–50 mL/kg/day. Other commonly used contraindications to advancement of enteral nutrition include an increase in stool output by >50% in 24 hours, stool pH <5.5, and strongly positive stool test for reducing substances.[17] Fecal-reducing substances >1% and fecal pH <5.5 usually indicate severe carbohydrate malabsorption. The presence of significant perineal dermatitis may also be a sign of a very high stool output.

Micronutrients

Fat malabsorption may be a significant problem in SBS patients with cholestasis. Supplementation with fat-soluble vitamins is needed to avoid or treat deficiencies associated with impaired fat absorption. Vitamin deficiency is not usually a problem when receiving parenteral nutrition as these vitamins are delivered directly into the bloodstream. Once a child with SBS has reached full enteral feeds and is off parenteral nutrition, adequacy of micronutrient absorption becomes a concern, so levels of vitamins, iron, magnesium, and zinc should be followed. Recommendations on micronutrient supplementation are presented in Table 8–16. Further dose adjustments may be needed based on serum vitamin levels. Fat-soluble vitamins can be continued for about 3 months after resolution of cholestasis, as normal bile flow may be delayed. Children who have lost a substantial portion of their distal ileum will require vitamin B_{12} supplementation. It can take several years for a vitamin B_{12} deficiency to develop, so regular long-term monitoring is needed. Appropriate vitamin B_{12} levels can be achieved by monthly injections. Other modes of vitamin B_{12} supplementation include intranasal applications and high oral doses. In humans, the essential fatty acids are linoleic acid and linolenic acid. In essential fatty acid deficiency, the trienoic:tetraenoic ratio can be measured, usually rising above 0.2. Normally, essential fatty acid deficiency can be avoided by providing premature infants with 0.6–0.8 g/kg/day and older children with 0.5–1 g/kg/day of intravenous lipids.

Supplements that may enhance intestinal adaptation (glutamine, growth hormone, and glycogen-like peptide) or slow intestinal transit (increased fiber intake) have been studied. Their benefits have not been confirmed, so they are occasionally used.[3]

Diarrhea

Diarrhea occurs commonly in SBS patients and can be from a combination of increased secretions, increased motility, and malabsorption. Other contributing factors include SBBO syndrome and gastric hypersecretion. Diarrhea can be initially controlled by restricting enteral intake, which reduces the osmotic component. Gastric hypersecretion can be addressed by use of an H2 receptor antagonist or a proton pump inhibitor, especially in the first few months after intestinal resection. Loperamide hydrochloride (Imodium) may be used to decrease stool frequency. Codeine and diphenoxylate hydrochloride (Lomotil) may also help slow the intestinal motility, but can be associated with side effects, including addiction, and can worsen bacterial overgrowth. Cholestyramine (Questran), a bile salt-binding resin, can be used to bind bile salts in patients with bile salt malabsorption.

Small Bowel Bacterial Overgrowth

As mentioned above, SBBO should be suspected in patients with worsening diarrhea, foul-smelling stools, flatulence, abdominal distention, and cramps. The diagnosis is often made based on clinical grounds and response to enteral antibiotic therapy. Confirmation (which is seldom necessary) requires a quantitative culture of aspirated small bowel fluid. The presence of $\geq 10^5$ colony-forming units of non-pharyngeal bacteria on culture is supportive of the diagnosis. Treatment of SBBO can resolve the presenting symptoms and also minimize bacterial translocation across the intestinal mucosa and resultant bacteremia. Antibiotics are often given in cycles of 5–10 days at the beginning of every month. In some patients, continuous alternating antibiotic cycles may be necessary to avoid development of resistant bacteria. Antibiotic choices include enteral metronidazole, gentamicin, neomycin, rifaximin, and trimethoprim-sulfamethoxazole.

Associated Liver Disease

Prolonged use of parenteral nutrition has been implicated in the development of cholelithiasis, cholestasis, and steatosis. Transient elevations of liver tests can be observed early with parenteral nutrition; however, with prolonged use, significant liver dysfunction can occur, with cholestasis progressing to cirrhosis and liver failure. Risk factors predisposing SBS patients to liver dysfunction include prolonged use of parenteral nutrition, reduced intestinal length, bacterial overgrowth, and interruption of the intrahepatic circulation after ileal resection. Other factors may include manganese and copper toxicity. Both of these metal ions are mainly eliminated with bile and can accumulate in the liver during cholestasis, possibly contributing to the liver injury.

A conjugated bilirubin level >2 mg/dL is often used to define parenteral nutrition-associated cholestasis.[18] Progressively worsening cholestasis has been associated with increased mortality. One report associated a conjugated bilirubin level of >4 mg/dL for at least 6 months after bowel resection with a 78% risk of mortality.[19] In fact, parenteral nutrition-associated liver disease with subsequent liver failure is a leading cause of death in patients with SBS.[20,21] In the absence of irreversible liver damage, liver tests tend to return to normal within 1–4 months after discontinuing parenteral nutrition.

Several strategies can be employed to prevent or treat parenteral nutrition-associated cholestasis. These include early introduction and advancement of enteral feeds, cycling and weaning parenteral nutrition, management of SBBO, and rapid and aggressive treatment of sepsis. It is very important to initiate enteral feedings whenever possible. Even small-volume trophic feeds can improve intestinal motility, reduce bacterial translocation, and improve bile flow. Restriction of manganese and copper intake in parenteral nutrition to avoid toxic hepatic accumulation should be considered.[22]

Intravenous lipid solutions have been implicated in liver dysfunction. Currently available lipid solutions in the United States are derived from soybean or soybean–safflower oil, and are rich in ω-6 fatty acids. There is increasing evidence that substituting soybean-based with fish oil-based lipid solutions (rich in ω-3 fatty acids) may reverse parenteral nutrition-associated cholestasis.[23,24] Cycling parenteral nutrition (providing the infusion over <24 hours/day) is thought to reduce hepatic complications. When cycling is performed over short periods, patients should be monitored for fluctuations in glucose levels. Advancing and tapering the infusion over 1 or 2 hours may avoid such fluctuations. Ursodeoxycholic acid, a naturally occurring hydrophilic bile acid, is often used to stimulate bile flow and displace toxic bile acids. Ursodeoxycholic acid at 20–30 mg/kg/day can be provided in two or three divided doses. In cases of advanced liver disease, intestinal or combined intestinal–liver transplantation may be the only life-saving alternative.

Pruritis, which is associated with reduced bile flow, can be a prominent symptom and difficult to treat. Available options include soothing topical creams and oral medications such as antihistamines, rifampin, phenobarbital, cholestyramine, and ursodeoxycholic acid. Further discussion on pruritus treatment can be found in Chapter 7. Table 20–4 provides general recommendations on the indications and dosing of commonly used medications in SBS patients.

Table 20–4.

Indications and Dosing of Commonly Used Medications

Medication (Reference)	Total Daily Enteral Dose (mg/kg/day)	Dosing Frequency (Per Day)	Indication	Possible Side Effects
Famotidine	0.5–1.2 (max 40 mg/day)	2	GERD, gastric hypersecretion	Constipation, diarrhea
Proton pump inhibitor	1–3	1–2	GERD, gastric hypersecretion	Abdominal pain, headache, diarrhea
Ursodeoxycholic acid[22]	15–30	3	Cholestasis, pruritus	Diarrhea, nausea, vomiting
Cholestyramine[22]	240	3	Pruritus, diarrhea	Constipation, nausea, vomiting, abdominal pain
Rifampin[25]	10 (max 600 mg/day)	2	Pruritus	Elevated liver tests, nausea, loss of appetite, urine discoloration
Metronidazole	20 (max 750 mg/day)	3–4	SBBO	Abdominal discomfort, loss of appetite, metallic taste, nausea and vomiting

GERD 5 gastroesophageal reflux disease; max 5 maximum dose; SBBO 5 small bowel bacterial overgrowth.

D-Lactic Acidosis

D-Lactic acidosis occurs in some patients with SBS due to colonic fermentation of undigested or partially digested carbohydrates. Certain bacterial species, mostly gram-positive anaerobes, such as lactobacillus and bifidobacterium, produce D-lactate that is subsequently absorbed. In humans, D-lactate accumulation can occur because of slow metabolism and clearance in addition to excessive production. D-Lactic acidosis may clinically manifest with recurrent episodes of weakness, clumsiness, slurred speech, confusion, somnolence, unsteady gait, or excessive irritability. The episodes are usually episodic, lasting hours to days. This has been described from a few months to many years after intestinal resection. The colon must be present for D-lactic acidosis to occur. Normally D-lactate is undetectable in blood, so a combination of a detectable D-lactate level, acidosis, and abnormal neurologic symptoms is highly suggestive of D-lactic acidosis. Treatment options can include a restricted carbohydrate diet to minimize substrate delivery to the colon, and enteral antibiotics, such as neomycin, kanamycin, or vancomycin.[26,27]

Cholelithiasis

Following ileal resection, the enterohepatic bile salt circulation is interrupted. Bile salt loss can exceed the liver's capacity to replenish losses, with a subsequent drop in the bile salt concentration. This can alter bile composition leading to increased saturation with cholesterol and subsequent gallstone formation. Biliary stasis and sludge formation, often associated with diminished oral/enteral intake, can also be contributing factors (see Figure 20–2).

Renal Stones

Patients with SBS with ileal resection are at risk of developing renal stones. Ileal resection can result in increased absorption of oxalate in the colon, which leads to hyperoxaluria and stone formation (see Figure 20–3). Such patients should be referred to for evaluation and management by a specialist. Treatment includes adhering to a low-oxalate diet, which excludes peanuts, pecans, tea, cocoa, wheat germ, soybeans, and spinach. Other medical approaches include using cholestyramine to bind bile salts and citrate to prevent further stone formation.[28]

Surgical Intervention

Several surgical procedures can be utilized in the management of SBS. These include the establishment of central venous access for delivery of parenteral nutrition, feeding tube placement for enteral nutrition, creation of ostomies, bowel-lengthening procedures, procedures to delay intestinal transit, and transplantation.

Two intestinal-lengthening surgeries are currently employed when dilated intestinal loops are present. The Bianchi procedure involves dividing the dilated segment longitudinally, creating two narrower segments that are

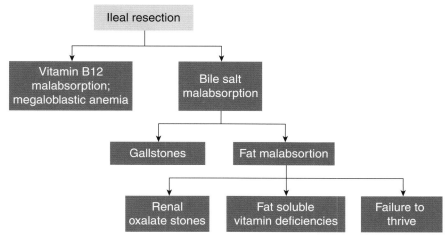

FIGURE 20–2 ■ Consequences of ileal resection.

anastomosed end-to-end (see Figure 20–4). The serial transverse enteroplasty (STEP) procedure involves application of a surgical stapler to the dilated loop at a right angle on alternating sides to create a zigzag longer and narrower intestinal segment (see Figure 20–5). The STEP procedure is simpler and requires no anastomoses. Indications for undergoing intestinal-lengthening surgery should include the presence of dilated intestinal loops and dependence on parenteral nutrition without evidence for further intestinal adaptation. Results from both lengthening procedures have been favorable by advancing enteral

nutrition, weaning parenteral nutrition and reversing its complications, and avoiding transplantation.[29]

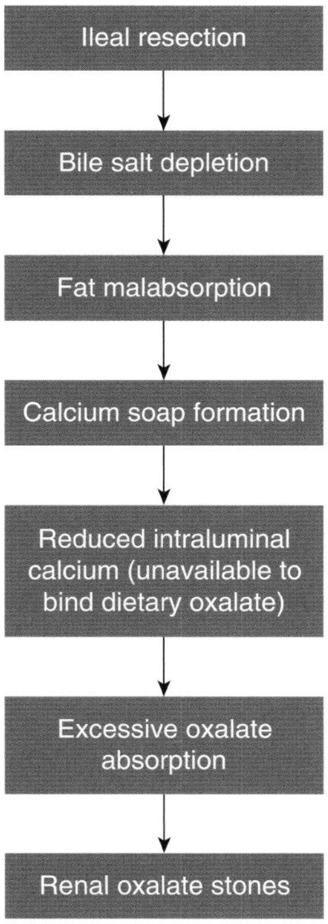

Transplantation is the last surgical option for SBS patients on prolonged parenteral nutrition who experience life-threatening complications such as liver failure. Other cited indications for transplantation include frequent episodes of severe dehydration despite parenteral nutrition and intravenous hydration and recurrent central line infections and thrombosis with progressive loss of vascular access.[30] Types of transplants offered include isolated intestinal, combined liver–intestinal, and multivisceral transplantation. Isolated liver transplantation is occasionally offered to a select population with liver failure in whom good bowel adaptation and eventual enteral autonomy are expected. Despite advances over the last decade, intestinal transplantation is still associated with a high risk of infection, multiorgan failure, rejection, and complications related to immunosuppression. The overall 3-year patient survival after intestinal transplantation is about 50%.[3] Medical and other surgical alternatives should therefore be maximally utilized prior to considering transplantation.

CONCLUSION

SBS is a complex and life-threatening disease affecting children with significant intestinal loss. Management includes meticulous nutritional support, with emphasis on early advancement of enteral feeds, weaning from parenteral nutrition, monitoring for complications, and addressing possible associated liver dysfunction. Significant liver dysfunction can lead to high morbidity and mortality in SBS patients. The early involvement of an experienced pediatric center can provide support from different subspecialists. Intestinal transplantation may be needed when other medical and surgical interventions have failed.

Ileal resection

↓

Bile salt depletion

↓

Fat malabsorption

↓

Calcium soap formation

↓

Reduced intraluminal calcium (unavailable to bind dietary oxalate)

↓

Excessive oxalate absorption

↓

Renal oxalate stones

FIGURE 20–3 ■ Oxalate stone formation.

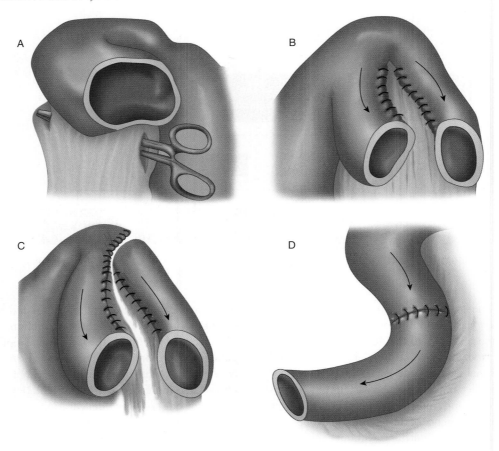

FIGURE 20-4 ■ Intestinal lengthening procedures: Bianchi procedure. (A) Split the mesentery; (B) divide the bowel lengthwise; (C) separate one half from the upstream bowel; (D) make end-to-end anastomosis.

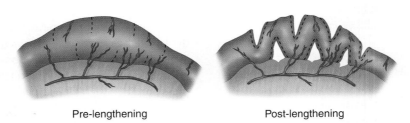

Pre-lengthening   Post-lengthening

FIGURE 20-5 ■ Intestinal lengthening procedures: serial transverse enteroplasty procedure.

REFERENCES

1. Cole CR, Hansen NI, Higgins RD, et al. Very low birth weight preterm infants with surgical short bowel syndrome: incidence, morbidity and mortality, and growth outcomes at 18 to 22 months. *Pediatrics.* 2008;122(3): e573–e582.

2. Goulet O, Ruemmele F. Causes and management of intestinal failure in children. *Gastroenterology.* 2006;130 (2 suppl 1):S16–S28.

3. Goulet O, Ruemmele F, Lacaille F, Colomb V. Irreversible intestinal failure. *J Pediatr Gastroenterol Nutr.* 2004;38(3):250–269.

4. Gourevitch D. The anatomy and physiology of the small bowel. In: Fielding JW, Hallissey MT, eds. *Upper Gastrointestinal Surgery.* London: Springer; 2005:39–44.

5. Vanderhoof JA, Young RJ. Enteral and parenteral nutrition in the care of patients with short-bowel syndrome. *Best Pract Res Clin Gastroenterol.* 2003;17(6): 997–1015.

6. Gupte GL, Beath SV, Kelly DA, Millar AJ, Booth IW. Current issues in the management of intestinal failure. *Arch Dis Child.* 2006;91(3):259–264.

7. Duro D, Kamin D, Duggan C. Overview of pediatric short bowel syndrome. *J Pediatr Gastroenterol Nutr.* 2008;47(suppl 1):S33–S36.

8. Crenn P, Messing B, Cynober L. Citrulline as a biomarker of intestinal failure due to enterocyte mass reduction. *Clin Nutr.* 2008;27(3):328–339.

9. Rhoads JM, Plunkett E, Galanko J, et al. Serum citrulline levels correlate with enteral tolerance and bowel length in infants with short bowel syndrome. *J Pediatr.* 2005;146(4):542–547.

10. Wessel JJ, Kocoshis SA. Nutritional management of infants with short bowel syndrome. *Semin Perinatol.* 2007;31(2):104–111.

11. Cordano A. Clinical manifestations of nutritional copper deficiency in infants and children. *Am J Clin Nutr.* 1998;67(5 suppl):1012S–1016S.

12. Elliott TS. The prevention of central venous catheter-related sepsis. *J Chemother.* 2001;13 Spec No 1(1):234–238.

13. Onland W, Shin CE, Fustar S, Rushing T, Wong WY. Ethanol-lock technique for persistent bacteremia of long-term intravascular devices in pediatric patients. *Arch Pediatr Adolesc Med.* 2006;160(10):1049–1053.

14. Vanderhoof JA. New and emerging therapies for short bowel syndrome in children. *J Pediatr Gastroenterol Nutr.* 2004;39(suppl 3):S769–S771.

15. Ziegler MM. Short bowel syndrome in infancy: etiology and management. *Clin Perinatol.* 1986;13(1):163–173.

16. Jakubik LD, Colfer A, Grossman MB. Pediatric short bowel syndrome: pathophysiology, nursing care, and management issues. *J Soc Pediatr Nurs.* 2000;5(3):111–121.

17. Vanderhoof JA. Short bowel syndrome. *Clin Perinatol.* 1996;23(2):377–386.

18. Drongowski RA, Coran AG. An analysis of factors contributing to the development of total parenteral nutrition-induced cholestasis. *JPEN J Parenter Enteral Nutr.* 1989;13(6):586–589.

19. Teitelbaum DH, Drongowski R, Spivak D. Rapid development of hyperbilirubinemia in infants with the short bowel syndrome as a correlate to mortality: possible indication for early small bowel transplantation. *Transplant Proc.* 1996;28(5):2699–2700.

20. Cooper A, Floyd TF, Ross AJ 3rd, Bishop HC, Templeton JM Jr, Ziegler MM. Morbidity and mortality of short-bowel syndrome acquired in infancy: an update. *J Pediatr Surg.* 1984;19(6):711–718.

21. Simmons MG, Georgeson KE, Figueroa R, Mock DL. Liver failure in parenteral nutrition-dependent children with short bowel syndrome. *Transplant Proc.* 1996;28(5):2701.

22. Btaiche IF, Khalidi N. Parenteral nutrition-associated liver complications in children. *Pharmacotherapy.* 2002;22(2):188–211.

23. Gura KM, Lee S, Valim C, et al. Safety and efficacy of a fish-oil-based fat emulsion in the treatment of parenteral nutrition-associated liver disease. *Pediatrics.* 2008;121(3):e678–e686.

24. Gura KM, Duggan CP, Collier SB, et al. Reversal of parenteral nutrition-associated liver disease in two infants with short bowel syndrome using parenteral fish oil: implications for future management. *Pediatrics.* 2006;118(1):e197–e201.

25. Yerushalmi B, Sokol RJ, Narkewicz MR, Smith D, Karrer FM. Use of rifampin for severe pruritus in children with chronic cholestasis. *J Pediatr Gastroenterol Nutr.* 1999;29(4):442–447.

26. Zhang DL, Jiang ZW, Jiang J, Cao B, Li JS. D-Lactic acidosis secondary to short bowel syndrome. *Postgrad Med J.* 2003;79(928):110–112.

27. Uribarri J, Oh MS, Carroll HJ. D-Lactic acidosis. A review of clinical presentation, biochemical features, and pathophysiologic mechanisms. *Medicine (Baltimore).* 1998;77(2):73–82.

28. Morton AR, Iliescu EA, Wilson JW. Nephrology: 1. Investigation and treatment of recurrent kidney stones. *CMAJ.* 2002;166(2):213–218.

29. Sudan D, Thompson J, Botha J, et al. Comparison of intestinal lengthening procedures for patients with short bowel syndrome. *Ann Surg.* 2007;246(4):593–601.

30. Torres C. Assessment of intestinal failure patients. In: Langnas A, Goulet O, Quigley E, Tappenden K, eds. *Intestinal Failure: Diagnosis, Management and Transplantation.* 1st ed. Malden, MA: Wiley-Blackwell; 2008:117–121.

CHAPTER 21

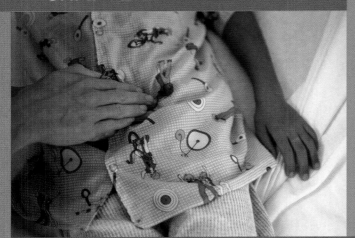

Surgical Emergencies

John Meehan

DEFINITIONS AND EPIDEMIOLOGY

The term "emergency" is subjective and therefore can be difficult to define, especially when considering all the complexities of caring for a sick child with a surgical problem. To the anxious parent, anything surgical may be an emergency. Healthcare providers often have differing perspectives on what is or is not an emergency. The topics in this chapter are all surgical issues that need intervention, most in a relatively short period of time. But some might be considered "urgencies" rather than true surgical emergencies. For example, most surgeons do not consider appendicitis and pyloric stenosis as true surgical emergencies. The infant with pyloric stenosis is often delayed hours, possibly even days, while undergoing the necessary fluid rehydration and resuscitation. Likewise, appendicitis can be temporized with IV antibiotics overnight and taken to the operating room the following morning. Conversely, malrotation with midgut volvulus and other causes of ischemic bowel are always surgical emergencies due to the impending irreversible effects of ongoing ischemia. Finally, there are many diagnoses that may fall over a wide spectrum of severity. Therefore, the clinical picture will often dictate the presence of an emergency more than the diagnosis. Many congenital and acquired pediatric surgical issues can progress to emergencies if the underlying problem has been present long enough. In a general sense, intervention for surgical emergencies and the less acute surgical urgencies fall into fur categories: *obstruction*, *ischemia*, *perforation*, and *bleeding*.

CLINICAL PRESENTATION AND TREATMENT

The first step in the evaluation and treatment of a patient with a possible surgical emergency is *resuscitation*. Fluid losses can be massive from bleeding and bowel obstructions, while enormous third spacing can occur from perforation and ischemia. Choice of fluid replacement depends on where the loss occurs but should be isotonic early in the resuscitation, using either lactated Ringer's (LR) solution or normal saline (NS). For most fluid losses and conditions where acidosis is present, LR is a better selection. It is the fluid replacement of choice for trauma, and many surgical problems can be compared to a trauma situation. LR contains electrolytes much closer to physiological serum chemistries than NS and also contains lactate for buffering. The lactate in LR does not contribute to the acidosis; in fact, it has the opposite effect. The lactate is rapidly converted to bicarbonate by the first-pass effect of the liver and will improve a patient's acidotic picture much more effectively than NS. Moreover, the pH of NS is acidic (5.0) and can worsen an underlying acidosis. Conversely, NS is a far better choice for upper GI fluid losses such as excessive emesis. Pyloric stenosis is the best example. In these patients, the emesis has progressed to such an extreme that a severe hypochloremic metabolic alkalosis results. The acidic nature and high chloride concentration (154 mEq/L) of NS make this fluid the ideal resuscitation fluid for upper GI losses.

DIAGNOSIS

Once resuscitation has been initiated, diagnostic workup can begin. Age is a key factor in determining where the problem is likely to be found. Bleeding is evaluated by upper or lower endoscopy or a radionucleotide scan. Possible obstruction or perforation is evaluated by plain film radiograph. In some cases, additional upper or lower GI contrast studies may be useful. Ultrasound may be useful in diagnosing some obstructive conditions where a mass may be involved such as intussusception. CT scans will show problems such as intussusceptions and enteric cysts causing obstruction but are not usually the first study of choice.

The differential diagnosis for a GI obstruction is large. Obstruction should not be considered a primary diagnosis, but rather the result of another diagnosis causing the obstruction. Once again, age at presentation helps to narrow the possibilities, many of which are exclusive to the first few weeks of life. Postoperative surgical adhesions still rank as one of the most common causes of obstruction in anyone with a prior abdominal surgical history. Other considerations include the location of the obstruction. Distal obstructions tend to cause significant abdominal distention while proximal obstructions may present with high-volume emesis and little or no abdominal distention. The color and frequency of emesis are helpful in narrowing down where an obstruction may have occurred. Moreover, the description and location of any overlying pain accompanied with a plain film radiographic may also point in the right direction early in the investigation.

Ischemia can occur from local mechanical issues such as twisting of the bowel to systemic functional conditions such as a low-flow state. It can be devastating once it begins because a vicious cycle may ensue. Bowel that has been compromised from low flow becomes more edematous and inflamed creating a third-spacing effect that draws in more fluid. As more fluid is drawn into the bowel wall, edema progresses, causing further mechanical compression of the vasculature and worsening ischemia. Coupled with the bacterial translocation and sepsis that often accompany a low-flow state, the ischemia can progress rapidly down a deteriorating route. Emergent intervention including aggressive fluid replacement is required. Failure to act quickly can lead to significant loss of bowel or death due to worsening acidosis, sepsis, and systemic circulatory collapse.

Perforation can result from obstruction, ischemia, or both. Distal colonic obstructions often lead to perforation of the cecum by the law of Laplace. Small bowel obstructions may lead to a perforation in a variety of locations proximally anywhere along the small bowel. Ischemic areas are especially susceptible to perforation due to weakened bowel wall strength. Other causes of perforation include trauma, foreign bodies, and ulceration (e.g., colonic ulceration due to acid production in a Meckel's diverticulum). Visceral perforations occasionally wall themselves off, but not before significant contamination has occurred. The patient with a hollow viscus perforation may have impressive peritoneal signs on physical exam. Gastric perforations, which tend to have low bacterial counts, may release huge quantities of air into the peritoneum, but the abdominal examination may not be as impressive as seen with small bowel or colon perforations.

Gastrointestinal Bleeding

Most GI bleeding is usually slow, chronic, or both, can be treated medically or endoscopically, and therefore rarely requires emergent surgical exploration. However, entities such as Meckel's diverticulum can result in massive bleeding that can best be managed surgically. Localization of any GI blood loss is critical before exploration is considered unless the patient is unstable. Most GI bleeds are localized through careful history and physical exam followed by endoscopy and imaging studies, as described in Chapter 6. For serious bleeding whose source remains elusive, exploring a GI tract through an open operation concurrently with luminal endoscopy by a gastroenterologist may be considered. Finally, emergent surgical exploration is reserved for situations where blood loss is high and standard diagnostic imaging modalities are either impossible or unsafe.

SPECIFIC CONDITIONS

Neonatal Gastric Perforation

Definitions and epidemiology

Neonatal gastric perforation can be spontaneous, ischemic, or traumatic. Nasogastric (NG) tube trauma is a common cause of iatrogenic perforation, especially in premature infants. The likelihood of this complication can be reduced using simple preventative means such as careful measurement and placement of an appropriate-sized NG tube. Other causes of iatrogenic perforations include barotrauma from bag-mask ventilation or other forms of positive pressure ventilation. Patients with a tracheoesophageal fistula are at particular risk and may require emergent decompression with a surgical G-tube before the fistula is dealt with. Ischemic perforation can result from birth asphyxia, sepsis, or necrotizing enterocolitis (NEC). The mechanisms may include impaired mucosal defenses secondary to poor perfusion or frank infarction of the gastric wall. Spontaneous perforation without obvious cause may happen, and usually occurs in newborns with no traumatic or ischemic histories.

Some of these babies are premature while others are simply small for gestation age.

Clinical presentation and diagnosis

A change in abdominal examination is common for these children when a gastric perforation occurs. The abdominal exam may only demonstrate a modest degree of tenderness, because the spilled gastric contents are not as irritating to the peritoneum as contents spilled from perforations in the large or small intestine. However, the volume of air released can be impressive. Plain film radiography often shows massive pneumoperitoneum. An excessively large volume of intra-abdominal air is a clue that suggests that a perforation may be gastric.

Treatment

Surgical management depends on the cause. Traumatic and spontaneous perforations do well with primary repair only. Ischemic perforations require debridement and resection of the devitalized tissues.

Gastric Volvulus

Definitions and pathogenesis

Gastric volvulus is a rare form of a proximal obstruction in children. Two variants of gastric volvulus exist: organoaxial and mesentericoaxial. Gastric volvulus is associated with congenital deficiencies in stomach fixation. Typically, the stomach is tethered by the gastrohepatic, gastrosplenic, and gastrophrenic ligaments as well as the retroperitoneal duodenum. Anomalies of the gastrohepatic and gastrosplenic ligaments allow for an organoaxial volvulus as the stomach rotates about its longitudinal axis. Abnormalities of the gastrophrenic and duodenal attachments may create a mesentericoaxial volvulus.

Clinical presentation

Both acute and chronic forms of volvulus may occur, with acute being significantly more common. The typical patient presents with severe epigastric pain. Patients may also have significant retching without emesis. The abdominal exam can be quite variable but gastric distention may be severe. A tender abdomen with peritoneal signs may suggest ischemia or perforation and emergent exploration is required. The diagnosis is suspected if a NG tube cannot be passed.

Diagnosis

Contrast radiologic evaluation may demonstrate significant gastric distention or the contrast may even fail to progress into the stomach and simply be retained in the esophagus because of an obstruction at the level of the GE junction. The organoaxial volvulus is the more common of the two types, but both can be hard to diagnose without a high degree of clinical suspicion.

Treatment

Emergent exploration is indicated in the acute setting to reduce the risk of ischemia. Operative treatment begins with reduction and may need to include resection of ischemic areas. Perforations are usually closed primarily whenever possible. From a historical standpoint, a gastrostomy had been advocated to help reduce the presumed risk of a subsequent volvulus but actual clinical data have not confirmed that placing a gastrostomy makes any difference in the recurrence rate. It is generally accepted that recurrent gastric volvulus should be treated with a gastropexy.

Hypertrophic Pyloric Stenosis (HPS)

Definitions and pathogenesis

HPS is an acquired condition that results in a thickened pyloric muscle layer that obstructs the gastric outlet. The incidence of HPS is around 0.86–3.96 per 1000 live births and is typically seen in infants between 3 and 6 weeks of age.[1] There is a significant male predominance, with a male to female ratio of 4:1.

Clinical presentation

Infants with HPS typically develop progressively worsening emesis after the first few weeks of life. Initially, symptoms are intermittent, which may lead to an early misdiagnosis of gastroesophageal reflux or formula intolerance. The diagnosis becomes clear when vomiting becomes more severe and is noted to be non-bilious and projectile. Significant dehydration occurs, and the loss of gastric HCl results in hypochloremic, hypokalemic metabolic alkalosis. In severe cases, hypoglycemia can precipitate seizures. Unconjugated hyperbilirubinemia is common. The hyperbilirubinemia often gets the attention of the physician, but is transient and does not warrant further attention if it resolves after the stenosis is repaired.

Diagnosis

Physical examination typically reveals an infant with significant dehydration including sunken eyes and fontanelles, decreased skin turgor, and dry mucus membranes. The classic finding on abdominal exam is the "olive sign" in the epigastrium. The olive is actually the thickened pylorus that can be easily palpated in the flaccid abdomen, but may be very difficult to find in the irritable or inconsolable infant. The exam is performed by placing two or three fingers lubricated with soap or lubricating jelly on the upper abdomen, slightly to the right of midline. The area is carefully palpated for a small oval mass while sliding the fingers inferiorly. A positive exam is 97% accurate and, if present, no further diagnostic studies are required.[2] However, the exam may be very difficult to perform in the irritable child, especially when the stomach is full of fluid. In this situation, consoling the child and examining when the stomach is empty create the best opportunity for palpating the pyloric mass. NG suction to empty the stomach or examining the child immediately after vomiting will improve the likelihood of a successful exam. After the NG suctioning has been completed, a small amount of sugar water can be given to the child by bottle while the examiner attempts to locate the pylorus. Allowing the child to have the sugar water is a very effective method and any volume consumed by the child can be easily removed by the NG tube once the diagnosis is confirmed.

Unfortunately, the art of the pyloric exam seems to be fading. More and more physicians immediately opt for an ultrasound, which is a very accurate method for diagnosis of HPS. Ultrasound is an additional expense and may not be readily available at all times of day or in all locations. However, it is a reliable diagnostic tool for the infants whose physical exam is indeterminate. Ultrasound-measured pyloric length of >17 mm or a muscle layer thickness of >4 mm has positive predictive value of 90% for infants 4 weeks of age or greater.[3] The barium upper GI series, once popular for diagnosing HPS, is used with much less frequency now, as it is notoriously inaccurate. Barium studies may still have utility in equivocal cases, but should be considered less reliable than either physical exam or ultrasound (see Figure 9–8).

Treatment

Proper preoperative resuscitation is critical before operative intervention is undertaken. Electrolyte disturbances can be severe and fatalities due to arrhythmias can occur if these infants are placed under anesthesia prior to replenishment of fluid and electrolytes. The resuscitation can take anywhere from 12 to 72 hours and electrolytes should be rechecked periodically. It cannot be overemphasized that there is no emergency to rush the child with HPS to the operating room. Severely dehydrated infants should receive repeated boluses of IV NS (20 mL/kg each) until vital signs are stabilized and good urine output is confirmed. After the emergent volume resuscitation is completed, 5% dextrose with 0.45% NaCl (1/2 normal) should be run at 1.5 times the calculated maintenance rate. Potassium should be added once urine output is achieved, using 20–40 mEq potassium/L of solution. Part of the electrolyte disturbance in these patients is a significant hypokalemia. Serum potassium measurements underestimate the

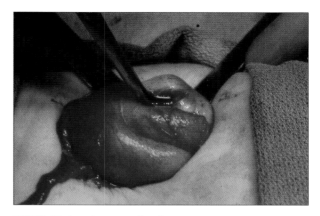

FIGURE 21–1 ■ Laparoscopic pyloromyotomy.

total body potassium deficit because the metabolic alkalosis will shift extracellular potassium intracellularly. All electrolyte derangements can be corrected with proper fluid replacement. Periodic checks of the electrolytes should be done during fluid resuscitation, in anticipation of performing surgery once the serum chloride is normalized and the serum bicarbonate is <30.

The classic operation for HPS is a *pyloromyotomy* (Figure 21–1). In open surgery, the procedure can be done through a right upper quadrant or an umbilical incision. Both approaches have their advocates and the choice between the two techniques was hotly debated among pediatric surgeons in the late 1990s, with no resolution. However, shortly after 2000, minimally invasive surgery (MIS) gained enormous popularity and the laparoscopic pyloromyotomy quickly replacing both open methods. Regardless of the approach, the key to the operation is a complete pyloromyotomy without perforation of the underlying mucosa. A longitudinal incision is made in the serosa of the pylorus all the way from antrum to pyloric–duodenal junction. Once the serosa is split, blunt spreading of the hypertrophic muscle is performed using a Ramstedt spreader. Care must be taken to avoid perforation of the mucosa, which is more likely to occur at the duodenal end of the myotomy. Fortunately, the risk of perforation is fairly low, with a rate of <3% in most series.[4] The pyloromyotomy needs to be long enough such that each half of the opened pyloric ring moves independently.

Feedings can be started relatively soon after the procedure. No feeding regimen has been shown to be superior over any other. There is significant disagreement over the ideal feeding regimen, with somewhat complicated protocols still in use. Recent studies indicate that feeding ad libitum within a couple of hours after surgery is tolerated just as well as the progressive feeding regimens, with multiple concentration and volume changes, that have been popular for decades.[5] The ad libitum method has the advantage of being much simpler to explain to residents, families, and staff.

Occasional emesis often occurs in the early postoperative period regardless of the chosen feeding regimen, but is not usually a cause for alarm. Persistent, high-volume emesis suggests an incomplete myotomy, which requires a return to the OR for completion. Intraoperative mucosal perforations recognized at the time of surgery can lead to peritonitis and sepsis. Initial signs and symptoms include abdominal tenderness, distention, and acidosis. This complication can be confirmed by contrast radiography and should be followed by emergent re-exploration when suspected. Fortunately, both incomplete myotomy and perforation are rare. The majority of patients go home within 24 hours following the surgery.

Malrotation

Definitions and epidemiology

Malrotation with midgut volvulus is a true surgical emergency. Once established, irreversible ischemia to the midgut can occur in just a few hours. Every physician must have malrotation in their differential diagnosis when evaluating children with sudden obstructive symptoms. Bilious emesis, the hallmark sign of malrotation, is assumed to be malrotation until proven otherwise.

Pathogenesis

Malrotation occurs due to a failure of the normal rotation and fixation of the bowel in the first 3 months of gestation. In the normal rotational process, the midgut herniates into the yolk sac during the fifth week of gestation. The superior mesenteric artery (SMA) serves as the blood supply for the midgut and is the main axis of its normal rotation. The rotation occurs in a counter-clockwise direction. Normally, after 270° of counter-clockwise rotation, the duodenojejunal region is tethered to the retroperitoneum in the expected "C-loop" orientation, with jejunum emerging into the peritoneum at the ligament of Treitz in the left upper quadrant. Concurrently, the ileocolic segment also rotates around the SMA, bringing the cecum down to the right lower quadrant. The normal mesentery of the midgut is tethered firmly along a broad retroperitoneal attachment from the ligament of Treitz to the cecum. For this reason, volvulus rarely happens in the properly rotated bowel.

Malrotated bowel did not complete this process, has no ligament of Treitz, and has a narrow pedicle of mesentery containing the SMA. This narrow attachment allows the bowel to twist around it easily, almost always in a clockwise fashion, resulting in volvulus. After twisting around the SMA enough times, the lumen becomes obstructed, usually causing bilious emesis, and

the vascular supply becomes compromised. The resulting intestinal ischemia can lead to a catastrophic loss of bowel.

Clinical presentation

The compromise of the SMA often leads to lactic acidosis and a rapidly worsening clinical picture. Patients may present in extremis with lethargy, dehydration, and profound acidosis. Physicians must have a very high index of suspicion in patients when evaluating the lethargic infant, whether typical bilious emesis is present or not. However, the symptom of bilious emesis is a very suggestive sign, and the possibility of malrotation must be emergently investigated. Any child with abdominal pain accompanied by vomiting must be investigated in the same manner.

Diagnosis

Standard abdominal plain films are of limited value in establishing the diagnosis of malrotation but may be useful for ruling out other concerns. The diagnosis is confirmed by an upper GI study and should be done emergently whenever the diagnosis is considered (see Figures 9–7 and 21–2). A full and complete C-loop must be seen in order to exclude the diagnosis. Malrotation without volvulus is also seen and may also present as an upper GI bowel obstruction. In these cases, retroperitoneal attachments known as Ladd's bands may be responsible for the obstruction, without the presence of a midgut volvulus. CT scans can also establish the diagnosis but are not the study of choice (Figure 21–3). A reversal of the

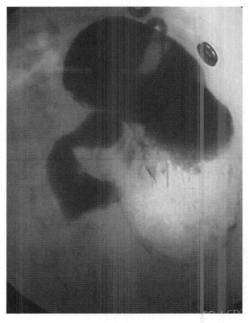

FIGURE 21–2 ■ Malrotation with midgut volvulus. Notice the cut-off sign in the duodenum and the lack of a complete C-loop.

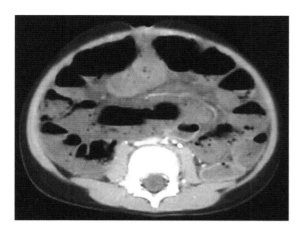

FIGURE 21–3 ▪ A CT scan showing a midgut volvulus was obtained in this patient who was lethargic with an unreliable abdominal exam. Of particular note, this patient never had a history of bilious emesis. The SMA and SMV are reversed in their usual orientation with the artery to the right of the vein indicating a twisting of the bowel. Also note the profound volume depletion in this patient with the collapse of the inferior vena cava.

normal relationship of the SMA and superior mesenteric vein (SMV) may be demonstrated. However, it should be emphasized that the upper GI is the gold standard for confirming the diagnosis of malrotation.

Treatment

Treatment for malrotation with midgut volvulus requires emergent and immediate exploration (Figure 21–4). Rapid resuscitation may be needed before induction of anesthesia, but should be done with great haste, as delay

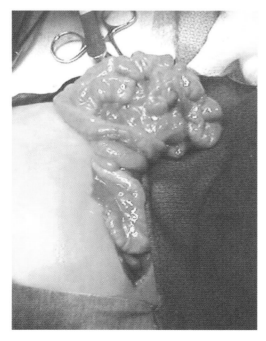

FIGURE 21–4 ▪ Intraoperative photograph of malrotation with midgut volvulus.

can lead to irreversible loss of the midgut. The operation is called a *Ladd's procedure*. The operation has four steps. The first step is to untwist the bowel. In the operating room, the direction of the twisted bowel may appear as a confusing mass to the surgeon. The simple rule is "turn back time," and untwist the bowel by rotating in a counterclockwise direction until the mesentery is flat and straight. Step two of the Ladd's procedure is to divide all the Ladd's bands and make the duodenum go straight caudad. There is no way to rotate the bowel to a normal anatomical configuration, so it needs to be laid down in a way that makes volvulus unlikely to recur. Step three is critical to the Ladd's procedure, widening the mesenteric base and pedicle. Scoring the peritoneum on one side of the pedicle frees the mesentery and allows it to be stretched and widened, thereby reducing the risk of a recurrent volvulus. The fourth and final step of the Ladd's procedure is an appendectomy, simply done as a preventative measure to avoid the confusing future possibility of appendicitis in someone whose appendix is not in the typical right lower quadrant. Once these four steps have been completed, the small bowel is laid down predominantly in the right side of the abdomen with the duodenum heading straight down and the mesentery flat and straight. The large bowel and cecum are placed in the left side of the abdomen.

Areas that are clearly necrotic or have perforated will require resection. The amount of bowel lost can be devastating. Areas that are ischemic but not necessarily necrotic can be watched intraoperatively for 30 minutes or more after the volvulus has been reduced. Bowel that may initially appear unsalvageable can often reperfuse. Administering fluorescein and using a Wood's lamp to visualize perfusion can also help distinguish bowel that is still viable (Figure 21–5). Since the reperfusion process may take several hours before it is complete, it is also reasonable to resect nothing immediately and to

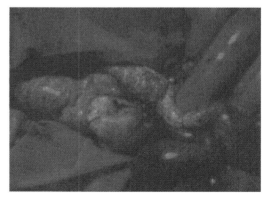

FIGURE 21–5 ▪ Bowel illuminated under a Wood's lamp following IV administration of flourescein. Notice the bowel that has the uptake of the fluorescent marker indicating viability. All other areas of the bowel are non-viable and require resection.

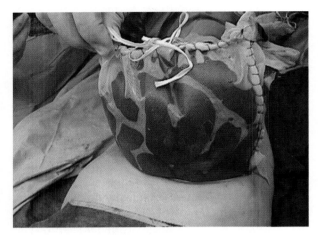

FIGURE 21–6 ■ Placing the non-viable bowel in a silo for planned second-look operation.

perform a second-look operation 24–48 hours later to better demarcate viable from non-viable bowel (Figures 21–6 and 21–7).

Another controversial situation arises with the asymptomatic patient with malrotation whose diagnosis is stumbled upon while investigating other issues. Although debated, most pediatric surgeons would recommend a Ladd's procedure for the asymptomatic malrotation on an elective basis. The risk of operative complications is small and usually minor in comparison to the devastating consequences of a potential midgut volvulus.

Minimally invasive surgery For the emergent situation patient with an acute volvulus, most surgeons would advocate an open procedure. However, MIS has become increasingly accepted in the non-volvulized elective patient.[6] Moreover, this operation has now even been performed robotically.[7] Proponents of the MIS technique note the faster return to normal preoperative activity, shorter hospital stays, less pain, and minimal

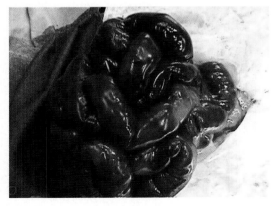

FIGURE 21–7 ■ Same bowel as in Figures 21–5 and 21–6 nearly 48 hours later. Note the demarcation of the viable and non-viable segments.

abdominal scarring. Opponents believe that open surgery will better reduce the risk of a recurrent volvulus by causing multiple adhesions. This debate will likely continue for quite some time until this question can be adequately studied.

Incarcerated Hernia

Definitions and epidemiology

A common cause of a bowel obstruction in small children is an incarcerated hernia. Examination of any patient with a presumed bowel obstruction must include a thorough genitourinary and abdominal inspection, specifically looking for presence of a hernia. Inguinal hernias are the type most likely to become incarcerated. Other possible hernia sites include umbilical, ventral, incisional, and internal. There are a number of other locations for possible hernias but these are exceedingly rare and will not be discussed in further detail.

Diagnosis

Incarcerated hernias are usually obvious on examination after a non-reducible mass is discovered. Relaxation of the patient is often difficult and repeated attempts at reduction fail, prompting a surgical consultation. Non-reducible bowel with resulting incarceration is a substantial risk for bowel ischemia and is considered a true surgical emergency.

Clinical presentation and treatment

Patients with an incarcerated *inquinal hernia* can present at any age. Signs and symptoms include a non-reducible groin mass, groin pain, emesis, and possibly even abdominal distention. Transillumination, while helpful in teenagers and adults for determining solid or fluid-filled scrotal masses, is worthless in the infant and small child. The small bowel of these young patients will transilluminate, giving a false sense of security to the examiner who assumes the transillumination is a sign of fluid and not bowel. Children with ischemic bowel progress to lethargy, dehydration, and acidosis. Even in these patients, an attempt at preoperative manual reduction is warranted; failure results in an immediate trip to the operating room. Patients with incarceration that is reduced in the clinic or emergency room should have their repair performed in the near future, but not necessarily emergently. There is a significant technical advantage to waiting a few hours or even days after a successful reduction to allow edema to resolve, thereby reducing the risk of injury to testicular vessels or the vas deferens. For the asymptomatic inguinal hernia, elective repair should be scheduled at a convenient date.

Umbilical hernias can incarcerate too, but this is a very rare event in young children. Incarcerations are more likely in teenagers or adults. Unlike inguinal hernias that never close and repair is always indicated, an umbilical hernia may close in the first few months or even years of life. Neonatal umbilical hernias usually close spontaneously with no intervention, although many families will tell the story of how Grandma cured someone by taping a large coin to their belly button for a few months! In reality, the hernia would have closed without the compressive dressing. The low risk of incarceration, coupled with the possibility of spontaneous closure, allows for the surgical treatment of an asymptomatic umbilical hernia to be deferred until patient is at least 3 or 4 years of age.

Incisional hernias (hernias occurring along a prior surgical incision) and ventral hernias (typically midline abdominal wall hernias occurring at a site other than the umbilicus) can also incarcerate, but this is exceedingly rare, and the hernias are usually not big enough to allow a bowel loop to become trapped. If an incarceration occurs, the omentum is usually the intra-abdominal component that is caught in these small hernias and may cause pain. Timing of surgical intervention should be predicated on the severity of the patient's symptoms.

Intussusception

Definition and epidemiology

Intussusception occurs when one segment of bowel invaginates into downstream intestine and is pulled further downstream by intestinal motility, very much like collapsing an old-fashioned hand-held telescope. This is most common in children 3 months to 3 years of age, with a peak incidence from 6 to 18 months of age. In young children, the affected area is ileocecal—the ileum telescopes into the cecum.

Pathogenesis

In most cases, a specific cause is never identified, but has been postulated to be related to lymphatic hyperplasia, which can serve as a lead point. The size difference of the ileocecal valve in relation to the terminal ileum has also been proposed as a possible mechanism. More proximal (ileoileal or jejunojejunal) intussusceptions may also occur, but are less common and often are caused by a pathological lead point. An example occurs in Henoch–Schlein purpura (HSP) patients due to bowel wall edema and hemorrhage, and requires operative reduction. Other potential lead points include angiomas, Meckel's diverticula, lipomas, and the appendix, but these account for only 2–8% of patients.

Clinical presentation

The signs and symptoms of intussusception can be variable. The classic triad of pain, vomiting, and bloody stools is present in less than one-third of patients.[8] The typical presentation is that of a 6–18-month-old child who cries inconsolably for a few minutes with legs drawn upward. The pain then suddenly disappears and the child seems fine, possibly even eating and playing normally, only to have the cyclical abdominal pain return a few minutes later. During these cycles, they may vomit or pass a bloody "current jelly" stool, consisting of mucous mixed with blood. Vomiting is a frequent symptom.

Diagnosis

Physical exam may be difficult to interpret. The intussuscepted, sausage-shaped mass is often palpated in the right upper abdomen and is a strong indicator for this diagnosis. However, sometimes the mass cannot be palpated. If the child is between bouts of colicky pain during the exam, the exam findings seem minimal and the described pain is out of proportion to the exam. A high index of suspicion is needed from the examiner in order to correctly identify the diagnosis.

Plain film radiographs often show paucity of gas in the right upper quadrant on AP view. This should immediately prompt a contrast or pneumatic enema to confirm the diagnosis as well as treat the problem (see Figure 9–10). When plain films are equivocal, an ultrasound may be beneficial (see Figure 9–9). CT scans will also demonstrate the diagnosis but are unnecessary as a first-line modality.

Treatment

Contrast reduction with air or barium is the first line of recommended treatment for stable patients and an ileocolic intussusception that has been present for 48 hours or less (Figure 21–8). After that time, it becomes increasingly difficult to reduce radiographically due to the edema and inflammation of such a prolonged course. In these cases, the surgeon and radiologist usually need to discuss utility of possible contrast reduction over an exploration.

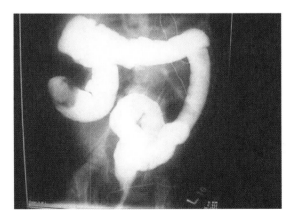

FIGURE 21–8 ■ Contrast enema of an intussusception.

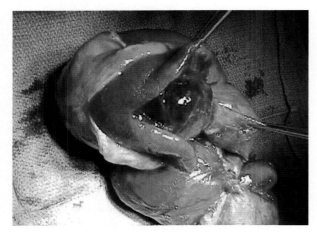

FIGURE 21–9 ■ Operative specimen from a resected intussusceptions. A bowel wall hematoma (arrow) served as a lead point in this specimen.

Children who have failed radiographic reductions or with profound acidosis may have ischemic bowel and warrant emergent exploration (Figure 21–9).

In the operating room, the intussusceptum (the bowel that has been invaginated and propelled distally) is gently squeezed out of the intussuscipiens (the distal bowel which has "swallowed" the proximal bowel) by starting distal to the palpable intussusceptum and pushing it back out proximally. The bowel is squeezed much in the manner of squeezing a tube of toothpaste until the intussuscepted bowel is forced back out. There has been an axiom in pediatric surgery that the intussusceptum should never be pulled out; it should be pushed out. This traditional teaching may not be as crucial as was once assumed: in the laparoscopic method of reduction, pulling the intussusceptum is much more readily accomplished technically than pushing it. With either technique, failure to reduce the bowel will necessitate a resection. Bowel that was successfully reduced but is perforated or necrotic will require resection. Re-intussusception can occur in patients that were reduced non-operatively and repeated episodes may warrant exploration searching for a lead point.

Adhesions

Definitions and pathogenesis

By far, the most common cause of a bowel obstruction in older children is adhesions from prior surgery. These are fibrous bands of scar tissue that can block adjacent loops of bowel by compression, or can serve as an abnormal anchor point causing twisting or traction on the bowel.

Diagnosis

Plain films are usually strongly suggestive, with dilated loops of bowel and air fluid levels above the blockage.

However, an ileus can look similar on plain films and the overall clinical picture must be correlated with the radiographic findings. One helpful distinguishing feature of an ileus over a true mechanical obstruction is the presence of air in the rectum on abdominal plain film, which is not usually present in a bowel obstruction. Some adhesions may only cause a partial bowel obstruction and conservative measures may suffice.

Treatment

NG tube decompression, IV fluids, and bowel rest may resolve the situation. However, signs or symptoms such as lethargy and acidosis may indicate ischemia and surgical intervention becomes emergent. Unclear cases can be treated with an attempt at non-operative management but plans for eventual exploration should be incorporated early in the plan.

Necrotizing Enterocolitis

Definitions and epidemiology

NEC is a condition characterized by spontaneous necrosis of segments of colon or small bowel, primarily in premature infants, resulting in symptoms of sepsis, intramural air, and often frank perforation.

Pathogenesis

The exact cause of NEC is still elusive but tends to be a disease predominately of low-birth-weight infants who are premature, rather than babies that are small for gestational age. Besides birth weight and prematurity, feedings have been strongly implicated as a contributor to the development of NEC.[9] The immaturity of the gut defenses in these premature babies is also likely to be a contributing factor. There is significant debate and large regional variability on the rate, timing, and osmolarity of feeds among many institutions. Recent evidence suggests that small-volume "trophic feeds" started immediately may have a protective effect.[10] Maternal prenatal cocaine use has been implicated in NEC because of its vasoconstrictive properties. Intestinal ischemia caused by low-flow states such as congenital heart disease, sepsis, and inadequate intravascular volume are all conditions that predispose to NEC.

Clinical presentation

Many of the initial findings are non-specific. A wide variety of signs and symptoms may develop including irritability, increased ventilator requirements, temperature instability, emesis, apnea, bradycardia, lethargy, hypoglycemia, fever, and shock. GI bleeding may occur grossly or can be occult. Physical exam may have obvious signs of peritonitis but can be unrevealing too. Abdominal distention may develop but not consistently. Abdominal wall erythema is an ominous sign that a severe inflammatory reaction is happening in the abdomen. Laboratory analysis often shows a noticeable drop in the platelet count and can be a harbinger of an impending NEC episode even before any signs or symptoms are witnessed. Likewise, the C-reactive protein may give one of the first clues to the degree of inflammation and a sudden increase may be another warning sign of NEC.

Diagnosis

Diagnostic imaging begins with a plain abdominal film. Abdominal distention is common in NEC, with radiographic findings of ileus or obstruction. *Pneumatosis intestinalis* is intramural gas in the wall of the bowel (Figure 21–10). The presence of pneumotosis on plain films is virtually pathognomonic of NEC. In some cases, the pneumotosis can be severe (see Figure 9–2). Portal venous gas is often an ominous sign (see Figure 9–3) but is not a guarantee that perforation or substantial bowel loss has occurred. Pneumoperitoneum is a clear sign of perforation and warrants immediate exploration.

Treatment

Medical management consists of immediate cessation of all feeds, bowel rest, TPN, IV antibiotics, an NGT, fluid resuscitation, maintaining perfusion of the gut with appropriate supportive measures, and correction of acidosis. No feedings are given for a minimum of

10 days, which may extend to 2 full weeks. Antibiotics are continued through for a minimum of 10 days and feedings are reinitiated at a very slow rate after the completion of the NPO status.

When medical treatment fails, surgery may be necessary. Indications for surgery are varied. Obvious perforation, with free air in the peritoneum, is an obvious indication for emergent intervention. Persistent dilated bowel loops that appear dilated and unchanged on sequential plain films over several days may suggest a local perforation and a walled-off abscess or fluid collection. Ultrasound that shows turbid intra-abdominal fluid also suggests perforation. The patient's overall status and response to therapy must to be analyzed in conjunction with these radiographic findings to determine the best course of action. Failure of medical management is another reasonable argument for surgical exploration.

The baby's overall fluid and cardiovascular status should be optimized before exploration commences including the use of broad-spectrum antibiotics. Neonates weighing <1 kg can be temporized by a bedside percutaneous drain. This is usually placed in the right lower quadrant because of the higher frequency of perforations in this region. This temporizing technique is a safe and effective alternative to taking extremely low-birth-weight, unstable infants to the operating room. About one-third of the patients treated in this manner will fail immediately and still require exploration. Another one-third will do well for quite some time but eventually require exploration for ongoing sepsis or delayed stricture formation. Interestingly, one-third will recover completely from this drainage procedure and never require any abdominal surgery.

Infants that are not candidates for the drainage procedure can undergo open exploration. The general plan should be to remove only those segments that are clearly necrotic or perforated. The surgeon should attempt to preserve as much bowel length as possible and to preserve the ileocecal valve whenever possible. Multiple segments of bowel may require resection, leaving the baby with significant loss of intestine, possibly resulting in short bowel syndrome.

NEC totalis is the complete or near complete loss of the bowel. This condition poses an ethical dilemma regarding the impending resection. These unfortunate patients will require massive resections if they are to survive the neonatal period but will be condemned to having short bowel syndrome and all the associated problems. Counseling, including options for lifelong TPN, bowel transplantation, or possible withdrawal of support is a difficult subject to discuss with new parents, but is an important part of the overall care of these unfortunate children.

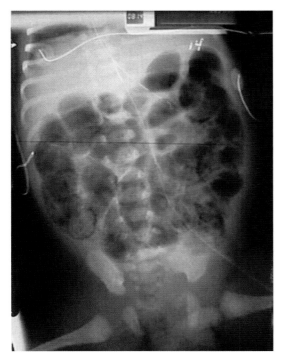

FIGURE 21–10 ■ Abdominal radiograph of a premature infant with NEC and severe pneumotosis intestinalis.

Meconium Plug, Meconium Ileus, and Small Left Colon Syndrome

Meconium plug syndrome

Meconium plug syndrome is characterized by inspissated meconium in the colon. Some neonates with this condition may be premature, but most are full term. The clinical presentation is significant abdominal distention in a newborn with failure to pass meconium. A simple rectal exam may deliver the inspissated meconium and relieve the obstruction. This may need to be repeated to completely relieve the obstruction. In cases where the obstruction is more proximal, a water-soluble contrast enema may be both diagnostic and therapeutic (Figure 21–11), establishing the diagnosis while also serving as a therapeutic modality by drawing fluid into the lumen of the bowel and evacuating the plug. Up to 10% of patients with meconium plug will have Hirschsprung's disease, so a suction rectal biopsy is recommended for all patients with meconium plug syndrome.

Small left colon syndrome

Approximately 40–50% of patients with *small left colon syndrome* are born to insulin-dependent diabetic mothers. The narrow caliber of the left colon is due to disuse caused by functional obstruction, and may not need surgical intervention. The obstruction is usually partial and occurs distal to the splenic flexure. The diagnosis is confirmed by contrast enema, which can also be

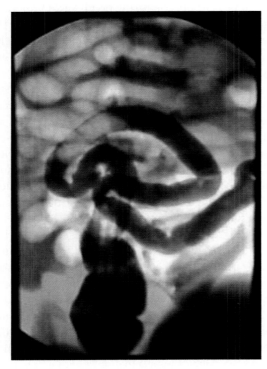

FIGURE 21–11 ■ Abdominal radiograph of meconium plug syndrome. The plug can be seen as a radiolucency in the lumen.

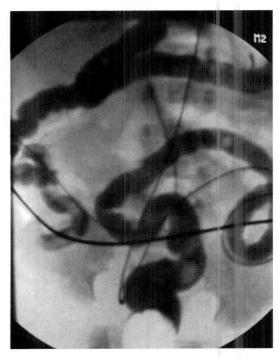

FIGURE 21–12 ■ Abdominal radiograph of meconium ileus. Notice the multiple pellets of meconium in the terminal ileum.

therapeutic in a similar fashion as meconium plug syndrome. Surgical intervention is sometimes required for patients who develop a proximal perforation from their obstructive process. These perforations are frequently found in the cecum during exploration.

Meconium ileus (Figure 21–12) and cystic fibrosis are discussed in Chapter 32. This form of bowel obstruction is caused by inspissated meconium in the ileum, and can often be treated with repeat water-soluble contrast enemas. These can hydrate inspissated meconium and result in evacuation (see Figure 9–4). Failed radiographic therapy may require urgent exploration. An enterotomy is made in the bowel and a dissolving solution such as 10% Mucomyst is instilled that easily breaks down the thick and tacky meconium in these patients. Perforation prior to exploration is a significant risk until the meconium has been evacuated and can result in an intense intra-abdominal inflammatory condition known as meconium peritonitis, which predisposes to adhesions for years afterward.

Foreign Body and Bezoars

Definitions and epidemiology

While many foreign bodies pass harmless through the GI tract, others can wreck havoc depending on their shape and the substance they are made of. Bowel obstruction or perforation can result. Bezoars are uncommon causes of obstruction but can be massive.

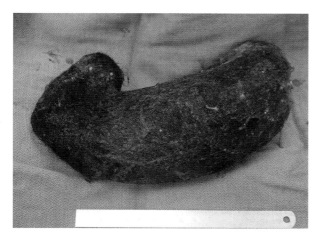

FIGURE 21-13 ■ The large cast of a gastric bezoar.

These unusual collections of hair or vegetable matter often collect in the stomach and create an enormous cast (Figure 21–13). Patients with bezoars secondary to ingestion of non-food items tend to have psychiatric illnesses.

Diagnosis

Patients with the known ingestion of a foreign body should be watched on an outpatient basis until the object passes in the stool. Serial plain films can follow the progression of radio-opaque objects. Foreign bodies that are retained and fail to progress should be removed before a complication occurs. Coins are the most commonly ingested foreign body and often lodge in the esophagus. Batteries are another commonly ingested foreign body and can lead to hollow viscus perforation. Sharp objects, such as the one shown in Figure 21–14, can also lead to perforation.

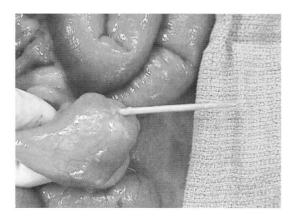

FIGURE 21-14 ■ This teenage boy was being explored for signs and symptoms consistent with appendicitis. On exploration, however, a toothpick was found transgressing across the terminal ileum resulting in a perforation. After surgery, the patient recalled swallowing a toothpick 2 weeks earlier.

Clinical presentation

The presenting symptoms may include emesis and inability to tolerate feeds except in very low volumes. Esophageal foreign bodies often cause chest pain and drooling. The patient may seem to have signs and symptoms of a bowel obstruction, yet the plain films show no evidence of an obstructive bowel gas pattern. Physical findings are often non-specific. For radiolucent objects, an upper GI contrast study may demonstrate the object.

Treatment

Foreign bodies that can be reached with an endoscope can usually be removed non-surgically. Surgical intervention is the only treatment for foreign bodies beyond the reach of an endoscope.

Appendicitis

Once always considered a surgical emergency, appendicitis is now handled in a variety of manners that ultimately may delay surgery for weeks. Besides the option for immediate surgery via an open or laparoscopic approach, surgery can be delayed for up to 24 hours with no appreciable impact on patient safety or outcome.[11] Moreover, perforated appendicitis can be effectively treated by non-operative initial management utilizing interventional radiology for drainage of an abdominal or pelvic abscess, followed by IV antibiotic coverage. Surgery is delayed for 4–6 weeks until inflammation has subsided, making the operation safer.

Definitions and epidemiology

The risk of appendicitis has been estimated to be between 6% and 10% over the lifetime of an individual. The peak age of incidence is between 10 and 12 years of age.[12]

Clinical presentation

The presentation is often quite variable, with right lower quadrant pain being the most common and repeatable symptom. Patients may have fevers and a general sense of feeling ill. They often initially experience periumbilical visceral pain that eventually migrates to the right lower quadrant as the overlying parietal peritoneum becomes inflamed. Emesis and anorexia usually develop. The speed with which the symptoms progress varies from just a few hours to several days. The diagnosis is often difficult to establish in the very young and, as a result, children under 3 years of age are almost always have a perforated appendix at diagnosis.[13]

Diagnosis

The diagnosis is typically made by a careful and thoughtful history and physical exam. If the history is fairly straightforward and the physical findings strongly

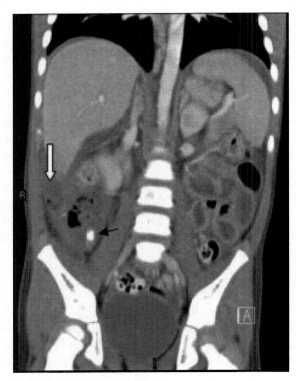

FIGURE 21–15 ■ Appendicitis. Note the bright appendicolith (black arrow) and the extraintestinal fluid and gas bubble in the adjacent abscess (white arrow).

support the diagnosis, then there is no need for additional imaging and surgery can be justified on the basis of the history and physical exam alone. Ultrasound and CT scan are very useful in equivocal cases (Figure 21–15).

Treatment

Surgery consists of a laparoscopic or open appendectomy. Children with on-perforated appendicitis usually go home within 24 hours and only require perioperative antibiotic coverage. Perforated appendicitis requires a longer course of antibiotics, typically 5–7 days, and patients are generally slow to resolve their ileus. Recurrent abscess formation is more common in perforated appendicitis and generally responds to a longer course of antibiotic coupled with drainage of large fluid collections, usually via percutaneous drains placed by an interventional radiologist. Small fluid collections usually respond to antibiotics alone.

SUMMARY

Emergent surgical intervention may be indicated for a wide variety of congenital and acquired conditions. The overall clinical picture may be the most important parameter in determining the haste with which surgical intervention is required. Resuscitation is a key element in the early

evaluation and treatment of most surgical problems and the patient's status should be reassessed frequently, with adjustments being made as required for optimal stabilization. Diagnosis and management may involve a number of important considerations before the patient is taken to the operating room. However, conditions in which bowel ischemia or perforation have already occurred or seem imminent are clear indications for emergent exploration.

REFERENCES

1. Pedersen RN, Garne E, Loane M, Korsholm L, Husby S, EUROCAT Working Group. Infantile hypertrophic pyloric stenosis: a comparative study of incidence and other epidemiological characteristics in seven European regions. *J Matern Fetal Neonatal Med.* 2008;21(9):599–604.
2. Godbole P, Sprigg A, Dickson JA, et al. Ultrasound compared with clinical examination in infantile hypertrophic pyloric stenosis. *Arch Dis Child.* 1996;75(4):335.
3. Forster N, Haddad RL, Choroomi S, Dilley AV, Pereira J. Use of ultrasound in 187 infants with suspected infantile hypertrophic pyloric stenosis. *Australas Radiol.* 2007;51(6):560–563.
4. Safford SD, Pietrobon R, Safford KM, Martins H, Skinner MA, Rice HE.A study of 11,003 patients with hypertrophic pyloric stenosis and the association between surgeon and hospital volume and outcomes. *J Pediatr Surg.* 2005;40(6):967–972 [discussion 972–973].
5. Kretz B, Watfa J, Sapin E. Our experience in "ad libitum" feeding after pyloromyotomy (review of 97 cases). *Arch Pediatr.* 2005;12(2):128–133.
6. Fraser JD, Aguayo P, Sharp SW, Ostlie DJ, St Peter SD. The role of laparoscopy in the management of malrotation. *J Surg Res.* 2009;156(1):80–82 [Epub May 3, 2009].
7. Meehan JJ, Sandler A. Pediatric robotic surgery: a retrospective review of a single institutional experience of 100 cases. *Surg Endosc.* 2008; 22(1):177–182 [Epub May 24, 2007].
8. Waseem M, Rosenberg HK. Intussusception. *Pediatr Emerg Care.* 2008;24(11):793–800 [review].
9. Schurr P, Perkins EM. The relationship between feeding and necrotizing enterocolitis in very low birth weight infants. *Neonatal Netw.* 2008;27(6):397–407 [review].
10. Sisk PM, Lovelady CA, Dillard RG, Gruber KJ, O'Shea TM. Early human milk feeding is associated with a lower risk of necrotizing enterocolitis in very low birth weight infants. *J Perinatol.* 2007;27(7):428–433 [Epub April 19, 2007; erratum in *J Perinatol.* 2007;27(12):808].
11. Partelli S, Beg S, Brown J, Vyas S, Kocher HM. Alteration in emergency theatre prioritisation does not alter outcome for acute appendicitis: comparative cohort study. *World J Emerg Surg.* 2009;4:22.
12. Addiss DG, Shaffer N, Fowler BS, et al. The epidemiology of appendicitis and appendectomy in the United States. *Am J Epidemiol.* 1990;132:910–925.
13. Nance ML, Adamson WT, Hedrick HL. Appendicitis in the young child: a continuing diagnostic challenge. *Pediatr Emerg Care.* 2000;16(3):160–162.

CHAPTER 22

Polyps and Tumors of the Intestines

Warren P. Bishop

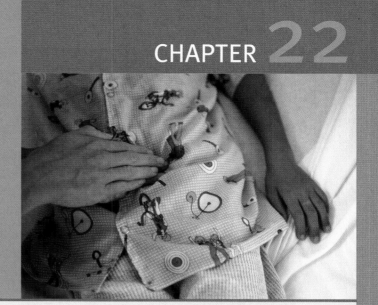

INTRODUCTION

An intestinal polyp is defined as a tissue mass that projects from the wall of the bowel into the lumen. It can be broadly classified into two main categories, neoplastic and non-neoplastic. Within each category, there are multiple potential types of lesions, some of which are associated with a syndrome including multiple polyps, some of which may carry a risk of cancer, and others which are less numerous and unlikely to cause future problems. The neoplastic polyps typically have an abnormal epithelial component resulting from abnormal proliferation. Non-neoplastic polyps can be either hamartomas, with involvement of all three germ layers, or inflammatory in nature.

A child with polyps typically presents with painless rectal bleeding, although larger polyps can be associated with pain if they cause obstruction, if motility-induced traction on the polyp results in stretching of mesenteric attachments, or if a polyp serves as a lead point for intussusception. Polyps may be encountered in any region of the intestine, although the region most commonly affected is the colon. They may occur sporadically, or there may be a strong familial component. It is therefore important to obtain a thorough family history of polyps and gastrointestinal cancers.

NON-NEOPLASTIC POLYPS

Juvenile Polyps

Definition and epidemiology

The most common of the intestinal polyps encountered in childhood is the *juvenile polyp*, a benign non-neoplastic tissue growth with a marked propensity for causing rectal bleeding.[1] These are relatively common, with most cases occurring before age 10 years and peaking at around ages 2–5 years. Isolated juvenile polyps are not associated with a genetic disorder and therefore not typically associated with a family history of polyps. If such history exists, other conditions must be suspected.

Pathogenesis

The etiology of isolated juvenile polyps is not well understood. In contrast to juvenile polyposis, in which multiple similar polyps occur throughout the GI tract (see below), there is no associated known gene mutation. Similar-appearing polyps (inflammatory polyps) are seen in children and adults with intestinal inflammation, and it is therefore likely that these lesions are in some way related to an inflammatory process. Long-term follow-up of patients with isolated juvenile polyps reveals no evidence of increased risk of intestinal malignancy,[2] which is in marked contrast to juvenile polyposis syndrome.

Clinical features

Children with juvenile polyps typically present with recurring episodes of small-volume, bright red rectal bleeding, not associated with any abdominal discomfort or significant anemia. Bleeding appears to be caused by intestinal contents moving across the friable surface of these polyps, causing mechanical trauma and resulting in bleeding. Occasionally, more brisk bleeding can occur if the head of the polyp is avulsed from its stalk, creating a very brief and hemodynamically insignificant higher volume bleeding episode.

At endoscopy, no lesions are found in the upper gastrointestinal tract, and fewer than five polyps are seen during colonoscopy. These polyps typically have a smooth surface and a deep red color with very friable

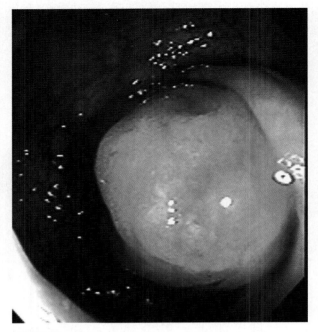

FIGURE 22–1 ▪ Juvenile polyp as seen in colon during colonoscopy.

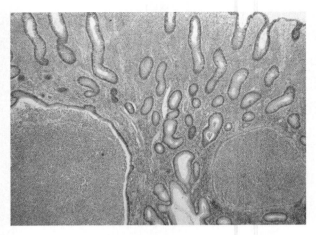

FIGURE 22–2 ▪ Histology of juvenile polyp. Note intense inflammation of lamina propria with cystic areas filled with inflammatory cells. Photo courtesy of Frank Mitros, MD.

surface, often covered with mucus (Figure 22–1). Juvenile polyps vary in size considerably, and are often quite large, sometimes >2 cm. There is frequently evidence of recent bleeding on the head of the polyp, which has a markedly friable surface. The colonic mucosa surrounding the polyp typically is mildly nodular in appearance, giving a "chicken skin"-like appearance.[3] Most of these polyps are easily removed during colonoscopy; even the larger ones can be removed piecemeal using a snare with electrocautery. After removal, bleeding ceases and seldom recurs. In young children, new polyps are occasionally found at repeat endoscopy, but new polyps are rarely seen in older children.

Differential diagnosis

The major potentially confusing condition is *juvenile polyposis syndrome*, described in detail below. Painless rectal bleeding may also be caused by other conditions, such as arteriovenous malformations, other types of polyps, Meckel's diverticulum, and inflammatory bowel disease. In the case of Meckel's diverticulum and arteriovenous malformations, the bleeding is often massive and hemodynamically significant, in contrast to the minor bleeding typically seen with juvenile polyps. Patients with rectal bleeding secondary to inflammatory bowel disease typically suffer from diarrhea and cramping along with the rectal bleeding, which is almost never the case with juvenile polyps.

Diagnosis

The diagnosis of rectal bleeding secondary to juvenile polyps depends on clinical suspicion, followed by colonoscopy and histological diagnosis. A complete colonoscopy should be performed, as polyps may be found throughout the length of the colon. Juvenile polyps are composed of cystic glands filled with mucus, with an intense inflammatory stroma and no smooth muscle elements. The surface epithelium may be slightly flattened but is otherwise normal. A degree of reactive atypia is often seen within the glands, probably due to the juxtaposition of epithelial elements with intense inflammation, but no true dysplasia is seen in these lesions.

The typical clinical presentation of recurrent, painless rectal bleeding that is not associated with diarrhea or weight loss should trigger colonoscopy. Because polyps may occur more proximal than the sigmoid colon, the patient should be adequately prepped and a full colonoscopy performed. All polyps should be removed with a snare and electrocautery, retrieved, and submitted for histopathological analysis. Accurate diagnosis depends on demonstration of the typical histological features described above (Figure 22–2).

Management

A child with typical juvenile polyps is managed by colonoscopy with snare removal of the polyps. Rarely, an extremely large polyp or one in a difficult-to-reach location may need to be removed surgically.[4] So long as bleeding stops, there are fewer than five polyps, there is no family history of polyposis, and histology is consistent with benign juvenile polyps, no further investigation or intervention is required. If bleeding does recur, repeat colonoscopy is indicated, and the possibility of juvenile polyposis syndrome should be considered.

Table 22–1.

Juvenile Polyposis Syndrome—Diagnostic Criteria

Diagnosis of JPS requires at least one of the following:
- >5 polyps in the colon and rectum
- Presence of any juvenile polyps in the stomach or small intestine
- Any number of juvenile polyps *with a family history of juvenile polyposis*

Juvenile Polyposis Syndrome

Definition and diagnosis

This syndrome consists of the presence of multiple juvenile polyps occurring throughout life and not limited to the colon and rectum. The diagnostic criteria for juvenile polyposis are listed in Table 22–1.[5,6] The diagnosis does not depend on the histological features, which typically are not distinguishable from isolated juvenile polyps. It must be remembered that a child with an initial diagnosis of simple juvenile polyp(s) may go on to meet criteria for juvenile polyposis syndrome. As a result, a child with a history of juvenile polyps who goes on to develop further symptoms of gastrointestinal bleeding or abdominal pain should be re-evaluated with colonoscopy and upper endoscopy.

Pathogenesis

Unlike typical juvenile polyps, about 30% of patients with a juvenile polyposis syndrome are found to have a gene mutation[7] (Table 22–2). Currently, two causative genes have been found to be involved: *MADH4* (also known as *SMAD4*) and *BMPR1A*. *MADH4* codes for a protein in TGF-beta signaling pathway. *BMPR1A* codes for a membrane receptor in the TGF-beta super family. When activated, the TGF-beta pathway tends to suppress epithelial cell proliferation. Obviously, other, as yet

Table 22–2.

Genetics of Non-neoplastic (Hamartomatous) Polyposis Syndromes

Syndrome	Gene	Chromosome
Juvenile polyposis	MADH4	18q21.1
Peutz–Jeghers syndrome	BMPR1A	10q22.3
Bannayan–Ruvalcaba– Riley syndrome	STK11	19p13.3
	PTEN	10q23.31
Cowden syndrome	PTEN	10q23.31

unidentified, mutations or other alterations affecting expression of these genes must be involved in pathogenesis of juvenile polyposis syndromes to account for the 70% of patients who do not have identifiable mutations. Despite this statistic, 85% of patients with juvenile polyposis report a family history of polyps.[8] Although 75% of patients will have an affected parent, approximately 25% of new cases are the result of a new gene mutation.

Clinical features

Children with juvenile polyposis syndrome have a very different course than patients with isolated juvenile polyps. Presenting symptoms are more severe than in isolated juvenile polyps, with prominent mucus present in the stools, and sometimes hypokalemia and hypoalbuminemia secondary to protein-losing enteropathy, as well as anemia from significant blood loss. These symptoms appear later than in isolated juvenile polyps, with a mean age at diagnosis of 18.5 years. The stomach is involved in 14%, the duodenum in 2%, and jejunum or ileum in 7%.[8] There is a tendency for juvenile polyps to occur throughout life in these patients. Some patients with the *MADH4* mutation also have hereditary hemorrhagic telangiectasia (HHT), a syndrome characterized by multiple systemic arteriovenous malformations, mucocutaneous telangiectasias, epistaxis, and risk of intracranial bleeding.[9]

A major concern is that patients with juvenile polyposis are at increased risk of gastrointestinal tract tumors, especially of the colon, stomach, and duodenum. A recent review of one Iowa kindred consisting of 29 affected individuals revealed that 11 developed colon cancer, 4 developed gastric cancers, 1 experienced cancer of the duodenum, and 1 had pancreatic cancer. This suggests a lifetime risk of gastrointestinal malignancies of around 55%.[10]

Management

Affected individuals should undergo both upper endoscopy and colonoscopy to identify and remove as many polyps as possible, as this will reduce the risk of bleeding and protein-losing enteropathy. In severe cases with numerous polyps (Figure 22–3), total colectomy or gastrectomy may be necessary. Screening colonoscopy recommendations for affected individuals and their children are listed in Table 22–3.[11]

Peutz–Jeghers Syndrome

Definitions and epidemiology

Peutz–Jeghers syndrome (PJS) is defined by the association between gastrointestinal polyps and abnormal pigmentation of the skin and oral mucosa. It is inherited in an autosomal dominant fashion. PJS is also frequently

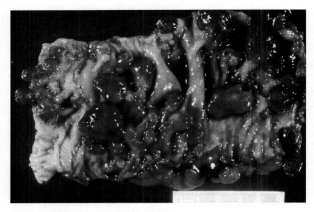

FIGURE 22–3 ■ Colon specimen from patient with severe juvenile polyposis requiring colectomy to control bleeding. Photo courtesy of Frank Mitros, MD.

sporadic, resulting from a new term line mutation. Affected individuals typically develop prominent freckle-like pigmentation around the mouth, lips, and on oral mucous membranes during the first decade of life, with appearance of rectal bleeding and abdominal pain secondary to polyps typically during the second decade of life. Polyps in this syndrome occur throughout the gastrointestinal tract, and are not limited to the colon and rectum.

Pathogenesis

PJS is caused by a variety of mutations in the *STK11* *(LKB1)* gene, one of which can be identified in around 90%[12] of affected patients. This gene codes for a serine–threonine kinase with tumor-suppressing activity as well as effects on cellular polarity and metabolism.

Clinical features

Affected individuals typically present with characteristic facial pigmentation and gastrointestinal symptoms. Although blood in the stools is frequently present, a more common presentation is abdominal pain and/or intestinal obstruction. Figure 22–4a shows typical facial pigmentation in a Peutz–Jeghers patient. Figure 22–4b demonstrates the associated pigmentation of the buccal mucosa. Typically, these pigmented spots tend to become less prominent or even fade away with age. Intestinal obstructive symptoms are caused by motility traction on the polyps, obstruction by the polyps themselves, or frequently by episodes of intussusception, with a polyp as a lead point. Onset of symptoms is most likely after 10 years of age, and the average age of diagnosis is 23 years for males and 26 years for females.[13]

Patients with this condition are at risk of gastrointestinal, pancreatic, breast, ovarian, cervical, and testicular malignancies. Sertoli cell tumors in males secrete estrogen, and this condition should therefore be suspected in males with prominent gynecomastia.

Diagnosis

Diagnostic criteria for PJS are listed in Table 22–4. In children of affected individuals, facial pigmentation alone is sufficient to make the diagnosis, whereas in other individuals the presence of typical polyps along

 Table 22–3.

Surveillance in Juvenile Polyposis Syndrome Patients

Clinical Status	Begin Surveillance at Age	Recommended Screening	Interval
Proband	Diagnosis	Molecular genetic testing (*MADH4, BMPR1A*)/genetic counseling	Once; if negative, may repeat as new testing becomes available
(1) All affected individuals and (2) all family members with known mutation	Diagnosis, or age 15 years	CBC, colonoscopy, upper endoscopy	Yearly until no new polyps are found, and then every 3 years
All at risk individuals with family history but: (a) no family genetic testing done or (b) family genetic testing uninformative	Age 15 years	CBC, colonoscopy, upper endoscopy	Yearly until no new polyps are found, and then every 3 years
Family members testing negative for known family mutation	Age 15 years	CBC, colonoscopy, upper endoscopy	Repeat endoscopic studies every 10 years if negative

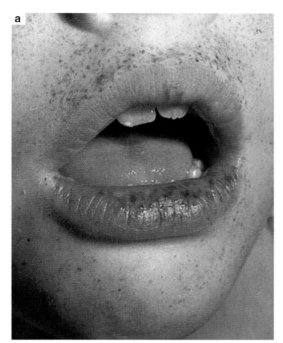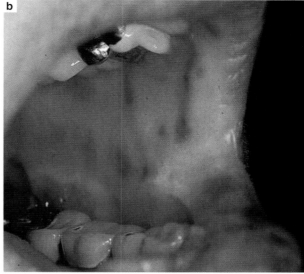

FIGURE 22–4 ■ (a) Facial pigmentation in Peutz–Jeghers syndrome. (b) Buccal pigmentation in Peutz–Jeghers syndrome. From: Wolff K, Goldsmith LA, Katz SI, Gilchrest BA, Paller AS, Leffell DJ. *Fitzpatrick's Dermatology in General Medicine*. 7th ed. 2008. Reproduced with permission.

with facial pigmentation is usually sufficient. Molecular genetic testing for *STK11 (LKB1)* mutations is an additional way to confirm the diagnosis. The polyps of PJS have a unique microscopic appearance, with prominent smooth muscle bundles branching in a tree-like pattern within the polyp. Figure 22–5 shows a typical histological appearance of a PJS polyp.

intestine. This should preferably be done using wireless capsule endoscopy,[14,15] compared to older techniques such as upper GI series with small bowel follow-through. These evaluations should be repeated every 2 years throughout life.

Management

After initial diagnosis, it is important to document the extent of intestinal involvement including both upper and lower endoscopy as well as examination of the small

Table 22–4.

Diagnosis of Peutz–Jeghers Syndrome

For individuals with histologically confirmed typical hamartomatous polyps, *one of the following* is required:
■ Family history consistent with autosomal dominant inheritance
■ Mucocutaneous pigmentation
■ Small bowel polyps
■ Mutation in the *STK11 (LKB1)* gene
For individuals with a family history of PJS, *only mucocutaneous pigmentation* is required

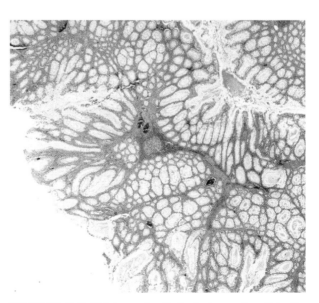

FIGURE 22–5 ■ Histology of a Peutz–Jeghers polyp. Note the arborizing strands of smooth muscle and minimal inflammation. Photo courtesy of Frank Mitros, MD.

Table 22–5.			
Surveillance of Peutz—Jeghers Syndrome Patients			
Cancer Type	Surveillance Test	Begin Screening	Screening iInterval
Gastric, small bowel, colon	Upper endoscopy, colonoscopy, and small bowel imaging	8 years	2 years
	Testicular exam, ultrasound Examination, mammography/MRI		
Testicular	Endoscopic ultrasound or CT, CA 19-9	Birth	1–2 years until age 12 years
Breast	Pelvic ultrasound and CA-125	18 years	6-Month exam, yearly imaging
Pancreas	Pelvic exam and	25 years	1–2 years
Ovaries	Pap smear	25 years	Yearly
Uterus and cervix		21 years	Yearly

Because individuals with PJS are at significant increased risk for a variety of cancers, they must be monitored closely. The overall increased risk of cancer is around 10-fold that of the general population, with up to 93% cumulative lifetime risk of cancer. Of these, about 29% patients experience cancer of the colon, 39% stomach, 13% small intestine, 36% pancreas, 9% testes, 54% breast, 21% ovary, and 10% cervix.[16] Screening recommendations for these conditions and for routine endoscopic surveillance of the intestine are detailed[13] in Table 22–5.

PTEN Hamartoma Syndromes

Definitions and epidemiology

Two syndromes associated with *PTEN* gene mutations are associated with intestinal polyps. These are *Bannayan–Ruvalcaba–Riley syndrome* (BRRS) and *Cowden syndrome* (CS). These are rare conditions with a prevalence estimated at 1 in 200,000. In BRRS, patients have macrocephaly, lipomas, and pigmented macules on the glans penis. CS patients have multiple hamartomas, with a high risk of both benign and malignant tumors of the breast, thyroid, and uterus.[17]

Pathogenesis

PTEN codes for a protein phosphatase that is able to remove phosphate from serine, threonine, and also tyrosine residues. PTEN specifically dephosphorylates phosphatidylinositol-3,4,5-triphosphate. Mutation of the gene results in increased resistance to apoptosis and favors cell proliferation.[18]

Clinical features

CS is characterized by facial trichilemmomas, papillomatous skin lesions, mental retardation, high risk of breast, thyroid, and endometrial cancer, acral and plantar keratoses, and macrocephaly, with intestinal hamartomas being a relatively minor and inconsistent finding. Manifestations of this disorder are often delayed in onset, with most patients developing characteristic features by the late 20s. Interestingly, there does not appear to be an increased risk of gastrointestinal cancer in this syndrome, despite the occurrence of gastrointestinal hamartomas.[19]

BRRS is characterized by a high incidence of gastrointestinal polyps, along with other features, including developmental delay, proximal myopathy, scoliosis, and joint hyperflexibility. Although initial reports indicated a low likelihood of associated malignancies in BRRS, it is now thought that affected individuals have the same cancer risk as those with CS.

Diagnosis

Diagnosis of the PTEN hamartomas syndromes is based on clinical criteria, as described above. The differential diagnosis includes juvenile polyposis syndrome and PJS. Identification of a *PTEN* mutation establishes the diagnosis with certainty, but a mutation is found in only about 80% of individuals who meet all other criteria for the diagnosis for CS.

Management

Comprehensive physical examination at diagnosis and yearly thereafter is mandatory. This exam should include skin, thyroid, breast examination, and annual endometrial biopsies in premenopausal women. Monthly breast self-examination should be performed, and annual mammography should begin at age 30 years, or 10 years younger than the earliest known familial cancer diagnosis. Colonoscopy is recommended beginning at age 50 years, as per American Cancer Society recommendations.[19]

NEOPLASTIC POLYPOSIS SYNDROMES

Familial Adenomatous Polyposis

Definitions and epidemiology

Familial adenomatous polyposis (FAP) is a syndrome associated with the appearance of multiple adenomatous polyps in the colon, with the inevitable development of colon cancer. The average age of cancer diagnosis in untreated individuals is 39 years. The prevalence of FAP is thought to be around 1 in 5–10,000 individuals.[20] Most patients develop polyps beginning at around the age of 16 years, but in some cases these appear much earlier, as young as age 7 years. By age 35 years, 95% of individuals have polyps. In some cases, an *attenuated phenotype* results in later development of fewer polyps and a later onset of colon cancer. Early diagnosis is essential in order to assure proper treatment and thereby avoid death from colon cancer. Surveillance for extracolonic manifestations is also critically important in these patients.

Pathogenesis

FAP is caused by mutations in the *APC* gene. This gene codes for a protein that functions as a tumor suppressor. Functions of the APC protein include indirect regulation of transcription of a number of cell proliferation genes via interaction with beta catenin,[21] leading to cellular adhesion and maturation with diminished proliferation and migration.[22] The overwhelming majority of *APC* mutations result in truncation of the protein, which clearly interferes with its functions.[23] Mutations in *APC* are therefore likely to result in dysregulation of all of the above processes, leading to development of cancer.

Studies of large numbers of FAP patients have begun to reveal correlations between the mutation site in the gene and the resulting phenotype, with the majority of severe cases associated with mutations occurring in the middle of the gene, between exon 1250 and 1464.[24] An attenuated form of FAP also exists, in which there are smaller numbers (<100) of colonic adenomas, with later onset of polyposis and cancer. These are not likely to be seen in childhood, and are associated with mutations in the far 5′ and 3′ regions of the gene.[20] It is therefore likely that knowledge of the specific mutation will prove clinically useful in decision-making regarding surgery and other therapies.

Diagnosis

In children with a family history of polyposis, it is very important to screen appropriately for the condition and to do so before any significant risk of adenocarcinoma occurs. Figure 22–6 is an algorithm that may be used to

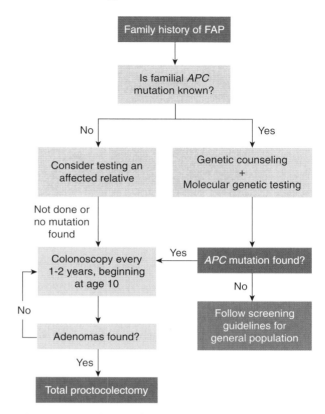

FIGURE 22–6 ■ Algorithm for the investigation of individuals with a family history of FAP.

guide the investigation of these children. Genetic counseling should be obtained in all cases, and children of affected individuals screened for the family mutation, if it is known. For those families that have not been tested or in whom a mutation could not be identified, colonoscopy for all vulnerable first-degree relatives (children and siblings) should be done every 1–2 years, beginning at age 10–12 years. Figure 22–7 shows the typical appearance of fully developed FAP in a colectomy specimen from a young adult.

In the instance of an individual being diagnosed with adenomatous polyposis in the absence of a family history, genetic testing for *APC* gene mutations should be performed, as up to 25% of cases are the result of new mutations.[25]

Clinical features

In classical FAP, large numbers of polyps develop quickly after beginning to appear during the second decade of life. In most cases, hundreds to thousands of polyps rapidly developed after onset of polyposis. Development of colon cancer is inevitable unless colectomy is performed in these patients. Cancer of the duodenum at the ampulla of Vater is the most common non-colonic site, occurring in up to 12% of cases.[26,27] Other cancers are rarely seen in this condition (<2% each), including

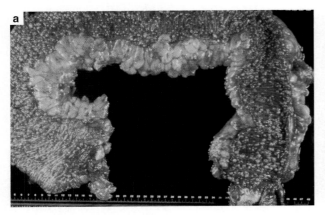
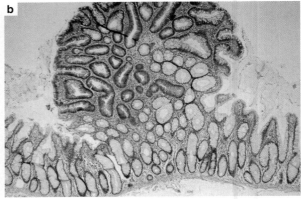

FIGURE 22–7 ■ (a) Thousands of colonic polyps in colon of patient with FAP. Photo courtesy of Frank Mitros, MD. (b) Small adenoma on mucosal biopsy of a patient with FAP. Photo courtesy of Frank Mitros, MD.

CNS medulloblastoma (*Turcot syndrome*), thyroid,[28] pancreas,[29] and hepatobiliary tumors.[30]

Various extraintestinal manifestations occur in many patients, including congenital hypertrophy of the retinal pigment epithelium (CHRPE) in about 40%.[31] When FAP includes prominent soft tissue tumors (desmoids tumors, fibromas, epidermoid cysts, and osteomas), the patient is said to have *Gardner syndrome*. Risk of Gardner syndrome is associated with mutations in codons 1395–1493, although many FAP patients have some extraintestinal manifestation.[32]

One important early manifestation of FAP in childhood is hepatoblastoma, which is highly (but not exclusively) associated with mutations 5′ to codon 1309. All reported cases of this tumor associated with familial APC mutations have occurred before the age of 10 years,[33] with a prevalence at least 750 times higher than expected in the general population, and occurring mostly in males.[33] In sporadic hepatoblastoma, not associated with any familial history of colon cancer, only about 10% are found to have a mutation of APC.[34] Surveillance for hepatoblastoma in children of FAP patients should be considered, and the risk of this may be a reason to consider early genetic screening when the family mutation is known.

Treatment

The only reliable treatment for FAP currently is total proctocolectomy.

OTHER NEOPLASMS OF THE GASTROINTESTINAL TRACT

Definitions and Epidemiology

Malignant tumors arising from the gastrointestinal tract are quite rare in childhood, accounting for only about 1.2% of all pediatric cancers.[35] Of these, the majority are

B-cell lymphomas, evenly divided between Burkitt's lymphoma and non-Burkitt's, non-Hodgkin's lymphoma, with adenocarcinomas, carcinoids, and leiomyosarcomas making up the remainder.[36] MALT lymphomas of the stomach associated with *Helicobacter pylori* have also been reported in children, as in adults.[37] Non-malignant tumors also occur, and include neurofibromas, ganglioneuromas, leiomyomas, and lipomas, as well as the various polyps described above.

Clinical Features

Patients with intestinal lymphomas present with weight loss, abdominal pain, anorexia, and diarrhea.[38] These features are often indistinguishable from inflammatory bowel disease, and are often misdiagnosed as this condition unless tumor tissue is obtained. These tumors can cause obstruction of the bowel due to mass effect or by serving as a lead point for intussusception; if either of these occurs, the tumor is identified at the time of surgery.

Carcinoid tumors are most commonly found in the appendix, but can occur throughout the GI tract. They most often present as acute appendicitis and are found incidentally at appendectomy. When they occur elsewhere in the gut, they can cause obstructive symptoms and gastrointestinal bleeding.[39] Most of these tumors are benign. Current opinion is that tumors <2 cm in size without evidence of metastasis can be adequately treated by simple excision, with verification of clear surgical margins.

Adenocarcinomas of the intestine in children most often occur spontaneously, without typical predisposing factors of FAP or ulcerative colitis. In these unfortunate children, the extreme rarity of this diagnosis virtually guarantees that metastasis will have occurred by the time of diagnosis. Patients most commonly present with the symptom of abdominal pain, typically without obvious rectal bleeding or change in bowel habits. Typically, because these symptoms are common and non-specific, the diagnosis is not suspected until very late in the course.[40]

Patients with benign tumors of the intestine typically present with abdominal pain, abdominal mass, intussusception, bleeding, or frank obstruction, depending on the nature, size, and location of the tumor.

Treatment

Treatment of lymphoma varies according to type; details are beyond the scope of this book. Primary excision should be the first priority, with various chemotherapy regimens used afterward. Patients with completely resectable disease have a very good prognosis of around 80% survival at 2 years, but, until recently, poor survival with metastatic disease. New therapies for B-cell lymphomas include targeted therapies with monoclonal antibodies, such as rituximab, directed at the CD-20 B-cell surface molecule. These are used either with standard chemotherapy regimens (such as cyclophosphamide, vincristine, and prednisone) or as a delivery vehicle for radioactive isotopes. These new therapies offer exciting new hope for intestinal lymphoma patients.[41]

Other intestinal tumors are also best managed by surgical excision, with subsequent therapy based on histology and presence or absence of metastatic disease.

REFERENCES

1. Corredor J, Wambach J, Barnard J. Gastrointestinal polyps in children: advances in molecular genetics, diagnosis, and management. *J Pediatr.* 2001;138(5):621–628.
2. Nugent KP, Talbot IC, Hodgson SV, Phillips RK. Solitary juvenile polyps: not a marker for subsequent malignancy. *Gastroenterology.* 1993;105(3):698–700.
3. Nowicki MJ, Subramony C, Bishop PR, Parker PH. Colonic chicken skin mucosa: association with juvenile polyps in children. *Am J Gastroenterol.* 2001;96(3):788–792.
4. Wiseman J, Emil S. Minimal access surgical management of large juvenile polyps in children. *J Pediatr Surg.* 2009;44(9):e9–e13.
5. Sachatello CR, Hahn IS, Carrington CB. Juvenile gastrointestinal polyposis in a female infant: report of a case and review of the literature of a recently recognized syndrome. *Surgery.* 1974;75(1):107–114.
6. Jass JR, Williams CB, Bussey HJ, Morson BC. Juvenile polyposis—a precancerous condition. *Histopathology.* 1988;13(6):619–630.
7. Pyatt RE, Pilarski R, Prior TW. Mutation screening in juvenile polyposis syndrome. *J Mol Diagn.* 2006;8(1):84–88.
8. Desai DC, Neale KF, Talbot IC, Hodgson SV, Phillips RK. Juvenile polyposis. *Br J Surg.* 1995;82(1):14–17.
9. Gallione CJ, Repetto GM, Legius E, et al. A combined syndrome of juvenile polyposis and hereditary haemorrhagic telangiectasia associated with mutations in MADH4 (SMAD4). *Lancet.* 2004;363(9412):852–859.
10. Howe JR, Mitros FA, Summers RW. The risk of gastrointestinal carcinoma in familial juvenile polyposis. *Ann Surg Oncol.* 1998;5(8):751–756.
11. Haidle JL, Howe JR. *Juvenile Polyposis Syndrome.* Bethesda, MD: National Institutes of Health; 2008. http://www.ncbi.nlm.nig.gov/br.fcgi?book=gene&part=jps.
12. de Leng WW, Jansen M, Carvalho R, et al. Genetic defects underlying Peutz–Jeghers syndrome (PJS) and exclusion of the polarity-associated MARK/Par1 gene family as potential PJS candidates. *Clin Genet.* 2007;72(6):568–573.
13. Giardiello FM, Trimbath JD. Peutz–Jeghers syndrome and management recommendations. *Clin Gastroenterol Hepatol.* 2006;4(4):408–415.
14. Lorenzo-Zuniga V, Moreno de Vega V, Manosa M, Domenech E, Boix J. The utility of wireless capsule endoscopy, as compared with barium contrast study, in a case of Peutz–Jeghers syndrome. *Acta Gastroenterol Belg.* 2006;69(4):423.
15. De Palma GD, Rega M, Ciamarra P, et al. Small-bowel polyps in Peutz–Jeghers syndrome: diagnosis by wireless capsule endoscopy. *Endoscopy.* 2004;36(11):1039.
16. Giardiello FM, Brensinger JD, Tersmette AC, et al. Very high risk of cancer in familial Peutz–Jeghers syndrome. *Gastroenterology.* 2000;119(6):1447–1453.
17. Blumenthal GM, Dennis PA. PTEN hamartoma tumor syndromes. *Eur J Hum Genet.* 2008;16(11):1289–1300.
18. Yin Y, Shen WH. PTEN: a new guardian of the genome. *Oncogene.* 2008;27(41):5443–5453.
19. Eng C. *PTEN Hamartoma Tumor Syndrome (PHTS).* Bethesda, MD: National Institutes of Health; 2009. http://www.ncbi.nlm.nih.gov/bookshelf/br.fcgi?book=gene&part=phts.
20. Nieuwenhuis MH, Vasen HF. Correlations between mutation site in APC and phenotype of familial adenomatous polyposis (FAP): a review of the literature. *Crit Rev Oncol Hematol.* 2007;61(2):153–161.
21. Rowan AJ, Lamlum H, Ilyas M, et al. APC mutations in sporadic colorectal tumors: a mutational "hotspot" and interdependence of the "two hits". *Proc Natl Acad Sci U S A.* 2000;97(7):3352–3357.
22. Hughes SA, Carothers AM, Hunt DH, Moran AE, Mueller JD, Bertagnolli MM. Adenomatous polyposis coli truncation alters cytoskeletal structure and microtubule stability in early intestinal tumorigenesis. *J Gastrointest Surg.* 2002;6(6):868–874 [discussion 75].
23. Hirschman BA, Pollock BH, Tomlinson GE. The spectrum of APC mutations in children with hepatoblastoma from familial adenomatous polyposis kindreds. *J Pediatr.* 2005;147(2):263–266.
24. Bertario L, Russo A, Radice P, et al. Genotype and phenotype factors as determinants for rectal stump cancer in patients with familial adenomatous polyposis. Hereditary Colorectal Tumors Registry. *Ann Surg.* 2000;231(4):538–543.
25. Davidson NO. Genetic testing in colorectal cancer: who, when, how and why. *Keio J Med.* 2007;56(1):14–20.
26. Kadmon M, Tandara A, Herfarth C. Duodenal adenomatosis in familial adenomatous polyposis coli. A review of

the literature and results from the Heidelberg Polyposis Register. *Int J Colorectal Dis.* 2001;16(2):63–75.

27. Wallace MH, Phillips RK. Upper gastrointestinal disease in patients with familial adenomatous polyposis. *Br J Surg.* 1998;85(6):742–750.

28. Truta B, Allen BA, Conrad PG, et al. Genotype and phenotype of patients with both familial adenomatous polyposis and thyroid carcinoma. *Fam Cancer.* 2003;2(2):95–99.

29. Elkharwily A, Gottlieb K. The pancreas in familial adenomatous polyposis. *JOP.* 2008;9(1):9–18.

30. Cetta F, Montalto G, Petracci M. Hepatoblastoma and APC gene mutation in familial adenomatous polyposis. *Gut.* 1997;41(3):417.

31. Tourino R, Conde-Freire R, Cabezas-Agricola JM, et al. Value of the congenital hypertrophy of the retinal pigment epithelium in the diagnosis of familial adenomatous polyposis. *Int Ophthalmol.* 2004;25(2):101–112.

32. Wallis YL, Morton DG, McKeown CM, Macdonald F. Molecular analysis of the APC gene in 205 families: extended genotype–phenotype correlations in FAP and evidence for the role of APC amino acid changes in colorectal cancer predisposition. *J Med Genet.* 1999;36(1):14–20.

33. Giardiello FM, Petersen GM, Brensinger JD, et al. Hepatoblastoma and APC gene mutation in familial adenomatous polyposis. *Gut.* 1996;39(6):867–869.

34. Aretz S, Koch A, Uhlhaas S, et al. Should children at risk for familial adenomatous polyposis be screened for hepatoblastoma and children with apparently sporadic hepatoblastoma be screened for APC germline mutations? *Pediatr Blood Cancer.* 2006;47(6):811–818.

35. Pickett LK, Briggs HC. Cancer of the gastrointestinal tract in childhood. *Pediatr Clin North Am.* 1967;14(1):223–234.

36. Ladd AP, Grosfeld JL. Gastrointestinal tumors in children and adolescents. *Semin Pediatr Surg.* 2006;15(1):37–47.

37. Wu TC, Chen LK, Lai CR. Primary gastric lymphoma associated with *Helicobacter pylori* in a child. *J Pediatr Gastroenterol Nutr.* 2001;32(5):608–610.

38. Al-Bahrani ZR, Al-Mondhiry H, Bakir F, Al-Saleem T. Clinical and pathologic subtypes of primary intestinal lymphoma. Experience with 132 patients over a 14-year period. *Cancer.* 1983;52(9):1666–1672.

39. Spunt SL, Pratt CB, Rao BN, et al. Childhood carcinoid tumors: the St Jude Children's Research Hospital experience. *J Pediatr Surg.* 2000;35(9):1282–1286.

40. Radhakrishnan CN, Bruce J. Colorectal cancers in children without any predisposing factors. A report of eight cases and review of the literature. *Eur J Pediatr Surg.* 2003;13(1):66–68.

41. Lim SH, Beers SA, French RR, Johnson PW, Glennie MJ, Cragg MS. Anti-CD20 monoclonal antibodies—historical and future perspectives. *Haematologica.* 2010 Jan;95(1):135–143.

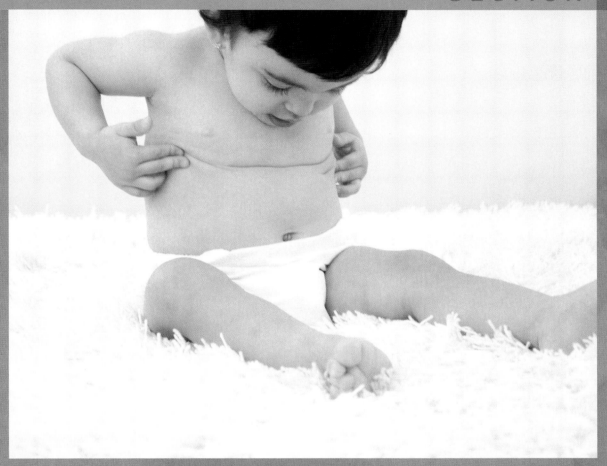

SECTION 4

Disorders of the Liver

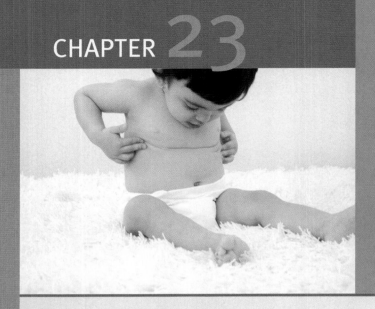

CHAPTER 23

Biliary Atresia

Melissa Leyva-Vega and
Barbara A. Haber

DEFINITIONS AND EPIDEMIOLOGY

Biliary atresia (BA) is a progressive idiopathic, necroinflammatory process involving the extrahepatic biliary tree, which can be either segmentally or entirely affected. As the disease progresses, there is obliteration of the extrahepatic bile duct lumen and obstruction to bile flow (Figure 23–1). The result is cholestasis and chronic liver damage. With time, the intrahepatic biliary system becomes increasingly involved. BA is the most common cause of neonatal jaundice for which surgery is indicated and the most common indication for liver transplantation in children.

Many different classifications of BA have been proposed over the years. One classification system focuses on the anatomy of the biliary tree. The most comprehensive is that used in the Japanese BA Registry

ABBREVIATIONS

BA: biliary atresia

BASM: biliary atresia splenic malformation

CXR: chest X-ray

DISIDA: diisopropyl iminodiacetic acid; hepatobiliary scintigraphy

ERCP: endoscopic retrograde cholangiopancreatography

HPE: hepatoportoenterostomy

MCT: medium-chain triglycerides

PPS: peripheral pulmonary stenosis

PTLD: post-transplant lymphoproliferative disease

US: ultrasound

The liver
Scarred bile bile duct remnant
Little/No flow of bile
Cystic duct
Pancreatic duct
No bile flows into the intestine
Abnormal gallbladder
Small intestine

FIGURE 23–1 ■ Schematic of BA. As the disease progresses there is obliteration of the extrahepatic biliary tree, leading to obstruction of bile flow. www.barcnetwork.org.

(Figure 23–2).[1] In this classification system there are three major types of atresia: *type I*, atresia of the common bile duct (10% of patients); *type II*, atresia of the hepatic ducts (2% of patients); and *type III*, atresia at the porta hepatitis (88% of patients). Within each type there are several subtypes, which will not be discussed here. The first two types of BA are sometimes labeled "correctable atresia," whereas type III corresponds to the so-called non-correctable type of atresia, and accounts for the majority of patients. However, with current hepatoportoenterostomy (HPE) techniques, most patients achieve at least some bile drainage, and thus the correctable versus non-correctable distinction is rarely used.

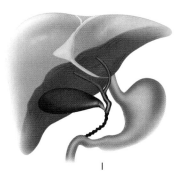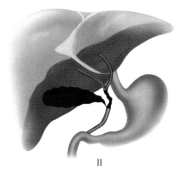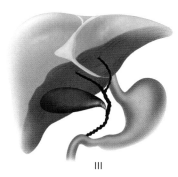

I   II   III

FIGURE 23-2 ■ Three major types of BA, based on anatomic findings.[1] This image was adapted from an image available at www.mayoclinicproceedings.com. The original image is found in reference #1. Type I (about 10%): atresia of the common bile duct. Type II (about 2%): atresia of the hepatic duct. Type III (over 88%): atresia at the porta hepatis.

Another classification system is based on the associated malformations and onset of jaundice. Many textbooks refer to embryonic and perinatal BA. In the former, there is typically onset of jaundice at birth and often multiple major malformations, the most common of which is heterotaxy. In the latter, jaundice appears several weeks after birth and there are usually no associated malformations. Perinatal BA accounts for 70–80% of all cases. Because there are so many exceptions to these patterns, new nomenclature systems have been proposed. Biliary atresia splenic malformation (BASM) is a term that specifically captures those previously termed "embryonic" who have heterotaxy. BASM applies to all infants with BA and either asplenia or polysplenia. The typical associated malformations include midline liver, malrotation, preduodenal portal vein, interrupted inferior vena cava, and cardiac malformations. Ten to 15% of all cases of BA have this categorization. Another 10–15% have major malformations in association with BA but do not fall into any stereotypical pattern. As our understanding of BA improves, it is likely that there will be an improved classification system.

BA occurs with an estimated frequency of 1 in 8000 to 1 in 20,000 live births, depending on the country. In the United States, there are 0.65–0.85 cases per 10,000 live births,[2] resulting in 250–400 new cases per year. The highest incidence occurs in Asians. In Taiwan, there are 1.46 cases per 10,000 live births. The female-to-male ratio is close to 1, and sexual predominance varies based on the study. BA appears to occur more frequently in certain racial groups in the United States. The most recent epidemiologic study of potential risk factors for BA identified 112 cases of BA using data from the National Birth Defects Prevention Study. This study found that patients with BA were more likely to be born to non-Hispanic black mothers than to non-Hispanic white mothers, OR = 2.29 (95th CI = 1.07 − 4.93).[3] Another study used a population-based birth defects surveillance system in Atlanta and identified 112 patients born with BA from 1968 to 1993

and also found higher rates of BA among non-white infants compared to white infants (0.96 versus 0.44 per 10,000 live births).[4] Caton et al. identified 369 BA cases from 1983 to 1998 in New York State and found that infants with BA were born to black mothers at an increased rate when compared to white mothers.[5] These reported racial differences in incidence may reflect genetic, socioeconomic, and/or environmental factors.

Studies looking at seasonal variations of BA have shown inconsistent results. The Atlanta study by Yoon et al. found seasonal clustering with a greater number of cases occurring from December to March.[4] In the New York Study, seasonal patterns varied by region, with infants in New York City more likely to be born in the spring, and infants from outside of the city more likely to be born in the period from September to November.[5]

Several epidemiologic studies have looked at gestational age, birth weight, and maternal age in BA patients. The findings from one study to the next are conflicting and therefore no definitive risk factors have been identified. For example, the Atlanta study found an increased incidence in term infants with low birth weights (<2500 g). On the other hand, The et al. found that patients with BA were more likely to have normal birth weight.[3] This study also found that infants with BA were more likely to be preterm (≤36 weeks). The largest and most comprehensive epidemiologic study used the Swedish national database, which included 99% of all children born in a 10-year period and identified 85 cases of BA.[6] They found that high maternal age (over 34 years of age), parity of at least 4, prematurity (22–32 weeks), and small for gestational age (SGA) were all associated with an increased incidence of BA. Although these findings are somewhat inconsistent between studies, the individual findings related to racial clustering, seasonal patterns, and birth weight have led researchers to investigate several possible environmental and genetic factors that may be involved in BA.

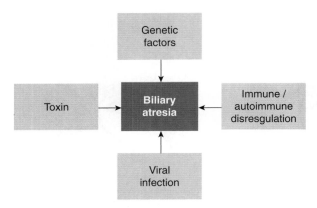

FIGURE 23–3 ■ There are several hypotheses regarding the pathogenesis of BA. The cause of BA is most likely multifactorial. Adapted from Sokol et al.[23]

PATHOGENESIS

The cause of BA is unknown, but is most likely multifactorial (Figure 23–3).[7,8] Some of the proposed mechanisms include: (1) defects resulting from a viral infection; (2) injury caused by toxin exposure; (3) immune or autoimmune dysregulation; (4) genetic predisposition. All four of these proposed etiologies may be involved, and there is some speculation that BA actually represents several different diseases all with the same common phenotype. This theory is supported by the fact that there is great variability in the timing of presentation, rate of disease progression, and phenotype, with the majority of patients having only BA and a minority having multiple other congenital anomalies.

Viral

Early reports of seasonal variation, with a predominance of cases in the winter months, suggested a viral etiology. However, as mentioned in the previous section, further studies looking at seasonality patterns are inconsistent. Nonetheless, various different viruses have been implicated, including reovirus, rotavirus, cytomegalovirus, and human papillomavirus. Of all these proposed viral etiologies, the evidence for reovirus is strongest. Identification of a specific viral agent is complicated by the fact that although a virus may trigger the first stage of inflammation in BA, by the time the patient has been diagnosed with BA, the virus may have cleared.

Toxin

Reports of increased incidence of BA in specific areas, mainly urban locations, suggest a possible toxin-mediated defect. The strongest evidence for a toxin as a possible etiology for BA comes from three reported outbreaks of BA in lambs in Australia in 1964, 1988, and 2007. During

gestation, the ewes that gave birth to affected lambs had grazed on lands that had recently been flooded. A significant number of offspring were thin, jaundiced, had acholic stools, and eventually died. The lambs had enlarged, firm, dark livers with shrunken gallbladders. These findings are consistent with BA. The proposed theory is that the pregnant ewes ingested a toxin when grazing on lands previously submerged. The toxin may have triggered BA. To date, a specific toxin has not been identified.

Immune

Mack et al. and Bezerra et al. suggest that immune or autoimmune dysregulation in response to an initial insult, such as a virus, leads to BA. Immunohistochemical staining of livers from infants with BA revealed increased CD4+ and CD8+ T lymphocytes as well as CD68+ Kuppfer cells, compared to normal controls.[9] In addition, increased production of pro-inflammatory cytokines, such as IL-2, IL-12, interferon-γ, and tumor necrosis factor-α, was found. Bezerra et al. demonstrated overexpression of interferon-γ RNA in the livers of infants with BA. In addition, his group used a rhesus rotavirus (RRV) model of BA and found that when interferon-γ knockout mice are inoculated with RRV, periductal inflammation develops, but the lumen of the bile ducts remains patent.[10] They therefore propose that interferon-γ may play a regulatory role in biliary obstruction.

Genetics

The role of genetics in the development of BA is currently of great interest. It is clear that BA does not follow Mendelian inheritance. For the most part, twin studies to date show discordance. However, there are multiple reports of recurrence of BA in the same families.[11–13] We know that the incidence of BA is higher in certain Asian populations, raising the possibility that there are unique polymorphisms among Asians resulting in susceptibility to BA. One study by Zhang et al. looked at gene expression profiles in liver tissue of perinatal BA compared to embryonic BA.[14] The two forms of BA had unique expression patterns, with the embryonic form showing over-expression of genes involved in regulatory functions and the perinatal form having over-expression of genes involved in metabolic functions.[14] The *CFC1* gene has been implicated in BASM. In one study the gene was analyzed in 10 patients with BASM.[15] Five of the 10 patients had a heterozygous transition in exon 5 of this gene. The frequency of this mutation was two times higher than in controls. The *inversin* gene has also been implicated in mice with BASM; however, this gene does not seem to be causative in humans. These examples suggest that genetics may play a role in BA. How much it actually contributes to the etiology of BA and how is yet to be determined. Schreiber and Kleinman proposed that perhaps BA is the result of a multi-hit pathologic process, in which a viral or toxic insult in a genetically predisposed individual leads to BA.[16]

CLINICAL PRESENTATION

Jaundice is the first sign of BA. All patients with BA have jaundice. Other signs and symptoms may occur, but vary from patient to patient (Table 23–1). Jaundice typically develops in the first weeks of life but it can also occur at birth. Some infants have acholic stools (Figure 23–4). The color of the stool may vary from day to day. Most infants have dark urine because of bilirubin excretion into the urine. In the majority of cases, infants with BA are born full term, have a normal birth weight, and initially thrive and seem healthy.

At the time of diagnosis, affected infants may or may not have hepatomegaly. Splenomegaly is a sign of portal hypertension and is less likely to be present. Similarly, coagulopathy and ascites rarely occur early in the disease process. Seventy to 80% of infants with BA have no other malformations. Of those with associated malformations, about half have BASM. Classically, these infants are jaundiced at birth; however, this is not always

Infant Stool Color Card

No. of Booklet : _____

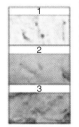

Abnormal

It is essential to observe your baby's stool color continuously after discharge from a nursery. If the stool color resembles the numbers 1~3 (white, clay-colored, or light yellowish), the possibility on your baby suffering from biliary atresia is higher. Please take this card and your baby to consult a dotor as quickly as possible. Regardless of what the stool color is, please bring this card to your doctor at 30 days of age for health check. If the baby cannot go back for health check, please fill in the number of the color resembling your baby's stool, along with the following blanks, and mail this card to our registry center.

Normal

The baby's stool color is most like No. _____
Date of this kind of stool _____

Name of the baby _____ Birthday _____
Name of the mother _____ Tel. _____
Address _____
The hospital or clinic where the baby was born
_____

If the number is No. 1~3, please inform us by fax immediately. We will provide the related information and help you out.

Fax: 02-2388-1798; Tel: 02-2382-0886

Infant Stool Color Card Registry Center

FIGURE 23–4 ■ English version of a Taiwanese stool card. When newborns are discharged from the hospital, parents are given a card like this and instructed that child should be evaluated if stool is acholic (panels 1–3). Reproduced with pemission from *Pediatrics*, vol. 117, pp. 1147–1154, Copyright © 2006 by the AAP.

Table 23–1.

Signs and Symptoms of BA

Sign/Symptom	Time of Onset	Comments
Jaundice	Early	Secondary to conjugated hyperbilirubinemia; may be difficult to assess in a dark-skinned infant
Acholic stools	Variable	Color may vary from day to day
Dark urine	Early	Occurs as a result of bilirubin excretion in the urine
		May make stool in diaper appear darker than it really is
Hepatomegaly	Variable	Patients may or may not have hepatomegaly
Splenomegaly	Late	Rarely present in first few months of life
Pruritus	Late	Rarely present in first few months of life
Ascites	Late	Rarely present in first few months of life

the case. The other half have BA associated with other malformations including several syndromes, for example, trisomy 18, trisomy 21, chromosome 22 aneuploidy, Martinez-Frias syndrome, Kabuki syndrome, CHARGE association, Mowat–Wilson syndrome, and caudal regression syndrome.

Differential Diagnosis

The differential diagnosis of conjugated hyperbilirubinemia in infancy is vast (Table 23–2). The most effective way to approach the evaluation of a cholestatic infant is to first look for those diagnoses that require urgent intervention, such as sepsis, metabolic disorders, and endocrinopathies. The most common causes of neonatal cholestasis are infection and parenteral nutrition toxicity. Once we exclude these two conditions, BA is at the top of the list. In one study of 1086 infants with conjugated hyperbilirubinemia referred over a 20-year period to King's College Hospital in London, about 35% had BA, 30% had idiopathic neonatal hepatitis, 17.4% had other hepatitis, 5.6% had Alagille syndrome, and 3.1% had a choledochal cyst. It should be noted that

Table 23–2.

Differential Diagnosis of Neonatal Cholestasis

Conditions requiring immediate intervention

Biliary atresia
Bacterial infection
■ Sepsis, urinary tract infection, tuberculosis, *Listeria, Treponema pallidum*
Hypothyroidism
Panhypopituitarism
Galactosemia
Glycogen storage disease
Fructosemia
Caroli's disease
Histiocytosis X
Ischemia secondary to congenital heart disease
Iatrogenic
Hypermethioninemia
Disorders of lipid metabolism (Wolman's disease, Niemann–Pick, Gaucher's)
Bile acid synthesis defects
Urea cycle disorders (arginase deficiency)
Hereditary tyrosinemia
Hereditary fructose intolerance

Conditions requiring supportive care

Other extrahepatic obstruction
■ Choledochal cyst, bile duct stricture or tumor, spontaneous perforation of the common bile duct, cholelithiasis, neonatal sclerosing cholangitis
Viral hepatitis
■ CMV, HIV, hepatitis B, EBV, HSV, enterovirus, echovirus, rubella, parvovirus, adenovirus, toxoplasmosis, syphilis, HIV, human herpesvirus 6, reovirus 3, paramyxovirus, varicella
Parenteral nutrition-associated cholestasis
Drugs
Extracorporeal membrane oxygenation (ECHMO)
Mitochondrial disease
Idiopathic neonatal hepatitis
Alpha-1 antitrypsin deficiency
Cystic fibrosis
Alagille syndrome
Nonsyndromic paucity of the interlobular bile ducts
Trisomy 21
Trisomy 17
Trisomy 18
Turner syndrome
Benign recurrent intrahepatic cholestasis (BRIC)
Cholestasis of North American Indian
Neonatal Dubin Johnson syndrome (MRP2 deficiency)
Progressive familial intrahepatic cholestasis
Congenital hepatic fibrosis and autosomal recessive polycystic kidney disease
North American Indian childhood cirrhosis
Peroxisomal disorders (Zellweger syndrome)
Neonatal iron storage disease
Neonatal lupus erythematosus

Conditions that require immediate interventions are listed first and in bold.

King's College is a tertiary care facility and therefore many of the more common causes of neonatal hepatitis, such as infections, TPN, and endocrinologic disease, are most likely not referred to this hospital.

DIAGNOSIS

In general, about 15% of all newborns have visible jaundice by 2 weeks of age. In the majority of cases, the jaundice is secondary to an elevated *unconjugated* bilirubin level as a result of breast milk jaundice or physiologic jaundice. Without laboratory evaluation, it is impossible to distinguish an infant with breast milk jaundice from a cholestatic infant. Therefore, all infants with jaundice after 2 weeks of age should have a fractionated bilirubin. Any infant with an elevated conjugated or direct bilirubin level, defined as a level >2 mg/dL and >20% of the total bilirubin level, requires a thorough evaluation, and is considered to have BA until proven otherwise.

It is critical to make a timely diagnosis of BA, because surgical intervention is most successful if performed early. Any infant with conjugated hyperbilirubinemia must be promptly referred to a pediatric gastroenterologist for further evaluation. The evaluation should be systematic and efficient (Figure 23–5). If the infant is young (i.e., 2–3 weeks of age), medical resources are readily available, and the family is reliable, then workup is started as an outpatient. However, if the infant is 4–5 weeks of age or older, the workup should be expedited, which might necessitate an inpatient stay. Ideally, the evaluation should be completed in a few days.

The evaluation should begin with some basic laboratory studies. A complete cell count (CBC) may reveal a low platelet count or a low white blood cell count (WBC), which commonly occur with advanced liver disease. An elevated WBC may indicate an infectious process. Aspartate aminotransferase (AST), alanine aminotransferase (ALT), gamma-glutamyl transpeptidase (GGT), and also alkaline phosphatase levels are sometimes helpful. A high GGT is seen with any cholestatic process, but in BA it is typically in the range of 100–300 IU/L. ALT and AST levels are variable, although in BA they are typically not more than 15 times the upper limit of normal. The levels of total bilirubin can vary, but, in general, it is rare to see levels over 20 mg/dL in BA unless there are other disease processes involved. Early on, most infants with BA are not coagulopathic. The newborn screen should be reviewed, since it may help exclude thyroid abnormalities, galactosemia, cystic fibrosis, and rare metabolic disorders. A catheterized urine culture should be obtained, because *E. coli* urinary tract infections can lead to elevated conjugated bilirubin levels. A low alpha-1 antitrypsin level is suggestive of alpha-1 antitrypsin deficiency. Alpha-1 antitrypsin pi typing is necessary to make the diagnosis of alpha-1 antitrypsin deficiency, but it takes longer to obtain this result than it does to obtain the result of an alpha-1 antitrypsin level. A sweat test should also be obtained in the initial evaluation phase although it should be noted that there have been cases where BA and cystic fibrosis co-exist.

Abdominal ultrasound (US) is a non-invasive way to exclude anatomic abnormalities, such as choledochal cyst. It can also reveal specific findings that, although not diagnostic for BA, may be supportive of the diagnosis, such as the triangular cord sign and lack of visualization of the gallbladder. The triangular cord represents the fibrous ductal remnant at the porta hepatitis. As BA progresses and the bile ducts become obliterated, the gallbladder eventually becomes atrophic, making it difficult to visualize on US.

Regardless of the US findings, many centers utilize hepatobiliary scintigraphy as part of the evaluation for BA. This test is also referred to as a diisopropyl iminodiacetic acid (DISIDA) scan. If there is excretion of the tracer in 24 hours, then BA is excluded. If the tracer is not excreted, then further evaluation is required. This test is not specific to BA, because other cholestatic diseases impaired excretion of the tracer. If BA is still suspected following the scan, the patient should have a liver biopsy. In some centers, a DISIDA scan is not performed; instead, all patients with suspected BA have a percutaneous liver biopsy. The liver biopsy may help exclude other diseases. For example, paucity of bile ducts could suggest Alagille disease. Bile duct proliferation on biopsy is supportive, but not diagnostic, of BA. Because the histologic changes in BA can mimic other diseases (e.g., TPN cholestasis and alpha-1 antitrypsin), it is extremely important that biopsies be read by an experienced pathologist in the context of the patient's history and workup. The absence of bile duct proliferation does not exclude BA if done early in the disease process. An inconclusive liver biopsy may require another liver biopsy in the near future if cholestasis persists. All patients suspected of having BA should have a cholangiogram, which is the gold standard in the diagnosis of BA. Most commonly, the cholangiogram is done intraoperatively, but it can also be done by interventional radiology. In this study, contrast is injected into the gallbladder to assess flow of bile into the duodenum in order to determine if there is patency of the common bile duct and that the hepatic ducts are also open. If the cholangiogram is done intraoperatively and the contrast does not excrete, the surgeon should perform a HPE at that time. If the cholangiogram reveals a patent biliary tree, then the abdomen is closed and the rest of the evaluation for neonatal cholestasis continues. Endoscopic retrograde cholangiopancreatography (ERCP) is technically very difficult to do in a neonate and is not typically part of the BA evaluation.

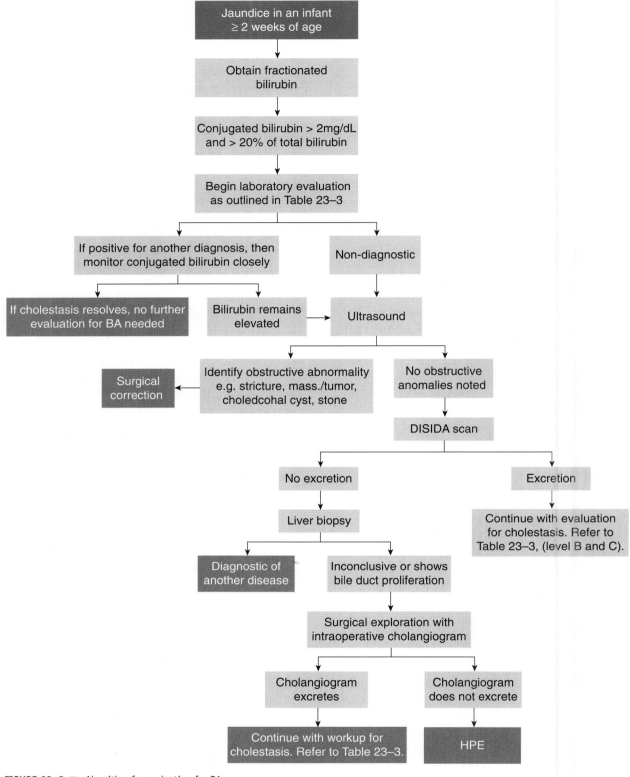

FIGURE 23–5 ■ Algorithm for evaluation for BA.

If a child is admitted for a BA workup, it is most efficient if he/she is also evaluated for other causes of cholestasis (Table 23–3) while completing a rapid evaluation for BA. Therefore, if it turns out that the patient does not have BA, the evaluation for other cholestatic diseases is already underway. Non-invasive procedures should be emphasized. A chest X-ray (CXR) may reveal butterfly vertebra or hemivertebra, which can be

Table 23–3.

Evaluation of Infant with Conjugated Hyperbilirubinemia (Conjugated Bilirubin >2 mg/dL and >20% of the Total Bilirubin Level)

Test	When to Order	Result Significance
CBC with differential	A	In advanced disease low platelets and low WBC
AST, ALT, GGT, ALP	A	In BA see a disproportionately high GGT
PT and PTT	A	Abnormal if PT >14 seconds and INR >1.5 Typically abnormal only in advanced BA. Usually mild, responds to vitamin K
Blood culture	A	
Newborn screen (galactosemia, thyroid, dysfunction, cystic fibrosis, metabolic diseases)	A	Normal in BA; however, the presence of other disease does not exclude BA
Complete abdominal US	A	+/− triangular cord sign in BA. +/− hepatomegaly in BA. Usually normal echotexture in BA Exclude choledochal cyst. Heterotaxia, asplenia, or midline liver is seen in BASM
DISIDA scan	A	Excretion of tracer into the bowel within 24 hours in general excludes BA. If tracer does not excrete, repeating the test with phenobarbital is not recommended. Instead, liver biopsy should be done next. If the test is done in the early phase of BA, there may be excretion of the tracer (although usually slow)
Percutaneous liver biopsy	A	In BA classically we see bile duct proliferation with bile plugs; however, the absence of this finding does not exclude BA. In its early phase, BA histology may be non-specific and similar to that of other diseases
Intraoperative cholangiogram	A	In BA see lack of flow of contrast into the small bowel
Alpha-1 antitrypsin level	A	Level is low in alpha-1 antitrypsin deficiency
Urine culture	A	Urinary tract infection can present as conjugated hyperbilirubinemia
Urine succinylacetone	B	Positive in tyrosinemia
Urine organic acids	B	Positive in organic acidemias
Urine bile acids	B	Abnormal in bile acid synthetic defects. Important to obtain prior to initiating ursodeoxycholic acid
Urine CMV PCR	B	Postnatally acquired CMV is common and identification of the virus should not preclude completing the workup for BA
Urine-reducing sugars	B	If positive in a recently fed infant, suspect galactosemia
CXR	B	Butterfly vertebra or hemivertebra is seen in Alagille syndrome. Dextrocardia, which is seen in BASM
Ophthalmologic exam	B	Exclude posterior embryotoxon, seen in Alagille syndrome
Plasma amino acids	C	Increased phenylalanine and methionine in tyrosinemia type I
Alpha-1 antitrypsin pi typing	C	ZZ phenotype develops cholestasis. MM is normal. MZ are generally asymptomatic. Liver biopsy shows PAS-positive, diastase-resistant globules in the cytoplasm of hepatocytes
Lactate/pyruvate	C	High lactate level and high lactate/pyruvate ratio are suggestive of a mitochondrial disorder
Sweat test	C	To evaluate for cystic fibrosis. Most newborn screens only test for the most common genetic defects in the CFTR gene
Cortisol	C	Low in hypopituitarism

A = first-line testing; B = second-line testing, non-invasive and can be done simultaneously to A, but results not required prior to cholangiogram; C = third-line testing, can be done after cholangiogram.

seen in Alagille syndrome. A CXR may also show dextrocardia, which is common in BASM. If a heart murmur of peripheral pulmonary stenosis (PPS) is heard on exam, one should consider Alagille syndrome and also obtain an echocardiogram. In addition, a number of urine tests should be obtained, including a urine culture, urine succinylacetone (present in tyrosinemia), urine organic acids (abnormal in organic acidemias and peroxisomal diseases), and urine bile acids (bile acid synthetic defects). An ophthalmologic exam by a pediatric ophthalmologist may reveal posterior embryotoxon, which is seen in Alagille syndrome. The rest of the evaluation for neonatal cholestasis is extensive, and is discussed in more detail in Chapter 7.

TREATMENT

Hepatoportoenterstomy

Once BA has been confirmed, surgical intervention should be the next step. Ideally the HPE should be done as soon as the diagnosis can be made. Current optimal timing is between 45 and 60 days of life. However, there is evidence showing that those who have surgery before 45 days[17] and even 30 days of age may have better outcomes. Schreiber and Kleinman found that the 4-year native liver survival rate in those patients who underwent HPE <30 days of age was 49%, whereas survival in those patients who underwent HPE between 31 and 90 days and >90 days was 36% and 23%, respectively.[16] In general, it appears that the earlier the HPE is done, the better.

Success is also dependent on the expertise of the center. For the most part, a center that does at least five cases a year has a better success rate. The most common type of HPE is the Kasai procedure (Figure 23–6). The procedure generally involves excision of obliterated extrahepatic ducts, creation of a Roux-en-Y loop using a portion of proximal jejunum, and apposition of the Roux limb to the transected porta hepatitis proximally and to the duodenum distally. The success of the procedure is defined by the presence of bile drainage. Bilirubin levels 3 months after HPE are most indicative of success of the procedure. Survival without transplantation at 24 months of age was 84% in patients whose bilirubin was <2 mg/dL at 3 months post-HPE and 16% in patients who had a bilirubin over 6 mg/dL at 3 months after HPE.[18] If there is failure of drainage, then the patient should be listed for transplant. Revision of a non-functioning HPE is generally not recommended. However, revision might be appropriate in certain circumstances. For example, if a previously successful HPE abruptly stops working, as determined by a sudden and persistent increase in bilirubin, there might be obstruction by developing scar tissue, or some other mechanical obstruction. Such patients might be a benefit from HPE revision. The focus of medical care following HPE is nutrition, prevention of cholangitis, and minimization of the sequelae of portal hypertension.[19]

Nutrition

Nutrition is one of the most important aspects of management post-HPE, especially in the first 2 years of life. BA patients have an extremely high caloric requirement and failure to thrive is often a major problem in the first year of life. This is due to a combination of factors, including malabsorption and increased needs. In addition, hepatomegaly and/or ascites may compress the stomach and cause a reduction in gastric capacity, making it difficult for the patient to consume adequate calories. There are several reasons why a patient with BA has malabsorption. First, there is usually inadequate bile flow into the intestine. Second, there is passive congestion of the intestine due to portal hypertension. In addition, because post-HPE patients do not have a gallbladder, even those with bile drainage do not benefit from the normal coordination of bile delivery with digestion of fats, which contributes further to malabsorption. Estimated caloric needs are about 150% that of a normal healthy young child. Because of poor intake caused by gastric compression and malaise, many infants and toddlers require nasogastric tube feeds to meet their caloric needs. Breast milk, formula, and food can be supplemented with medium-chain triglyceride (MCT) oil in the first year of life. MCT oil is useful because it is calorically rich and is readily absorbed without micellar solubilization. It is important to monitor growth very closely and maximize caloric intake as much as possible after surgery. In addition, all children should receive fat-soluble vitamins. Vitamin levels should be monitored frequently, that is, several times in the first year, starting at the first month after HPE, in order to adjust supplements appropriately. Maintaining adequate growth and nutrition is crucial to the patient's overall outcome post-HPE. In patients who go on to require liver transplantation following HPE, poor growth has been associated with increased mortality post-transplantation and increased risk of graft failure.[20]

Medications

All patients should receive antibiotics during the first year of life in order to prevent cholangitis (Table 23–4). The incidence of cholangitis in BA is between 40% and 90%, with the majority of patients experiencing at least one episode prior to 2 years of age.[21] Although cholangitis frequently occurs in the first year after HPE, it can occur at any time, with some papers describing cholangitis as a complication encountered during pregnancy among those living with native liver into adulthood. Trimethoprim with sulfamethoxazole is preferred, but neomycin can be used as an alternative.

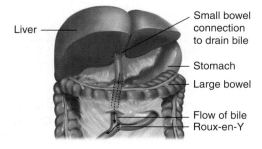

FIGURE 23–6 ■ Kasai hepatoportoenterostomy involves excision of the bile ducts and anastomosis of a limb of jejunum to the liver. Distal duodenum is anastomosed to the jejunal limb to create a Roux-en-Y. www.barcnetwork.org.

Table 23–4.

Recommended Dosages for Medications Used in Management of BA

Medication	Dosage
Ursodiol	20–30 mg/kg/day divided BID
Trimethoprim/ sulfamethoxazole	4 mg (TMP)/kg/day divided Q12 hours
Neomycin*	25 mg/kg/day divided Q8 hours
Vitamin A	3000 units orally QD for infants
Vitamin E (alpha-tocopherol)	15–25 units/kg QD for infants
Vitamin D (ergocaliferol)	4000 units QD for infants
Vitamin K (phytonadione)	2.5 mg three times per week for infants

Neomycin can be used as an alternative in allergic patients.

Ursodiol, originally a Chinese folk remedy found in bear gallbladders, has become standard therapy for many liver diseases. Its benefits included choleresis and a hepatoprotective effect. A recent study documented improvement of liver enzymes in children with BA, but little else specific to BA has been published. Studies are currently underway looking at the role of steroid therapy. Although steroids may improve bilirubin drainage in the early postoperative period, it is unclear if steroids are helpful in improving the long-term outcome.[22] In general, it is acceptable to use acetaminophen as an antipyretic if needed, as long as it is dosed appropriately. Ibuprofen is discouraged because of platelet dysfunction and risk of bleeding.

Management of Portal Hypertension

Portal hypertension may progress rapidly, necessitating liver transplantation. Those who do not require transplantation in the first 2 years of life may have slowly progressive cirrhosis that results in significant portal hypertension in the teen years or early adulthood. If portal hypertension leads to variceal bleeds, these can often be controlled with sclerotherapy or banding. In young adults, various interventions may be used to manage portal hypertension, such as transjugular intrahepatic portosystemic shunts (TIPS) and splenic shunts. Beta-blockers are another option for young adults. Some centers perform surveillance endoscopies to look for varices in patients known to have portal hypertension even if they have not had a variceal bleed. Other centers begin routine surveillance endoscopies only after the patient has had his/her first bleed. There are no data indicating whether one approach is better than the other.

Management of Ascites

The presence of significant ascites is an indication for liver transplantation. Ascites can be managed in the interim with a combination of diuretics, β-blockers, paracentesis, and salt and/or water dietary restriction.

Liver Transplantation

Liver transplantation is reserved for those who fail HPE. In general, it is best to delay transplantation as long as children are relatively healthy to allow for maximal growth, because there are certain advantages to performing a transplant in older and larger children. Not only is it technically easier to perform surgery on a larger child, but there are also fewer complications, such as a lower risk of post-transplant lymphoproliferative disease (PTLD) in older children. One should consider evaluation at a liver transplant center in patients with signs of end-stage liver disease including progressive cholestasis, failure to thrive despite enteral nutrition, worsening coagulopathy, repeated gastrointestinal bleeds (secondary to portal hypertension), repeated episodes of cholangitis, significant ascites, and the presence of bile lakes or bilomas within the liver.

PROGNOSIS

Overall survival in all BA patients who undergo HPE is 90%. The chance of retaining the native liver post-HPE is approximately 50% at 24 months of age.[18] These data vary from center to center, and depend largely on age at time of Kasai, experience of the center, and the presence of other malformations.[23,24] In one recent Swedish study, the 4-year survival with the native liver was 75% in patients who underwent HPE before 46 days, 33% in patients who underwent HPE between 46 and 75 days, and 11% in patients operated on after 75 days ($p = 0.02$).[25] McKiernan et al. found that when HPE was successful, 80% of patients were alive without liver transplantation at 13 years.[26] However, the overall chance of surviving into adulthood with a native liver is only approximately 20%.[27,28] It does appear that the rate of liver damage is much slower for those who make it past the first 2 years of life.

We do not have a good sense of long-term outcomes of patients who survive into adulthood with their native livers, in part because HPE was introduced in the 1970s in the United States, and only a decade earlier in Japan. Therefore, the survivors among these first patients have only just reached middle age. Lykavieris et al. looked at 63 patients who underwent Kasai operation and were alive with their native liver at 20 years of age or more.[28] All but two had signs of cirrhosis. Although growth and nutrition can be challenging in the first 1–2 years follow-ing HPE, growth failure is actually an uncommon occurrence among children who have successful HPE and establish sufficient bile drainage. In fact, Lykavieris et al. found that the adult height in BA survivors was average or above average. They also reported on the quality of life in 52 patients who survived with their native livers into adulthood. They found that 21 were regularly employed, 17 were university students, 21 were married or in stable relationships, 7 females gave birth to 9 children, and 3 male patients fathered 6 children.

Patients who require transplantation, in general, do very well. Recent national data suggest the 1-year patient and liver-graft survival rates for pediatric patients undergoing liver transplantation for BA are 92.1% and 83.6%, respectively.[28]

In general, children born today with BA can expect to live to adulthood with either their own liver or a transplanted liver.

REFERENCES

1. Ohi R, Masaki N. The jaundiced infant: biliary atresia and other obstructions. In: O'Neill J, ed. *Pediatric Surgery.* St. Louis: Mosby; 1998:1465–1482.
2. Tiao MM, Tsai SS, Kuo HW, Chen CL, Yang CY. Epidemiological features of biliary atresia in Taiwan, a national study 1996–2003. *J Gastroenterol Hepatol.* 2008;23:62–66.
3. The NS, Honein MA, Caton AR, Moore CA, Siega-Riz AM, Druschel CM. Risk factors for isolated biliary atresia, National Birth Defects Prevention Study, 1997–2002. *Am J Med Genet A.* 2007;143A:2274–2284.
4. Yoon PW, Bresee JS, Olney RS, James LM, Khoury MJ. Epidemiology of biliary atresia: a population-based study. *Pediatrics.* 1997;99:376–382.
5. Caton AR, Druschel CM, McNutt LA. The epidemiology of extrahepatic biliary atresia in New York State, 1983–98. *Paediatr Perinat Epidemiol.* 2004;18:97–105.
6. Fischler B, Haglund B, Hjern A. A population-based study on the incidence and possible pre- and perinatal etiologic risk factors of biliary atresia. *J Pediatr.* 2002;141:217–222.
7. Haber BA, Russo P. Biliary atresia. *Gastroenterol Clin North Am.* 2003;32:891–911.
8. Mack CL, Sokol RJ. Unraveling the pathogenesis and etiology of biliary atresia. *Pediatr Res.* 2005;57:87R–94R.
9. Mack CL, Falta MT, Sullivan AK, et al. Oligoclonal expansions of CD4+ and CD8+ T-cells in the target organ of patients with biliary atresia. *Gastroenterology.* 2007;133:278–287.
10. Bezerra JA. The next challenge in pediatric cholestasis: deciphering the pathogenesis of biliary atresia. *J Pediatr Gastroenterol Nutr.* 2006;43(suppl 1):S23–S29.
11. Cunningham ML, Sybert VP. Idiopathic extrahepatic biliary atresia: recurrence in sibs in two families. *Am J Med Genet.* 1988;31:421–426.
12. Smith BM, Laberge JM, Schreiber R, Weber AM, Blanchard H. Familial biliary atresia in three siblings including twins. *J Pediatr Surg.* 1991;26:1331–1333.
13. Kobayashi K, Kubota M, Okuyama N, Hirayama Y, Watanabe M, Sato K. Mother-to-daughter occurrence of biliary atresia: a case report. *J Pediatr Surg.* 2008;43:1566–1568.
14. Zhang DY, Sabla G, Shivakumar P, et al. Coordinate expression of regulatory genes differentiates embryonic and perinatal forms of biliary atresia. *Hepatology.* 2004;39:954–962.
15. Davit-Spraul A, Baussan C, Hermeziu B, Bernard O, Jacquemin E. CFC1 gene involvement in biliary atresia with polysplenia syndrome. *J Pediatr Gastroenterol Nutr.* 2008;46:111–112.
16. Schreiber RA, Kleinman RE. Genetics, immunology, and biliary atresia: an opening or a diversion? *J Pediatr Gastroenterol Nutr.* 1993;16:111–113.
17. Chardot C, Carton M, Spire-Bendelac N, Le Pommelet C, Golmard JL, Auvert B. Prognosis of biliary atresia in the era of liver transplantation: French national study from 1986 to 1996. *Hepatology.* 1999;30:606–611.
18. Shneider BL, Brown MB, Haber B, et al. A multicenter study of the outcome of biliary atresia in the United States, 1997 to 2000. *J Pediatr.* 2006;148:467–474.
19. Haber BA, Erlichman J, Loomes KM. Recent advances in biliary atresia: prospects for novel therapies. *Expert Opin Investig Drugs.* 2008;17:1911–1924.
20. Utterson EC, Shepherd RW, Sokol RJ, et al. Biliary atresia: clinical profiles, risk factors, and outcomes of 755 patients listed for liver transplantation. *J Pediatr.* 2005;147:180–185.
21. Luo Y, Zheng S. Current concept about postoperative cholangitis in biliary atresia. *World J Pediatr.* 2008;4:14–19.
22. Davenport M, Stringer MD, Tizzard SA, McClean P, Mieli-Vergani G, Hadzic N. Randomized, double-blind, placebo-controlled trial of corticosteroids after Kasai portoenterostomy for biliary atresia. *Hepatology.* 2007;46:1821–1827.
23. Sokol RJ, Shepherd RW, Superina R, Bezerra JA, Robuck P, Hoofnagle JH. Screening and outcomes in biliary atresia: summary of a National Institutes of Health workshop. *Hepatology.* 2007;46:566–581.
24. Davenport M, Caponcelli E, Livesey E, Hadzic N, Howard E. Surgical outcome in biliary atresia: etiology affects the influence of age at surgery. *Ann Surg.* 2008;247:694–698.
25. Wildhaber BE, Majno P, Mayr J, et al. Biliary atresia: Swiss national study, 1994–2004. *J Pediatr Gastroenterol Nutr.* 2008;46:299–307.
26. McKiernan PJ, Baker AJ, Lloyd C, Mieli-Vergani G, Kelly DA. British paediatric surveillance unit study of biliary atresia: outcome at 13 years. *J Pediatr Gastroenterol Nutr.* 2009;48:78–81.
27. Altman RP, Lilly JR, Greenfeld J, Weinberg A, van Leeuwen K, Flanigan L. A multivariable risk factor analysis of the portoenterostomy (Kasai) procedure for biliary atresia: twenty-five years of experience from two centers. *Ann Surg.* 1997;226:348–353 [discussion 53–55].
28. Lykavieris P, Chardot C, Sokhn M, Gauthier F, Valayer J, Bernard O. Outcome in adulthood of biliary atresia: a study of 63 patients who survived for over 20 years with their native liver. *Hepatology.* 2005;41:366–371.

CHAPTER 24

Viral Hepatitis

José R. Romero and
Judith A. O'Connor

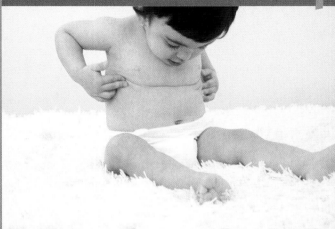

Infectious hepatitis is a syndrome characterized by injury (inflammation or death) to hepatocytes. The process may be self-limiting or may lead to fibrosis, cirrhosis, and neoplastic changes. Clinically, the hepatocellular insult is manifested by elevation of serum aminotransferases (alanine aminotransferase (ALT) and aspartate transaminase (AST)). Typically, the alphabetically designated hepatitis viruses (A–G) and, in particular, hepatitis viruses A, B, and C are those generally considered by the clinician when evaluating a child with hepatitis (Table 24–1). However, many other viral agents such as Epstein–Barr virus (EBV), cytomegalovirus (CMV), coxsackieviruses, echoviruses, West Nile virus,

etc., have the potential to infect the liver and cause clinical or subclinical hepatitis (Table 24–1). This chapter will focus on the hepatitis A, B, and C viruses, the major causes of viral hepatitis in children.

DEFINITIONS AND EPIDEMIOLOGY

Hepatitis A Virus

Hepatitis A virus (HAV) is a small nonenveloped RNA virus in the genus *Hepatovirus* within the *Picornaviridae* family.[1] Transmission of HAV occurs predominantly via

Table 24–1.

Viruses Associated with Hepatitis

Virus	Taxonomy	Genome
Hepatitis A	*Picornaviridae*	RNA
Hepatitis B	*Hepadnaviridae*	DNA
Hepatitis C	*Flaviviridae*	RNA
Hepatitis D	*Deltavirus*	RNA
Hepatitis E	*Hepevirus*	RNA
Hepatitis G	*Flaviviridae*	RNA
Human immunodeficiency virus	*Retroviridae*	RNA
Cytomegalovirus	*Herpesviridae*	DNA
Epstein–Barr virus	*Herpesviridae*	DNA
Herpes simplex viruses types 1 and 2	*Herpesviridae*	DNA
Enteroviruses	*Picornaviridae*	RNA
▪ Coxsackieviruses A and B		
▪ Echoviruses		
▪ Numbered enteroviruses		
Adenoviruses	*Adenoviridae*	DNA
West Nile virus	*Flaviviridae*	RNA

a fecal–oral route. Because the majority of HAV infections in children result in subclinical disease, children play a major role in the transmission of the virus within communities. Outbreaks of hepatitis A occurring in child care centers are well known to occur. Common-source outbreaks through the ingestion of contaminated food or water have also been well documented. Transmission of HAV via transfusion of blood or blood products occurs occasionally when donors are sampled during the viremic phase of the infection. High-risk groups for the acquisition of HAV infection include travelers to developing countries, men who have sex with men, users of injection and noninjection drugs, and individuals working with nonhuman primates.

With the advent of recommendations for vaccination of high-risk individuals and children residing in states with a high prevalence of HAV infection, followed by the more recent recommendation of routine vaccination of all children ≥1 year of age, the incidence of hepatitis A infections in the United States has decreased significantly.[2] In 2007, the reported incidence of hepatitis A infection was 1 case per 100,000 persons in the United States. During that year, the lowest rates of infection occurred among children <5 years of age. Taking into account asymptomatic infections and underreporting, it was estimated that 25,000 new cases of hepatitis A occurred that year.[3] This represented the lowest incidence ever recorded.

Hepatitis B Virus

Hepatitis B virus (HBV) is a DNA virus in the *Hepadnaviridae* family.[4] Replication of HBV occurs in an asymmetric manner, using an RNA intermediate and subsequent reverse transcription to give rise to the viral DNA genome.[5] Error-prone replication occurs due to the lack of proofreading activity of the viral polymerase and gives rise to genetic heterogeneity in HBV. Phylogenetic analysis of HBV isolates indicates the existence of eight HBV genotypes, designated A–H (Table 24–2).[4,6,7] The

Table 24–2.	

Hepatitis B Genotypes[17]

Genotype	Geographic Regions
A	North America, Western Europe, Central Africa
B	China, Indonesia, Vietnam, Taiwan
C	East Asia, Korea, China, Japan, Taiwan, Polynesia, Vietnam
D	Mediterranean area, Middle East, India
E	Nigeria, West Africa
F	Alaska, Polynesia
G	North America, France
H	Central America

eight HBV genotypes exhibit a characteristic geographic distribution, and have a correlation with clinical and, in adults, therapeutic outcomes (Figure 24–1).[6]

Transmission of HBV may occur via mucosal or percutaneous exposure to infected blood or body fluids through injection drug use, blood or blood product transfusion, sexual contact, or during delivery. Today, transfusion-associated transmission is a rare event as a result of screening of blood donors and blood products. Nonsexual transmission may occur in settings of extended interpersonal contact such as those in households of individuals with chronic hepatitis B infection.[3]

Geographic areas of high endemicity (i.e., ≥8%) for HBV infection are shown in Table 24–3.[8] In endemic regions of the world, maternal–fetal transmission is the principal mode of acquisition of HBV. Maternal HBe antigenemia has been shown to be a risk factor for vertical transmission of HBV.[9] Approximately 90% of infants born to mothers who are hepatitis Beantigen (HBeAg) positive will become chronically infected.[8] Approximately 5–15% of maternal–fetal transmission occurs as

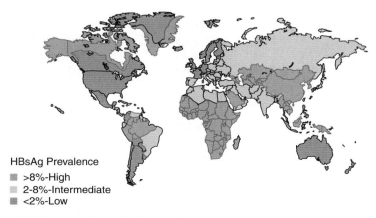

HBsAg Prevalence
■ >8%-High
■ 2-8%-Intermediate
■ <2%-Low

FIGURE 24–1 ■ Global distribution of chronic Hepatitis B infection.

Table 24-3.

Geographic Regions of High Hepatitis B Endemicity[8]

Geographic Region	Specific Countries or Exceptions
Africa	Exceptions: Algeria, Egypt, Libya, Tusia
South Asia	Exceptions: Afghanistan, Bangladesh, Bhutan, India, Malaysia, Maldives, Nepal
Western Pacific	Exceptions: Australia, Guam, Japan, New Zealand
Middle East	Jordan, Saudi Arabia
Eastern Europe and Former Soviet Union	Albania, Azerbaijan, Bulgaria, Croatia, Georgia, Kazakhstan, Kyrgyzstan, Tajikistan, Turkmenistan, Uzbekistan
Western Europe	Malta
North America	Alaska Native populations, indigenous populations of Northern Canada and Greenland
South America	Amazonian areas of Bolivia, Brazil, Colombia, Peru, Venezuela

Table 24-4.

Hepatitis C Genotypes

Genotype	Geographic Regions
1	United States, Europe
2	United States, Europe
3	India, Far East, Australia
4	Africa, Middle East
5	South Africa
6	Hong Kong, Vietnam, Australia

a result of transplacental (congenital) infection with remaining 85–95% occurring at the time of delivery.[10]

In the U.S. recommendations for HBV vaccination of high-risk individuals, universal vaccination of all children and adolescents coupled with screening of pregnant women for HBV infection and prophylaxis of high-risk newborns has contributed to a significant reduction in the incidence of HBV infection. In 2007 the overall incidence of hepatitis B infections in the United States was 1.5 cases per 100,000 persons, the lowest ever recorded. The rate of hepatitis B infectionv

among children and adolescents <15 years was 0.02 cases per 100,000 persons. After correction for asymptomatic cases and underreporting, it was estimated that 43,000 new infections occurred in 2007. That same year, only 83 cases of perinatal HBV transmission were reported. The Centers for Disease Control and Prevention estimate that, although perinatal HBV infection is a reportable disease, the number of actual reported cases represented <10% of the true number of cases.

Hepatitis C Virus

Hepatitis C virus (HCV) is an RNA virus in the family *Flaviviridae*.[11] Error-prone replication of the RNA genome by the viral polymerase gives rise to significant viral heterogeneity in the form of viral quasispecies as well as genotypic diversity. Phylogenetic analysis has identified six genotypes of HCV (Table 24–4).[12] The genomic heterogeneity of HCV displays a geographic distribution and plays a role in the pathogenesis of infection, response to therapy, and host immune evasion (Figure 24–2).

Hepatitis C, 2003
Some of the world's poorest areas suffer most from the disease

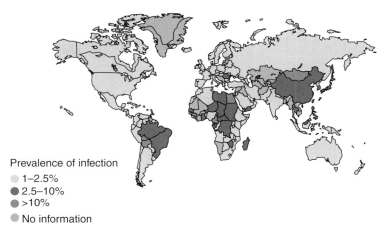

Prevalence of infection
- 1–2.5%
- 2.5–10%
- >10%
- No information

FIGURE 24–2 ■ Global prevalence of Hepatitic C infection.

Transmission of HCV occurs primarily through percutaneous exposure. However, in some cases, mucosal exposure has also been shown to lead to infection. Transmission via blood and blood product transfusion has been significantly reduced by screening of blood donors and HCV inactivation of plasma-derived products.

HCV infection is the most common blood-borne infection in the United States. Previous studies of the seroprevalence of HCV infection in American children 6–11 years of age documented it to be 0.2% and for those aged 12–19 years 0.4%.[13] In 2007, HCV infections among children continued to be rare.[3] The incidence of HCV infection in older individuals was 0.5 cases per 100,000 persons for persons 25–39 years and for those ≥40 years 0.3 cases per 100,000 persons.

Unlike HBV maternal–fetal transmission occurs in only 5% of cases. However, rates of vertical transmission may be as high as 19% in women co-infected with the human immunodeficiency virus (HIV) (reviewed in[14]). This increased rate of transmission may be due to higher levels of hepatitis C viremia seen in HIV co-infected women. Although conflicting data regarding the level of viremia necessary for perinatal transmission of HIV exist, ample evidence suggests that in non-HIV-infected women viremia should be considered a risk factor for vertical transmission. Additional risk factors favoring vertical transmission include infant of female gender, prolonged rupture of membranes, obstetrical procedures (amniocentesis and fetal scalp monitoring), and exposure to maternal blood (maternal vaginal or perineal lacerations).[14]

Breastfeeding, in the absence of cracked or bleeding nipples, does not increase the rate of perinatal transmission of HCV. As such, recommendations for the avoidance of breastfeeding by HCV-infected women are unwarranted. Lastly, the mode of delivery and HCV genotype have not been shown to be correlated with increased maternal–fetal transmission rates.[14]

PATHOGENESIS

Hepatitis A

HAV is a single-stranded, positive-sense RNA virus in the genus *Hepatovirus.*[1] It is transmitted via the fecal–oral route. The virus replicates within the cytoplasm of the hepatocytes and is excreted in bile resulting in fecal shedding. Virus may be found in blood (viremia) soon after infection. This viremia persists throughout the period of hepatic enzyme elevation. HAV is cleared via host humoral immune response.

Infected individuals are most contagious during the 2-week period prior to the onset of jaundice or, in

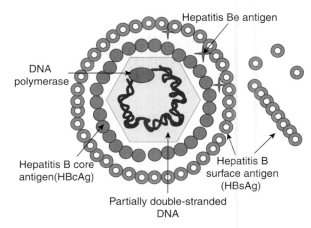

FIGURE 24–3 ■ Structure of the Hepatitis B virus.

anicteric children, the elevation of liver enzymes. Shedding in children is significantly longer than in adults and may last for up to 10 weeks after the onset of clinical illness. Infants may be prolific shedders of HAV, with virus present in their stool for up to 6 months after infection. Chronic infection with HAV does not occur.

Hepatitis B

HBV is an enveloped, 40–45 nm in diameter, virus containing a loosely coiled, partially double-stranded DNA genome[15,16] (Figure 24–3). The viral genome measures approximately 3.2 kb and codes for three structural and four nonstructural viral proteins: S, L, and M, and polymerase, core, e, and X, respectively (Table 24–5).

The envelope of the virion is derived from the hepatocyte membrane and contains three virally derived surface proteins: S, also known as the hepatitis B surface antigen (HBsAg), L, and M. The viral membrane surrounds the viral nucleocapsid that is composed of the hepatitis B core protein or hepatitis Bc antigen (HBcAg). The nucleocapsid, in turn, encloses the partially double-stranded circular DNA viral genome as well as the viral DNA polymerase and several host cell proteins.

The viral replication cycle begins with binding of the virion, presumably via the L protein, to an, as of yet, unidentified host cell protein on the hepatocyte membrane. Subsequent fusion of HBV envelope and host cell membrane results in entry of the viral nucleocapsid core to the cell cytoplasm. The viral cores are transported to the cell nucleus where the HBV DNA genome is released, repair of the single-stranded gap is performed by host cell enzymes, and the genome is converted to a covalently closed circular DNA molecule (cccDNA). Viral genome then serves as a template for the generation of pregenomic and subgenomic RNA transcripts by the host cell's RNA polymerase II.

Table 24–5.

Hepatitis B Virus Proteins[4]

Protein	Comment	Principal Antigens	Host Antibody
S (small, HBsAg)	Constituent of the intact viral envelope	HBsAg	Anti-HBs
M (medium)	Constituent of the intact viral envelope		
L (large)	Constituent of the intact viral envelope. May interact with host cell receptor		
C (core, HBcAg)	Forms the nucleocapsid of the mature virion	HBcAg	Anti-HBc
Polymerase	Responsible for reverse transcription		
e (HBeAg)	Truncated derivative of the core (C) protein. May modulate host immune response	HBeAg	Anti-HBe
X	Functions as a transcriptional activator. Implicated in a proposed mechanism of carcinogenesis		

HBsAg = hepatitis B surface antigen; HBcAg = hepatitis B core antigen; HBeAg = hepatitis B e antigen.

HBV RNA transcripts are transported from the nucleus to the cytoplasm where subgenomic-length transcripts are translated to yield the viral proteins essential to the HBV life cycle (Table 24–5). Core proteins assemble to form the nucleocapsid in the cytoplasm and a single molecule of pregenomic RNA is incorporated within the nascent core. The HBV reverse polymerase transcribes the nucleocapsid-associated pregenomic RNA to DNA. However, generation of cccDNA is not completed until the virus infects another cell or nascent nucleocapsid containing partially double-stranded DNA and is transported back to the nucleus of the cell to maintain the pool intranuclear DNA template. The majority of mature cores bud into the ER membrane, which is studded with HBV surface proteins (S (HBsAg), L, and M), thus forming the mature virion's envelope. Fully formed virions are then exported from the cell. Viral replication does not result in lysis of the host cell.

The host immune response to HBV infection is age-related and mediates the clinical presentation and outcome of infection. In immunocompetent adults, a robust CD8$^+$ cytotoxic T-lymphocyte-mediated response results in clearance of the viral infection in >95% of all patients.[17] Following a period of unchecked replication, during which HBV serum titers exceed 10^9 copies/μL (>10^{12} copies/mL), a rapid fall in viral titer occurs. The fall in serum viral concentration occurs prior to the occurrence of hepatic injury or cellular infiltration of the liver. This phase of noncytolytic clearance is believed to be the result of cytokine-mediated inhibition of HBV replication without associated hepatocellular injury. In simian and murine models, HBV-specific CD8$^+$ cytotoxic T-lymphocytes are important during this phase of the immune response to HBV. Important cytokines mediating this phase of the host immune response are interferon-gamma, tumor necrosis factor-alpha, and interferon alpha/beta: which are all produced by CD8$^+$ cytotoxic T-lymphocytes.

The development of clinical hepatitis, manifested by an increase in serum aminotransferases, follows the noncytolytic clearance of HBV for the serum. This period is characterized by cytolytic clearance of HBV accompanied by maximal CD4$^+$ and CD8$^+$ T-lymphocyte responses. Hepatic infiltration by HBV-specific and nonspecific T-lymphocytes, neutrophils, natural killer cells, monocytes, and macrophages occurs as a result of chemokine recruitment to the liver. During this phase of acute hepatitis, it is believed that much of the hepatocellular damage is due to nonantigen-specific inflammatory responses. The ultimate outcome of the combination of noncytolytic and cytolytic responses is the prevention of infection of hepatocytes and the elimination of those already infected. In addition to the host's cell-mediated immune response, the immune system's humoral arm also plays a role in clearing HBV. Antibodies to HBsAg aid in viral clearance and prevention of infection of hepatocytes.

In stark contrast to the vigorous response to HBV exhibited by the adult immune system, intrauterine or immediate postnatal exposure to HBV proteins produces a state of immunologic tolerance that prevents clearance of the infection in the majority of infants. Hepatitis B-specific CD4$^+$ and CD8$^+$ T-lymphocyte responses are diminished in comparison to those seen during the adult response. In animal models of chronic HBV infection, the persistence of viral antigens leads to a functional decline of HBV-specific cytotoxic T cell responses and, ultimately, T-cell elimination.[17] The clinical outcome of this immunotolerant state is chronic HBV infection, so much so that 90% of prenatally infected infants develop chronic hepatitis.

Several HBV proteins have been associated with the development of chronic infection.[17,18] HBeAg, which is derived from the nucleocapsid protein, is essential in the development of chronic infection. In the transgenic murine model of HBV, HBeAg contributes to the poor T-lymphocyte and antibody response to the core protein. Additionally, in the same model, HBeAg can cross the placenta and induce neonatal tolerance.[18] Toll-like receptor 2 expression and function on monocytes, Kupffer cells, and hepatocytes is down-regulated in patients with HBeAg-positive chronic hepatitis.[17] In contrast, patients with HBeAg-negative chronic hepatitis exhibit up-regulation of Toll-like receptor 2.

HBsAg is present in noninfectious filamentous and spherical particles produced during viral replication. These viral particles serve to bind anti-HBs antibodies, thus diverting them from neutralization of infectious HBV virions.[17] Additionally, HBsAg may contribute to low CD8$^+$ T-lymphocyte response and CD8$^+$ T-lymphocyte depletion.[18]

Lastly, HBV X protein can inhibit cellular proteasome activity when it is over-expressed. As such, it has the potential to inhibit antigen processing and presentation.[18]

Hepatitis C

HCV is an enveloped, single-stranded, positive-sense RNA virus classified within the *Flaviviridae* family.[11] The virion is approximately 50 nm in diameter (Figure 24–4). The RNA is 9.6 kb in length and codes for

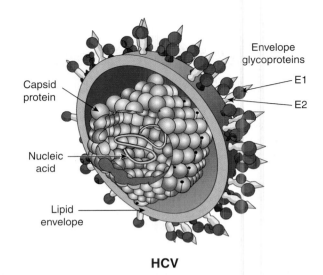

FIGURE 24–4 ■ Structure of the Hepatitis C virus.

four structural proteins (core (C), E1, and E2) as well as seven nonstructural proteins (p7, NS2, NS4A, NS4B, NS5A, NS5B, and F/ARFP) (Table 24–6).[11,19] Immediately preceding and following the single open reading frame of the viral genome are long untranslated regions (UTR), designated 5′ UTR and 3′ UTR, respectively. These regions are essential for viral translation and replication.

The replication cycle of HCV remains to be fully elucidated. Although several cellular surface proteins have been identified that can bind HVB envelope

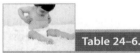

Table 24–6.

Hepatitis C Virus Proteins[19]

Protein	Function	Comment
Core (C)	Viral capsid protein	Together with HCV RNA genome forms the viral nucleocapsid. Implicated in carcinogenesis, apoptosis, immunomodulation, liver steatosis
E1	Constituent of viral envelope	Forms heterodimer with E2
E2	Constituent of viral envelope	Forms heterodimer with E1. May be major viral protein that interacts with cell receptor. E2 hypervariable region evades host humoral response to HCV. Inhibits host interferon and NK cell responses to HCV
p7	Cation channel	Essential for formation of infectious virus
NS2	Protease	Essential for viral assembly
NS3	Protease, RNA helicase	Protease activity requires NS4A. Inhibits host interferon response to HCV
NS4A	Protease cofactor	A cofactor for NS3. Inhibits host interferon response to HCV
NS4B	Putative replication complex scaffold protein	Essential to formation of the membranous web
NS5A	Replication and assembly regulatory protein	May be important in directing replication or viral assembly depending on degree of phosphorylation. May play a role in evading host interferon response
NS5B	RNA-dependent RNA polymerase	Responsible for − and + strand RNA synthesis
F/ARFP	Unknown	Arises from a +1 codon frameshift of the core-encoding region of the HCV genome

proteins, the definitive cellular receptor(s) for HCV has not been identified. Viral internalization appears to occur via clathrin-mediated endocytosis.

After internalization and release of the HCV genome from the viral capsid, translation begins in a cap-independent manner in which the HCV 5′ UTR interacts with the 40S ribosomal unit without the need for the canonical cap-dependent initiation factors. The 40S ribosomal unit is directed to the viral polyprotein start codon (AUG). Formation of the 80S then ensues and translation of viral open reading frame ensues. The nascent viral polyprotein is co- and post-translationally processed to yield the structural and nonstructural viral proteins. Viral replication is believed to occur at a membrane-anchored complex derived from the endoplasmic reticulum. The NS4B protein is essential in the formation of the scaffold for replication. Fully assembled virus containing genomic RNA is believed to be exported from the cell via the secretory pathway.

CLINICAL PRESENTATION

Hepatitis A

The incubation period for hepatitis A ranges from 15 to 50 days with an average time of 28 days.[2,20] The onset of HAV infection is typically abrupt and consists of nonspecific signs and symptoms that include fever, malaise, anorexia, nausea, vomiting, abdominal discomfort or pain, and diarrhea. During this phase of the illness, serum aminotransferase levels are generally elevated. Approximately 1 week after the onset of symptoms, patients may develop jaundice, as a result of conjugated hyperbilirubinemia, in association with choluria (dark urine secondary to bilirubinemia). Mild hepatomegaly and hepatodynia may be detected on abdominal palpation and percussion of the right upper quadrant, respectively.

The probability of developing symptomatic HAV infection is inversely related to age. Approximately 70% of infections incurring in children <6 years of age are asymptomatic. If illness does occur, it is typically anicteric in nature. In older children and adults, infections are typically symptomatic with jaundice occurring in >70% of cases.

In children, the infection is generally self-limited with signs and symptoms typically lasting <2 weeks. Prolonged or relapsing disease of up to 6-month duration may occur in 10–15% of individuals with symptomatic infection; however, chronic infection does not occur. The overall case fatality ratio is approximately 0.3–0.6% but may be three times higher in adults >50 years of age. Among children <14 years of age, the reported case fatality rate is 0.3%. Acute liver failure occurs in <1% of cases and is more common with individuals with underlying chronic liver disease. This underscores the need to assure that children with any type of chronic hepatitis including HBV or HCV are immunized against HAV.

Hepatitis B

The incubation period for HBV infection ranges from 45 to 160 days, with an average of approximately 90 days following postnatal infection. Subclinical HBV infection is common, and more so in children. The risk of developing clinically evident hepatitis varies with age, such that 90% of infections in infants and children are asymptomatic.[21,22] This is contrasted with adult-acquired HBV infection in which 30–50% of patients have icteric disease.[23]

In older postnatally infected children, the clinical manifestations of acute hepatitis B may include nonspecific constitutional symptoms such as fatigue, anorexia, and nausea. These may be followed by jaundice and choluria.[8,22] In children old enough to express themselves, right upper quadrant tenderness or discomfort may be reported. Biochemical evidence of hepatocellular inflammation is present in the form of elevation of serum aminotransferase levels, in particular ALT, and serum bilirubin concentration.

The risk of developing chronic hepatitis is inversely related to the individual's age of time of infection. More than 90% of infants who acquire HBV infection perinatally will develop chronic disease.[8] In children infected after birth and up to 5 years of age, chronic infection occurs in between 25% and 30% of cases.[24] Older children develop chronic HBV infection in only 5–7% of cases. Progression to chronic infection has been reported to occur in <5% of acutely infected adults.[23,25]

Chronic hepatitis is characterized by persistence of HBsAg for >6 months, elevation (persistent or fluctuating) of serum aminotransferase levels, and the presence of >10^5 copies/mL of HBV DNA in serum.[26] Chronic hepatitis B may be divided into three phases: (1) immune tolerant phase, (2) immune activation phase, and (3) low or nonreplicative (inactive carrier) phase.[17,23,24] During the immune tolerant phase, which is generally seen only in children who have acquired HBV infection congenitally or perinatally, high titers of HBV (>10^9 copies/μL) are present in serum and HBsAg is readily detectable in serum. Hepatitis B-specific T-lymphocyte responses are minimal or undetectable. A minimal hepatocellular inflammatory response to the infection results in normal serum ALT concentrations. On liver biopsy there is, at most, evidence of minimal inflammation without evidence of fibrosis. Liver disease does not progress during this phase. As discussed previously, immune tolerance is believed to be the result of the inability of the host immune system to recognize viral antigens and may last for two decades.[23] As a result, the majority of children with chronic HBV infection are asymptomatic.[27] Spontaneous viral clearance during this phase is low.

Phase 2 is the immune active phase and is characterized by elevated or fluctuating levels of serum aminotransferases, hepatic inflammation, and falling levels of HBV DNA in serum.[17,23] This phase arises as a result of the development of host hepatitis B-specific T-lymphocyte responses that clear virally infected hepatocytes. Liver biopsy may show evidence in inflammation and hepatocellular necrosis. This phase may last from months to years. Individuals who remain in this phase for prolonged periods (years to decades) are at the highest risk for development of hepatocellular carcinoma (HCC).[23] During this phase some patients may develop antibodies to HBeAg. The rate of spontaneous HBeAg disappearance (seroconversion) in children younger than 3 years of age is <2% per year.[27] In children older than 3 years of age, spontaneous annual seroconversion rates are 4–5%.

During the inactive carrier, or nonreplicative, phase of chronic HBV infection, serum aminotransferase levels are normal and HBV DNA levels are low or even undetectable using sensitive polymerase chain reaction (PCR) assays.[17,23] Serologically, these patients exhibit HBsAg in their serum in association with loss of HBeAg and development of anti-HBe. Regression of hepatic fibrosis may be seen during this phase. During this phase 1–2% of patients per year will clear HBsAg. However, up to 30% of patients may relapse to the immune active phase of infection.

Loss of HBeAg is not synonymous with clearance of HBV DNA from the blood.[28] In some, high levels of HBV DNA and elevation of ALT persist.[17] In these patients a mutation in the viral genome results in an inability to produce HBeAg.[29] Thus, it is important to note that clearance of HBeAg may not be protective against the development of HCC.[24]

Death from HCC or cirrhosis occurs in 15–40% of individuals with chronic HBV infection.[17,22] The risk of HCC is 100 times greater among chronically infected individuals as compared to those who are noncarriers.[28] The risk for the development of HCC can be further stratified by HBeAg status in HBsAg patients, being greatest for those who are both HBsAg and HBeAg positive. Additional risk factors for development of HCC include high viral load (>10^5 copies/mL) and genotype (i.e., genotype C).[17]

Extrahepatic manifestations (Table 24–7) associated with acute and chronic HBV infection[17,30] occur in 1–10% of adults[22] and are due to the deposition of circulating immune complexes in various tissues. HBV-associated nephropathy is more common in children than adults. Membranous glomerulonephritis is the most common form. Liver disease may be mild or absent and about 30–60% will develop spontaneous remission with HBeAg seroconversion. Gianotti–Crosti syndrome, or papular acrodermatitis, is a distinct skin manifestation of acute HBV infection in children.

Table 24–7.

Extrahepatic Manifestations of Hepatitis B Infection

Clinical Condition	Comment
Serum sickness-like syndrome	Seen with acute hepatitis. Often precedes jaundice. Clinical features: fever, skin rash, and polyarthritis
Polyarteritis nodosa	Associated with chronic hepatitis. Multisystem involvement: fever, proteinuria, pericarditis, congestive heart failure, hypertension, abdominal pain, GI bleeding, vasculitic skin lesions, neurological disorders
Glomerulonephritis ■ Membranous ■ Mesangial proliferative ■ Membranoproliferative	More commonly seen in children. Membranous glomerulonephritis is most common in children. Membranoproliferative more common in adults
Papular acrodermatitis (Gianotti–Crosti syndrome)	More commonly seen in acute hepatitis of children. Skin lesions: maculopapular, erythematous, nonpruritic. Involves the face and extremities
Essential mixed cryoglobulinemia	Association with HBV is controversial
Peripheral neuropathy, Guillain–Barre syndrome	

Hepatitis C

After an acute exposure, HCV RNA is detected in serum as early as 2 weeks following exposure, whereas HCVAb is usually not present until 8 weeks after exposure. Less than 30% of patients acutely infected with HCV experience symptoms of fever, malaise, abdominal pain, or jaundice. Children, like adults acutely infected with HCV, are generally asymptomatic but are more likely to spontaneously clear the infection, with 25% of infected neonates and 28% of acutely infected children clearing HCV virus in 7–10 years, respectively.[33]

Chronically infected patients are usually asymptomatic; however, fatigue is a common complaint in teenagers and adults. Patients with symptoms of anorexia, weight loss, abdominal pain, hepatomegaly, and splenomegaly generally have advanced liver disease. Unlike chronic HBV infections, chronic hepatitis C results in serum aminotransferase levels that can be normal despite significant hepatic necroinflammatory damage.

Extrahepatic manifestations of chronic HCV are rare, occurring in <2% of infected patients, and occur predominately in adults. Cryoglobulinemia is the most common and serious complication and is, in itself, an indication for treatment. Symptoms include rashes (purpura, vasculitis, or urticaria), arthropathy, myopathy, kidney disease, and neuropathy. Cryoglobulins, rheumatoid factor, and decreased complement levels are identified in serum. Other nonhepatic manifestations include glomerulonephritis and porphyria cutanea tarda.

Cirrhosis develops in 10–20% of chronically affected adults usually after at least two decades of infection. Once cirrhosis develops, the risk of HCC is 1–4% per year. Disease severity and rate of disease progression is influenced by age at acquisition, duration of infection, and alcohol ingestion. Most children who are chronically infected have mild to moderate inflammation on liver biopsy. Cirrhosis occurs in about 5%, and some children will present with end-stage liver disease requiring transplantation. Although rare, cases of HCV-associated HCC have been reported in pediatric patients. Most patients, however, are asymptomatic and are typically identified by positive blood screening of high-risk groups, or incidentally during evaluation of abdominal pain, elevated serum aminotransferase levels, or blood donation.

DIAGNOSIS

The diagnosis of HAV, HBV, and HCV is based on identification of viral-specific antigens, host-specific antibody formation, or viral RNA or DNA in serum. Most patients with HAV are anicteric, with symptoms of an acute viral syndrome. Patients with chronic HBV and

Table 24–8.

Common Causes of Chronic Hepatitis

Infectious hepatitis
■ Hepatitis B
■ Hepatitis C
■ HIV
Autoimmune hepatitis
Alpha-1-antitrypsin deficiency
Wilson's disease
Nonalcoholic steatohepatitis
Drug-induced liver disease

HCV usually have normal growth and development and appear clinically well. All patients with HBV and HCV should be screened for HIV as well as other causes of chronic liver disease, as these conditions are not mutually exclusive and all may be acquired in the same manner during high-risk behaviors or exposures (Tables 24–8 and 24–9). In addition, patients should be

Table 24–9.

Laboratory and Radiographic Evaluation for Chronic Hepatitis

Hepatitis B surface antigen (HBsAg) and core antibody (HBcAb)
■ If positive
  ■ Hepatitis B e antigen (HBeAg) and antibody (HBeAb)
  ■ Hepatitis B virus DNA
  ■ Hepatitis D virus antibody (HDVAb)
Hepatitis C antibody (HCVAb)
■ If positive
  ■ HCV viral RNA
Hepatitis A antibody
HIV antibody
Routine complete chemistry panel
■ Aminotransferase levels, alkaline phosphatase, total and direct bilirubin, total protein, albumin, blood urea nitrogen, and creatinine, serum electrolytes
Prothrombin time and international normalized ratio (INR)
Complete blood count
Quantitative immunoglobulin levels
Alpha-fetoprotein level
Alpha-1-antitrypsin level
Autoimmune hepatitis panel
Copper
Ceruloplasmin
Fasting lipid profile
Abdominal ultrasound

screened for evidence of malignancy with a serum alpha-fetoprotein (AFP) and an abdominal ultrasound.

Hepatitis A

The diagnosis of hepatitis A infection is established using serologic testing for IgM antibodies to the capsid proteins of HAV.[20] Serum anti-HAV IgM becomes detectable 5–10 days before the onset of symptoms. IgM antibodies to HAV typically become undetectable within 6 months after infection, although reports of individuals testing positive for anti-HAV IgM >1 year after infection exist. Anti-HAV IgM is replaced by anti-HAV immunoglobulin (IgG) that confers lifelong protection against HAV infection. Individuals vaccinated against HAV will have anti-HAV IgG in their serum.

Hepatitis B

The diagnosis of HBV infection relies on the detection of HBV antigens and host-specific antibodies (Table 24–10).[17,26] The presence of circulating HBV DNA defines active infection.

HBsAg is a component of the surface envelope of HBV. This protein is the first viral protein to appear in the blood after infection with HBV. It may present as early as 1 week after infection but typically becomes detectable 6–10 weeks after exposure. The host response to HBsAg, in the form of anti-HBsAg, generally clears this viral protein in 4–6 months. The persistence of

HBsAg for >6 months defines a chronic infection. Anti-HBsAg persists for life and provides immunity to all HBV genotypes.

HBcAg is associated with intact virions as a component of the nucleocapsid protein. It does not circulate freely in the serum and cannot be detected in serum using standard diagnostic assays. Host anti-HBc IgM is present in sera shortly after the appearance of HBsAg. IgM anti-HBc may persist for as long as 2 years after HBV infection. During the course of HBV infection, IgM anti-HBc is eventually replaced by IgG anti-HBc. Prior to the advent of the currently available assays for the detection of HBsAg and anti-HBs, some patients were noted to have a period of time (or window) during which neither HBsAg nor anti-HBs could be detected in serum. During this "window period" the presence of IgM anti-HBc was used to diagnose acute HBV infection. If contemporary assays are used, the "window period" rarely occurs.[26]

Isolated detection of anti-HBc may occur in up to 5% of healthy blood donors and up to 42% of HIV-infected individuals.[26] The presence of anti-HBc without evidence of circulating HBsAg or anti-HBs may occur in certain settings, such as: (1) during a chronic HBV infection; (2) as anti-HBs levels fall below the limit of detection of assays following a resolved HBV infection occurring in the distant past; (3) as a false-positive result; and (4) during the "window period." For patients in whom isolated anti-HBc is detected, sera should be tested for HBV DNA to identify an occult chronic HBV infection.

HBeAg is derived from the precursor protein to the core protein. It may be found in the serum of infected

Table 24–10.

Interpretation of Hepatitis B Serologic and Nucleic Acid Detection Assays[17,26]

Clinical Status	HBsAg	Anti-HBs	HBeAg	Anti-HBe	Anti-HBc IgM	Anti-HBc Total	HBV DNA	ALT
Immunized	−	+	−	−	−	−	−	Normal
Incubation ("window") period	−	−	−	−	+	−	+/−	Normal
Acute infection	+		+		+	+/−	+	Increased
Resolved infection	−	+	−	+	−	+	0 or low (10^1–10^2) copies/mL	Normal
Chronic—immune tolerant phase	+	−	+	−	−	+	>10^7 copies/mL	Normal
Chronic—HBeAg (+)	+	−	+	−	−	+	>10^5 copies/mL	Increased
Chronic—HBeAg (−) (inactive carrier)	+	−	−	+	−	+	0 to <10^5 copies/mL	Normal
Chronic—HBeAg (−) (precore mutant)	+	−	−	+	−	+	>10^5 copies/mL	Fluctuating

individuals 6–12 weeks after infection. Its presence is associated with high levels of HBV viremia. Serum levels of HBeAg decline with the development of host anti-HBe. The presence of HBeAg for >3–4 months after infection may be a harbinger of chronic infection. Some patients chronically infected with HBV may lack the presence of HBeAg in serum as a result of a mutation in the HBV genome that inhibits its production.[29]

Hepatitis B viral DNA can be detected in the serum of infected individuals using a variety of molecular methods. Detection of HBV DNA by PCR is not necessary for the diagnosis of HBV infection, but is used to follow treatment response. The upper and lower limits of detection of these assays vary, depending on the methodology used to detect the HBV DNA.[17,26] The more sensitive PCR assays demonstrate that the presence of HBV DNA in serum may persist for years after clearance of HBsAg and the development of anti-HBs and possibly for life.[17] Persistence of HBV may place the patient at risk for reactivation of disease in the future if significant immunosuppression occurs.

Hepatitis C

There are two types of diagnostic assays that detect HCV infection: serologic assays that detect virus-specific antibody to HCV (HCVAb) and molecular assays that detect viral nucleic acid. These tests identify infection but do not assess disease severity or prognosis.

Identification of HCVAb is the initial step in diagnosing HCV infection. There are two enzyme immunoassays (EIAs) and one enhanced chemiluminescence immunoassay (CIA) approved by the U.S. Food and Drug Administration (FDA) for clinical use. False-positive results are more likely when the test is used in populations with a low prevalence of HCV. False negatives may occur in patients with severe immunosuppression, HIV co-infection, solid organ transplant, hypogammaglobulinemia, or hemodialysis. Previously, a recombinant immunoblot assay (RIBA) was developed as a supplemental assay to improve specificity and confirm positive EIA tests. The specificity for current EIAs for HCVAb is >99% and RIBA testing is no longer recommended.[34]

HCV viral RNA can be identified by commercially available real-time PCR-based assays and transcription-mediated application (TMA) assays. Viral load is referred to as international unit (IU) rather than copies. Sensitivities of available assays are excellent, identifying levels of HCV at 10–50 IU/mL with >98% accuracy.[33] Patients with a positive HCVAb should have HCV-PCR to identify active infection. HCV genotyping and liver biopsy are not needed for diagnosis but are important in determining prognosis and indications for treatment.

Screening tests for HCV are recommended in infants born to HCV-infected mothers. Testing for HCVAb should be postponed, as passively transferred maternal antibodies can persist in the newborn up to 18 months of age. If early diagnosis is desired, HCV-PCR may be obtained at 1–2 months of age. False-negative testing can occur due to low viral load. Current recommendations are to withhold testing for HCV by PCR until after 6 months of age to improve sensitivity. If a negative test is obtained earlier, it should be repeated between 6 and 12 months of age. Other patient populations that should be screened include adolescent patients with high-risk behavior, adoptees or emigrants from HCV-endemic areas, and children with unexplained elevated serum aminotransferase levels.

PREVENTION AND TREATMENT

In keeping with the old adage, "an ounce of prevention is worth a pound or cure," nothing could be truer when approaching infectious hepatitis. Education and avoidance of risk of exposure is the first step in prevention of infection. Vaccines and virus-specific IgG are available for prevention and prophylaxis of HAV and HBV. Unfortunately, other than education and avoidance of risk, no effective biologic preventative treatment is available for HCV.

Hepatitis A

The first step in prevention is careful rinsing of fruits and vegetables from endemic areas, and frequent hand washing when handling food products. As the majority of children have an anicteric illness, careful hand washing after diaper changes in children with signs and symptoms of acute viral gastroenteritis is effective. HAV vaccination is indicated for all children >1 year of age, nonimmune adults and children visiting endemic areas, high-risk individuals, and patients with chronic infectious and noninfectious liver disease. HAV vaccine is given in two separate injections, with >94% and 100% of patients developing immunity after a single and second injection, respectively. Post-exposure prophylaxis with a single IM dose of HAV-IgM is indicated if given within 2 weeks of exposure in a non-HAV immune patient.

Patients who develop symptomatic hepatitis from HAV rarely require more than supportive therapy. Hospitalization may be needed to treat dehydration resulting from nausea, vomiting, or diarrhea. In the rare instance of acute liver failure, hospitalization in a liver transplant center is required as recovery is not guaranteed. Although uncommon, recurrent HAV has been reported in patients transplanted for liver failure secondary to HAV.

Hepatitis B

In the United States, adaptation of universal vaccination of all children and adolescents, coupled with prenatal maternal screening for HBV and prophylactic treatment of high-risk newborns, is the primary preventive strategy. Children immigrating or adopted from endemic regions of the world represent the most common source of childhood infection in the United States and should be screened for chronic infection. All household contacts of patients with chronic HBV should be immunized. Patients with HBV should be immunized against HAV. Children diagnosed with chronic HBV should not have restrictions in school attendance or physical activity.

Patients diagnosed with chronic HBV need to be followed closely for the development of sequelae. In adult studies, 35% of chronically infected patients will develop progressive disease manifested by cirrhosis, portal hypertension, or HCC. In children, cirrhosis and HCC are rare but can occur. Serum aminotransferases should be attained at least every 6 months. Serum HBeAg, HBeAb, AFP, and abdominal ultrasound should be performed annually. If serum AST becomes elevated, the frequency of monitoring should be at least every 3 months. Patients who have a persistent AST >1.5 times the upper limit of normal and no spontaneous seroconversion should be considered for liver biopsy and treatment. In children, the duration for monitoring AST elevation and seroconversion is not defined, and should be managed individually taking in patient age, age of acquisition, and AST elevation into consideration, as spontaneous seroconversion can occur.

The goal for treatment is immunity, but unfortunately most patients treated for chronic HBV fail to develop HBsAb; thus, the aim for current treatment regimens is viral eradication to prevent the development of disease progression and HCC. End of treatment measures thus focus on viral eradication, HBeAg seroconversion (HBeAb production), and HBsAg seroconversion. End of treatment response (ETR) is the result of the above measures at the conclusion of therapy and a durable response is a sustained ETR after a defined period following the end of therapy.

Seven treatments are currently approved for adult patients with chronic HBV infection in the USA and include both interferons (interferon and peginterferon) and nucleoside or nucleotide analogs (Table 24–11). In children, approved treatments for chronic HBV currently include: alpha-interferon or lamivudine for children >2 years, adefovir for children >12 years, and entecavir and telbivudine for children >16 years of age. Current and complete reviews in the management of chronic HBV in adults[1] and children[2] have been recently published. In both adult and pediatric studies, response rates are improved if patients are in the immune active phase of infection. Most children with chronic HBV infection are in the immune tolerant phase and have a decreased response to interferons and oral agents. They respond poorly to current treatment regimes.

Alpha-interferon is the only licensed antiviral in the United States that has both immunomodulatory and antiviral activity against HBV. Unfortunately, poor clinical response (21% over placebo), three times per week intramuscular dosing requirement, high side-effect

Table 24–11.

Treatment for Chronic Hepatitis B Infection

Medication	Age Group	Dose	Advantages	Disadvantages
Alpha-interferon	>2 years	6 MU/m² three times a week for 16–24 weeks	No resistance, short duration	IM delivery side effects
Lamivudine	>2 years	3 mg/kg/day (100 mg maximum dose), continue until 6 months after HBeAg seroconversion	Oral delivery, liquid formulation, minimal side effects	Drug resistance high, 20% in 2 years
Adefovir	>12 years	10 mg/day, continue until 6 months after HBeAg seroconversion	Oral delivery, minimal side effects, effective against lamivudine-resistant HBV	Low potency, drug resistance 2% at 2 years
Entecavir	>16 years	0.5 mg/day, continue until 6 months after HBeAg seroconversion	Oral delivery, minimal side effects, high potency	Less effective against lamivudine-resistant HBV
Telbivudine	>16 years	600 mg/day	Oral delivery, minimal side effects, high potency	Drug resistance high, 21% at 2 years

profile, and multiple contraindications to therapy have led to general disuse. Pediatric studies have been somewhat more encouraging, with a HBeAg seroconversion rate of 23% and HBsAg seroconversion of 10%. Factors associated with a higher rate of seroconversion include female gender, AST >2 times normal, low HBV DNA level, younger age, and active inflammation on liver biopsy. Long-term studies have shown that untreated children eventually experience a rate of HBeAg seroconversion that tends to overlap with that of treated children, suggesting that interferon does not increase HBsAg seroconversion rate but may simply accelerate spontaneous clearance. As with adults, poor response, dosing requirement, side-effect profile, and contraindications have led to general disuse. Studies investigating combination therapy with lamivudine or prednisone did not show improved response when compared to interferon monotherapy.

A resurgence of interest in interferon therapy in adults with chronic HBV using peginterferon has occurred in the last 5 years. Initial studies show a 30% response rate with a 40% sustained response. Initial studies using combination peginterferon and lamivudine did not improve initial or sustained response rates. No studies using peginterferon in children have been published.

Oral nucleoside and nucleotide analogs have dramatically changed the management of chronic HBV in adults. These medications are taken orally and range in virologic potency, side-effect profile, and susceptibility to development of viral resistance. Initial treatment was for 1–2 years; however, low durability of response has prompted prolonged treatment. The degree of viral suppression correlates to the degree of histological, biochemical, and serologic improvement. Studies have shown these medications need to be taken for at least 18 months if viral eradication and HBeAg seroconversion occurs, but therapy can be indefinite if detectable HBV DNA or HBeAg persists. Medications should be taken for at least 6 months following HBeAg seroconversion. HBV DNA resurgence will invariably occur if medications are discontinued in the absence of HBeAg seroconversion. Additionally HBV DNA resurgence can occur even after HBeAg seroconversion; therefore, patients must be monitored long term.

In children treated with 3 mg/kg (100 mg maximum) lamivudine daily, clearance of HBeAg and HBV DNA at 52 weeks occurred in 23% of patients compared to 13% of controls. If baseline AST was more than twice normal, the response rate improved to 31%. HBsAg loss occurred in 3% of patients, and HBeAg seroconversion was durable for 3 years in 82% of patients. Unfortunately, resistance to lamivudine is common, with adult studies showing 10–30% after 1 year of treatment and up to 70% by 5 years of treatment.

Adefovir dipivoxil is a nucleotide analog and was the second oral agent to be introduced. Adefovir has a high safety profile and low resistance profile, but is less potent than the other oral agents. Another advantage to adefovir is the absence of cross-reactivity with lamivudine and other nucleoside-induced resistance. In a large multisite, randomized, double-blind, placebo-controlled study of adefovir in children with chronic HBV viral eradication and HBeAg seroconversion was, unfortunately, limited only to adolescent patients.

Entecavir and tenofovir are both approved therapies for chronic HBV in adults and are undergoing clinical trials in children. Entecavir has a high potency, low resistance profile, and is well tolerated. Tenofovir is a nucleotide analog similar to adefovir but is more potent. Tenofovir, like Adefovir, is effective in treating lamivudine-resistant HBV. Because telbuvidine has a cross-resistance with lamivudine and 2-year resistance profile of 21%, it has not emerged as a treatment of choice of chronic HBV.

Various combinations of nucleotide analog drugs have been studied in adults, and such therapy is indicated for HBV-drug resistance, decompensated cirrhosis, HIV co-infection on retroviral therapy, and post-liver transplantation. In pediatric patients, combination therapy should be individualized, taking into account the risks and benefits.

Indications for treatment in pediatric patients should be individualized. To improve response rates, it is currently recommended that patients should be in the active immune phase for at least 6 months without HBeAg seroconversion and have evidence of active inflammation and fibrosis on liver biopsy. Treatment is also indicated for a special subgroup of patients that include those with co-morbid conditions requiring chemotherapy or immunosuppressive agents. Ideally, treatment should be started at least 6 months prior to the initiation of immunosuppression and continued for at least 6 months following completion of immunosuppression. Patients should have necessary support to insure compliance. There are currently no data to support or refute treatment of children in the immune tolerant phase with normal or minimally elevated aminotransferase levels and minimal or no evidence of inflammation on liver histology. As spontaneous seroconversion is common, and response rates are poor, watchful waiting remains an option for clinicians treating children with chronic HBV without evidence of active inflammation.

Hepatitis C

Unfortunately, there are no effective prophylactic regimes for HCV infection except for the use of universal precautions, screening of donor blood products, and avoidance of exposure with shared intravenous needles. As in chronic HBV, treatment regimens were developed in the adult population and then extended to pediatric patients. The goal of therapy is to prevent complications and death from HCV infection. Treatment response is defined as virologic clearance. There are several types of virologic responses, the most important being a sustained virologic response (SVR), defined as the absence of HCV RNA in serum, by sensitive PCR, 24 weeks after discontinuation of treatment. This is generally interpreted as a "cure," although in the presence of cirrhosis HCC has been reported to occur.

An ETR is the absence of HCV RNA after 24 or 48 weeks of therapy, depending on genotype. An ETR is necessary for an SVR, but is not predictive. Undetectable HCV RNA after the first 4 weeks of treatment is called a rapid virologic response (RVR) and is positive predictor of achieving a SVR. Complete absence or detection of $>2 \log_{10}$ reduction of serum HCV RNA from baseline at 12 weeks of therapy is an early virologic response (EVR). Failure to achieve an EVR is the most accurate negative predictor for achieving a SVR. Patients not achieving EVR are considered to be null responders and treatment should be discontinued. Patients who achieve EVR, but never clear viral RNA from serum, are considered to be partial responders.

The initial standard of care for adult and pediatric patients was interferon plus ribavirin. This has been replaced with peginterferon and ribavirin. Peginterferon consists of alpha-interferon covalently linked to polyethylene glycol, which confers an extended half-life, allowing once weekly administration and improved SVR.

There are two commercially available pegylated alpha-interferons, 2a and 2b, which have equal efficacy, side effects, and safety profiles. Both are FDA approved for treatment of adults with chronic HCV. In adults, pretreatment predictors of response include genotypes 2 and 3, and viral load $<600,000$ IU/mL.

Current guidelines recommend that adult patients with genotype 1 should be treated for a 48-week course of combination therapy. Ribavirin and peginterferon doses are adjusted per body weight with both preparations. Patients defined as null responders at 12 weeks should have therapy discontinued. Patients with a partial response should continue therapy and be retested at 24 weeks. If HCV RNA remains positive at 24 weeks, therapy should be discontinued, while those that become negative between 12 and 24 weeks should be considered for extension of treatment to 72 weeks. Patients who complete 48 or 72 weeks of therapy should have HCV RNA measured 24 weeks after completion of therapy. Patients with genotype 2 and 3 should receive combination peginterferon with standard dosing of 800 mg ribavirin daily for 24 weeks and retested for HCV RNA 24 weeks after therapy. Retreatment of null responders with the same or alternate peginterferon is not recommended. Null responders who were treated with nonpegylated combination therapy can

be treated with peginterferon combination therapy as described above. Newer treatments using triple combination therapy with standard peginterferon and ribavirin plus novel HCV protease inhibitors are undergoing clinical trials and offer promising results.

Currently only peginterferon alpha-2b is approved for children >2 years of age.[34] Recommended dosing is 60 µg/m^2 IM weekly, in combination with ribavirin, 15 mg/kg, for 48 weeks. In two large studies results were similar or improved compared to adult studies and a SVR was achieved in 49–59% of patients with genotype 1. In both studies SVR was achieved in 100% of patients with genotype 3.[35,36] There are insufficient data, however, to recommend a 24-week course of treatment in children with genotype 2 or 3 infection, and length of treatment for these patients should be individualized.[34]

The decision to treat should be individualized based on genotype, evidence of inflammation, psychologic factors, and support mechanisms for compliance. Children over the age of 3 years with active inflammation on histology and elevated serum aminotransferases should be offered treatment regardless of genotype. Because of the improved response rate for children with genotype 2 or 3, treatment should be offered to children over 3 years of age with these genotypes, even without evidence of active inflammation or elevated aminotransferase levels. Children with genotype 1 who have minimal inflammation and normal or minimally elevated aminotransferase levels should have an individualized approach. Treatment can be offered but response rates and side effects should be clearly discussed as the risks may outweigh the benefits in these patients. Careful observation while waiting for new drug development remains an option.

SUMMARY

Acute viral hepatitis is usually self-limited. Exceptions include both hepatitis B and hepatitis C, which are the leading causes of chronic infectious hepatitis worldwide. Most adults acutely infected with HBV will recover, while over 90% of infants infected in the perinatal period will develop chronic infection. This is in contrast to HCV, in which only 5% of perinatally exposed infants develop chronic infection, yet 50–85% of exposed adults develop chronic infection. Cirrhosis and HCC are complications of chronic HCV and HBV infection and are a significant cause of morbidity and mortality in chronically infected adults. Treatment goals are to clear virus and decrease disease progression and complications of infection. The pediatric patient is unique due to an apparent immune tolerance to prenatally acquired infection. Although rare, complications of cirrhosis and HCC have been reported in pediatric patients.

REFERENCES

1. Stanway G, Brown F, Christian P, et al. Family *Picornaviridae*. In: Fauquet CM, Mayo MA, Maniloff J, Desselberger U, Ball LA, eds. *Virus Taxonomy. Eighth Report of the International Committee on Taxonomy of Viruses.* London: Elsevier/Academic Press; 2005:757.

2. Centers for Disease Control and Prevention. Prevention of hepatitis A through active or passive immunization: recommendations of the Advisory Committee on Immunization Practices (ACIP). *MMWR.* 2006;55(RR-7):1–23.

3. Centers for Disease Control and Prevention. Surveillance for acute viral hepatitis—United States, 2007. *MMWR.* 2009;58(SS-3):1–28.

4. Mason WS, Burrell CJ, Casey J, et al. Family *Hepadnaviridae*. In: Fauquet CM, Mayo MA, Maniloff J, Desselberger U, Ball LA, eds. *Virus Taxonomy. Eighth Report of the International Committee on Taxonomy of Viruses.* London: Elsevier/Academic Press; 2005:373–384.

5. Summers J, Mason WS. Replication of the genome of a hepatitis B-like virus by reverse transcription of an RNA intermediate. *Cell.* 1982;29(2):403–415.

6. Dienstag JL. Hepatitis B infection. *N Engl J Med.* 2008;359(14):1486–1500.

7. Ghany MG, Doo EC. Assessment and management of chronic hepatitis B. *Infect Dis Clin North Am.* 2006 Mar;20(1):63–79.

8. American Academy of Pediatrics. Hepatitis B. In: Pickering LK, Baker CJ, Lons SS, McMillan JA, eds. *Red Book: 2006 Report of the Committee on Infectious Diseases.* 27th ed. Elk Grove Village, IL: American Academy of Pediatrics; 2006:335–355.

9. Stevens CE, Beasley RP, Tsui J, Lee WC. Vertical transmission of hepatitis B antigen in Taiwan. *N Engl J Med.* 1975;292(15):771–774.

10. Stevens CE, Toy PE, Tong MJ, et al. Perinatal hepatitis B virus transmission in the United States: prevention by passive–active immunization. *JAMA.* 1985;253(12):1740–1745.

11. Theil H-J, Collett MS, Gould EA, et al. Family *Flaviviridae*. In: Fauquet CM, Mayo MA, Maniloff J, Desselberger U, Ball LA, eds. *Virus Taxonomy. Eighth Report of the International Committee on Taxonomy of Viruses.* London: Elsevier/Academic Press; 2005:981–1008.

12. Simmonds P. Genetic diversity and evolution of hepatitis C virus—15 years on. *J Gen Virol.* 2004;85(Pt 11):3173–3188.

13. American Academy of Pediatrics. Hepatitis C virus infection. Committee on Infectious Diseases. *Pediatrics.* 1998;101:481–485.

14. Indodfi G, Resti M. Perinatal transmission of hepatitis C virus infection. *J Med Virol.* 2009;81(5):836–843.

15. Seeger C, Mason WS. Hepatitis B biology. *Microbiol Mol Biol Rev.* 2000;64;51–68.

16. Mason WS, Burrell CJ, Casey J, et al. Family *Hepadnaviridae*. In: Fauquet CM, Mayo MA, Maniloff J, Desselberger U, Ball LA, eds. *Virus Taxonomy. Eighth Report of the International Committee on Taxonomy of Viruses.* London: Elsevier/Academic Press; 2005;373–384.

17. Thompson, AJV, Bell AJ, Locarnni SA. Hepatitis B virus. In: Richman DD, Whitley RJ, Hayden FG, eds. *Clinical Virology.* 3rd ed. Washington, DC: American Society for Microbiology Press; 2009:673–707.

18. Weiland SF, Chisari FV. Stealth and cunning: hepatitis B and hepatitis C viruses. *J Virol.* 2005;79(15):9369–9380.

19. Rotman Y, Liang TJ. Hepatitis C virus. In: Richman DD, Whitley RJ, Hayden FG, eds. *Clinical Virology.* 3rd ed. Washington, DC: American Society for Microbiology Press; 2009:1215–1240.

20. American Academy of Pediatrics. Hepatitis A. In: Pickering LK, Baker CJ, Lons SS, McMillan JA, eds. *Red Book: 2006 Report of the Committee on Infectious Diseases.* 27th ed. Elk Grove Village, IL: American Academy of Pediatrics; 2006:326–335.

21. McMahon BJ, Alward WL, Hall DB, et al. Acute hepatitis B virus infection: relation of age to the clinical expression of disease and subsequent development of the carrier state. *J Infect Dis.* 1985;151(4):599–603.

22. Slowik MK, Jhaveri R. Hepatitis B and C viruses in infants and young children. *Semin Pediatr Infect Dis.* 2005;16(4):296–305.

23. Tram TT, Martin P. Hepatitis B: epidemiology and natural history. *Clin Liver Dis.* 2004;8(2):255–266.

24. McMahon BJ. Epidemiology and natural history of hepatitis B. *Semin Liver Dis.* 2005;25(suppl 1):3–8.

25. Sherlock S. The natural progression of hepatitis B. *Postgrad Med J.* 1987;63(suppl 2):7–11.

26. Servoss JC, Friedman MD. Serologic and molecular diagnosis of hepatitis B virus. *Infect Dis Clin North Am.* 2006;20(1):47–61.

27. Chang MH. Natural history of hepatitis B virus infection in children. *J Gastroenterol Hepatol.* 2002;5(suppl):E16–E19.

28. Ganem D, Prince AM. Hepatitis B virus infection—natural history and clinical consequences. *N Engl J Med.* 2004(11);350:1118–1129.

29. Brunetto MR, Giarin MM, Oliveri F, et al. Wild-type and e antigen-minus hepatitis B viruses and course of chronic hepatitis. *Proc Natl Acad Sci U S A.* 1991;88(10):4186–4190.

30. Han SH. Extrahepatic manifestations of chronic hepatitis B. *Clin Liver Dis.* 2004;8(2):403–418.

31. Hoofnagle JH. NIH Consensus Development Conference: management of hepatitis B, Oct 20–22, 2008. *Hepatology.* 2009;49(5):S1.

32. Kurbegov AC, Sokol RJ. Hepatitis B therapy in children. *Expert Rev Gastroenterol Hepatol.* 2009;3(1):39–49.

33. Yeung LT, To T, King SM, et al. Spontaneous clearance of childhood hepatitis C virus infection. *J Viral Hepat.* 2007;14:797–805.

34. Ghany MG, Strader DB, Thomas DL, et al. AASLD practice guidelines. Diagnosis, management and treatment of hepatitis C: an update. *Hepatology.* 2009;49(4):1335–1374.

35. Jara P, Hierro L, de la Vega A, et al. *Pediatr Infect Dis J.* 2008;27(2):142–148.

36. Wirth S, Pieper-Boustani H, Lang T, Ballauff A, Kullmer U, Gerner P, Wintermeyer P, Jenke A. Peginterferon alfa-2b plus ribavirin treatment in children and adolescents with chronic hepatitis C. *Hepatology.* 2005 May;41(5):1013–1018.

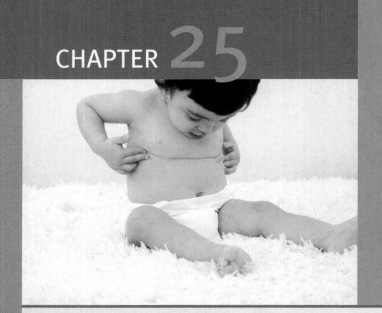

CHAPTER 25

Wilson's Disease

Karan McBride Emerick

DEFINITIONS AND EPIDEMIOLOGY

Wilson's disease is a human copper storage disease. Wilson's results in the accumulation of toxic levels of copper in mainly the liver and secondarily in other organs such as the kidneys, brain, and cornea. The disease is caused by a mutation in the *ATP7B* gene, which codes for a protein that facilitates the incorporation of copper into proteins (such as ceruloplasmin) and also the transportation of copper into vesicles that allow it to be secreted in bile.[1] The critical effect of a mutation in *ATP7B* is diminished copper secretion into bile, which leads to excess copper accumulation in the hepatocyte. The disease related to this defect therefore involves toxicity to the liver with clinical disease that may range from abnormal liver function tests to fulminant hepatic failure and cirrhosis.

Wilson's is an autosomal recessive disease with an estimated incidence of 1:30,000 live births internationally.[2] The most common presentation is in the second decade of life with hepatic or hematologic symptoms (40–60%). The remaining patients present with neurologic (~30%) or psychiatric (10%) symptoms in their third or fourth decade.[2]

PATHOGENESIS

In normal human copper metabolism, the dietary intake and absorption of copper is in excess of physiologic needs. The estimated daily copper requirement for an adult is 1.3–1.7 mg, whereas the normal daily Western copper intake is 2–5 mg of copper.[3,4] The estimated efficiency of copper absorption in the stomach and small intestine is approximately 40–60%. Therefore, the amount of copper absorbed by the intestine and retained

in the body must be regulated to prevent accumulation of excess copper—which is toxic. The main regulatory system for maintaining copper balance in the body is the excretion of up to 80% of absorbed copper in the bile[5,6] (Figure 25–1). Up to 1.2–1.7 mg/day of copper is excreted in the bile daily.[6,7] There are also several chemical factors that impair intestinal copper absorption, such as excess zinc or ascorbic acid.[8–10]

Dietary copper is absorbed into the small intestine epithelial cells where it complexes either to the protein metallothionein or to amino acids for transport into the portal circulation. Metallothionein also forms complexes with zinc and cadmium, though less strongly than copper. Zinc stimulates metallothionein synthesis in the intestinal cell. In doing so, it promotes retention of metallothionein-bound copper in the enterocyte that will then be excreted in the feces when the enterocyte is shed.[11] It is on this basis that zinc was postulated to reduce intestinal copper absorption and became a modality of treatment for Wilson's.

Once in the portal circulation, the copper complexes to albumin or amino acids with only a small fraction remaining "free." A copper transporter (hCTR) for albumin-bound copper then transports the copper into the hepatocyte.[12,13] There it interacts with several proteins that direct the copper to chaperones for incorporation into essential proteins (such as ceruloplasmin, copper/zinc superoxide dismutase, and cytochrome *c* oxidase), or into lysosomes for biliary excretion.

In 1993, it was discovered that Wilson's disease was caused by a mutation in the *ATP7B* gene, on chromosome 13, which resulted in absent or reduced function of a copper–chaperone protein, ATP7B.[14] ATP7B is a metal-transporting P-type ATPase, located on the trans-Golgi complex of the hepatocyte.[15] The ATP7B protein is

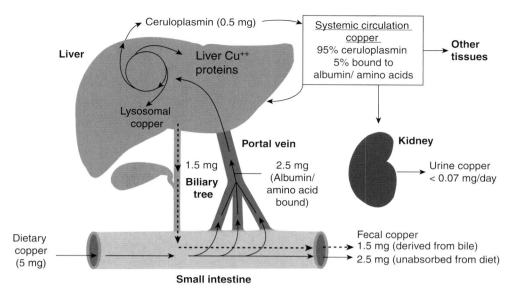

FIGURE 25–1 ■ Copper metabolism in humans (adapted from Ref.[7]).

necessary for transport of copper into vesicles that form lysosomes for excretion into the bile. It also functions in the incorporation of copper into ceruloplasmin. Ceruloplasmin, a copper-containing globulin, is secreted into the systemic circulation from the liver. The functions of ceruloplasmin include the mobilization of iron from tissues (by oxidizing ferrous iron for transfer into transferrin) and the transport of copper to other tissues. The absence or diminished function of ATP7B results in accumulation of copper in the hepatocyte due to both impaired copper excretion into bile and inability to incorporate copper into ceruloplasmin.[14] The production of ceruloplasmin without attached copper (apoceruloplasmin), which has a shorter half-life than ceruloplasmin, results in decreased levels of ceruloplasmin in the blood of Wilson's patients. It is this dynamic that has made measurement of serum ceruloplasmin the primary screening test for Wilson's.[16]

Ultimately, the excess retained copper in the hepatocytes of Wilson's patients leads to toxic injury to the cell and eventually spillage of copper into the circulation, where it may be deposited in other organs such as the brain, cornea, and kidneys. The relative quantity of copper that overflows into the circulation may be measured by determining the copper content of a 24-hour urine collection. In Wilson's disease, this value usually will be double normal levels of urinary copper of <40 μg of copper/24 hours. This is the basis of 24-hour urine collection as the supporting follow-up diagnostic test to the serum ceruloplasmin level for diagnosing Wilson's.

The mechanism of toxicity of copper at the cellular level may be a combination of several different copper-sensitive processes that include inhibition of cytosolic enzymes and pro-oxidant effects that damage plasma membrane function and alter oxidative phosphorylation in mitochondria. Evidence of abnormal mitochondrial ultrastructure in hepatocytes of patients with Wilson's disease supports the theory that mitochondria are one of the affected organelles in copper toxicity.[17] There is also evidence to suggest that the mechanism of hepatocyte death in Wilson's disease is via apoptosis that may explain the typical mild elevation in the transaminases associated with hepatitis in Wilson's disease.[18]

CLINICAL PRESENTATION

One of the challenges of diagnosing Wilson's disease is the wide spectrum of clinical presentations. Wilson's patients with hepatic symptoms could present with anything from isolated asymptomatic elevated transaminase levels to liver failure. Wilson's patients with a neurologic presentation can experience symptoms ranging from declining school performance to frank psychosis (Table 25–1). The youngest patient ever reported to present with liver involvement due to Wilson's disease was 3 years old; therefore, this disorder is not usually considered on the differential of neonatal or infantile liver disease.[19] The most common clinical presentation for Wilson's disease is a hepatic presentation between 10 and 20 years of age (40–60%). The second most common presentation is with primarily neurologic (34%) or psychiatric (10%) symptoms between the ages of 20–40 years[2,20] (Figure 25–2). Occasionally, Wilson's patients are diagnosed based on the finding of hemolytic anemia.

Although Wilson's disease always begins with liver involvement, many patients may be asymptomatic and

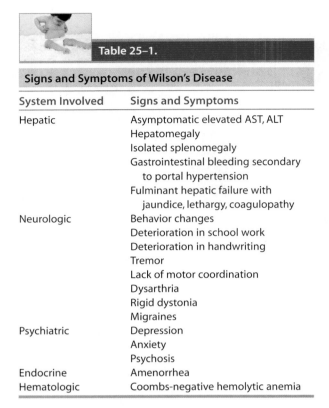

Table 25–1.

Signs and Symptoms of Wilson's Disease

System Involved	Signs and Symptoms
Hepatic	Asymptomatic elevated AST, ALT
	Hepatomegaly
	Isolated splenomegaly
	Gastrointestinal bleeding secondary to portal hypertension
	Fulminant hepatic failure with jaundice, lethargy, coagulopathy
Neurologic	Behavior changes
	Deterioration in school work
	Deterioration in handwriting
	Tremor
	Lack of motor coordination
	Dysarthria
	Rigid dystonia
	Migraines
Psychiatric	Depression
	Anxiety
	Psychosis
Endocrine	Amenorrhea
Hematologic	Coombs-negative hemolytic anemia

patients can be diagnosed in the presymptomatic phase of the disease by obtaining a screening ceruloplasmin, 24-hour urine for copper, or genetic testing if the screening is ambiguous.

The pathophysiology of the disease predicates the development of clinical symptoms caused by storage of excess copper in various organs. Initially the excess copper is stored in the liver. Once the liver is saturated, the copper is circulated in a free form (non-ceruloplasmin-bound) and begins to accumulate in the central nervous system, cornea, kidneys, and endocrine organs. This progression explains the typical mode of presentation during childhood as hepatic disease. Only about 17% of patients under 10 years of age are found to have neuropsychiatric symptoms at presentation, whereas in patients presenting after 18 years of age, 74% experience neurologic manifestations.[2,20] It is usually after 10 years of age that patients may manifest evidence of involvement of the other organ systems such as renal, hematologic, and endocrine (Figure 25–2).

One of the most widely recognized extrahepatic manifestations of Wilson's disease is the characteristic Kayser–Fleischer (K-F) ring in the ocular cornea[21] (Figure 25–3). The K-F ring is a green-brown-colored ring at the edge of the cornea caused by copper accumulation. The appearance of the ring is due to the reflection of light from the copper granules deposited there. The ring is usually present at the superior pole of the cornea first and then may progress to the inferior pole and finally circumferentially. Slit-lamp exam

therefore go undiagnosed until they present at 20–30 years of age with advanced hepatic or neurologic disease. The symptoms of Wilson's disease are rarely apparent before 5 years of age. Siblings of known Wilson's

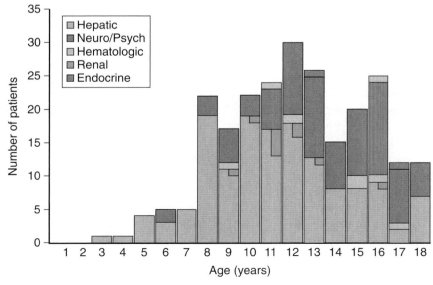

FIGURE 25–2 ■ Histogram of age of distribution of initial mode of clinical presentation in children and adolescents with Wilson's disease. Split vertical bars represent combined clinical presentation (adapted from Ref.[44], 3rd ed.).

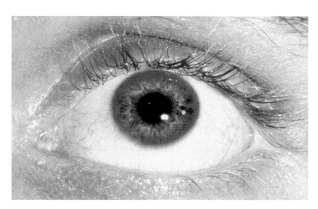

FIGURE 25–3 ■ Kayser–Fleischer ring. Copper deposited in Descemet's membrane can form a brown ring at the junction of the cornea with the sclera, encircling the iris. This patient has an intense Kayser–Fleischer ring, seen easily with the naked eye. In many cases, these are more subtle, observable only with a slit lamp microscope. Used with permission from Fauci et al. *Harrison's Principles of Internal Medicine*, 17th ed. © 2008 The McGraw-Hill Companies, Inc.

by an ophthalmologist is the best way to determine the presence of K-F rings. The K-F ring has no impact on visual acuity, and treatment with chelation therapy can lead to complete disappearance of the rings. The K-F ring is present in the vast majority of Wilson's patients who present with neurologic symptoms with few exceptions (about 5%).[22] Children with Wilson's generally present with hepatic symptoms initially, and therefore rarely have K-F rings. It is important to note that K-F rings may also occur in other liver diseases that have reduced biliary excretion; therefore, an isolated finding K-F rings is not pathognomonic of Wilson's disease. In particular, K-F rings due to secondary copper overload may be seen in primary biliary cirrhosis, intrahepatic cholestasis, or chronic hepatitis.[23,24] Another ophthalmologic finding of Wilson's is deposits of copper in the anterior and posterior lens capsule called a "sunflower cataract."[25] These, too, do not interfere with vision and can resolve with chelation therapy.

The neuropsychiatric presentation of Wilson's is the first indication of disease in 40–45% of patients older than 20 years of age.[2,20] The youngest patient recorded with neurologic onset was 6 years old.[2] The symptoms of neurologic involvement of Wilson's are usually related to dysfunction of the basal ganglia, cerebellum, and corticospinal and corticobulbar pathways. These symptoms are often motor abnormalities associated with cerebellar or extrapyramidal injury.[26] They may include tremor, coordination defects, dystonia, or choreiform movements.[27–29] Sensory function and intelligence are generally unaffected in Wilson's dis-

ease. In up to 10–25% of Wilson's disease patients, the initial manifestation may be a psychiatric disturbance. The symptoms can include dementia, neuroses, schizophrenia, psychosis, or antisocial behavior. It is therefore important for psychiatrists to consider this diagnosis when evaluating psychiatric symptoms, especially if the patient has a history of liver disease. A screen that includes a plasma ceruloplasmin level and an ophthalmology examination for K-F rings would be prudent.[30]

The renal dysfunction that results from copper accumulation in the kidneys includes proximal renal tubular dysfunction, and decreased glomerular filtration rate.[31] The renal tubular dysfunctional is manifested by presence of blood, protein, glucose, phosphate, and amino acids in the urine and decreased ability to acidify the urine.[19] Renal stones can be seen in up to 16% of Wilson's patients. The patients with the most severe hepatic disease, that is, presentation with fulminant hepatic failure or end-stage liver disease, may develop renal insufficiency as well.

The primary hematologic manifestation of Wilson's is intravascular hemolysis. The hemolysis may be caused by the oxidative stress resulting from sudden releases of copper from the liver. This damages red cell membranes via lipid peroxidation. Wilson's patients may present with transient hemolysis in the absence of any hepatic or neuropsychiatric symptoms. Hemolysis is the presenting complaint in 15% of patients.[32,33] If a patient presents with the combination of hemolysis and liver failure, the prognosis is poor because of possible associated renal failure secondary to hemoglobinuria.[34,35]

The hepatic disease of Wilson's can present as one of the following four clinical subtypes: acute hepatitis, fulminant hepatic failure, chronic active hepatitis, and cirrhosis.[36] However, it is also common to diagnose Wilson's disease during investigation of elevated transaminases found on health screening in asymptomatic children. The presentation of acute hepatitis typically consists of jaundice, nausea, fatigue, dark urine, and pale stools. These patients will typically be tested for common infectious conditions such as hepatitis A, B, and C and Epstein–Barr virus (Table 25–2). If these are negative and the patient spontaneously improves, no further workup may occur. However, other clues to the possibility of Wilson's disease include the presence of low serum uric acid (due to renal losses), low serum alkaline phosphatase (mechanism unknown), or a hemolytic anemia.[2]

Chronic hepatitis in Wilson's disease usually manifests in young adulthood with generalized symptoms of liver disease. Frequently cirrhosis is present at the time of diagnosis.[2] Patients may have malaise,

Table 25–2.

Differential Diagnosis of Hepatic Presentation of Wilson's Disease

Presentation	Asymptomatic Elevation of AST and ALT	Chronic Hepatitis	Fulminant Hepatic Failure
Common conditions	Drug toxicity Medications for ■ Attention deficit disorder ■ Seizures ■ Psychiatric disease	Infectious hepatitis (B, C)	Drugs and toxins ■ Acetaminophen ■ Isoniazid ■ Valproate ■ Propylthiouracil ■ Halothane ■ Amanita
	Nonalcoholic steatohepatitis Viral infection ■ Non-A–G ■ Infectious hepatitis B, C Hypothyroidism	Nonalcoholic steatohepatitis	Viral hepatitis non-A–G
Rare conditions	Wilson's disease Autoimmune hepatitis Primary sclerosing cholangitis Alpha 1 antitrypsin deficiency	Wilson's disease Autoimmune hepatitis Primary sclerosing cholangitis Alpha 1 antitrypsin deficiency	Wilson's disease Autoimmune hepatitis Ischemia/hypoperfusion Erythrophagocytic lymphohistiocytosis
	Celiac disease Muscle disease	Cystic fibrosis Rheumatologic disease: ■ Systemic lupus erythmatosis ■ Juvenile rheumatoid arthritis	Budd–Chiari

fatigue, anorexia, and amenorrhea as well as jaundice, edema, ascites, and/or clubbing. The overall clinical picture of chronic Wilson's disease is typical of chronic hepatitis of any etiology, except that the Wilson's patients may have lower transaminases levels and alkaline phosphatase comparatively.[37] Because the clinical presentation is nonspecific, it is important that all patients with chronic hepatitis be screened for Wilson's with ceruloplasmin levels and possibly 24-hour urine copper measurements.

When Wilson's disease presents as fulminant hepatic failure, the typical course begins with an episode of jaundice that then progresses to severe hepatic insufficiency with coagulopathy, and then encephalopathy and possibly coma.[38,39] The patient becomes very jaundiced because of the accompanying hemolysis, and may also develop renal failure and will ultimately die without liver transplantation. Several clues that help to identify Wilson's as the cause of the failure include: Coombs-negative hemolytic anemia, relatively low serum transaminases for the presence of liver failure, and a low serum alkaline phosphatase. An ophthalmologic exam that confirms the presence of K-F rings can also help to confirm the diagnosis, although in the younger patients who have no neuropsychiatric symptoms, it is unlikely

that these will be found. Wilson's disease patients who present with fulminant liver failure virtually never recover despite chelation or plasmapheresis. It is therefore recommended that patients with this presentation be urgently referred for liver transplantation.[38,40–42] Acute liver failure can also develop in stable Wilson's patients on chelation therapy who then abruptly discontinue their medication. The resultant liver failure is postulated to be due to a release of a large amount of free copper. This is due to loss of coupling of the copper to the chelating agent or to another protein that rendered it nontoxic. All patients must be told repeatedly that copper chelation therapy is life-long and that discontinuation could be fatal.

DIFFERENTIAL DIAGNOSIS

The differential diagnosis of each possible presentation of Wilson's would be prohibitively lengthy. However, in the pediatric population, the initial presentation is usually hepatic in nature and carries a more limited differential, as listed in Table 25–2. An algorithm for laboratory investigation of possible Wilson's disease is given in Figure 25–4.

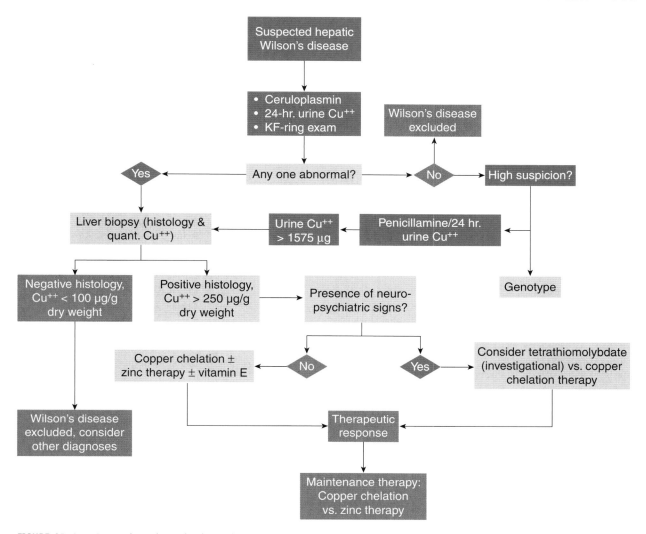

FIGURE 25–4 ■ Approach to the evaluation and treatment of a pediatric patient with presentation of liver disease and suspected Wilson's disease (adapted from Ref.[44], 3rd ed.).

DIAGNOSIS

No single laboratory test is adequate to diagnose Wilson's disease. The diagnosis is made using a combination of clinical history, physical exam, and key laboratory tests (Table 25–3; Figure 25–4). The testing used to confirm the diagnosis may also vary depending on the clinical presentation. For example, a patient presenting with mental status changes might undergo ophthalmologic evaluation as an early diagnostic test given that K-F rings are virtually always present when neurologic or psychiatric symptoms develop.

In cases with evident liver disease, whether it is elevated transaminases or fulminant liver failure, the recommended approach is to start the screening with a serum ceruloplasmin (Figure 25–4).[43] If the ceruloplasmin is low (<20 mg/dL), then further testing with a 24-hour urine copper excretion is needed because no single test will confirm Wilson's. An elevated urine copper >100 µg/24 hours is highly suggestive of the copper overload of Wilson's, although there can be overlap with other chronic liver diseases that result in copper overload such as chronic active hepatitis or cholestatic cirrhosis.[44] The final confirmatory test would be measurement of hepatic copper concentration via liver biopsy.[45] Normal hepatic copper content is <50 µg copper/g dry weight of liver, whereas in Wilson's disease it is virtually always >250 µg/g dry weight of liver. The characteristic histologic findings of Wilson's disease seen on light microscopy include glycogenated nuclei and hepatic steatosis. The steatosis may be microvesicular initially and then evolve into a macrovesicular pattern.[2] The histology is supportive but the copper content is diagnostic.

Table 25–3 describes testing for Wilson's and a few conditions under which the testing may be falsely positive in non-Wilson's patients.[44] Clinical factors may also interfere with collecting diagnostic data such as oliguric

Table 25–3.

Diagnostic Testing for Wilson's Disease

Diagnostic Test	Diagnostic Value for Wilson's Disease	Factors Associated with False-positive Results
Serum ceruloplasmin	<20 mg/dL	Massive protein losses Protein malnutrition Hepatic insufficiency
24-Hour urine copper excretion	>100 µg/24 hours	Contamination by exogenous copper Chronic active hepatitis Cholestatic cirrhosis Nephrotic syndrome
24-Hour urine copper excretion after penicillamine challenge (500 mg orally at start of collection and 12 hours into collection)	1575 µg/24 hours	Acute persistent hepatitis A
Ophthalmologic exam	Presence of Kayser–Fleischer rings	Chronic cholestatic disease
Hepatic copper concentration (normal <50 µg copper/g dry weight)	>250 µg copper/g dry weight of liver tissue	Chronic hepatitis Chronic cholestatic disease Primary sclerosing cholangitis
Genotyping	Two disease-causing mutations in ATP7B	Laboratory error

renal failure or severe coagulopathy that prohibits liver biopsy at presentation. If the diagnosis is still unclear after the testing above, or if a liver biopsy cannot be performed safely, molecular genetic testing is available.[46] Sequencing the entire coding region of *ATP7B* can demonstrate a disease-causing mutation in about 98% of cases. Due to the high mortality associated with the severe acute presentation of Wilson's, it is critical that referral to specialists for supportive and life-saving care be prompt (Table 25–4). Because of the possibility that siblings may have presymptomatic Wilson's disease, all brothers and sisters of affected individuals should also be evaluated for biochemical evidence of the condition. If the proband's mutation is known, screening for this may also be considered.

TREATMENT

The treatment of Wilson's disease consists of first removing the excess stored copper from the body with copper chelation, followed by measures to prevent re-

Table 25–4.

When to Refer Wilson's Patients to Specialists

Presentation	Symptoms	Referral
Primary hepatic failure with insufficiency	Jaundice, coagulopathy, lethargy, hepatic coma, renal failure	Transplantation center urgently
Secondary hepatic failure with insufficiency	Due to cessation of chelation therapy—jaundice, coagulopathy, lethargy, hepatic coma, renal failure	Transplantation center urgently
Renal failure	Usually in the setting of liver failure	Transplantation center urgently
Neuropsychiatric symptoms	Motor abnormalities: bradykinesia, cogwheel rigidity, ataxia, tremor Cognitive impairment, organic personality syndrome	Ophthalmologist for slit-lamp exam
Coombs-negative hemolytic anemia with liver dysfunction	Hemolysis is poor prognostic factor	Transplantation center urgently

Table 25–5.

Medications Used to Treat Wilson's Disease

Medication	Dosage	When to Use
D-Penicillamine	*START*: 20 mg/kg/day (up to 2.0 g/day), 3 doses/day between meals *Maintenance*: 10–20 mg/kg/day (up to 1.0 g/day) *Oral pyridoxine 25–50 mg/day*	Initial and maintenance therapy
Trientine	Same dosing as D-penicillamine	May be first choice as initial therapy or after patient failed D-penicillamine
Zinc acetate	25–50 mg three times per day between meals	Maintenance after successful chelation or during pregnancy
Ammonium tetrathiomolybdate	120–200 mg/day	Investigational drug
Vitamin E	400–1200 IU/day (2–3 doses per day with meals)	Adjunctive therapy

accumulation. These include a low-copper diet and possibly zinc therapy (Table 25–5). Copper chelation requires the use of approved agents—either D-penicillamine or trientine. These medications are indicated in the care of any Wilson's patient who presents with stable liver disease.[47] Chelation therapy is not recommended for Wilson's patients who present with fulminant hepatic failure or with complications of cirrhosis such as portal hypertensive bleeding, ascites, or encephalopathy. Historical evidence supports that patients who present with failure do not recover with chelation therapy. Other attempts to remove the excess copper released from dying hepatocytes, including plasmapheresis, hemodialysis, and hemofiltration, are not effective. Rapid referral to a liver transplant center is recommended in those cases.[38,48,49]

D-penicillamine (β-β-dimethylcysteine) is a metabolite of penicillin that chelates copper.[50–52] It is believed to detoxify copper by complexing directly with it, thereby making free copper less available to injure the hepatocytes. There is controversy whether D-penicillamine reduces the copper content of the liver or mainly detoxifies the free copper. The occurrence of fulminant hepatic failure in Wilson's disease patients who discontinue chelation after many years of successful treatment suggests that D-penicillamine may form a nontoxic copper–penicillamine complex, only some of which is excreted in the urine.[44] At the cessation of D-penicillamine, it is believed that a large amount of free copper can be released from the previously formed complex and causes large-scale injury. It is for this reason that Wilson's patients are constantly reminded that their copper chelation therapy must never be stopped as it could be fatal.[1]

D-Penicillamine can also cause an antipyroxidine effect, and therefore all patients instituting treatment should also receive 25 mg of pyridoxine daily. The dosing of D-penicillamine in older children and adults is 1 g daily, usually given by mouth in four divided doses, given 30 minutes before or 2 or more hours after meals. In young children, the dose is 20 mg/kg/day rounded to the nearest 250 and divided into three doses. The dosing is recommended to begin at one-quarter or one-half of the full dose, with increases to full dose over 2 weeks.[44]

Penicillamine can cause both toxic and allergic reactions. Early side effects can include fever, skin rash, lymphadenopathy, and pancytopenia due to bone marrow suppression. For this reason, a complete blood cell count, urinalysis, and renal and liver blood tests should be done weekly after initiation of therapy. If after several weeks the patient has no side effects, then the monitoring can be scheduled every 3 months for a year and then every 6 months thereafter. An annual 24-hour urinary copper excretion is one of the most informative analyses to measure effectiveness of chronic therapy. If appropriate chelation is being achieved, the initial urinary copper may exceed several grams of copper per day. This value should decline over months to years of treatment. Copper excretion typically falls to 200–500 µg/24 hours. Compliance with the medication may be monitored by comparing urine copper secretion over time. A sudden significant increase in copper excretion may suggest a lapse in medication followed by a recent resumption of therapy. A significant and sudden fall in copper excretion (i.e., <200 µg/24 hours) may suggest poor compliance with medication. Calculation of free serum copper may also help to determine compliance. Sudden rises in free copper >20 µg/dL may suggest noncompliance, whereas effective therapy should be associated with levels between 5 and 15 µg/dL[47]:

Free copper = [3 × serum ceruloplasmin (mg/dL)] − total serum copper (µg/dL)

Late toxic effects of D-penicillamine may include proteinuria and nephrotic syndrome, Goodpasture's syndrome, optic neuritis, agranulocytosis, thrombocytopenia, myasthenia gravis, and anaphylactic reactions.[53–57] There are also late reactions to D-penicillamine that are related to the interference with the cross-linking of collagen and elastin. These side effects may include cutis laxa (a weakening of the subcutaneous tissue), aphtous stomatitis, systemic sclerosis-like lesions, and pemphigoid lesions of the mouth and skin. Treatment of these side effects can include very brief discontinuation of the D-penicillamine until the lesions resolve. D-Penicillamine may be then restarted using premedication with prednisone (0.5 mg/kg/day) 2–3 days before resuming treatment at a reduced dose and working up to the treatment dose again. Alternatively, trientine (triethylene tetramine dihydrochloride) therapy may be substituted for D-penicillamine for any toxic reaction or may be used as the initial copper-chelating drug.

Trientine was approved for use in copper chelation in 1985, as an alternative to D-penicillamine.[51,58–60] However, because of its significantly lower side-effect profile, trientine has become the preferred first-line treatment for Wilson's in many centers. Trientine chelates copper by forming a stable complex with copper through its four nitrogen atoms in a planar ring. The dosing is similar to D-penicillamine at 1–2 g daily in three divided doses, given prior to meals, for adolescents and adults. The main toxicities include bone marrow suppression, nephrotoxicity, and skin and mucosal lesions. The monitoring schedule for use of trientine is therefore similar to that discussed above for D-penicillamine. There appears to be no cross-reactivity between toxic reactions to penicillamine and trientine.

An alternate drug, ammonium tetrathiomolybdate, has been proposed for use as initial therapy in patients with neurologic symptoms.[61,62] It is still in investigational trials; however, it has been demonstrated to slow or halt neurologic progression in the short term when compared to trientine.

In addition to copper chelation, Wilson's disease patients need to prevent re-accumulation of copper by limiting their dietary copper intake. This mainly involves the avoidance of high-copper foods such as mushrooms, shellfish, liver, nuts, chocolate, and legumes. Along with a low-copper diet, the use of zinc has been proposed as maintenance or adjunctive therapy for Wilson's.[63,64] Zinc inhibits intestinal copper absorption of copper and may also increase metallothionein binding of copper in the liver.[65] Zinc therapy has a slower onset of action than chelating agents; therefore, it is generally not used as initial or primary therapy for symptomatic patients or in combination with a chelating agent. It has been used as a single follow-up therapy for patients who have already undergone chelation therapy with good results. It has also been used in presymptomatic siblings to avoid the potential side effects of the chelating agents. Zinc (1 mg/kg/dose of elemental zinc given three times a day) may be administered as zinc acetate or sulfate and is given between meals. Zinc therapy also merits close monitoring for evidence of hepatocellular injury (elevated transaminases and bilirubin, serum albumin, and blood-clotting studies) to assure appropriate control of copper accumulation and to reinforce the importance of compliance. Patients have developed fulminant liver failure after the discontinuation of zinc therapy.

Antioxidant use, such as α-tocopherol (vitamin E), has been considered, but has not been thoroughly tested. The basis of this treatment is the observation of oxidative injury to copper-overloaded hepatocytes in terriers and Wilson's patients.[66] Dosing may be 400–1200 IU/day given in divided doses with meals.

Liver transplantation is a life-saving therapy in Wilson's patients who present initially with fulminant hepatic failure, or in liver failure due to discontinuation of chelation therapy or in cirrhotic patients who have decompensated despite medical therapy. The initial presentation of Wilson's disease with liver failure is often associated with a Coombs-negative hemolytic anemia and may progress to include renal failure. Attempts to salvage the patient with chelation therapy, hemodialysis, or antioxidant therapy have historically been futile, so this clinical presentation requires prompt referral to or transfer to a liver transplantation center. Survival post-transplant has been reported to be 73% at 5 years, with a poorer outcome for those with fulminant hepatic failure. To help determine criteria for referral for liver transplantation, Nazer et al. developed a prognostic index based on a combination of serum bilirubin, serum AST, and prolongation of the prothrombin time.[67] Each category was graded from 1 to 4 for a total of 12 possible points. A patient with seven or more points would likely have a fatal course and therefore required transplantation. Patients with six or less points usually would survive with medical therapy. This index was shown to have a sensitivity of 87% and specificity of 98% when applied to pediatric patients.

REFERENCES

1. Walshe JM. Wilson's disease. *Lancet.* 2007;369(9565):902.
2. Scheinberg IH, Sternlieb I, eds. *Wilson's Disease.* Philadelphia: WB Saunders; 1984.
3. Klevay LM. Deficiency, intake and the dietary requirement for copper. *J Neurol Sci.* 2009 Oct 15;285(1–2):272
4. Klevay LM, Reck SJ, Jacob RA, Logan GM Jr, Munoz JM, Sandstead HH. The human requirement for copper. I. Healthy men fed conventional, American diets. *Am J Clin Nutr.* 1980;33(1):45–50.
5. Frommer DJ. Defective biliary excretion of copper in Wilson's disease. *Gut.* 1974;15(2):125–129.

6. van Berge Henegouwen GP, Tangedahl TN, Hofmann AF, Northfield TC, LaRusso NF, McCall JT. Biliary secretion of copper in healthy man. Quantitation by an intestinal perfusion technique. *Gastroenterology.* 1977;72(6):1228–1231.

7. Sokol RJ. Copper storage diseases. In: Kaplowitz N, ed. *Liver and Biliary Diseases.* Baltimore: Williams and Wilkins; 1992:322–333.

8. Van den Berg GJ, Yu S, Lemmens AG, Beynen AC. Ascorbic acid feeding of rats reduces copper absorption, causing impaired copper status and depressed biliary copper excretion. *Biol Trace Elem Res.* 1994;41(1–2):47–58.

9. Gonzalez BP, Nino Fong R, Gibson CJ, Fuentealba IC, Cherian MG. Zinc supplementation decreases hepatic copper accumulation in LEC rat: a model of Wilson's disease. *Biol Trace Elem Res.* 2005;105(1–3):117–134.

10. Reeves PG, Briske-Anderson M, Johnson L. Physiologic concentrations of zinc affect the kinetics of copper uptake and transport in the human intestinal cell model, Caco-2. *J Nutr.* 1998;128(10):1794–1801.

11. Sturniolo GC, Mestriner C, Irato P, Albergoni V, Longo G, D'Inca R. Zinc therapy increases duodenal concentrations of metallothionein and iron in Wilson's disease patients. *Am J Gastroenterol.* 1999;94(2):334–338.

12. Lee J, Pena MM, Nose Y, Thiele DJ. Biochemical characterization of the human copper transporter Ctr1. *J Biol Chem.* 2002;277(6):4380–4387.

13. Klomp AE, Tops BB, Van Denberg IE, Berger R, Klomp LW. Biochemical characterization and subcellular localization of human copper transporter 1 (hCTR1). *Biochem J.* 2002;364(Pt 2):497–505.

14. Schilsky ML. Identification of the Wilson's disease gene: clues for disease pathogenesis and the potential for molecular diagnosis. *Hepatology.* 1994;20(2):529–533.

15. Bacon BR, Schilsky ML. New knowledge of genetic pathogenesis of hemochromatosis and Wilson's disease. *Adv Intern Med.* 1999;44:91–116.

16. Cauza E, Maier-Dobersberger T, Polli C, Kaserer K, Kramer L, Ferenci P. Screening for Wilson's disease in patients with liver diseases by serum ceruloplasmin. *J Hepatol.* 1997;27(2):358–362.

17. Sokol RJ, Twedt D, McKim JM Jr, et al. Oxidant injury to hepatic mitochondria in patients with Wilson's disease and Bedlington terriers with copper toxicosis. *Gastroenterology.* 1994;107(6):1788–1798.

18. Strand S, Hofmann WJ, Grambihler A, et al. Hepatic failure and liver cell damage in acute Wilson's disease involve CD95 (APO-1/Fas) mediated apoptosis. *Nat Med.* 1998;4(5):588–593.

19. Wilson DC, Phillips MJ, Cox DW, Roberts EA. Severe hepatic Wilson's disease in preschool-aged children. *J Pediatr.* 2000;137(5):719–722.

20. Walshe J. The liver in Wilson's disease. In: Schiff L, Schiff ER, eds. *Diseases of the Liver.* Philadelphia: JB Lippincott; 1982:1037–1050.

21. Harry J, Tripathi R. Kayser–Fleischer ring. A pathological study. *Br J Ophthalmol.* 1970;54(12):794–800.

22. Demirkiran M, Jankovic J, Lewis RA, Cox DW. Neurologic presentation of Wilson disease without Kayser–Fleischer rings. *Neurology.* 1996;46(4):1040–1043.

23. Fleming CR, Dickson ER, Hollenhorst RW, Goldstein NP, McCall JT, Baggenstoss AH. Pigmented corneal rings in a patient with primary biliary cirrhosis. *Gastroenterology.* 1975;69(1):220–225.

24. Fleming CR, Dickson ER, Wahner HW, Hollenhorst RW, McCall JT. Pigmented corneal rings in non-Wilsonian liver disease. *Ann Intern Med.* 1977;86(3):285–288.

25. Deguti MM, Tietge UJ, Barbosa ER, Cancado EL. The eye in Wilson's disease: sunflower cataract associated with Kayser–Fleischer ring. *J Hepatol.* 2002;37(5):700.

26. Sudmeyer M, Saleh A, Wojtecki L, et al. Wilson's disease tremor is associated with magnetic resonance imaging lesions in basal ganglia structures. *Mov Disord.* 2006;21(12):2134–2139.

27. Hefter H, Roick H, von Giesen HJ, et al. Motor impairment in Wilson's disease. 3: the clinical impact of pyramidal tract involvement. *Acta Neurol Scand.* 1994;89(6):421–428.

28. Hefter H, Arendt G, Stremmel W, Freund HJ. Motor impairment in Wilson's disease, II: slowness of speech. *Acta Neurol Scand.* 1993;87(2):148–160.

29. Hefter H, Arendt G, Stremmel W, Freund HJ. Motor impairment in Wilson's disease, I: slowness of voluntary limb movements. *Acta Neurol Scand.* 1993;87(2):133–147.

30. Scheinberg IH, Sternlieb I. Treatment of the neurologic manifestations of Wilson's disease. *Arch Neurol.* 1995;52(4):339–340.

31. Zhuang XH, Mo Y, Jiang XY, Chen SM. Analysis of renal impairment in children with Wilson's disease. *World J Pediatr.* 2008;4(2):102–105.

32. Balkema S, Hamaker ME, Visser HP, Heine GD, Beuers U. Haemolytic anaemia as a first sign of Wilson's disease. *Neth J Med.* 2008;66(8):344–347.

33. Grudeva-Popova JG, Spasova MI, Chepileva KG, Zaprianov ZH. Acute hemolytic anemia as an initial clinical manifestation of Wilson's disease. *Folia Med (Plovdiv).* 2000;42(2):42–46.

34. Degenhardt S, Blomhard G, Hefter H, et al. A hemolytic crisis with liver failure as the first manifestation of Wilson's disease. *Dtsch Med Wochenschr.* 1994;119(42):1421–1426.

35. Christl SU, Flieger D, Keller R, Stremmel W, Fischbach W. Acute liver failure and hemolysis in a 16-year-old woman. First manifestation of Wilson's disease. *Med Klin (Munich).* 2005;100(9):579–582.

36. Gill HH, Shankaran K, Desai HG. Wilson's disease: varied hepatic presentations. *Indian J Gastroenterol.* 1994;13(3):95–98.

37. Schilsky ML. Diagnosis and treatment of Wilson's disease. *Pediatr Transplant.* 2002;6(1):15–19.

38. Markiewicz-Kijewska M, Szymczak M, Ismail H, et al. Liver transplantation for fulminant Wilson's disease in children. *Ann Transplant.* 2008;13(2):28–31.

39. Sevmis S, Karakayali H, Aliosmanoglu I, et al. Liver transplantation for Wilson's disease. *Transplant Proc.* 2008;40(1):228–230.

40. Marecek Z. Acute liver failure due to Wilson's disease. *Med Sci Monit.* 2001;7(suppl 1):68–71.

41. Matsui Y, Sugawara Y, Yamashiki N, et al. Living donor liver transplantation for fulminant hepatic failure. *Hepatol Res.* 2008;38(10):987–996.

42. Medici V, Mirante VG, Fassati LR, et al. Liver transplantation for Wilson's disease: the burden of neurological and psychiatric disorders. *Liver Transpl.* 2005;11(9):1056–1063.

43. Merle U, Eisenbach C, Weiss KH, Tuma S, Stremmel W. Serum ceruloplasmin oxidase activity is a sensitive and highly specific diagnostic marker for Wilson's disease. *J Hepatol.* 2009 Nov;51(5):925–930.

44. O'Connor J, Sokol R. Copper metabolism and copper storage disorders. In: Suchy F, Sokol R, Balistreri W, eds. *Liver Disease in Children.* New York: Cambridge University Press; 2007:626–660.

45. Ferenci P, Steindl-Munda P, Vogel W, et al. Diagnostic value of quantitative hepatic copper determination in patients with Wilson's Disease. *Clin Gastroenterol Hepatol.* 2005;3(8):811–818.

46. Sundaresan S, Eapen CE, Shaji RV, Chandy M, Kurian G, Chandy G. Screening for mutations in ATP7B gene using conformation-sensitive gel electrophoresis in a family with Wilson's disease. *Med Sci Monit.* 2007;13(3):CS38–CS40.

47. Roberts EA, Schilsky ML. Diagnosis and treatment of Wilson disease: an update. *Hepatology.* 2008;47(6):2089–2111.

48. Pabon V, Dumortier J, Gincul R, et al. Long-term results of liver transplantation for Wilson's disease. *Gastroenterol Clin Biol.* 2008;32(4):378–381.

49. Chan PC, Chen HL, Ni YH, et al. Outcome predictors of fulminant hepatic failure in children. *J Formos Med Assoc.* 2004;103(6):432–436.

50. Walshe JM. Hepatic Wilson's disease: initial treatment and long-term management. *Curr Treat Options Gastroenterol.* 2005;8(6):467–472.

51. Schilsky ML. Treatment of Wilson's disease: what are the relative roles of penicillamine, trientine, and zinc supplementation? *Curr Gastroenterol Rep.* 2001;3(1):54–59.

52. Walshe JM. Penicillamine: the treatment of first choice for patients with Wilson's disease. *Mov Disord.* 1999;14(4):545–550.

53. Kocturk S, Oktay G, Guner G, Pekcetin C, Gure A. Effect of D-penicillamine on rat lung elastin cross-linking during the perinatal period. *Cell Biochem Funct.* 2006;24(2):167–172.

54. Rath N, Bhardwaj A, Kar HK, Sharma PK, Bharadwaj M, Bharija SC. Penicillamine induced pseudoxanthoma elasticum with elastosis perforans serpiginosa. *Indian J Dermatol Venereol Leprol.* 2005;71(3):182–185.

55. Becuwe C, Dalle S, Ronger-Savle S, et al. Elastosis perforans serpiginosa associated with pseudo-pseudoxanthoma elasticum during treatment of Wilson's disease with penicillamine. *Dermatology.* 2005;210(1):60–63.

56. Tang MB, Chin TM, Yap CK, Ng SK. A case of penicillamine-induced dermopathy. *Ann Acad Med Singapore.* 2003;32(5):703–705.

57. Svetel M, Sternic N, Pejovic S, Kostic VS. Penicillamine-induced lethal status dystonicus in a patient with Wilson's disease. *Mov Disord.* 2001;16(3):568–569.

58. Brewer GJ, Askari F, Dick RB, et al. Treatment of Wilson's disease with tetrathiomolybdate: V. Control of free copper by tetrathiomolybdate and a comparison with trientine. *Transl Res.* 2009;154(2):70–77.

59. Brewer GJ. Novel therapeutic approaches to the treatment of Wilson's disease. *Expert Opin Pharmacother.* 2006;7(3):317–324.

60. Kobayashi S, Kodama H, Inuzuka R, Mori Y, Yanagawa Y. Combination treatment with penicillamine and trientine in a patient with Wilson's disease. *Pediatr Int.* 2005;47(5):589–591.

61. Brewer GJ. The use of copper-lowering therapy with tetrathiomolybdate in medicine. *Expert Opin Investig Drugs.* 2009;18(1):89–97.

62. Brewer GJ, Dick RD, Johnson V, et al. Treatment of Wilson's disease with ammonium tetrathiomolybdate. I. Initial therapy in 17 neurologically affected patients. *Arch Neurol.* 1994;51(6):545–554.

63. Brewer GJ. Zinc acetate for the treatment of Wilson's disease. *Expert Opin Pharmacother.* 2001;2(9):1473–1477.

64. Cacic M, Percl M, Jadresin O, Kolacek S. The role of zinc in the initial treatment of Wilson's disease in children. *Lijec Vjesn.* 2000;122(3–4):77–81.

65. Friedman LS, Yarze JC. Zinc in the treatment of Wilson's disease: how it works. *Gastroenterology.* 1993;104(5):1566–1568.

66. Fryer MJ. Potential of vitamin E as an antioxidant adjunct in Wilson's disease. *Med Hypotheses.* 2009 Dec;73(6):1029–1030.

67. Nazer H, Ede RJ, Mowat AP, Williams R. Wilson's disease: clinical presentation and use of prognostic index. *Gut.* 1986;27(11):1377–1381.

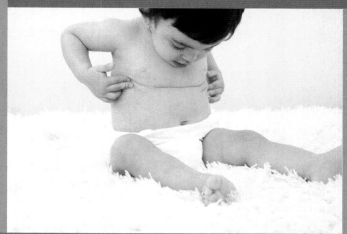

Alpha-1-antitrypsin Deficiency

Jeffrey H. Teckman

CHAPTER 26

DEFINITION AND EPIDEMIOLOGY

The classical, most common form of alpha-1-antitrypsin (a1AT) deficiency is caused by homozygosity (ZZ) for the autosomal co-dominant Z mutant allele of a1AT.[1] This is referred to as "PIZZ" in World Health Organization nomenclature.[2] ZZ homozygotes may be as common as 1 in 2000 births in many North American and European populations, although the disease is under-recognized and many patients go undiagnosed. The mutant Z gene is especially common in populations derived from Scandinavian or British Isles gene pools (Figure 26–1).

a1AT is a glycoprotein primarily synthesized in the liver, which is normally secreted into the serum where its function is to inhibit non-specific, neutrophil protease-induced host tissue injury.[3–5] The protein product of the mutant Z gene accumulates within hepatocytes rather than being efficiently secreted. The result is a "deficient" level of a1AT in serum. ZZ homozygous adults have a markedly increased risk of developing emphysema by a loss-of-function mechanism in which insufficient circulating a1AT is available in the lung to inhibit connective tissue breakdown by neutrophil proteases. Within the hepatocyte, the accumulated a1AT mutant Z protein may attain an altered conformation in which many a1AT mutant Z molecules aggregate to form large polymers. ZZ homozygous children and adults may develop liver disease and hepatocellular carcinoma because the intracellular accumulation of a1AT mutant Z protein triggers cell death and chronic liver injury.[6,7] There are many other, uncommon a1AT alleles, other than the normal, wild-type M and the most common disease-associated Z allele. Most of the other alleles are not associated with liver disease, with the notable exception of the S mutant allele which when present in a compound heterozygote

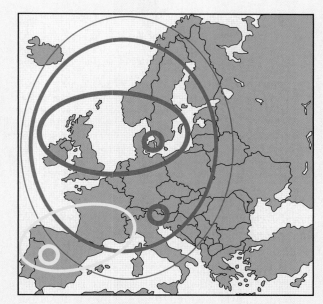

FIGURE 26–1 ■ Political map of Western European Nations overlaid with indicators of relatively increased a1AT mutant gene frequencies. Red lines circumscribe areas of original populations of high frequency of the a1AT mutant Z gene and yellow lines areas of a1AT mutant S gene high frequency. Thicker lines denote areas of highest frequency in original populations in Scandinavia, especially Denmark, and the Iberian Peninsula.

with Z, a so-called SZ heterozygote, can cause liver and lung disease in some patients.

PATHOGENESIS

The critical step in the pathophysiology of a1AT deficiency is retention and accumulation of the newly synthesized mutant Z protein molecule within the endo-

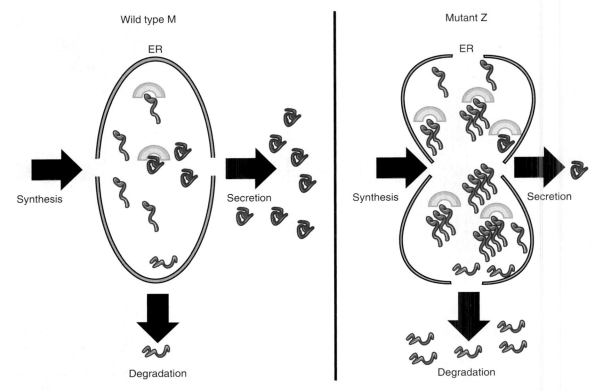

FIGURE 26–2 ■ Conceptual model of a1AT mutant Z intracellular retention. The wild-type, normal M a1AT gene is appropriately transcribed and translated and the nascent polypeptide chain (blue wavy line) enters the endoplasmic reticulum (ER) lumen of the hepatocyte. In the ER, a group of proteins known as "chaperones" (yellow semicircles) binds to the polypeptide and assists in folding into the final, secretion-competent conformation (red knot). A few molecules do not fold properly and are directed to degradation pathways for recycling into their constitutient amino acids. In the case of a1AT mutant Z, the nascent polypeptide chain also enters the ER lumen, but very few of the peptides attain the secretion-competent conformation. Some of the a1AT mutant Z molecules polymerize (groups of blue wavy lines) and the rest are directed to degradation pathways. The accumulation of the misfolded a1AT mutant Z polypeptides distorts the ER structure and triggers cell injury pathways.

plasmic reticulum (ER) of hepatocytes (Figure 26–2).[8,9] The liver synthesizes large quantities of a1AT protein every day. During biosynthesis, the a1AT mutant Z gene is appropriately transcribed, and then the nascent mutant Z polypeptide chain is assembled on the ribosome and translocated into the ER lumen in the usual way. However, in the ER the mutant Z protein molecule folds slowly and inefficiently into its final, secretion-competent conformation. The mutant Z molecule may attain a variety of abnormal conformations including a unique state in which multiple molecules aggregate to form large protein polymers.[8] A system of proteins within the ER, termed the "quality control" apparatus, recognizes these mutant Z molecules as abnormal and directs them to a series of proteolytic systems rather than allowing progression down the secretory pathway. The result of these processes is that approximately 85% of a1AT mutant Z protein molecules are retained within the liver cell, rather than secreted into the serum.[1]

For reasons that are still unclear, a small proportion of the mutant Z protein molecules retained within the liver cells escape degradation and remain within the

hepatocytes for an extended period of time. Some of these intracellular a1AT mutant Z protein polymers form large inclusions in the hepatocytes, called "globules," which are visible under light microscopy on liver biopsy in some, but not all, hepatocytes (Figure 26–3). The accumulation of this abnormal, mutant Z protein triggers an intracellular injury cascade causing some hepatocytes to die, and a regenerative response in the remaining cells to repair the damage resulting in chronic liver disease (Figure 26–4). Although all ZZ patients exhibit intrahepatic accumulation of the mutant Z protein, not all patients develop liver disease. This observation strongly suggests a large influence of other genetic or environmental disease modifiers of the liver disease, although research into specific candidate factors is still ongoing. The "deficient" serum level of a1AT, resulting from the lack of secretion from the liver, leaves the lungs vulnerable to injury from neutrophil proteases during periods of inflammation (pneumonia) or from environmental exposures, especially cigarette smoking. Physical–chemical studies have shown that the a1AT mutant S protein can heteropolymerize intracellularly only when it is co-expressed with the mutant Z protein,

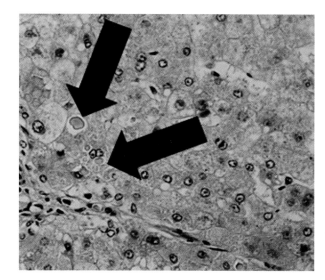
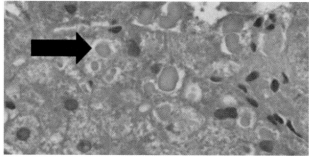

FIGURE 26–3 ■ Photomicrographs of human ZZ liver stained with H&E. Human ZZ liver with eosinophilic inclusions ("globules") of a1AT mutant Z polymerized protein visible within some hepatocytes (arrows) at low magnification (left) and high magnification (right).

Hypothetical injury pathway

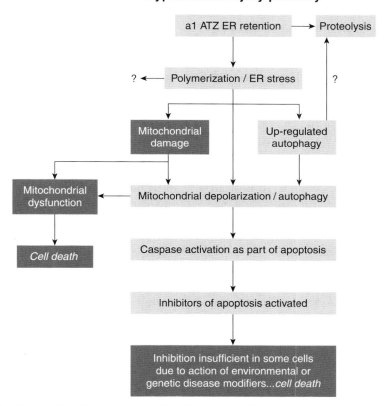

FIGURE 26–4 ■ Hypothetical hepatocellular injury pathway in ZZ a1AT deficiency. The a1AT mutant Z protein is appropriately synthesized, but then retained in the ER of hepatocytes rather than being secreted. Quality control processes within the cells direct most of the mutant Z protein molecules into intracellular proteolysis pathways. However, some of the mutant Z protein molecules escape proteolysis and may attain a unique, polymerized conformation forming long-lived inclusions in the endoplasmic reticulum (ER) membranes. It is unclear how effectively these protein polymers can be degraded by the cell. In a small population of hepatocytes with the largest accumulated burden of mutant protein, this accumulation results in activation of a variety of cellular responses. Autophagy, a process of intracellular vacuolar proteolysis, may be up-regulated possibly resulting in more effective removal of a1AT protein polymers from the cell. However, autophagy can also be involved in damage to mitochondria. Mitochondria may be damaged directly, or may be involved in activation of caspases and the ER stress arm of the intrinsic pathway of apoptosis. Hepatocellular death may result from mitochondrial dysfunction, or from an uninhibited apoptotic cascade. Given the variable nature of clinical liver injury between individuals with the same genotype, and the usually slow disease progression, there are likely to be important environmental and genetic disease modifiers affecting the rate and magnitude of the hepatocellular death cascade. Some new evidence suggests that this pathway is most active in the small proportion of hepatocytes with the greatest intracellular burden of a1AT mutant Z protein (i.e., the largest globules).

which may explain the occurrence of liver injury in SZ patients when liver disease is known to be absent in SS individuals.[10,11]

CLINICAL PRESENTATION

The presentation of liver disease in ZZ a1AT deficiency can be highly varied and non-specific, ranging from chronic metabolic hepatitis to cirrhosis to rare occurrences of fulminant hepatic failure (Table 26–1).[2,3,12] In the neonatal period, the typical presentation is one of neonatal cholestasis, also called the "neonatal hepatitis syndrome," and may include the symptoms and signs of jaundice, abdominal distention, pruritis, poor feeding, poor weight gain, hepatomegaly, and splenomegaly. Laboratory evaluation may reveal elevated total and conjugated (direct) bilirubin, elevated serum AST and ALT, hypoalbuminemia, or coagulopathy due to vitamin K deficiency or to liver synthetic dysfunction. There are rare reports of severe vitamin K-deficient coagulopathic hemorrhage as the presenting feature of a1AT deficiency in infants, presumably resulting from impaired vitamin K absorption during sub-clinical neonatal cholestasis. Occasionally infants come to medical attention through evaluation of what is thought to be an unusually prolonged period of physiology jaundice. The typical evaluation of a neonate with jaundice and an elevated conjugated (direct) bilirubin begins with non-invasive tests designed to identify biliary atresia, a1AT deficiency, cystic fibrosis, and congenital infection, which are generally indistinguishable without specific testing. Occasionally infants escape specific testing until the diagnosis is suggested by the results of a liver biopsy, or when biliary atresia is first suspected but later ruled out by a demonstration of extrahepatic biliary continuity.

Liver biopsy findings may be highly variable in infants including giant cell transformation, lobular hepatitis, significant steatosis, fibrosis, hepatocellular necro-

Table 26–1.
Liver-related Clinical Presentations and Indications for Testing for a1AT Deficiency
Infant: cholestatic jaundice
Infant or child: unexplained failure to thrive or poor feeding
Any age: unexplained, including asymptomatic, hepatosplenomegaly, or elevated AST/ALT
Any age: unexplained liver disease, cirrhosis, or hepatocellular carcinoma

sis, bile duct paucity, or bile duct proliferation.[3,12] Differentiation from biliary atresia or from other liver diseases of infancy by liver biopsy alone may be difficult. Globular, eosinophilic inclusions in some but not all hepatocytes are usually seen under conventional H&E stain, which represent dilated ER membranes engorged with polymerized a1AT mutant Z protein (Figure 26–3).[13] Staining with periodic acid-Schiff (PAS) followed by digestion with diastase, a technique which labels glycoproteins red, is used to highlight the red "globules" ("PAS-positive") within hepatocytes on a neutral background (Figure 26–5). Significant accumulations of PAS-positive material are not usually seen in normal hepatocytes. Examination of liver biopsies for PAS-positive globules should be done with caution, however, as similar structures have sometimes been described in other liver diseases, such as hepatitis B infection and alcoholic liver disease. Furthermore, the globules are not present in all hepatocytes or can be small and "dust-like," and they are occasionally absent in very young infants. Although life-threatening liver disease can occur in the first few months or years of life, prospective, population-based studies indicate that 80% of ZZ patients presenting with neonatal cholestasis are healthy and free of chronic disease by age 18 years.[14]

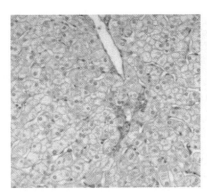
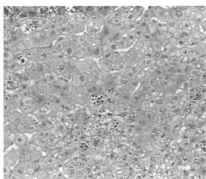
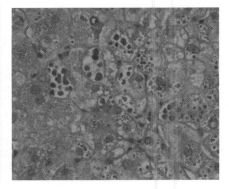

FIGURE 26–5 ■ Photomicrograph stained with PAS with diastase digestion of liver from a normal, MM liver and from ZZ, a1AT-deficient liver. Human liver stained with periodic acid-Schiff (PAS) with diastase digestion from normal MM liver and from ZZ liver at low and high magnifications. Arrows show inclusions within hepatocytes of eosiniphillic and "PAS-positive" (red) globules composed of polymerized a1AT mutant Z protein.

The best, prospective data on the natural history of a1AT deficiency are the landmark study by Sveger and colleagues who screened 200,000 newborns in Sweden in the 1970s and identified 127 PIZZ who are still followed as a study cohort.[2] These data suggest that the overall risk of life-threatening liver disease in childhood may be as low as 3–5%. The Swedish study is the best unbiased, population-based cohort data available, although there is concern that the outcomes reported might not be fully representative of a less homogenous genetic population, such as North America, which may carry a different and broader array of modifier genes. A smaller newborn screening series from the United States based in the state of Oregon, which has not been consistently followed up, also suggested a low rate of life-threatening childhood liver disease, as has a Canadian cohort.[1]

In toddlers and older children, ZZ a1AT deficiency may present as asymptomatic chronic hepatitis, failure to thrive, possibly with poor feeding, or as isolated hepatomegaly. Some children come to medical attention when asymptomatic hepatomegaly or splenomegaly is detected during routine medical check-ups. The occurrence of these various problems ranged from 15% to 60% in prospectively identified infant cohorts, although many of these patients may escape medical attention without newborn screening.[15] Many children appear to be completely healthy, without evidence of liver injury, except for mild and usually clinically insignificant elevations of serum AST or ALT. Occasionally, children with previously unrecognized chronic liver disease and cirrhosis present with ascites, gastrointestinal bleeding, or hepatic failure. There has also been a common observation that some children with severe liver disease in the first few months or years of life may enter a "honeymoon period" with few signs or symptoms and normal growth, before a period of renewed progressive injury and decompensation as teenagers. The pathophysiology of this pattern is unknown. However, even ZZ children with established cirrhosis may remain stable and grow and develop normally for a decade or more before beginning a process of decompensation.[12,16] The liver biopsy findings in later childhood often become more classical with easy-to-identify, large globules in many but not all hepatocytes, steatosis, and significant lobular inflammation and fibrosis. Hepatocellular carcinoma has been described in ZZ children, but it appears to be exceedingly rare.

There are little firm data on the incidence or the rate of progression of significant liver injury in ZZ adults, although many authorities believe the development of life-threatening disease to be uncommon in young and middle-aged adults. Liver disease in adults may present as chronic hepatitis, with or without cirrhosis, and the risk of clinically significant disease may increase with advancing age.[4] The biochemical and histopathologic findings may be similar to those of adult alcoholic liver disease, which may lead to diagnostic confusion. There are many anecdotal reports of ZZ patients misdiagnosed as alcoholic based on nonspecific enzyme elevations and on a1AT intrahepatic globules being improperly identified on liver biopsy. There appears to be an increased risk of hepatocellular carcinoma in ZZ adults, although the magnitude of the risk is unclear.[4] Liver biopsy findings in adults may include lobular inflammation, variable hepatocellular necrosis, fibrosis, cirrhosis, steatosis, and PAS-positive, diastase-resistant globules in some, but not all, hepatocytes in nearly every patient.[12] It is likely that the rate of significant liver injury increases in older ages. Autopsy studies suggest that sometimes clinically unapparent, but histologically significant liver injury and cirrhosis may be present in 40% of elderly ZZ adults.[4]

Individuals who are heterozygous for a1AT, carrying one normal, wild-type M allele and one mutant Z allele ("PIMZ" or "MZ"), are generally considered asymptomatic and healthy "carriers."[2] However, data from retrospective, referral center studies report groups of patients with chronic liver disease, such as cryptogenic cirrhosis, sometimes in association with concurrent viral hepatitis, that have a significantly higher frequency of the MZ heterozygous state than would be expected simply by chance alone.[2] Limited but unselected population-based studies have thus far failed to confirm this increased risk. There are also anecdotal case reports of rare MZ adults developing liver disease, although the possible genetic or environmental influences on the development of this injury remain controversial. MZ children appear to be completely healthy, and even in adults an MZ phenotype result is not readily accepted as the cause of otherwise unexplained liver disease without extensive further evaluation. At present there is no basis for any change in health care or monitoring for MZ individuals, other than the usual care recommended for the general population. It is most likely that the MZ state acts as a genetic modifier to increase the severity of liver injury if another liver disease, such as viral hepatitis, is present. There is also the suggestion of a possible increased risk of asthma, or other adult lung conditions in MZ heterozygotes, although this is controversial and still being investigated.

The destructive, emphysematous lung disease associated with ZZ a1AT deficiency takes several decades to develop and therefore is only found in adults. Smoking and occupational lung exposures greatly increase the risk of adult lung disease. Although emphysema does not develop in children, childhood exposure to secondhand smoke, or to other respiratory irritants, appears to be significantly associated with the development of emphysema later in life. ZZ children are, however, at increased risk of severe childhood asthma, which typically responds to conventional therapy. There are anecdotal reports of rare, but more severe problems with lung function in ZZ children, and sometimes these patients appear to report increased respiratory symptoms associated with intercurrent illnesses.

DIFFERENTIAL DIAGNOSIS

The differential diagnosis of a1AT deficiency is quite broad, and varies with age and with variable symptoms of liver versus lung disease (Table 26–2).[1] Liver disease most commonly becomes symptomatic in childhood or in late adulthood, and lung disease most commonly becomes symptomatic in middle adulthood. Some patients remain asymptomatic and healthy throughout life and likely never come to medical attention. The signs and symptoms of liver disease related to a1AT deficiency are similar to many other conditions ranging from congenital anomalies (biliary atresia) to metabolic conditions (cystic fibrosis or Wilson's disease) to infection (hepatitis A, B, or C or Epstein–Barr virus). Therefore, the differential diagnosis of a1AT deficiency in the neonate is the same as is generally considered in the neonatal hepatitis syndrome. In infants and children the differential diagnosis includes many common acquired conditions, as well as atypical presentation of rare metabolic conditions. a1AT deficiency rarely presents as lung

disease in childhood. If any lung symptoms are present at all in childhood, it is usually as a typical case of childhood asthma. In adults, by far the most common condition in the differential diagnosis of a1AT deficiency is smoking-related emphysema, and rare conditions would include atypical cystic fibrosis.

DIAGNOSIS

The gold standard for the diagnosis of a1AT deficiency is the "phenotype" (PI or PI-type) of the a1AT protein present in a sample of the patient's serum as determined by isoelectric focusing gel electrophoresis, although new, PCR-based tests on DNA from a patient's peripheral blood leukocytes are also recognized as equally powerful to determine a diagnostic "genotype."[1,2] Testing for a1AT deficiency by one of these methods is indicated in a wide variety of clinical situations when there is an unexplained liver abnormality (Table 26–1), because of the protean manifestations and ages of presentation of this disease. There is no lengthy diagnostic algorithm. If there is evidence of liver disease, and one of the more common causes is not readily identified, then testing for a1AT deficiency with one of the gold standard tests should be considered, with the simultaneous determination of a serum a1AT level (Table 26–2). The DNA-based genotype tests only detect the normal, wild-type M, mutant Z,

Table 26–2.

Differential Diagnosis of Liver Disease Related to a1AT Deficiency

Age at Presentation	Most Common Conditions	Rare Conditions
Neonate	Biliary atresia	Tyrosenemia
	Cystic fibrosis	Niemann–Pick
	Ideopathic neonatal hepatitis	Other aminoacidurias
	Congenital infection	Alagille syndrome
	Hypothyroidism	Galactosemia
	Acute viral hepatitis	Other rare metabolic—genetic conditions
	Congenital anomalies of abdominal vasculature	
Infant–child–teen	Viral hepatitis	Wilson's disease
	Malignancy (hematologic–hepatic)	Budd–Chiari
	Toxic hepatitis (acetaminophen)	Gaucher's disease
	Autoimmune hepatitis	Hereditary fructose intolerance
		Portal vein thrombosis, or other acquired abdominal vascular lesion
		Trauma (hepatic–splenic)
		Other rare metabolic–genetic conditions
Adulthood	Viral hepatitis	Wilson's disease
	Alcoholic hepatitis	Budd–Chiari
	Autoimmune hepatitis	Trauma (vascular, liver–spleen)
	Toxic hepatitis (acetaminophen)	Malignancy

and mutant S alleles, but not other rare variants which can only be evaluated by a phenotype test in a reference laboratory. A liver biopsy is not required to establish the diagnosis of a1AT deficiency. However, liver biopsy may be useful as an assessment of the degree of liver injury, the rate of progression, or to investigate the possible presence of other liver diseases. The phenotype gel analysis is technically demanding and is therefore best performed in an experienced reference laboratory. Some clinicians advise the use of a serum a1AT level as a screening test and then perform the gold standard test if the result is outside the normal range. This approach should be interpreted with caution, however, as a1AT is an acute phase reactant and even a ZZ patient will have modest increases in serum level during times of systemic inflammation. Although a ZZ patient would not be expected to ever produce a level in the normal range, the author has seen SZ patients with liver disease occasionally having a1AT levels reported in the normal range during episodes of systemic inflammation. The best approach, which is used in some experienced reference laboratories, is to compare the a1AT serum level to the phenotype or genotype result to see if they are consistent, as a check on diagnostic confusion (Table 26–3). Care should also be taken not to obtain serum for a level or phenotype if the patient has recently had a plasma transfusion, as is sometimes used to treat patients with severe liver disease. After a plasma transfusion the phenotype test may erroneously report the plasma donor's a1AT status. In such a situation, one of the DNA-based tests should be used.[2,3,12]

Over 100 other rare mutations in the a1AT gene have been described.[2] Some of these gene products yield a normal M result on the phenotype test but when present in the heterozygous state with a Z allele can accumulate within the liver and have been associated with liver disease.[1] Such patients are usually recognized by a profoundly low a1AT level in peripheral blood that is not in keeping with the phenotype result. Similarly, a genotype result only showing one copy of the mutant Z allele, but combined with a profoundly low (less than 30% of the lower range) a1AT blood level, indicates the need for further analysis. Consultation with an expert at a reference laboratory is usually needed to resolve incompatable or inconclusive test results, and sometimes involves gene sequencing.

TREATMENT

There is no specific treatment for the liver disease associated with a1AT deficiency. However, the general supportive measures typically used in many liver diseases are generally applied. Management focuses on preventing the complications of chronic liver disease, such as bleeding, ascites, pruritis, malnutrition, fat-soluble vitamin deficiency, infection, malignancy, and growth disturbances, or attenuating the systemic repercussions if they do occur.[2,3,12] Typically the evaluation will involve a center that specializes in pediatric hepatology, although most patients do well with minimal intervention. Infants with cholestatic jaundice often benefit from so-called "elemental" formulas with a high proportion of MCT oil to optimize fat and energy absorption in the setting of impaired bile flow. Supplementation with additional fat-soluble vitamins is sometimes needed in this same setting, and will sometimes require specialized watermiscible formulations when cholestasis and liver failure in an infant is progressive. Some clinicians routinely prescribe ursodeoxycholic acid, although there are no studies of the use of this agent in a1AT deficiency. It may be useful to relieve cholestatic itching, or in mild cases, to improve bile flow. Some authorities cite the antiapoptotic effects of ursodeoxycholic acid documented in in vitro studies as being theoretically able to inhibit the pro-apoptotic effects of a1AT mutant Z intracellular retention as justification. Studies in animal models of a1AT deficiency liver disease suggest that non-steroidal anti-inflammatory drugs (NSAIDs) may increase liver injury by increasing accumulation of a1AT mutant Z protein within the liver. There has been no study of the effect of NSAIDS in ZZ humans. Typically, acetaminophen in recommended dosages used occasionally for intercurrent illnesses is safe, even in patients with chronic liver disease. Therefore, some clinicians favor acetaminophen for patients with a1AT deficiency over NSAIDS, although there are insufficient human data to support a consensus.

Many patients have normal health and can be monitored conservatively with infrequent visits to a physician knowledgeable in liver disease. Monitoring for progressive liver disease requires careful attention

Table 26–3.

a1AT Phenotypes (Also True for Genotypes) and their Typical, Corresponding a1AT Serum Levels

Phenotype	Level (µM)*
PIMM	20–48
PIMZ	12–35
PISS	15–33
PISZ	8–19
PIZZ	2.5–7.0
Null–null	0.0

*Convert micromolar to milligrams per deciliter by multiplying by conversion factor of 5.2.

to many aspects of the patients' health status. This includes repeated questioning for liver-related symptoms such as pruritis and fatigue, among others, and repeated extensive physical examination to monitor for hepatosplenomegaly, or for other less obvious signs of liver disease. Laboratory tests should not exclusively focus on serum transaminase levels, as some patients with cirrhosis can have normal or nearly normal ALT and AST. Bilirubin levels, coagulation, and fat-soluble vitamin levels should occasionally be examined. There is an increased risk of hepatocellular carcinoma in older adults with a1AT deficiency, although there are also rare reports of tumors in children. Out of concern for hepatocellular carcinoma, some clinicians employ routine, but infrequent, screening imaging such as liver ultrasound. However, some patients with significant degrees of liver injury, and even cirrhosis, can remain stable for many years with very little intervention. If life-threatening liver disease does develop, then liver transplantation is commonly employed with excellent success rates. Exogenous a1AT replacement has no effect on the development of liver disease since liver injury is related to the accumulation of the a1AT mutant Z protein within hepatocytes, not a lack of circulating antiprotease activity.

There is no evidence that smoking or lung exposures are related to the development of liver disease. However, some studies suggest that exposure to second-hand smoke and environmental air pollutants in childhood is an important risk factor for the development a1AT deficiency-associated adult emphysema.[2] Studies indicate that identification of a1AT-deficient patients as children dramatically reduces their incidence of smoking as adults and therefore decreases morbidity and mortality from lung disease.[17] Therefore, ZZ children and their household contacts are urgently cautioned against smoking, even if they come to medical attention primarily because of liver disease. Children with ZZ a1AT deficiency generally do not develop clinically detectable emphysema, although they may be at increased risk for childhood asthma that typically responds to conventional treatment.[18] ZZ children are commonly referred to an adult pulmonologist at age 18 years for a baseline evaluation, unless asthma or other respiratory symptoms are present necessitating referral to a lung specialist in childhood.

It is commonly accepted that individuals who are compound heterozygotes for the mutant S and the mutant Z alleles of a1AT (SZ) may develop liver disease identical to ZZ patients, including PAS-positive, diastase-resistant globules on liver biopsy. However, the magnitude of the risk of disease in SZ patients is not well documented, and may be lower than the risk of liver disease in ZZ patients. SZ patients are generally monitored and treated identically to ZZ patients. The S allele is also common in North American and Western European populations.

a1AT deficiency is a common metabolic liver disease that can affect adults and children. The clinical manifestations are highly variable, with many patients remaining healthy or exhibiting only mild biochemical abnormalities until late in life. Accumulation of the mutant Z protein within hepatocytes activates an intracellular injury cascade that damages liver cells. Genetic and environmental disease modifiers are thought to be important, but are still poorly described, although exposure to cigarrette smoke is known to be a critical risk factor for the adult lung disease. Treatment options are limited, and are primarily focused on supportive measures, although avoidance of cigarette smoke is strongly recommended to preserve future health even in children.

REFERENCES

1. Teckman JH. Alpha1-antitrypsin deficiency in childhood. *Semin Liver Dis.* 2007;27:274–281.
2. Sveger T. Liver disease in 1 antitrypsin deficiency detected by screening of 200,000 infants. *N Engl J Med* 1976;294: 1316–1321.
3. Teckman JH, Lindblad D. Alpha-1-antitrypsin deficiency: diagnosis, pathophysiology, and management. *Curr Gastroenterol Rep.* 2006;8:14–20.
4. Eriksson S. Alpha-1-antitrypsin deficiency: natural course and therapeutic strategies. In: Boyer JL, Blum HE, Maier K-P, Sauerbruch T, Stalder GA, eds. *Falk Symposium 115: Liver Cirrhosis and its Development.* Dordrecht: Kluwer Academic Publishers; 2001:307–315.
5. Perlmutter DH, Brodsky JL, Balistreri WF, Trapnell BC. Molecular pathogenesis of alpha-1-antitrypsin deficiency-associated liver disease: a meeting review. *Hepatology.* 2007; 45:1313–1323.
6. Lindblad D, Blomenkamp K, Teckman J. Alpha-1-antitrypsin mutant Z protein content in individual hepatocytes correlates with cell death in a mouse model. *Hepatology.* 2007; 46:1228–1235.
7. Eriksson S. Discovery of alpha 1-antitrypsin deficiency. *Lung.* 1990;168(suppl):523–529.
8. Lomas DA, Mahadeva R. Alpha1-antitrypsin polymerization and the serpinopathies: pathobiology and prospects for therapy. *J Clin Invest.* 2002;110:1585–1590.
9. Carrell RW, Lomas DA. Alpha1-antitrypsin deficiency—a model for conformational diseases. *N Engl J Med.* 2002;346:45–53.
10. Mahadeva R, Chang WS, Dafforn TR, et al. Heteropolymerization of S, I, and Z alpha1-antitrypsin and liver cirrhosis. *J Clin Invest.* 1999;103:999–1006.
11. Teckman JH, Perlmutter DH. The endoplasmic reticulum degradation pathway for mutant secretory proteins alpha1-antitrypsin Z and S is distinct from that for an unassembled membrane protein. *J Biol Chem.* 1996;271:13215–13220.
12. Perlmutter DH. Alpha-1-antitrypsin deficiency: diagnosis and treatment. *Clin Liver Dis.* 2004;8:839–859, viii–ix.

13. An JK, Blomenkamp K, Lindblad D, Teckman JH. Quantitative isolation of alpha1AT mutant Z protein polymers from human and mouse livers and the effect of heat. *Hepatology*. 2005;41:160–167.

14. Sveger T, Eriksson S. The liver in adolescents with alpha 1-antitrypsin deficiency. *Hepatology*. 1995;22:514–517.

15. Sveger T. Liver disease in alpha1-antitrypsin deficiency detected by screening of 200,000 infants. *N Engl J Med*. 1976;294:1316–1321.

16. Greene CM, Miller SD, Carroll T, et al. Alpha-1 antitrypsin deficiency: a conformational disease associated with lung and liver manifestations. *J Inherit Metab Dis*. 2008;31: 21–34.

17. Piitulainen E, Sveger T. Respiratory symptoms and lung function in young adults with severe alpha(1)-antitrypsin deficiency (PiZZ). *Thorax*. 2002;57:705–708.

18. Eden E, Hammel J, Rouhani FN, et al. Asthma features in severe alpha1-antitrypsin deficiency: experience of the National Heart, Lung, and Blood Institute Registry. *Chest*. 2003;123:765–771.

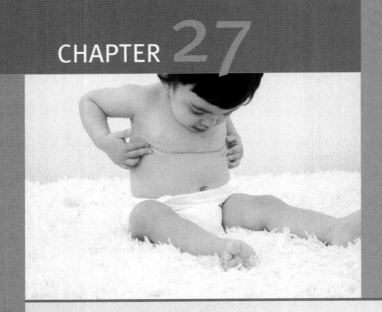

Autoimmune Liver Disorders

Tyler M. Burpee and Karen F. Murray

There are three liver diseases in which an autoimmune mechanism is primarily responsible for damage to the liver: autoimmune hepatitis (AIH), autoimmune sclerosing cholangitis (ASC), and de novo AIH after liver transplant. This chapter will review each of these three topics.

AUTOIMMUNE HEPATITIS

Definitions and Epidemiology

This disorder has been alternately called a variety of terms, including active chronic hepatitis, chronic active hepatitis, chronic aggressive hepatitis, lupoid hepatitis, plasma cell hepatitis, and, most commonly, autoimmune chronic active hepatitis. In 1992, the International Autoimmune Hepatitis Group (IAIHG) recommended AIH as the most appropriate and least redundant term for this disease.[1]

AIH is characterized by inflammatory liver histology, circulating non-organ-specific autoantibodies, and elevated levels of IgG, all in the absence of a known etiology. Two types of AIH have been described, with the distinction made according to differing profiles of the circulating autoantibodies. Type 1 or classic AIH is characterized by the presence of smooth muscle antibody (SMA) and/or anti-nuclear antibody (ANA), whereas type 2 AIH is positive for anti-liver kidney microsomal type 1 antibody (anti-LKM-1). There are several other antibodies, discussed below, which can also be present (Table 27–1).

AIH affects both children and adults. Type 1 AIH, which accounts for roughly two-thirds of cases, has a bimodal age distribution. One incidence peak is between

Table 27–1.

Classification of Autoantibodies in Autoimmune Hepatitis

Type	Autoantibodies
Type 1 AIH	Anti-smooth muscle
	Anti-nuclear
	Anti-actin
	Anti-SLP/LP
	Atypical pANCA
Type 2 AIH	Anti-LKM-1
	Anti-LC1

AIH = autoimmune hepatitis; SLP/LP = anti-soluble liver/liver pancreas antigen; pANCA = perinuclear antineutrophil cytoplasmic antibodies; anti-LKM-1 = liver kidney microsomal type 1 antibody; LC1 = liver cytosol-1.

10 and 20 years of age, with the second between 45 and 70 years of age.[2] Type 2 AIH generally presents at a younger age, often between the ages of 2 and 14 years, though not infrequently in infancy.[3,4] In both types 1 and 2 AIH, females represent roughly 75% of cases.[4] The exact prevalence in children is unknown.

Pathogenesis

A paradigm for the pathogenesis of AIH centers upon the concept that in a genetically susceptible host, exposure to an environmental agent can trigger a cascade of events, ultimately resulting in a chronic hepatic necroinflammatory response, leading to fibrosis and cirrhosis.[5]

The search for genetic predisposing factors has focused to a large extent on the genes encoding human leukocyte antigens, located in the major histocompatibility complex. In Caucasians, type 1 AIH is strongly associated with the HLA-DR3 serotype and with HLA-DR4.[6-8] HLA-DR3-associated disease is more commonly found in the early onset, severe form of disease, resulting more frequently in liver transplantation.[9] HLA-DR4, in contrast, is more common in Caucasians with late-onset disease and appears to be associated with a higher incidence of extrahepatic manifestations and a better response to corticosteroids.[7,8]

Liver damage is believed to be orchestrated by CD4-positive T lymphocytes recognizing a self-antigenic peptide. To trigger an autoimmune response, this peptide must be presented to an uncommitted T helper (Th0) cell by an antigen-presenting cell via an HLA class II molecule. Depending on the microenvironment, this T helper cell then adapts either a Th1 or Th2 phenotype, initiating a series of immune reactions that culminates in an inflammatory attack on the liver. Impairment in the immunoregulatory system, described in AIH, allows this attack to be perpetuated. Recent evidence points to a reduction in the number of regulatory T cells (T-regs) in patients with AIH, and their reduction relates to the stage of disease, with a greater reduction at the time of diagnosis than during drug-induced remission.[10]

The autoantigens responsible for initiating this inflammatory response have not been definitively identified. Candidates include the asialoglycoprotein receptor (a liver-specific membrane protein highly expressed in periportal hepatocytes)[11] and CYP2D6 (cytochrome P450IID6).[12]

The presumed environmental agent that triggers the immune system to react to an autoantigen is as of yet unknown. Several viruses have been implicated, including measles virus, hepatitis viruses, herpes simplex virus, cytomegalovirus, and Epstein–Barr.[13] Drugs are another potential candidate, with reports of oxyphenisatin, methyldopa, nitrofurantoin, diclofenac, minocycline, and possibly statins inducing liver damage that mimics AIH.[14,15]

Clinical Presentation

AIH can present with a variety of clinical manifestations, ranging from silent elevation of liver enzymes to fulminant hepatic failure. Asymptomatic patients may come to attention during routine blood screening for a variety of reasons, when an elevated aminotransferase level may be the only clue to the presence of underlying liver disease. At the other extreme, patients may present with acute liver failure, characterized by profound jaundice, an elevated prothrombin time, and aminotransferase levels in the thousands. Fortunately, such a presentation is somewhat infrequent.[4] The most common

presentation is that of acute hepatitis, with non-specific symptoms such as malaise, nausea/vomiting, anorexia, and abdominal pain progressing to include jaundice, dark urine, and pale stools. Many of these patients will have cirrhosis at the time of initial biopsy, indicating that subclinical disease had existed for some time. Second, patients may present with a more insidious onset, characterized by progressive fatigue, relapsing jaundice, headache, and anorexia, lasting from months to years. Third, as 40–80% of patients will have cirrhosis at the time of diagnosis,[4,16,17] some patients may present with complications from unknown portal hypertension, such as bleeding from esophageal varices. Lastly, AIH patients may present with manifestations from other autoimmune disorders, including thyroid disease, diabetes mellitus, ulcerative colitis, celiac, and Behçet's disease. Type 2 AIH can be part of the autoimmune polyendocrinopathy–candidiasis–ectodermal dystrophy syndrome, an autosomal recessive genetic disorder in which the liver disease is reportedly present in roughly 20% of cases.[18]

Physical findings range from a normal physical examination to the presence of hepatomegaly, splenomegaly, stigmata of chronic liver disease, and/or jaundice.

Laboratory values vary, but aminotransferase values are typically more significantly elevated than bilirubin, γ-glutamyl transferase, and alkaline phosphatase. Occasionally, a more cholestatic picture is noted, though this should alert the clinician to the possibility of other conditions, including extrahepatic biliary obstruction, viral hepatitis, or primary sclerosing cholangitis. One characteristic laboratory feature of AIH, although not universally present, is an elevation in serum globulins, particularly IgG.

Table 27–2 summarizes the presenting characteristics for 52 pediatric AIH patients that presented to a single tertiary referral center over a 20-year period.[4]

Differential Diagnosis

The differential diagnosis for AIH depends on its mode of presentation. With the acute presentation, the clinical picture resembles that of acute viral hepatitis (e.g., hepatitis A–E, cytomegalovirus, and Epstein–Barr virus), Wilson disease, or drug-induced hepatitis if relevant. When AIH presents as chronic hepatitis or cirrhosis, the differential diagnosis again includes viral hepatitis (hepatitis B/D, or C), Wilson disease, and drug-induced liver disease, but additionally, one must consider alpha-1-antitrypsin deficiency, non-alcoholic steatohepatitis, primary sclerosing cholangitis, and iron overload syndromes (Table 27–3). Of note, distinguishing AIH from chronic hepatitis C requires the analysis for hepatitis C RNA, as some patients with AIH develop a non-specific antibody response, potentially leading to false-positive

Table 27–2.

Clinical and Laboratory Features in 52 Patients with Autoimmune Hepatitis

Features	Type 1 AIH (*n* = 32)	Type 2 AIH (*n* = 20)
Demographics		
Age at diagnosis (years), median (range)	10 (2–15)	7 (0.8–14)
Female (%)	24 (75)	15 (75)
Clinical presentation (%)		
Acute hepatitis	16 (50)	13 (65)
Insidious onset	12 (38)	5 (25)
Fulminant hepatitis	1 (3)	5 (25)
Cirrhosis on biopsy	18/26 (69)	5/13 (38)
Laboratories at presentation (range)		
Total bilirubin (mg/dL)	3.6 (0.4–27)	11 (0.8–45.2)
AST (IU/L)	632 (81–2,500)	1146 (93–2,440)
GGT (IU/L)	126 (11–871), *n* = 26	91 (36–299), *n* = 17
Alkaline phosphatase (IU/L)	376 (131–1,578)	377 (102–1,677)
Albumin (g/dL)	3.2 (2.0–4.3)	3.8 (2.5–5.4)
International normalized ratio	1.6 (1–2.5)	1.6 (1–8.6)
Immunoglobulin G (mg/dL)	2800 (1340–7330)	2100 (1020–4000)
ANA titer	120 (10–5,120)	NA
SMA titer	160 (10–2,560)	NA
LKM-1 titer	NA	640 (40–10,4000), *n* = 19
Anti-LSP titer	1000 (0–3,300), *n* = 21	1250 (0–2,400), *n* = 7
Anti-ASGPR titer	0 (0–1,500), *n* = 21	200 (0–750), *n* = 7

AST = aspartate aminotransferase; GGT = gamma-glutamyl transpeptidase; ANA = anti-nuclear antibody SMA = smooth muscle antibody; LKM-1 = liver kidney microsomal type 1 antibody; LSP = liver-specific lipoprotein; ASGPR = asialoglycoprotein receptor; n = number; NA = not applicable.

Table 27–3.

Differential Diagnosis for Autoimmune Hepatitis

Common conditions
Autoimmune hepatitis/primary sclerosing cholangitis overlap
    syndrome (autoimmune sclerosing cholangitis)
Wilson disease
Viral hepatitis (hepatitis A, B, C, or delta, cytomegalovirus,
    Epstein–Barr virus, herpes viruses)
Steatohepatitis
    Non-alcoholic
    Alcoholic
Alpha-1-antitrypsin deficiency (variable penetrance)
Primary sclerosing cholangitis
Iron overload

Rare conditions
Drug-induced hepatitis
Graft-versus-host disease
Systemic lupus erythematosus
Primary biliary cirrhosis
Granulomatous hepatitis

hepatitis C antibodies. Additionally, ANA, SMA, and LKM-1 autoantibodies are commonly elevated in those with chronic hepatitis C.

As the signs and symptoms of AIH are non-specific, it is important to consider this diagnosis in any child presenting with unexplained liver disease.

Diagnosis

The diagnosis of AIH requires both the presence of classic features and the absence of other conditions that can resemble AIH (Table 27–4).[1,19] Elevated transaminases are a universal finding. Increased levels of IgG are typical, though not universal (Table 27–2). The presence of autoantibodies (ANA, SMA, and LKM-1) is characteristic. Liver biopsy is mandatory to establish the diagnosis. The typical histology includes a dense mononuclear and plasma cell infiltrate of the portal areas that expands into the liver lobule; destruction of the hepatocytes at the periphery of the lobule with erosion into the limiting plate ("interface hepatitis"); connective tissue collapse resulting from hepatocyte death and expanding from the portal area into the lobule ("bridging collapse"); and hepatic regeneration with "rosette" formation (Figure 27–1). Other potential disorders with similar presentations, as discussed in the preceding section "Differential Diagnosis", must be ruled out prior to arriving on the diagnosis (Figure 27–2).

Table 27–4.

Diagnostic Criteria for Autoimmune Hepatitis

Requisites	Definite	Probable
No genetic liver disease	Normal α1-antitrypsin phenotype Normal ceruloplasmin, iron, and ferritin levels	Partial α1-antitrypsin deficiency Non-specific serum copper, ceruloplasmin, iron, and/or ferritin abnormalities
No acute viral infection	No markers of current infection with hepatitis A, B, and C viruses	No markers of current infection with hepatitis A, B, and C viruses
No toxic or alcohol injury	Daily alcohol $<$25 g/day and no recent use of hepatotoxic drugs	Daily alcohol $<$50 g/day and no recent use of hepatotoxic drugs
Laboratory features	Predominant serum aminotransferase abnormality Globulin, γ-globulin, or immunoglobulin G $\geq$1.5 times normal	Predominant serum aminotransferase abnormality Hypergammaglobulinemia of any degree
Autoantibodies	ANA, SMA, or anti-LKM-1 $\geq$1:80 in adults and $\geq$1:20 in children; no AMA	ANA, SMA, or anti-LKM-1 $\geq$1:80 in adults or other autoantibodies*
Histologic findings	Interface hepatitis No biliary lesions, granulomas, or prominent changes suggestive of another disease	Interface hepatitis No biliary lesions, granulomas, or prominent changes suggestive of another disease

ANA = antinuclear antibodies; SMA = smooth muscle antibodies; LKM-1 = liver kidney microsomal type 1 antibodies; AMA = antimitochondrial antibodies. Reprinted with permission from Ref.[22].

**Includes perinuclear anti-neutrophil cytoplasmic antibodies and the not generally available antibodies to soluble liver antigen/liver pancreas, actin, liver cytosol type 1, and asialoglycoprotein receptor.*

The IAIHG set forth a detailed scoring system for the diagnosis of AIH for research purposes.[19] Given its complexity, a simpler scoring system was recently published and validated in adults, using only autoantibodies, IgG, histology, and exclusion of viral hepatitis.[20] This has not yet been adapted to children.

The detection of autoantibodies is crucial for both the diagnosis and differentiation of AIH types. The presence of ANA and SMA, which characterize type 1 AIH, is practically mutually exclusive to that of LKM-1, which characterizes type 2 AIH. In the rare instances where they are both present, the clinical course is similar to that of type 2 AIH.[21] Other autoantibodies may exist.

FIGURE 27–1 ■ Histologic findings in autoimmune hepatitis. Hematoxylin and eosin-stained micrograph (×200 power), demonstrating characteristic interface hepatitis and portal inflammation with plasma cells and lymphocytes.

FIGURE 27–2 ■ Diagnostic algorithm for autoimmune hepatitis. AT = antitrypsin; HCV = hepatitis C virus; RNA = ribonucleic acid; HBSAg = hepatitis B surface antigen; ANA = anti-nuclear antibody; SMA = smooth muscle antibody; anti-LKM-1 = liver kidney microsomal type 1 antibody; AIH = autoimmune hepatitis.

Circulating anti-soluble liver/liver pancreas antigen or anti-actin antibodies are at times present in type 1 AIH, though testing for them is not available in most clinical laboratories. Anti-liver cytosol-1 antibodies can be present in type 2 AIH, either alone or in conjunction with LKM-1.[5] Additionally, not all cases of AIH will have any detectable autoantibodies. Rare seronegative individuals whose picture otherwise fits with the diagnosis of AIH may be labeled cryptogenic chronic hepatitis until conventional autoantibodies appear later in the course of the disease or autoantibodies that are not generally available are tested.[22]

The presence of autoantibodies alone is not absolutely specific for the diagnosis of AIH, as they can be present at low titers in adults with other diseases, including Wilson disease,[23] non-alcoholic steatohepatitis,[24] and viral hepatitides.[25,26] In otherwise healthy children, however, this is quite rare. In keeping with this, low titers of 1:20 for ANA and SMA and 1:10 for anti-LKM-1 are clinically relevant.

Treatment

Unless presenting with fulminant liver failure, AIH is typically exquisitely responsive to immunosuppression, and treatment should be initiated quickly. The goal of treatment is to reduce or eliminate liver inflammation, induce disease remission, and prolong survival.

Immunosuppression is the basis for treatment of AIH, with the treatment being divided into two phases: (1) induction of remission (defined as a lack of symptoms, normalization of IgG levels and aminotransferases, negative or low-titer autoantibodies, and histologic resolution of inflammation) and (2) maintenance of remission.

Traditionally, corticosteroids have been the mainstay of treatment. Therapy is usually started with prednisone 2 mg/kg/day (maximum 60 mg/day), which is then gradually decreased over a period of 4–8 weeks if there is progressive normalization of the aminotransferase levels. The patient is then maintained on the minimal dose required to sustain normal aminotransferase levels, typically 2.5–5 mg/day.[5,27] Alternate-day or pulsed steroid regimens have not proven beneficial.[5] Laboratories are monitored weekly during the initial 6–8 weeks of therapy, in order to facilitate frequent dose adjustments and avoid excessive steroid exposure. Relapse during therapy is common, affecting roughly 40% of patients. This requires a temporary increase in the steroid dose.

To facilitate the decrement in steroid dosing azathioprine is usually commenced at a starting dose of 0.5 mg/kg/day, after a few weeks of steroid treatment. In the absence of toxicity, this is increased up to a maximum of 2–2.5 mg/kg/day until remission is achieved. It is advisable to use caution initially, as azathioprine can be hepatotoxic, particularly in severely jaundiced patients. The measurement of thiopurine methyltransferase (TPMT) activity before initiating therapy with azathioprine has been reported to predict an individual's drug metabolism and help prevent toxicity,[5] though a recent report shows that neither TPMT activity nor genotype predicts azathioprine hepatotoxicity in AIH, which appears instead to be related to the degree of liver fibrosis.[28] Measurement of the azathioprine metabolites 6-thioguanine and 6-metylmercaptopurine may be useful to monitor for drug toxicity and non-adherence,[29] though the ideal therapeutic levels for AIH have not been established.

More recent treatment protocols have shown that cyclosporine A can induce remission in 70% of treatment in naïve children without the need for high-dose steroids. The cyclosporine A is used as monotherapy for 6 months, followed by low-dose prednisone and azathioprine.[30] Remission at 5-year follow-up was 95%. Controlled trials comparing this protocol to the standard steroid treatment regimen are lacking.

Roughly 10% of patients do not enter remission with standard therapy. In this group, mycophenolate mofetil at a dose of 20 mg/kg twice daily is successfully used.[31] If toxicity is encountered (headache, diarrhea, nausea, dizziness, hair loss, and neutropenia), then the use of calcineurin inhibitors (cyclosporine A or tacrolimus) should be considered. The possibility of non-adherence should not be overlooked when assessing a non-responsive patient.

In those that respond to immunosuppressive therapy, the prognosis is generally good, with most patients surviving long term with excellent quality of life on low-dose medication. The measurement of IgG levels can serve as a reliable, objective, and inexpensive measure of disease control. The question of when to discontinue therapy is, however, a difficult one. In general, treatment should be continued for at least 3 years. Prior to stopping immunosuppression, aminotransferases should be persistently normal for at least 12 months, IgG levels should be normal, and autoantibody titers should be low or negative. A liver biopsy should demonstrate histologic resolution of inflammation. As relapses appear common during or immediately before puberty, discontinuation at this time should be avoided. Gregorio et al.[4] reported that 20% of children with AIH type 1 were able to successfully and permanently stop treatment, whereas this was rarely achieved in those with type 2 AIH.

Those with acute hepatic failure or end-stage liver disease should be referred for liver transplantation. Post-liver transplantation, recurrent AIH may develop in roughly 20% of cases,[32] even years post-transplant.

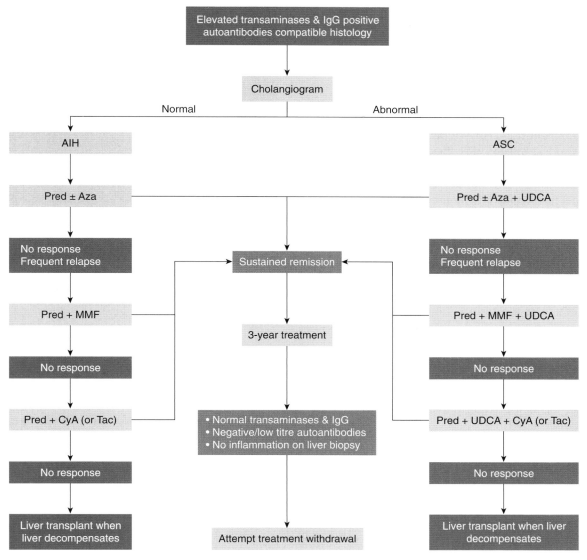

FIGURE 27–3 ■ Flowchart for treatment decision making in children with autoimmune liver disease.

As such, maintenance of immunosuppression, inclusive of steroids, at a higher dose than is typical is generally recommended.

Figure 27–3 summarizes a decision-making flowchart for the treatment of children with autoimmune liver disease.

AUTOIMMUNE SCLEROSING CHOLANGITIS

Definition and Epidemiology

Sclerosing cholangitis is a progressive hepatobiliary disease of unknown etiology, characterized by chronic inflammation and fibrosis of the intrahepatic and/or extrahepatic bile ducts. In both children and adults, an overlapping syndrome between AIH and sclerosing cholangitis has been described.[33] In a prospective study, Gregorio et al.[34] found 27 out of 55 children (49%) who presented with clinical and/or laboratory features characteristic of AIH had evidence of sclerosing cholangitis when assessed by cholangiography at presentation. Fifty-five percent were girls. This autoantibody-positive sclerosing cholangitis has been termed ASC. The current IAIHG criteria do not allow distinction between AIH and ASC. It appears to be as prevalent as type 1 AIH in childhood.

Pathogenesis

It is unclear if ASC is a distinct entity from AIH or a different aspect of the same underlying disease. Little is known regarding its distinct pathophysiology.

Clinical Presentation

Patients with ASC present similarly to those with typical AIH. In the aforementioned prospective study,[34] 50% of ASC patients presented with symptoms of acute hepatitis and 18% with symptoms of chronic hepatitis. The remaining 32% presented without jaundice and were referred for either hepatosplenomegaly or abnormal liver function tests. Forty-four percent of those with ASC also had inflammatory bowel disease, as opposed to 18% of those with typical AIH. More than 75% of children with ASC had greatly increased IgG levels. All patients fulfilled the criteria for the diagnosis of "definite" or "probable" AIH established by the IAIHG[19] and six patients with an abnormal cholangiogram had histologic features more compatible with AIH than sclerosing cholangitis.[34] In fact, the diagnosis of ASC was only possible because of the characteristic cholangiographic studies. This illustrates the difficulty in distinguishing ASC from AIH.

Differential Diagnosis

Given the similar presentations, the differential diagnosis for ASC overlaps with that of typical AIH (Table 27–3). Cholangiography is required to distinguish between the two disorders.

Diagnosis

The diagnosis of ASC rests on demonstrating characteristic multifocal stricturing and dilation of intrahepatic and/or extrahepatic bile ducts on cholangiography, in the setting of positive autoantibodies. Conventionally this has been done using endoscopic retrograde cholangiopancreatography (ERCP), though there may be an emerging role for magnetic resonance cholangiopancreatography (MRCP) (Figure 27–4). A percutaneous liver biopsy may be supportive of the diagnosis but will often show features indistinguishable from AIH. Given the frequent association with inflammatory bowel disease, this should be investigated and treated appropriately, even in the absence of symptoms.

Treatment

Children with ASC respond to the same immunosuppressive treatment as described above for typical AIH.[34] Contrary to data in adults with primary sclerosing cholangitis, treatment normalized the liver tests in nearly 90% of patients. Ursodeoxycholic acid (UDCA), a hydrophilic bile acid, has been reported to be of value in the treatment of adults with primary sclerosing cholangitis, presumably via protection of cholangiocytes against cytotoxic hydrophobic bile acids, stimulation of

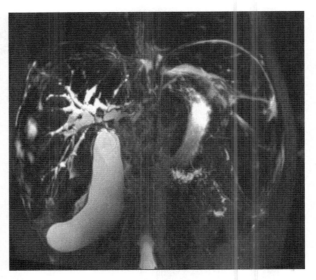

FIGURE 27–4 ■ Cholangiographic findings in autoimmune sclerosing cholangitis. Coronal magnetic resonance cholangiopancreatography (MRCP) image demonstrating characteristic multifocal strictures and dilation of intrahepatic bile ducts.

hepatobiliary secretion, protection of hepatocytes against bile acid-induced apoptosis, and induction of antioxidants.[35] As such, its use is advocated in children with ASC, though extensive data are lacking. High-dose UDCA therapy (20–30 mg/kg) was reported to be associated with higher adverse events in adults with primary sclerosing cholangitis,[36] so doses not exceeding 15 mg/kg/day are prudent. Figure 27–3 schematically represents a decision-making flowchart in the treatment of children with autoimmune liver disease.

Just as in typical AIH, the measurement of serum IgG levels and autoantibody titers can be used to monitor disease activity.[37]

DE NOVO "AUTOIMMUNE" HEPATITIS AFTER LIVER TRANSPLANT

Definition and Epidemiology

After liver transplant for causes distinct from AIH, a form of late graft dysfunction not attributable to recognized causes such as rejection, infection, or vascular/biliary complications may occur. Like typical AIH, it is characterized by increased levels of IgG and positive autoantibodies (ANA, SMA, or atypical LKM-1). This de novo AIH after liver transplant has been described in both adults and children.[38–42] One center reported an incidence of 2% during 1 year of monitoring 471 pediatric liver transplant patients.[38] None had previous autoimmune liver disease.

Pathogenesis

It is unclear whether the hepatic damage in this condition is the consequence of rejection or an autoimmune injury, perhaps precipitated by exposure to certain drugs and/or infections. Episodes of cellular rejection appear to predispose to its development.[43,44] Tacrolimus or cyclosporine A given to rodents post-bone marrow transplant can result in a "paradoxical" autoimmune syndrome, where these drugs interfere with the maturation of T lymphocytes and promote the appearance of autoaggressive T-cell clones.[45–47] A similar pathophysiology may be involved in children with de novo AIH after liver transplant.

Clinical Presentation

Patients present with elevated liver enzymes post-transplant, in a manner indistinguishable from other causes. One series reported a median post-transplant period of 24 months (range 6–45 months).[48]

Differential Diagnosis

Other causes of graft dysfunction, including rejection, infection, vascular, and/or biliary complications, and recurrent disease (e.g., HCV infection) must be considered.

Diagnosis

The diagnosis rests on the discovery of autoantibodies (ANA, SMA, and LKM-1) and the absence of other causes of abnormal liver function tests post-transplant. Characteristic histologic findings include chronic hepatitis with lymphocytes and plasma cells, bridging collapse, and perivenular cell necrosis, without evidence for acute or chronic rejection.[48]

Treatment

Patients with de novo AIH after liver transplant typically respond to the conventional AIH treatment of prednisolone and azathioprine. Increasing the level of maintenance cyclosporine or tacrolimus is not effective.

REFERENCES

1. Johnson PJ, McFarlane IG. Meeting report: International Autoimmune Hepatitis Group. *Hepatology*. 1993;18:998–1005.
2. Granito A, Muratori L, Pappas G, et al. Clinical features of type 1 autoimmune hepatitis in elderly Italian patients. *Aliment Pharmacol Ther*. 2005;21:1273–1277.
3. Homberg JC, Abuaf N, Bernard O, et al. Chronic active hepatitis associated with antiliver/kidney microsome antibody type 1: a second type of "autoimmune" hepatitis. *Hepatology*. 1987;7:1333–1339.
4. Gregorio GV, Portmann B, Reid F, et al. Autoimmune hepatitis in childhood: a 20-year experience. *Hepatology*. 1997;25:541–547.
5. Krawitt EL. Autoimmune hepatitis. *N Engl J Med*. 1996;334:897–903 [see comment].
6. Strettell MD, Donaldson PT, Thomson LJ, et al. Allelic basis for HLA-encoded susceptibility to type 1 autoimmune hepatitis. *Gastroenterology*. 1997;112:2028–2035.
7. Czaja AJ, Carpenter HA, Santrach PJ, Moore SB. Significance of HLA DR4 in type 1 autoimmune hepatitis. *Gastroenterology*. 1993;105:1502–1507.
8. Czaja AJ, Strettell MD, Thomson LJ, et al. Associations between alleles of the major histocompatibility complex and type 1 autoimmune hepatitis. *Hepatology*. 1997;25:317–323.
9. Scully LJ, Toze C, Sengar DP, Goldstein R. Early-onset autoimmune hepatitis is associated with a C4A gene deletion. *Gastroenterology*. 1993;104:1478–1484.
10. Longhi MS, Ma Y, Bogdanos DP, Cheeseman P, Mieli-Vergani G, Vergani D. Impairment of CD4(+)CD25(+) regulatory T-cells in autoimmune liver disease. *J Hepatol*. 2004;41:31–37.
11. Lohr H, Treichel U, Poralla T, Manns M, Meyer zum Buschenfelde KH. Liver-infiltrating T helper cells in autoimmune chronic active hepatitis stimulate the production of autoantibodies against the human asialoglycoprotein receptor in vitro. *Clin Exp Immunol*. 1992;88:45–49.
12. Lohr HF, Schlaak JF, Lohse AW, et al. Autoreactive CD4+ LKM-specific and anticlonotypic T-cell responses in LKM-1 antibody-positive autoimmune hepatitis. *Hepatology*. 1996;24:1416–1421.
13. Vento S, Cainelli F, Ferraro T, Concia E. Autoimmune hepatitis type 1 after measles. *Am J Gastroenterol*. 1996;91:2618–2620.
14. Nietsch HH, Libman BS, Pansze TW, Eicher JN, Reeves JR, Krawitt EL. Minocycline-induced hepatitis. *Am J Gastroenterol*. 2000;95:2993–2995.
15. Graziadei IW, Obermoser GE, Sepp NT, Erhart KH, Vogel W. Drug-induced lupus-like syndrome associated with severe autoimmune hepatitis. *Lupus*. 2003;12:409–412.
16. Saadah OI, Smith AL, Hardikar W. Long-term outcome of autoimmune hepatitis in children. *J Gastroenterol Hepatol*. 2001;16:1297–1302.
17. Ferreira AR, Roquete ML, Penna FJ, Toppa NH, Castro LP. Type 1 autoimmune hepatitis in children and adolescents: assessment of immunosuppressive treatment withdrawal. *J Pediatr (Rio J)*. 2005;81:343–348.
18. Ahonen P, Myllarniemi S, Sipila I, Perheentupa J. Clinical variation of autoimmune polyendocrinopathy–candidiasis–ectodermal dystrophy (APECED) in a series of 68 patients. *N Engl J Med*. 1990;322:1829–1836.
19. Alvarez F, Berg PA, Bianchi FB, et al. International Autoimmune Hepatitis Group Report: review of criteria for diagnosis of autoimmune hepatitis. *J Hepatol*. 1999;31:929–938.
20. Hennes EM, Zeniya M, Czaja AJ, et al. Simplified criteria for the diagnosis of autoimmune hepatitis. *Hepatology*. 2008;48:169–176.

21. Vergani D, Alvarez F, Bianchi FB, et al. Liver autoimmune serology: a consensus statement from the committee for autoimmune serology of the International Autoimmune Hepatitis Group. *J Hepatol.* 2004;41:677–683.

22. Czaja AJ, Freese DK, American Association for the Study of Liver Disease. Diagnosis and treatment of autoimmune hepatitis. *Hepatology.* 2002;36:479–497.

23. Dhawan A, Taylor RM, Cheeseman P, De Silva P, Katsiyiannakis L, Mieli-Vergani G. Wilson's disease in children: 37-year experience and revised King's score for liver transplantation. *Liver Transpl.* 2005;11:441–448.

24. Cotler SJ, Kanji K, Keshavarzian A, Jensen DM, Jakate S. Prevalence and significance of autoantibodies in patients with non-alcoholic steatohepatitis. *J Clin Gastroenterol.* 2004;38:801–804.

25. Gregorio GV, Jones H, Choudhuri K, et al. Autoantibody prevalence in chronic hepatitis B virus infection: effect in interferon alfa. *Hepatology.* 1996;24:520–523.

26. Gregorio GV, Pensati P, Iorio R, Vegnente A, Mieli-Vergani G, Vergani D. Autoantibody prevalence in children with liver disease due to chronic hepatitis C virus (HCV) infection. *Clin Exp Immunol.* 1998;112:471–476.

27. Mieli-Vergani G, Vergani D. Autoimmune hepatitis in children. *Clin Liver Dis.* 2002;6:623–634.

28. Heneghan MA, Allan ML, Bornstein JD, Muir AJ, Tendler DA. Utility of thiopurine methyltransferase genotyping and phenotyping, and measurement of azathioprine metabolites in the management of patients with autoimmune hepatitis. *J Hepatol.* 2006;45:584–591.

29. Rumbo C, Emerick KM, Emre S, Shneider BL. Azathioprine metabolite measurements in the treatment of autoimmune hepatitis in pediatric patients: a preliminary report. *J Pediatr Gastroenterol Nutr.* 2002;35:391–398.

30. Alvarez F, Ciocca M, Canero-Velasco C, et al. Short-term cyclosporine induces a remission of autoimmune hepatitis in children. *J Hepatol.* 1999;30:222–227.

31. Mieli-Vergani G, Bargiota K, Samyn M, Vergani D. Therapeutic aspects of autoimmune liver disease in children. In: Dienes H, Leuschner U, Lohse A, Manns M, eds. *Autoimmune Liver Diseases—Fault Symposium.* Dordrecht, the Netherlands: Springer; 2005:278–282.

32. Duclos-Vallee JC, Sebagh M, Rifai K, et al. A 10 year follow up study of patients transplanted for autoimmune hepatitis: histological recurrence precedes clinical and biochemical recurrence. *Gut.* 2003;52:893–897.

33. McNair AN, Moloney M, Portmann BC, Williams R, McFarlane IG. Autoimmune hepatitis overlapping with primary sclerosing cholangitis in five cases. *Am J Gastroenterol.* 1998;93:777–784 [see comment].

34. Gregorio GV, Portmann B, Karani J, et al. Autoimmune hepatitis/sclerosing cholangitis overlap syndrome in childhood: a 16-year prospective study. *Hepatology.* 2001;33:544–553.

35. Paumgartner G, Beuers U. Ursodeoxycholic acid in cholestatic liver disease: mechanisms of action and therapeutic use revisited. *Hepatology.* 2002;36:525–531.

36. Lindor KD, Kowdley KV, Luketic VA, Harrison ME, McCashland T, Befeler AS, Harnois D, Jorgensen R, Petz J, Keach J, Mooney J, Sargeant C, Braaten J, Bernard T, King D, Miceli E, Schmoll J, Hoskin T, Thapa P, Enders F. High-dose ursodeoxycholic acid for the treatment of primary sclerosing cholangitis. *Hepatology.* 2009 Sep;50(3): 808–814.

37. Gregorio GV, McFarlane B, Bracken P, Vergani D, Mieli-Vergani G. Organ and non-organ specific autoantibody titres and IgG levels as markers of disease activity: a longitudinal study in childhood autoimmune liver disease. *Autoimmunity.* 2002;35:515–519.

38. Andries S, Casamayou L, Sempoux C, et al. Posttransplant immune hepatitis in pediatric liver transplant recipients: incidence and maintenance therapy with azathioprine. *Transplantation.* 2001;72:267–272.

39. Duclos-Vallee JC, Johanet C, Bach JF, Yamamoto AM. Autoantibodies associated with acute rejection after liver transplantation for type-2 autoimmune hepatitis. *J Hepatol.* 2000;33:163–166.

40. Heneghan MA, Portmann BC, Norris SM, et al. Graft dysfunction mimicking autoimmune hepatitis following liver transplantation in adults. *Hepatology.* 2001;34:464–470.

41. Hernandez HM, Kovarik P, Whitington PF, Alonso EM. Autoimmune hepatitis as a late complication of liver transplantation. *J Pediatr Gastroenterol Nutr.* 2001;32:131–136.

42. Salcedo M, Vaquero J, Banares R, et al. Response to steroids in de novo autoimmune hepatitis after liver transplantation. *Hepatology.* 2002;35:349–356.

43. D'Antiga L, Dhawan A, Portmann B, et al. Late cellular rejection in paediatric liver transplantation: aetiology and outcome. *Transplantation.* 2002;73:80–84.

44. Miyagawa-Hayashino A, Haga H, Egawa H, et al. Outcome and risk factors of de novo autoimmune hepatitis in living-donor liver transplantation. *Transplantation.* 2004;78:128–135.

45. Bucy RP, Xu XY, Li J, Huang G. Cyclosporin A-induced autoimmune disease in mice. *J Immunol.* 1993;151:1039–1050.

46. Cooper MH, Hartman GG, Starzl TE, Fung JJ. The induction of pseudo-graft-versus-host disease following syngeneic bone marrow transplantation using FK 506. *Transplant Proc.* 1991;23:3234–3235.

47. Hess AD, Fischer AC, Horwitz LR, Laulis MK. Cyclosporine-induced autoimmunity: critical role of autoregulation in the prevention of major histocompatibility class II-dependent autoaggression. *Transplant Proc.* 1993;25:2811–2813.

48. Kerkar N, Hadzic N, Davies ET, et al. De-novo autoimmune hepatitis after liver transplantation. *Lancet.* 1998;351:409–413.

49. Mieli-Vergani G, Heller S, Jara P, et al. Autoimmune hepatitis. *J Pediatr Gastroenterol Nutr.* 2009;49:158–164.

CHAPTER 28

Metabolic and Drug-induced Liver Disease

Judith A. O'Connor

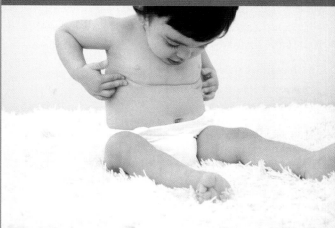

DEFINITIONS AND EPIDEMIOLOGY

Metabolic liver disease has traditionally referred to diseases that result from inborn errors of metabolism. These disorders are due to a single enzyme defect that affects the synthesis or catabolism of a carbohydrate (CHO), protein, or lipid. These defects in metabolism can result in either liver failure or cirrhosis, with or without injury to other tissues, or relative sparing of the liver with primary toxicity to other organ systems (Table 28–1). Metabolic disorders that arise in the liver with primary toxicity to other organ systems are not addressed in this chapter. This chapter approaches metabolic-induced liver disease not only from the traditional approach, those resulting from a single enzyme defect, but also as a genetic susceptibility induced by a trigger, such as a drug or a metabolic derangement associated with visceral obesity (nonalcoholic fatty liver disease (NAFLD)).

Taken individually, single enzyme defects are rare, although as a group they constitute at least 10% of pediatric liver transplantations. Wilson's disease, alpha-1-antitrypsin deficiency (A1AT), and cystic fibrosis are the most common inherited metabolic conditions that affect the liver and are discussed individually in this textbook. Fortunately, in children most drug-induced liver disease (DILI) remains uncommon, although certain pediatric patient populations are at increased risk. NAFLD is becoming a worldwide problem of childhood and is the most common cause of liver disease in this age group. The increase in prevalence parallels the epidemic of obesity.[1] This chapter will address the following three categories of metabolic liver disease in separate sections: inherited metabolic-induced liver disease, DILI, and obesity-induced NAFLD.

INHERITED METABOLIC-INDUCED LIVER DISEASE

Pathogenesis

Enzymatic disorders that cause liver disease include disorders of CHO, protein, lipid/microsomal, and bile acid synthesis. Because the pathogenesis of these disorders is directly related to the metabolic pathway where the defect occurs, each class of disorders is addressed separately.

Clinical Presentation

Clinical manifestations of inherited metabolic liver disease result from the location of the enzyme defect, by either the loss of substrate or accumulation of abnormal byproducts. The approach to the child with a suspected metabolic defect is guided by the age of presentation, physical exam, and biochemical abnormalities. Patients can present acutely with evidence of liver failure or as a chronic presentation of liver dysfunction (Tables 28–2 and 28–3). Defects that present as a life-threatening event are more common in the neonate, but can present in infancy or childhood. The importance of the onset of neurologic deterioration in a newborn infant has been categorized by Saudubray et al.[2] In the neonate, neurologic symptoms resulting rapidly after a variable symptom-free period indicate a toxic cause. Alternatively, the absence of a symptom-free period associated with delayed evolution of coma suggests an energy-deficient type of defect. Symptoms are protean and can mimic a variety of disorders. Unexplained symptoms or failure to respond to routine measures should raise the suspicion of a metabolic disease.

Table 28–1.

Inborn Errors of Metabolism Causing Liver Disease

Metabolic Defect	Disease
Carbohydrate disorders	
Galactose metabolism	
Galactose transferase	Galactosemia
Galactose-4-epimerase	Galactosemia
Fructose metabolism	
Fructose dysphosphatase	Hereditary fructose intolerance (HFI)
Fructokinase	Fructosemia
Glycogen metabolism	
Glucose-6-phosphatase	Glycogen storage disease type 1 (GSD-I)
Debranching enzyme	Glycogen storage disease type 3 (GSD=III)
Branching enzyme	Glycogen storage disease type 4 (GSD-IV)
Protein disorders	
Tyrosine metabolism	
Fumarylacetoacetate hydrolase	Hereditary tyrosinemia type 1 (TT1)
Lipid disorders	
Cholesterol metabolism	
Lysosomal acid lipase	Wolman's/cholesterol ester storage
Cholesterol transport	Niemann–Pick type C (NPC)
Bile acid disorders	
Bile acid synthesis	
Sterol nucleus modification	3B hydroxy, 5B reductase, 7a hydroxylase
Side-chain shortening	Zellweger, Refsum, neonatal ALD
Bile acid transport	
FICI/*ATP8B1*	PFIC-1
BSEP/*ABCB11*	PFIC-2
MDR3/*ABAB4*	PFIC-3
Unclassified disorders	
Alpha-1-antitrypsin deficiency	Chapter 26
Alagille syndrome	
Cystic fibrosis	Chapter 32
Drug induced	
Nonalcoholic fatty liver disease (NAFLD)	
Wilson's disease	Chapter 25

Abbreviations: PFIC = progressive familial intrahepatic cholestasis; 3B = 3-beta-hydroxysteroid oxidoreductase; 5B = delta 4,3-oxysteriod-5B reductase; 7a = oxysterol-7-a-hydrolase; ALD = adrenol leukodystrophy.

History

Diet is one of the most important historical facts to ascertain, and should include current diet, recent changes, introduction of new foods, or avoidance of a

Table 28–2.

Metabolic-induced Liver Disease; Neonatal–Infant Clinical Presentation

Acute presentation
- Acute liver failure
- Seizures
- Sepsis

Acute or chronic presentation
- Coma
- Hypoglycemia
- Jaundice
- Lethargy
- Vomiting

Chronic presentation
- Failure to thrive
- Hepatomegaly
- Hepatosplenomegaly
- Hypotonia

Table 28–3.

Metabolic-induced Liver Disease; Child–Adolescent Clinical Presentation

Acute presentation
- Acute liver failure
- Seizures
- Hypoglycemia
- Jaundice
- Vomiting

Chronic presentation
- Cholestasis
- Chronic seizures
- Development delay
- Growth failure
- Hepatomegaly
- Hepatosplenomegaly
- Mental retardation
- Pruritus
- Recurrent liver failure
- Recurrent sepsis
- Recurrent/cyclic vomiting

particular food. In addition, the frequency of feeds and length of fasting should be explored. Associated signs and symptoms may include vomiting, diarrhea, lethargy, seizures, growth failure, and recurrent infections. Family history of spontaneous abortions, stillbirth, early childhood death, developmental delay, or mental retardation is worrisome for metabolic liver disease.

Table 28–4.

Metabolic Liver Disease; Alternative of Misdiagnoses in the Neonate–Infant

Acute liver failure
Cerebral vascular accident
Congenital heart disease
Intestinal ischemia
- Intussusception
- Necrotizing enterocolitis (NEC)
- Obstruction
- Volvulus
Seizures
Sepsis
Sudden infant death

Physical Examination

Most patients with metabolic liver disease will have some degree of hepatomegaly, with or without splenomegaly. Depending on the disorder there may be jaundice, or hepatic synthetic dysfunction with ascites and a coagulopathy. Most patients will have some degree of growth failure. Neurologic status will depend on the particular enzymatic defect.

Differential Diagnosis

The differential diagnosis varies by age of presentation and acute versus chronic symptoms. Noninherited causes are listed in Tables 28–4 and 28–5.

Diagnosis

Suspicion of a metabolic condition is the key to diagnosis. In all children who present with unexplained liver

dysfunction, a sample of blood and urine should be obtained at presentation. Serum and urine samples can be stored to be analyzed at a later date, as indicated by the patient's clinical course. Key laboratory studies need to be obtained at presentation, when the patient is ill, as many laboratory values will normalize with supportive treatment (Tables 28–6 and 28–7).

Table 28–6.

Initial Biochemical Evaluation in Patients with Hepatic Dysfunction

Blood
- CBC
- Prothrombin time (PT)/international normalized ratio (INR)
- Glucose
- Electrolytes
- Calcium
- Phosphorus
- Magnesium
- Blood gas
- Ammonia
- Uric acid
- Lactic dehydrogenase (LDH)
- Creatinine phosphokinase (CPK)
- Lactic/pyruvic acid ratio (L:P)
- Serum ketone bodies
- Stored specimen

Urine
- Ketones
- Reducing substance
- Glucose
- Culture
- Stored specimen

Table 28–5.

Metabolic-induced Liver Disease; Alternative or Misdiagnoses in the Child–Adolescent

Autism
Cerebral palsy
Cerebral vascular accident
Cyclic vomiting syndrome
Development delay
Drug/toxic ingestion
Nonaccidental trauma
Reye's syndrome
Seizures
Sepsis

Table 28–7.

Specialized Biochemical Evaluation for Metabolic-induced Liver Disease on Stored Blood and Urine Samples

Blood
- Quantitative amino acids
- Carnitine/acylcarnitine profile
- Lipid profile
- Free fatty acids

Urine
- Quantitative amino acids
- Organic acids
- Succinyl acetone

DISORDERS OF CARBOHYDRATE METABOLISM

There are many known disorders of carbohydrate metabolism, but only three classes of these cause significant liver injury. These include disorders of fructose and galactose metabolism and certain glycogen storage diseases (GSDs) (Figure 28–1). All are inherited in an autosomal recessive mode. As opposed to disorders of lipid and protein metabolism, disorders of CHO can be either prevented by prenatal diagnosis or treated with modest dietary restriction.[3]

Disorders of Galactose Metabolism

There are three disorders of galactose metabolism that have traditionally been referred to as *galactosemia*. Each disorder is a result of a specific enzyme deficiency. Transferase deficiency and epimerase deficiency result in liver disease. Consequences of transferase deficiency are more severe than the relatively rare epimerase deficiency. Galactokinase deficiency results in cataracts, but does not cause liver disease.

Transferase deficiency galactosemia was first described in 1935 and affects 1 in 30,000–50,000 live births. Symptoms result from a deficiency of the enzyme

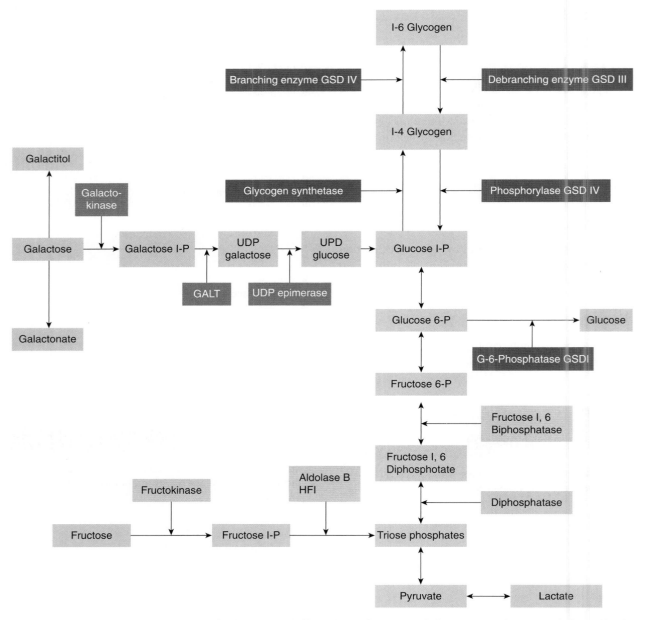

FIGURE 28–1 ■ Carbohydrate metabolism. Red = glycogen metabolism; yellow = fructose metabolism; green = galactose metabolism. *Abbreviations*: GSD = glycogen storage disease; HFI = hereditary fructose intolerance; GALT = galactose-1-phosphate uridyl transferase.

galactose-1-phosphate uridyl transferase (GALT), which catalyzes conversion of galactose-1-phosphate (Gal-1-P) to uridine diphosphate galactose (UDP-galactose) and glucose-1-phosphate (Figure 28–1). UDP-galactose is then converted to UDP glucose by UDP-galactose-4-epimerase. The gene is mapped to chromosome 9p18, and >150 mutations have been identified. Toxicity has been attributed to the metabolic byproducts of galactose: Gal-1-P and galactitol. Although the exact mechanism is unknown, liver toxicity has been attributed to the accumulation of Gal-1-P, while accumulated galactitol causes cataract formation.

Patients with GALT deficiency present in early infancy. Some patients present within the first day or two of life with a severe, fulminant illness. The most common presentation is a subacute illness with vomiting, diarrhea, and growth failure within a few days after the infant has received breast milk or a lactose-containing formula. This is followed by jaundice and hepatomegaly. Some patients are identified while being evaluated for obstructive jaundice. The liver disease is progressive and patients can present with liver failure. Hemolytic anemia has also been observed. There is a strong association of *E. coli* sepsis and galactosemia, such that this diagnosis should be considered in any infant with *E. coli* sepsis, and galactose should be removed from the diet until the diagnosis has been excluded. Cataracts may be present at birth if the mother has consumed a large amount of milk products during pregnancy, or may develop postnatally. Commercially available formula preparations that are lactose-free may mask the symptoms until months or years later when cataracts, developmental delay, or hepatomegaly develop.

Laboratory findings include hypoglycemia, hyperchloremic acidosis, and elevated blood and urine galactose levels. A positive urine reducing substance in the absence of glucosuria is suggestive but is neither sensitive nor specific. False-negative results can occur if there is inadequate lactose intake. Reducing substances will clear from the urine within days after lactose has been removed or intravenous hydration has been administered. False positives can occur with severe liver dysfunction and some medications. Various degrees of liver dysfunction, aminoaciduria, and proteinuria have been identified. Diagnosis is made by measuring GALT activity in red blood cells. Prenatal diagnosis can be made by measuring enzymatic activity cells obtained by amniocentesis. Most patients are detected by newborn screening programs.

Treatment is elimination of all dietary galactose. This is a lifelong task and older patients need to pay attention to additives in prepared foods. Sources of hidden galactose include soybeans, legumes, tomatoes, coffee, and processed meats or organ meats such as liver, kidney, and brain. Fruit or fruit juices made from apples,

oranges, kiwi, or watermelons also contain galactose. Galactose-free diet results in reversal of acute symptoms, normal growth, and recovery of liver function. Long-term intellectual development is unclear with many patients developing various degrees of learning disabilities, and neurologic defects.

Ovarian failure has been described in up to 65% of women with galactosemia. As a result of dietary restrictions and ovarian failure, osteoporosis is also a frequent complication.

UDP galactose-4-epimerase deficiency galactosemia is a rare disorder that was discovered incidentally from screening programs in Switzerland. Patients have elevated levels of Gal-1-P, but normal levels of GALT. The clinical presentation varies from a benign condition to that similar to GALT galactosemia.[4]

Disorders of Fructose Metabolism

There are three disorders of fructose metabolism: hereditary fructose intolerance (HFI), fructose diphosphatase deficiency, and essential fructosuria, of which only the first two cause hepatic injury (Figure 28–1). The initial step in fructose metabolism is the phosphorylation of fructose to fructose-1-phosphate by fructokinase. Absence of this enzyme results in benign essential fructosuria.

HFI occurs in about 1 in 20,000 live births. First recognized in 1957, it is caused by a deficiency of fructose-1-phosphate aldolase (aldolase B). Aldolase B is present in liver, kidneys, and muscle. There are two other isoenzymes, aldolase A in muscle and aldolase C in brain, which are unaffected in this disorder. Aldolase B has been sequenced and mapped to chromosome 9q13-32. More than 20 mutations have been described. Aldolase B is the second step in fructose metabolism catalyzing the conversion of fructose-1-phosphate to produce D-glyceraldeyde and dihydroxyacetone phosphate (triose-phosphate). Accumulation of fructose-1-phosphate results in hypoglycemia secondary to impaired glycogenolysis (inhibition of glycogen phosphorylase) and impaired gluconeogenesis as the triose-phosphates is not produced for substrate. Additionally, formation and accumulation of fructose-1-phosphate results in ATP and GTP depletion, impairing protein synthesis.

Patients with HFI remain completely asymptomatic on breast milk or sucrose-free formula. Symptoms occur with the introduction of sucrose-containing formulas, sucrose- or fructose-containing foods, or medications prepared in a sucrose base. Symptoms vary depending on the amount, duration, and age of exposure. Infants most commonly have poor feeding, vomiting, sweating, and hypoglycemia. A large exposure may result in signs of liver failure (hepatomegaly, ascites, and coagulopathy) and renal tubular dysfunction (renal tubular acidosis and hypophosphatemia). Occasionally, older children may be diagnosed due to a profound aversion to dietary "sweets."

Laboratory abnormalities include hypoglycemia, hypophosphatemia, hypokalemia, hypoalbuminemia, and elevated aminotransferase and prothrombin time. Anemia, thrombocytopenia, and hyperuricemia may be present while serum ammonia is usually normal. Urinalysis reveals increased reducing substances, proteinuria, aminoaciduria, organic aciduria, and fructosuria.

Diagnosis can be made by enzyme analysis of intestinal or preferably liver tissue or targeted DNA analysis. Negative results from targeted sequencing do not completely eliminate the diagnosis; however, targeted DNA sequencing is a useful tool to screen siblings. Complete gene sequencing is available as a research tool.

Initial treatment is supportive care. Long-term treatment is based on dietary restriction with complete avoidance of fructose and sucrose with special attention to food additives and medications. Sorbitol should be avoided, as it is metabolized to fructose. Lifelong abstinence of these sugars results in normal intelligence with reversal of growth failure and organ dysfunction, although hepatomegaly may persist.

Fructose-1,6-biphosphate deficiency (FDP) was first described in 1970. FDP deficiency is a heterogeneous disorder of gluconeogenesis. FDP catalyzes the conversion of fructose-1,6-biphosphate to triphosphates, as a substrate for gluconeogenesis. Patients with FDP differ from those with HFI, as their symptoms (hypoglycemia and lactic acidosis) can be precipitated not only by fructose consumption, but also with fasting. Euglycemia depends on appropriate glucose intake or adequate hepatic glycogen stores. In periods of prolonged fasting, or limited hepatic glycogen, as in the neonate, gluconeogenic precursors will accumulate and hypoglycemic lactic acidosis will occur.

Symptoms usually occur in the first few days of life with hypoglycemia, hyperventilation, and metabolic acidosis. Irritability, seizures, coma, hypotonia, and hepatomegaly are often observed. Abnormal laboratory studies include elevated serum lactate, ketones, alanine, and uric acid. In contrast to HFI, liver and kidney abnormalities are not observed. The fasting-induced hypoglycemia can be confused with GSD type Ib. Diagnosis is based on measuring enzymatic activity in liver tissue. Treatment focuses on avoiding prolonged fasting. Fructose, sucrose, and sorbitol should be avoided, but strict dietary avoidance is not required.

Disorders of Glycogen Metabolism

GSD is a group of disorders first described by von Gierke in 1929. Ten types of GSD have been described based on a specific enzyme deficiency in glycogen synthesis or degradation. Type I, III, IV, VI, and IX primarily affect the liver, but only I, III, and IV cause significant hepatic injury (Figure 28–1). In most types of GSD, there is increased glycogen content in liver, muscle, or both. In some cases, the glycogen content may be normal or less than normal; however, the molecular structure may be altered. Although each type of GSD results from a specific enzyme defect, determination of the specific type cannot be made by clinical presentation alone.

Glycogen metabolism is controlled by two enzymes, glycogen synthetase and phosphorylase, both of which exist in active and inactive states. Glycogen synthesis is inhibited by phosphorylase and cyclic AMP (cAMP). Following a meal, increased blood glucose inactivates phosphorylase, halting glycogenolysis and stimulating glycogen production. During periods of fasting, glucagon-mediated increases in cAMP result in activation of phosphorylase and deactivation of glycogen synthesis, stimulating glycogenolysis (Figure 28–2).

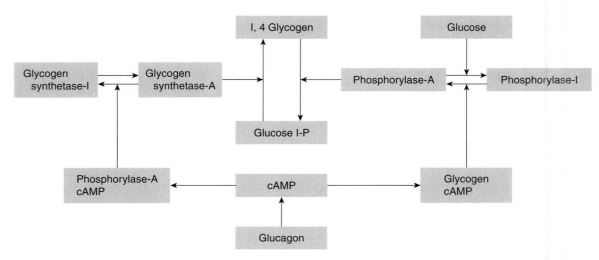

FIGURE 28–2 ■ Metabolic pathway for regulation of glycogen synthesis and glycogenolysis. I = inactive; A = active; cAMP = cyclic adenosine monophosphate.

Glycogen storage disease type I (GSD-I) is also referred to as von Gierke's disease and results from a deficiency of glucose-6-phosphatase. Glucose-6-phosphatase is located in the endoplasmic reticulum and catalyzes the terminal step in both glycogenolysis and gluconeogenesis (Figure 28–1). GSD-I is estimated to occur in approximately 1 in 100,000 live births and accounts for 25% of all GSDs. GSD I has three different clinical forms: type Ia, Ib, and Ic. GSD-Ib and -Ic are clinically similar to GSD-Ia, but, during testing of tissue extracts, have normal glucose-6-phosphatase activity in disrupted microsomes but not in intact microsomes.

The enzyme is composed of a catalytic subunit and three transporter subunits, T1, T2, and T3. Defects in the catalytic unit result in GSD-Ia. The gene has been mapped to chromosome 17q21 and is found in the liver, kidney, and intestine. GSD-Ib results from a defect in transporter subunit T1, which has been localized to chromosome 11q23.3. The gene product is *microsomal glucose-6-phosphate translocator*, which is found in liver, kidney, and leukocytes. GSD-Ic results from defects in transporter subunit T2 that is a microsomal phosphate and pyrophosphate transporter localized to chromosome 11q23.3-24.2. It is found in liver, kidney, and pancreas.

GSD-Ia is considered the classic form of the disease, representing 90% of all GSD-I cases. Patients present with severe hypoglycemia and hepatomegaly, and because the enzyme is also found in the kidney, renal enlargement may be noted. This defect affects both glycogenolysis and gluconeogenesis; thus, symptoms occur when fasting >3–4 hours. Symptoms may occur in the first few weeks of life or later, when feeding frequency decreases. It often presents when infants begin to sleep through the night or when fasting is caused by illness. When infants are fed on demand rather than on a rigid schedule, the diagnosis may be delayed. In addition to hepatomegaly, these children have growth failure, Cushingoid facies, and delayed motor development. Laboratory tests reveal profound hypoglycemia, metabolic acidosis, and elevated serum lactic and uric acid. Triglycerides are markedly elevated, up to 6000 mg/dL, while serum aminotransferases are modestly elevated and bilirubin is normal. There may be hypophosphatemia, dyslipidemia, and platelet dysfunction. Adolescent and adult patients may develop hepatic adenomas or carcinomas, nephrolithiasis, nephropathy, and gouty arthritis.

Diagnosis is suspected based on clinical and laboratory findings. Histologic examination of liver tissue stained with periodic acid-Schiff (PAS) reveals swollen hepatocytes with microvesicular fat, but minimal inflammatory infiltrate. Electron microscopy reveals glycogen-filled hepatocytes. The diagnosis is confirmed by absence of enzymatic activity in fresh or frozen liver tissue.

Management of infants with GSD-1 requires continuous glucose delivery. This can be done by daytime feeds every 2–3 hours and nocturnal feeds every 3 hours. The goal is to maintain serum glucose >70 and <120 mg/dL. If frequent feeding is not possible, continuous gastric feeds using a complete, low-lipid formula can be utilized. After the first months of life, serum glucose level can be maintained by taking uncooked cornstarch (2 g/kg) orally every 4–6 hours, depending on age and activity. Successful dietary management is reflected in sustained growth and correction of biochemical abnormalities. Patients should be monitored every 3 months for normalization of serum glucose, uric acid, lipids, and serum aminotransferase levels. Once biochemical markers have stabilized, the frequency can be decreased to every 6 months. Annual evaluation should also include an alpha-fetoprotein (AFP) level and liver ultrasound to assess for adenoma or tumor formation. Liver transplantation is curative and has been performed for patients with progressive adenomas or isolated hepatic carcinomas; however, dietary management is preferred.

GSD-Ib is clinically similar to GSD-Ia, except that patients have neutrophil dysfunction and neutropenia, which may be cyclic in nature. Patients with GSD-Ib often have recurrent infections and older patients have an increased incidence of inflammatory bowel disease. Diagnosis is based on clinical suspicion, classic laboratory abnormalities found in GSD-Ia, and normal glucose-1-phosphatase enzyme activity of frozen liver tissue. Complete gene sequencing is available if indicated by a strong clinical suspicion. Treatment is the same as GSD-Ia with the goal to maintain glucose homeostasis. Use of recombinant granulocyte colony-stimulating factor for recurrent infections due to neutropenia has been advocated. There should be a high degree of suspicion for inflammatory bowel disease in patients with gastrointestinal symptoms.

Glycogen storage disease type III (GSD-III), first recognized in 1952, also known as Forbe's disease, is a defect in debranching enzyme (Figure 28–1). Estimated incidence is approximately 1 in 100,000 live births and has been reported in all ethnic groups. Debranching enzyme is composed of two catalytic subunits, oligo-1,4-1,4-glucan transferase and amylo-1,6-glucosidase. The transferase molecule moves short 1,4-1,4-glucose subunits produced by phosphorylase to other short subunits. Amylo-1,6-glucosidase degrades the branch points. The enzyme has been localized to chromosome 1p21 and is found in liver and muscle. Two distinct isoforms exist: GSD-IIIa, where there is absence of enzyme activity in both liver and muscle, and GSD-IIIb, which affects only the liver. GSD-IIIa occurs in about 85% of affected patients. Absence of debranching enzyme results in accumulation of abnormal glycogen with excessive 1,6-branched points.

Patients with GSD-III can tolerate longer fasts than patients with GSD-I, because glucose can still be still cleaved from the outer branches by phosphorylase and, as opposed to GSD-I, gluconeogenesis remains intact. In infancy and early childhood, physical examination cannot readily distinguish patients with GSD-III from GSD-I. Patients with GSD-III tend to present at a later age with profound hepatomegaly, growth failure, and Cushingoid facies. Laboratory findings include fasting ketotic hypoglycemia, elevated triglycerides, hyperlipidemia, and modest elevation of transaminase levels. In contrast to GSD-I, serum lactate and uric acid are usually normal. Patients with GSD-III have a heterogeneous presentation and clinical course. Patients with GSD-IIIa can develop muscle weakness in the third to fourth decade of life; some develop cardiomegaly, while others have subclinical symptoms apparent only on ECG. Additionally fibrosis, cirrhosis, splenomegaly, and adenomas can develop in some patients.

Examination of liver tissue will reveal swollen hepatocytes with fibrous septa and less fat than GSD-I. Electron microscopy demonstrates hepatocytes contain a large amount of atypical-appearing glycogen. Diagnosis is based on enzyme analysis of frozen liver tissue. Some patients with GSD-III may also have decreased levels of glucose-6-phosphatase, phosphorylase, and phosphorylase kinase. Patients with GSD-IIIa will also have increased glycogen content and decreased enzyme activity in muscle.

Treatment is the same, but not as stringent, as for GSD-I, utilizing a high-starch diet. The goal is to prevent hypoglycemia, correct metabolic abnormalities, and restore normal growth. Patients with GSD-IIIa need to have annual cardiac evaluations. Due to the risk of adenomas, annual AFP level and liver ultrasound has been advocated. Liver transplantation has been reported for progressive adenoma formation or cirrhosis, but remains investigative as it will not correct or prevent myopathy or cardiomyopathy.

Glycogen storage disease type IV (GSD-IV) is a rare form of glycogenosis, also known as Anderson's disease. First described in 1952, it has since been demonstrated to result from a defect in branching enzyme (1,4-glucan; 1,4-glucan-6-glucosyltransferase) activity (Figure 28–1). Abnormal enzyme activity causes accumulation of glycogen with unbranched, long outer chains that has poor solubility, similar to amylopectin. The gene has been localized to chromosome 3p14.

Clinical presentation is heterogeneous. Classically, most patients with GSD-IV are normal at birth, developing failure to thrive, hepatosplenomegaly, and cirrhosis by 18 months of age. Liver failure occurs early, with death before 5 years of age. Approximately 50% of patients with GSD-IV have neuromuscular involvement. GSD-IV can also present with a nonprogressive form of liver disease, multiple combinations of hepatic and myopathic involvement, and primary neuromuscular and cardiopathic forms.

Unlike other types of GSD, hypoglycemia is not a prominent feature unless liver failure is present. In the absence of liver failure, serum aminotransferase levels are three to six times normal, while electrolytes, lactic acid, uric acid, and cholesterol levels are normal. Liver biopsy specimens show hepatocytes containing PAS-positive deposits, with displaced nuclei and micronodular cirrhosis. Ultrastructural studies show glycogen particles, fibrils, and granular material, which can also be seen in cardiac, skeletal, and neurologic muscle. The diagnosis is made by measuring branching enzyme activity in liver, muscle, or cultured fibroblasts. Prenatal diagnosis can be made with mutation analysis or enzyme activity level in cultured amniocytes or chorionic villi.

There is no medical treatment for GSD-IV other than supportive care. Liver transplantation offers the only effective therapy for individuals with progressive liver disease; however, the outcome is variable. Some liver transplant patients have demonstrated resorption of extrahepatic deposits while others have succumbed to cardiac failure.

Disorders of Protein Metabolism

Hereditary tyrosinemia type I (TTI) was first reported in 1957. It is inherited in an autosomal recessive mode. The incidence is <1 in 100,000 live births, although there is an increased incidence in French Canadians (1.4 in 1000). Hereditary tyrosinemia is the only inborn error of amino acid metabolism that results in permanent liver injury. The disease is due to a defect in fumarylacetoacetate hydrolase (FAH), which is the last enzyme in the tyrosine degradation pathway (Figure 28–3). Hepatocellular and renal tubular injury result from an accumulation of fumarylacetoacetate and maleylacetoacetate. Succinylacetone is one of the byproducts of these metabolites and is a diagnostic marker of tyrosinemia. Succinylacetone is also an inhibitor in the porphobilinogen pathway. The gene has been mapped to chromosome 15q23-25.

Acute and chronic forms of tyrosinemia exist, and both can be seen in the same family. The acute form presents in the first few months of life with hepatic dysfunction while the chronic form presents later. Presentation at an early age worsens the prognosis. Symptoms include failure to thrive, vomiting, diarrhea, irritability, hepatosplenomegaly, jaundice, bleeding diathesis, and ascites. Untreated children die of liver failure within the first 2 years of life. Neurologic crisis results from disruption of porphobilinogen synthesis by succinylacetone, and some patients may be misdiagnosed as having porphyria. There is an increased incidence of hepatocellular carcinoma

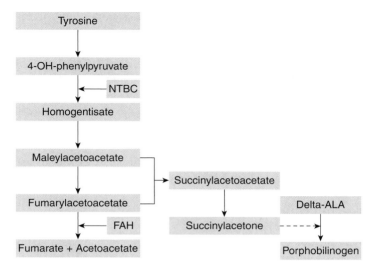

FIGURE 28-3 ■ Tyrosine degradative pathway. *Abbreviations*: FAH = fumarylacetoacetate hydrolase; NTBC = 2-(2-nitro-4-trifluoromethylbenzoyl)-1,3-cyclohexanedione; delta-ALA = delta-aminolevulinic acid.

(HCC), as fumarylacetoacetate and maleylacetoacetate are alkylating agents that cause damage to DNA. Laboratory studies reveal marked increase in synthetic dysfunction out of proportion to aminotransferase levels. AFP level is often markedly elevated. Diagnosis is suggested by identifying elevated blood or urine succinylacetone, and confirmed by full or targeted gene sequencing.

Prior to 1992, treatment included dietary restriction of tyrosine and phenylalanine and obligatory liver transplantation. The introduction of 2-(2-nitro-4-trifluoromethylbenzoyl)-1,3-cyclohexanedione (NTBC), which blocks the second step in tyrosine degradation, has markedly reduced the number of patients requiring transplantation and is now the first line of management (Figure 28–3). Patients are given a diet reduced to 25 mg/kg of tyrosine and phenylalanine with a goal of maintaining plasma tyrosine level below 400 mcmol/L. In addition to diet, NTBC is initiated at 1 mg/kg/day in two divided doses and titrated to achieve a plasma NTBC level or >50 mcmol/L and no detectable urinary or blood succinylacetone. The major side effect is corneal ulceration. Because HCC can occur in NTBC-treated patients, hepatic ultrasonography and serum AFP levels should be monitored. Liver transplantation is indicated for patients with acute liver failure not responding to medical management, progressive cirrhosis, and hepatic adenoma or carcinoma.

DISORDERS OF LIPID METABOLISM

This is a group of disorders that arises from defects in cholesterol metabolism, defects in fatty acid oxidation (FAO), or disorders of mitochondrial function. These patients are usually asymptomatic until metabolically stressed with an acute infection, surgery, or trauma. The hepatic presentation is that of acute liver failure; however, once supportive care is given, the liver dysfunction reverses and chronic liver disease rarely develops. Comprehensive reviews of these disorders are available elsewhere.[5,6] This chapter will focus on defects in cholesterol metabolism causing liver disease.

Disorders of Cholesterol Metabolism

Peripheral cells can synthesize free cholesterol and cholesterol esters; however, most intracellular cholesterol is derived from exogenous sterols, absorbed from the diet and circulating as low-density lipoproteins (LDL). These particles are enriched with cholesterol esters. LDL receptors on hepatocytes bind circulating LDL and form endosomes, which remain metabolically inactive until fusion with lysosomes. Lysosomal acid lipase cleaves cholesterol ester from the LDL. The free cholesterol is then transported out of the lysosome for use by the cell. There are three disorders of cholesterol metabolism that cause hepatic injury. *Wolman's disease* and *cholesterol ester storage disease* (CESD) result from defects in lysosomal acid lipase. Niemann–Pick type C (NPC) results from a disorder of cholesterol transport. Accumulation of cholesterol esters or unesterified cholesterol in lysosomes results in symptoms that include hepatosplenomegaly, growth failure, neurologic symptoms, and, not infrequently, jaundice.

Wolman's disease and CESD are extremely rare conditions that are inherited in an autosomal recessive mode. The defective gene product, lysosomal acid lipase, had been mapped to chromosome 10q24-25. These diseases have been described as separate entities, but may represent the acute and chronic forms of defective lysosomal acid lipase, with the severity of the phenotype reflecting the degree of residual enzymatic activity. Wolman's disease was first described in 1956 and is a lethal condition. Most patients die from nutritional failure by 2–3 months of age, presenting with vomiting, diarrhea, and hepatosplenomegaly. Adrenal calcification is always present and is a hallmark of this disorder. Biochemical abnormalities include anemia, elevated serum bilirubin and aminotransferase levels, and steatorrhea. Liver histology reveals marked steatosis, swollen histocytes with foamy cytoplasm, and increased fibrosis or cirrhosis. Diagnosis depends on the clinical picture, presence of adrenal calcification, and identification of deficient acid hydrolase in cultured leucocytes or fibroblasts. There is a case report of successful stem cell transplantation for this condition.[7]

CESD was first described in 1963 and is a milder defect of lysosomal acid lipase. Patients present in early childhood with hepatosplenomegaly and hyperlipidemia and can be confused with GSD. In contrast to GSD, however, recurrent hypoglycemia or lactic acidosis does not occur. Liver histology reveals increased fat content and dense fibrous bands. Diagnosis is made by determination of acid hydrolase activity in leukocytes or cultured fibroblasts. Inhibitors of 3-hydroxy-3-methylglutaryl-coenzyme-A reductase ("statins") may improve the degree of hepatomegaly as well as lower cholesterol/triglyceride levels. Although this condition is relatively benign, liver transplantation is indicated for progressive cirrhosis.

NPC is a lysosomal lipid storage disease that is inherited in an autosomal recessive mode. The incidence is approximately 1:20,000 to 1:50,000 live births. Based on phenotypic characteristics, it is grouped with Niemann–Pick types A and B, but is metabolically distinct. Niemann–Pick types A and B result from defects in the *SMP1* gene that encodes sphingomyelinase. NPC is due to defects in the *NPC1* or *NPC2* gene disrupting intracellular cholesterol transport; thus, unesterified cholesterol and lipids accumulate in lysosomes of various tissues. Over 95% of NPC is a result from defects in the *NPC1* gene that has been localized to chromosome 18q11-12. The *NPC2* gene is localized to 14q24.3.

Clinical presentation is highly variable; three types are described by age of onset. Approximately 20–30% of patients present in early infancy with growth failure and splenomegaly, with or without hepatomegaly. Up to 65% of these children will have liver dysfunction, cholestasis, or neonatal hepatitis. Approximately 10% will progress to cirrhosis and liver failure. In childhood or adolescence, symptoms of progressive neurodegeneration dominate, including ataxia, supranuclear vertical gaze palsy, dystonia, progressive speech deterioration, and seizures. Death, most commonly from

pulmonary infections, occurs in early childhood to the third decade of life.

Laboratory findings and liver histology are nonspecific. The diagnosis is suspected on identification of lipid-laden macrophage cells, which appear "foamy" microscopically, in liver or bone marrow specimens. NPC is confirmed by biochemical testing measuring cholesterol esterification coupled with positive filipin staining in cultured fibroblasts. Treatment is supportive. Unfortunately, liver transplantation does not halt progressive neurologic degeneration.

Disorders of Bile Acid Metabolism

Disorders of bile acid metabolism include defects in bile acid synthesis and transport. Hepatic *de novo* bile acid synthesis results from a series of enzymatic steps within the cytosol, mitochondria (sterol nucleus modification), and peroxisome (side-chain shortening). Single enzyme defects result in accumulation of toxic bile acid metabolites. Defects involving side-chain shortening are seen as one of the features of generalized peroxisomal defects. Three of these disorders, *Zellweger syndrome*, *neonatal adrenoleukodystrophy*, and *infantile Refsum disease*, have prominent liver disease and form a spectrum of overlapping features. Liver transplantation is not indicated, as neurologic dysfunction is progressive.

Three distinct disorders involving sterol nucleus modification and liver disease have been identified (Table 28–8). Infants present with progressive jaundice, liver dysfunction, and growth failure. Many patients will present with normal bile acid and gamma-glutamyl transpeptidase (GGT) levels. Diagnosis is made by exclusion of common disorders and identification of abnormal bile acids in blood or urine by fast atom bombardment ionization mass spectrometry (FAB-MS) or more recently by electrospray mass spectrometry technique. Treatment is oral administration of primary bile acids

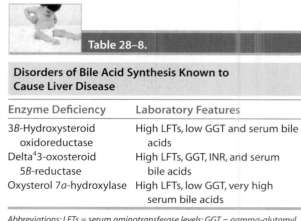

Table 28–8.

Disorders of Bile Acid Synthesis Known to Cause Liver Disease

Enzyme Deficiency	Laboratory Features
3*B*-Hydroxysteroid oxidoreductase	High LFTs, low GGT and serum bile acids
Delta[4]3-oxosteroid 5*B*-reductase	High LFTs, GGT, INR, and serum bile acids
Oxysterol 7*a*-hydroxylase	High LFTs, low GGT, very high serum bile acids

Abbreviations: LFTs = serum aminotransferase levels; GGT = gamma-glutamyl transpeptidase.

Table 28–9.			
Progressive Familial Intrahepatic Cholestasis			
Features	PFIC-1	PFIC-2	PFIC-3
Clinical	Progressive cholestasis, diarrhea, growth failure, severe pruritus	Rapidly progressive, cholestasis, pruritus, growth failure	Late-onset cholestasis, portal hypertension, cholelithiasis
Histology	Cholestasis	Giant cell hepatitis	Bile duct proliferation
Biochemical	Low GGT, high serum acids	Low GGT, high serum bile acids	High GGT, low serum bile acids
Treatment	Biliary diversion, liver	Biliary diversion	UDCA, liver transplantation

Abbreviations: GGT = gamma glutamyl transpeptidase; UDCA = ursodeoxycholic acid.

and the dose is titrated by monitoring the disappearance of the abnormal bile acid. In rapidly progressive disorders, liver transplantation has been curative.[8]

Disorders of Bile Acid Transport

Three syndromes of *progressive familial intrahepatic cholestasis* (PFIC) have been described clinically. These syndromes represent a heterogeneous group of hepatocellular cholestatic disorders, usually presenting in early infancy, with the potential to progress to liver failure and death. Advances in molecular and genetic studies have identified three genes, each encoding canalicular proteins involved in bile transport mechanisms. Defects in these genes are inherited in an autosomal recessive mode and result in abnormalities of bile secretion that are responsible for the three clinical syndromes (Table 28–9). PFIC syndromes have been well studied.[9,10] Diagnosis is suspected based on clinical presentation, elimination of other conditions, and typical laboratory and histologic findings. A novel "jaundice chip" has been developed to diagnose mutations for inherited disorders of intrahepatic cholestasis.[11]

Progressive intrahepatic cholestasis type 1 (PFIC-1), also called *Byler's disease,* was first described in 1965 in the Amish descendents of Joseph Byler. Defects in the *FIC1 (ATP8B1)* gene result in diminished bile excretion across the canalicular membrane. The gene is localized to chromosome 18q21-22 and expressed in hepatocytes and small intestine. Defects in the gene result in a spectrum of clinical phenotypes, ranging from severe cholestasis progressing to liver failure, PFIC-1, to a relatively mild condition of intermittent pruritus with or without jaundice, known as *benign recurrent intrahepatic cholestasis* (BRIC-1).

Children with PFIC-1 present in the first year of life with growth failure, diarrhea, pruritus, and jaundice. Laboratory tests reveal elevated serum conjugated bilirubin and aminotransferase levels; however, despite severe cholestasis, the *GGT level is normal.* Stool studies

show severe steatorrhea. Liver histology is nonspecific but has marked intracellular cholestasis. Electron microscopic studies show markedly abnormal biliary duct canaliculi filled with coarsely particulate amorphous bile. Untreated this is a progressive disorder resulting in death from liver failure, bleeding, and malnutrition. There is heterogeneity in response to treatment with some patients responding to oral cholestyramine or ursodeoxycholic acid (UDCA), or biliary diversion. Liver transplantation is indicated for severe intractable pruritus or liver failure and has successfully resolved cholestasis and pruritus; however, some patients suffer from chronic diarrhea.

Progressive familial intrahepatic cholestasis type-2 (PFIC-2) was previously referred to as Byler's syndrome, as these patients had a similar clinical presentation, but were unrelated to the Byler family. This condition results from mutations in the canalicular bile salt export pump (BSEP). The gene *(ABCB11)* is localized to chromosome 2q24 and the product is expressed almost entirely in hepatocyte canalicular membrane. Similar to PFIC-1, disease severity is correlated with the degree of BSEP expression.

Children with PFIC-2 present in the neonatal period. In contrast to PFIC-1, these patients do not have diarrhea but have a much more rapidly progressive course. Pruritus and growth failure are the dominant features until cirrhosis and end-stage liver disease develop. Laboratory studies are similar to PFIC-1 with elevated serum aminotransferase and bile acid levels, and a normal GGT level. Compared to PFIC-1, liver histology has increased lobular and portal fibrosis, inflammation, and giant cell transformation. Patients should be monitored for the development of HCC. Similar to PFIC-1, PFIC-2 is terminal if untreated and clinical response to treatment is variable. Liver transplantation is indicated for chronic liver failure, HCC, and intractable pruritus.

Progressive familial intrahepatic cholestasis type-3 (PFIC-3) is clinically similar to PFIC-1 and PFIC-2, but can be distinguished from these disorders by an elevated serum GGT level. PFIC-3 is caused by mutations in the multidrug-resistance 3 P-glycoprotein *(MDR3/ABAB4)* gene, resulting in disruption of canalicular phospholipid transport. The gene has been localized to chromosome7q21-26. As with the other types of PFIC, the clinical course is a result of the severity of the mutation and ranges from a benign course with recurrent cholelithiasis to progressive biliary cirrhosis and end-stage liver disease.

Patients with PFIC-3 have significant clinical variability, with age of diagnosis ranging from 1 to 20 years of age. Symptoms include growth failure, cirrhosis, jaundice, and pruritus, although the pruritus is less than that seen with PFIC-1 and -2. Clinical course is most consistent with biliary cirrhosis. Laboratory findings that distinguish PFIC-3 from the other types of PFIC include an elevated GGT and an absent serum lipoprotein X (LPX). Liver histology reveals extensive bile duct proliferation and periportal fibrosis that can evolve into biliary cirrhosis. Treatment with UDCA has been successful; liver transplantation is indicated for end stage secondary to biliary cirrhosis.

DRUG-INDUCED LIVER DISEASE

Definitions and Epidemiology

DILI in children is generally considered uncommon as compared to that reported to occur in adults. The reason for this observation in children is unclear and may due to the relative infrequent use of medications and/or the lack of risk factors such as alcohol consumption, tobacco use, and obesity. Indeed, in children with cancer or neurologic disease, where multidrug use is common, drug-induced liver injury occurs more frequently. Developmental changes in hepatic drug metabolism and immune response may be sufficiently different in children than adults and confer a degree of protection from drug toxicity. Drug metabolism has been shown to vary depending on age and sex, with advanced age or female sex being independent risk factors for drug-induced hepatotoxicity.

Pathogenesis

Hepatic drug metabolism, or biotransformation, can be divided into two broad phases (Figure 28–4). In phase I, enzymes of the cytochrome P-450 system activate the parent compound via hydroxylation, dealkylation, and dehalogenation, usually producing a more polar intermediate. In phase II, the active hydrophilic metabolite is conjugated to an endogenous substrate by glucuronsyl-, sulfo-, *N*-acetyl-, and glutathione *S*-transferases (GSH)

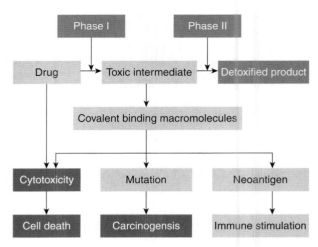

FIGURE 28–4 ■ Drug metabolism and potential causes of drug-induced liver injury (DILI).

and by epoxide hydrolase. This conjugation usually completes the process of biotransformation and the compound can then be excreted in bile or urine. Phase I reactions commonly result in a highly reactive toxic metabolite that is inactivated by phase II reactions before cell damage occurs. Hepatotoxicity results from an imbalance of these two phases. Factors that can influence this balance include age, fasting or undernutrition, co-administered drugs, and enzyme polymorphisms. These polymorphisms have been shown to exist in both phases of biotransformation and alter the balance of the reactions.

Toxicity has been categorized as resulting from an intrinsic or idiopathic response. An intrinsic toxin results directly from the compound and causes a predictable dose-dependent response in most people. Idiopathic reactions are the most common and include both contingent hepatotoxins and immunoallergic hepatotoxins. These reactions occur sporadically and are not predictable or dose-dependent. Contingent hepatotoxins cause liver injury in susceptible individuals when circumstances favor an imbalance between the production of a toxic metabolite and its detoxification. This imbalance can result from enzyme induction (medication/alcohol), enzyme depletion (fasting/malnutrition), or inborn genetic defects or polymorphism. Drugs that elicit an immune response are most likely a result of the individual's immunogenetic makeup.

Hepatotoxicity is often a result of cytotoxity; however, the mechanism of hepatocyte death is unknown, and is probably dependent on the individual toxin. Because hepatocytes in Rappaport zone 3 (in the vicinity of central veins) have the highest concentration of cytochrome P-455, zonal necrosis is often seen in DILI. Cytotoxicity can also be directed to other cells in the liver such as bile duct cells, stellate cells, and endothelial

Table 28–10.

Common Medications Associated with Pediatric Drug-induced Liver Disease (DILI)

Injury Type	Drug
Hepatocellular	Acetaminophen (zonal necrosis)
	Halothane
	Isoniazid
	Methyldopa
	Phenytoin
Cholestatic	Cyclosporine
	Estrogens
Hepatocellular/cholestatic	Amoxicillin
	Azathioprine
	Chlorpromazine
	Erythromycin (macrolides)
	Nitrofurantoin
Steatosis	
Macrovesicular	Amiodarone
	Nonalcoholic (metabolic syndrome)
Microvesicular	Tetracycline
	Valproic acid
Vascular	
Peliosis	Estrogens/androgens
Hepatic vein thrombosis	Estrogens
Veno-occlusive disease	Alkaloids *(Senecio)*
	Busulfan
	Thioguanine
Adenoma/malignant tumor	Anabolic steroids
	Estrogens

cells. Toxicity is not limited to cell death, but can be a result of interference of bile formation, accumulation of fat, fibrosis, and carcinogenesis. Toxicity can be either acute or chronic, and reversible or progressive. This section will focus on the most common causes of DILI in children (Table 28–10).[12,13]

Clinical Presentation

The clinical spectrum of disease is a result of the specific hepatotoxin and includes clinical hepatitis, fatty liver, vascular changes, and adenoma/malignant tumor formation (Table 28–10). Clinical hepatitis has been categorized into three patterns: hepatocellular, cholestatic, and mixed (hepatocellular/cholestatic), with and without immunoallergic features. In patients with an immune-allergic component, there is fever, inflammation of other organs, morbilliform rash, myocarditis, pancreatitis, renal dysfunction, and lymphadenopathy. Laboratory findings also include eosinophilia and atypical lymphocytosis.

Hepatocellular (hepatitic) pattern of injury is the most common and results from hepatocyte apoptosis/necrosis. In many cases, there is an asymptomatic elevation in serum aminotransferase levels; however, when severe, symptoms are similar to acute viral hepatitis. Patients complain of anorexia, fatigue, abdominal pain, nausea, and vomiting. Laboratory features include marked elevation of serum aminotransferases, with a normal/near-normal alkaline phosphatase. Serum bilirubin levels are variable; however, an extreme elevation is a negative prognostic factor. Imaging studies show either a normal liver or, more commonly, diffuse homogeneous hepatomegaly without bile duct dilatation. In most cases, there is no specific therapy beyond identifying and stopping the drug. Medications used in children that cause this type of injury include phenytoin, methyldopa, isoniazid, halothane, and acetaminophen. Most patients will recover once the toxin has been removed, although in rare situations an autoimmune hepatitis is triggered. This is not true for acetaminophen overdose, which is an intrinsic toxin, and specific treatment is discussed below.

Cholestatic pattern of injury presents with complaints of jaundice and itching. Nausea, vomiting, and anorexia are prominent when symptoms are severe. Laboratory features include a marked elevation of alkaline phosphatase, GGT, and total and direct bilirubin, with preservation of synthetic function and relatively normal serum aminotransferase levels. Imaging studies are normal, without ductal dilation or evidence of cholecystitis. Liver histology reveals intracellular cholestasis, bile plugs, and the absence of biliary inflammation and bile lakes. The clinical course differs from the hepatocellular pattern, as jaundice and pruritus can linger up to 6 months after removal of the toxin. Pediatric drugs causing cholestatic injury include estrogens and cyclosporine. In addition to removal of the toxin, patients can be treated with UDCA to enhance bile flow.

Hepatocellular–cholestatic (mixed) pattern of injury involves feature of both types of injury. In general, patients present with nausea, vomiting, and anorexia, with the more severe cases having jaundice and pruritus. Laboratory features are variable with elevations of all liver tests, but usually not to the same extremes as seen in the hepatitic or cholestatic patterns. The same is true for liver histology. Drugs used in children that cause a mixed injury pattern include macrolide antibiotics, azathioprine, nitrofurantoin, and chlorpromazine. Treatment is similar to the other patterns: recognizing and removing the toxin and symptomatic treatment for pruritus. The typical disease course is also intermediate, being longer than that for hepatocellular injury, but shorter than the course for pure cholestatic pattern.

Fatty liver pattern of injury (steatotic) occurs in two main types: microvesicular, or small fat droplets, and macrovesicular, or large fat droplets. In macrovesicular steatosis there is usually a microvesicular component as well. Macrovesicular steatosis results from drugs that produce phospholipidosis, alcohol, and also liver disease associated with the metabolic syndrome (MetS; see below). Microvesicular steatosis is principally due to mitochondrial toxicity, leading to a deficiency in mitochondrial beta-oxidation of free fatty acids (FFA) and a critical compromise of mitochondrial ATP production. Patients present with nausea, anorexia, and vomiting. Confusion or coma due to elevated serum ammonia can be present. Laboratory features include marked hyperammonemia, lactic acidosis, elevated serum aminotransferases, and minimal elevation of alkaline phosphatase or GGT levels. Serum bilirubin levels reflect the severity of toxicity. Imaging studies are usually normal and liver histology reveals microvesicular steatosis with minimal inflammatory infiltrate. Pediatric drugs associated with microvesicular steatotic injury pattern include valproic acid (VPA) and tetracycline. The usual course is rapid improvement after the toxic has been removed; however, liver transplantation should be considered in patients with higher grades of encephalopathy.

History

Children with malignancies and seizure disorders are at increased risk of DILI and a heightened level of suspicion is warranted. In all cases, a through history of current or recent medications includes reviewing medication preparation, dose, and frequency of administration. The use of herbal preparations, illicit drugs, and xenobiotics needs to be ascertained. Evidence for recent infection or infectious exposures must be explored. Family history should include documentation of chronic liver disease, autoimmune conditions, early childhood/neonatal death, and stillbirths or spontaneous abortions.

Differential Diagnosis

The differential diagnosis of suspected hepatotoxicity includes acute viral hepatitis, acute ischemic liver injury, autoimmune hepatitis, congestive hepatitis, and hepatic decompensation due to Wilson's disease. Consideration of alternative causes of the cholestatic pattern includes biliary obstruction from gallstones, tumor, strictures, pancreatic disease, and autoimmune disorders such as primary biliary cirrhosis and primary sclerosing cholangitis. The differential diagnosis for the mixed condition includes all of the above. The differential diagnosis for steatotic pattern of injury includes Reye's syndrome and inborn or acquired defects in mitochondrial fatty acid metabolism or ATP production.

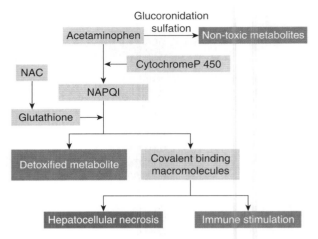

FIGURE 28–5 ■ Acetaminophen metabolism. *Abbreviations*: NAPQI = *N*-acetyl-*p*-benzoquinoneimine; NAC = *N*-acetylcysteine.

Specific Drug Hepatotoxicities in Children

Acetaminophen-induced liver disease results in a predictable injury. Acetaminophen is a hydroxylated compound and does not require phase I activation prior to conjugation (Figure 28–5). In therapeutic doses, acetaminophen is sulfated and glucuronidated by phase II detoxification. In an overdose, phase II pathways are saturated, and excess acetaminophen undergoes biotransformation by hepatic cytochrome P450 enzymes to produce the electrophilic intermediate, *N*-acetyl-*p*-benzoquinoneimine (NAPQI). At low rates of production, NAPQI is detoxified by S-conjugation with GSH. At high rates of production, GSH is depleted, and it is assumed that NAPQI becomes covalently bound to intracellular proteins, resulting in loss of cell function and cell death secondary to free radical-induced lipid peroxidation or an inappropriate stimulation of an immune response. Toxicity resulting from a single large dose is distinctive. Nausea and vomiting occur immediately, followed by an asymptomatic interval of 12–24 hours, during which serum aminotransferase levels are increasing. Liver injury appears clinically in 2–4 days with the onset of jaundice, markedly elevated aminotransferases, and a developing coagulopathy, ultimately leading to liver failure and coma. Serum bilirubin, although elevated, is less so than in other causes of acute liver failure and can be a clue to recognizing acetaminophen-induced ALF. Treatment with *N*-acetylcysteine (NAC) acts by providing a substrate for glutathione production. Treatment must be given early as NAC will not reverse toxic effects once they have occurred. Treatment is most effective if given within 10 hours of ingestion; however, late administration of NAC has been associated with improved survival. Utilization of NAC can be determined using a semilogarithmic graph plotting plasma acetaminophen concentration against time; however, if there is any doubt of usefulness, NAC should be given anyway. Treatment can be administered for either 20 hours intravenously or 72 hours orally. Although compared to adults and adolescents children appear to be relatively resistant to acetaminophen-induced liver disease, they can definitely develop hepatotoxicity. The estimated threshold dose is between 120 and 150 mg/kg. Positive prognostic factors include normal clotting factors and aminotransferase levels 48 hours after treatment. Liver transplantation is indicated for progressive liver failure and all patients with significant toxicity should be transferred to a transplant center.

Children can also develop acetaminophen-induced liver disease by receiving repeated administration of an inappropriate dose over several days. This is often termed a therapeutic misadventure, and can result from shortening of the dosing frequency, inappropriate measuring device, or substitution of a different preparation. The toxic dose is estimated to be about 90 mg/kg. Clinically, the patient presents with acute liver failure for which other causes are usually suspected. Diagnosis requires a detailed drug history. Detecting serum acetaminophen 24 hours past the last dose, or demonstrating the presence of acetaminophen protein adducts, formed by NAPQUI–glutathione, is suggestive of the diagnosis. The nomogram for treatment of acute overdose with NAC does not apply, and these children should be treated immediately and transferred to a liver transplant center.

Phenytoin-induced liver injury results from an unpredictable response to normal dosing. Although considered rare, it is second only to acetaminophen in reported incidents of pediatric drug-induced hepatotoxicity. Most patients present with hepatitis and immunoallergic features of fever, rash, lymphadenopathy, and other organ involvement. Laboratory features include leukocytosis, atypical lymphocytosis, eosinophilia, elevated serum aminotransferases, and variable bilirubin levels. Severe cases can progress to liver failure. The mechanism of toxicity has not been completely defined but felt to result from abnormal metabolism of a toxic byproduct. Treatment consists of withdrawing the drug and, possibly, intravenous methylprednisolone, 2 mg/kg/day, to reverse the allergic features.

VPA-induced liver disease can be mild or severe. Fortunately, mild disease is the most common and is associated with an asymptomatic elevation of serum aminotransferases or ammonia. It is dose related and resolves with dose reduction. Serious liver disease is probably related to polypharmacy and individual genetic factors. A distinctive risk factor for VPA hepatotoxicity is that, unlike other DILIs, it is more common in children than adults. Identifiable risk factors include an age <2 years, treatment with multiple anticonvulsants, and

coexistent medical problems such as congenital abnormalities, mental retardation, developmental delay, and an intercurrent infection. In children with these risk factors, the incidence of fatal hepatotoxicity is 1 in 600.

Serum aminotransferase levels should be monitored for the first 6 months of treatment and with any dose escalation. A three-fold increase in serum level should prompt drug cessation. Associated symptoms of fever, nausea, vomiting, and abdominal pain are worrisome. Patients that develop progressive liver dysfunction and poor seizure control will probably develop irreversible liver failure. The defective detoxification pathway is not known, but it appears that mitochondria are the target organelle. Liver histology shows microvesicular steatosis and abnormal mitochondria. Similar to Reye's syndrome, serum carnitine is low. Prophylactic use of L-carnitine is recommended for children taking VPA and for asymptomatic hyperammonemia.

NONALCOHOLIC-INDUCED LIVER DISEASE

Definitions and Epidemiology

NAFLD is a condition characterized by abnormal lipid deposition in hepatocytes in the absence of excessive alcoholic consumption. It represents a spectrum of conditions ranging from fatty liver without inflammation (hepatosteatosis) to fatty liver with necroinflammation (steatohepatitis). Nonalcoholic steatohepatitis (NASH) can progress to fibrosis and cirrhosis, causing portal hypertension and liver failure. NASH can coexist with other causes of fatty liver disease and, when present, can exacerbate disease activity.

NAFLD is rapidly becoming the most common cause of elevated serum aminotransferase levels in children and the increase in prevalence parallels the obesity epidemic. The prevalence of pediatric NAFLD is unknown, but is estimated to be 8% of adolescents and increases to approximately 20% of obese children. The prevalence increases with age and degree of obesity, and is affected by ethnicity. Hispanic children have a higher prevalence than Caucasian or African American children, respectively. There is a significant association with type 2 diabetes mellitus (DM-2) and features of the MetS: insulin resistance, hypertriglyceridemia, hypertension, and visceral obesity. MetS has been reported in up to 66% of children with NAFLD and is considered the hepatic manifestation of MetS.[14]

Pathogenesis

The obesity epidemic is attributed to overconsumption of dense-calorie foods containing saturated or hydrogenated fats and high glycemic index carbohydrates, coupled with a sedentary lifestyle. Pathogenesis of NAFLD and NASH has not been defined, but is clearly associated with obesity. The current concept for the development of NAFLD/NASH is centered on a "two hit hypothesis" involving fat deposition in hepatocytes and a genetic predisposition. Fats accumulate in adipose tissue and inappropriately in liver and muscle as FFA and triglycerides. Insulin resistance promotes gluconeogenesis, glycogenolysis, and FFA release from adipose tissue. Unregulated FFA uptake by hepatocytes increases triglyceride synthesis and impairs FFA oxidation, resulting in increased hepatocyte lipid. Progression to NASH is felt to result from genetic factors causing an increased susceptibility of hepatocytes to oxidative stress.

Clinical Presentation

Most children are asymptomatic and identified by elevated serum aminotransferases obtained after screening for obesity-related co-morbidities. Some children have right upper quadrant or epigastric abdominal pain and are identified with fatty liver by ultrasound or abnormal aminotransferase levels. Fatigue, malaise, and sleep apnea may be associated symptoms. More than 90% of children will have central obesity. Some children are identified due to the presence of acanthosis nigricans.

History

NAFALD/NASH is an insidious disease as there are few to no signs or symptoms of chronic liver disease. There is an absence of jaundice, acholic stools, pruritus, anorexia, ascites, and variceal hemorrhage. Patients may have symptoms related to MetS such as hypertension, DM2, dyslipidemia, obstructive sleep apnea, or polycystic ovary syndrome. Family history is notable for obesity, DM2, hypertension, dyslipidemia, and cardiovascular disease. A careful history exploring medication exposure should be obtained. There is a negative family history for chronic liver disease.

Physical Examination

Over 90% of patients will be obese. Hepatomegaly, usually without splenomegaly, is common but can be difficult to appreciate due to the central distribution of fat. Acanthosis nigricans is present in up to 45% of children. Blood pressure should be obtained with an appropriate-sized cuff. There is an absence of jaundice, scleral icterus, ascites, and peripheral edema.

Differential Diagnosis

Although NAFLD/NASH is associated with obesity, the presence of obesity does not exclude other disorders associated with fatty liver; thus, the diagnosis should include an evaluation for other disorders associated with fatty liver disease. In adolescents, alcohol consumption should be investigated. Other causes of fatty liver disease include autoimmune hepatitis, A1AT, Wilson's disease, drug toxicity, FAO defects, lipodystrophy, and infectious causes: hepatitis B and C, EBV, and CMV.

Diagnosis

Although some patients may have normal serum aminotransferases, in most patients they will be elevated. In particular, the alanine aminotransferase (ALT) is significantly elevated and the ALT:aspartate transaminase (AST) ratio will be 1 or greater. Evidence of MetS with elevated fasting serum glucose, insulin, and triglycerides and exclusion of other causes of fatty liver disease is supportive evidence. Abdominal imaging may confirm fatty infiltration and exclude other causes of elevated aminotransferases.

Abdominal ultrasound is relatively inexpensive, noninvasive, and easy to perform. Presence of fat causes the liver to appear bright when compared to the kidney or spleen. Ultrasound, however, does not quantify the amount of fat or fibrosis and can be difficult to perform in patients with central obesity. Other imaging modalities include computed tomography (CT), magnetic resonance imaging (MRI), and MR spectroscopy. These have the advantage of being quantitative. CT has the disadvantage of radiation exposure, while MRI and MRS are relatively expensive. Most importantly, none of these imaging studies can differentiate benign steatosis from NASH, nor can the grade of inflammation be determined. Transient elastography is a new noninvasive technique designed to differentiate the stage of hepatic fibrosis. In children with NAFLD, this technique has been shown to accurately discriminate the presence of any degree of fibrosis from none; however, differentiation of grade 1 and 2 fibrosis was less certain.[15] This technique has not yet been validated as a screening tool.

Currently, liver biopsy provides the only way to definitely distinguish benign steatosis from NASH. It provides quantitative information on the amount of steatosis, inflammation, and fibrosis. Interestingly, histologic features differ in adults and children and are referred to as type 1 or 2 NASH, respectively. In type 1 (adult) NASH, there is macrovesicular steatosis with ballooning degeneration and/or perisinusoidal fibrosis in the absence of portal fibrosis. In type 2 NASH, which is unique to children, the fibrosis and inflammation is primarily in the portal tracts, with *absence* of ballooning degeneration and perisinusoidal fibrosis. In addition, an overlap pattern has been described, containing findings from both types. This observation suggests that there is a spectrum of disease patterns. In children, the majority will have type 2 or the overlap pattern.

Currently the diagnosis of NAFLD can be inferred by clinical and laboratory features. The decision of when to perform a liver biopsy in children is controversial. In children the primary rational for biopsy is to confirm the diagnosis and discriminate NASH from benign steatosis. Some centers diagnose NAFLD with clinical and laboratory features alone, and reserve biopsy for patients whose serum aminotransferases are >2.5 times normal, ALT:AST ratio >1, exhibit an inhomogeneous hepatic parenchyma on liver ultrasound, or who were treated empirically, but failed to resolve laboratory abnormalities.

Treatment

Current therapeutic regimens are based on recognition and treatment of co-morbidities, reversal of insulin resistance, and utilization of hepatoprotective agents. All treatment regimens are based on weight reduction and exercise. Weight loss should be approximately 1 lb/week, as rapid weight loss may exacerbate NAFLD. Patients should increase physical activity to at least 20 minutes of sustained activity at least three times a week, but preferably more. Unfortunately it is diet and lack of exercise that caused NAFLD and MetS; thus, treatment requires a significant lifestyle change, which is challenging to enforce.

Lifestyle changes require a new approach to eating habits and daily activities. Multidisciplinary centers providing education and assistance in nutrition and fitness are ideal. In younger children, family commitment to these changes is essential. One of the most important changes is choosing foods with a low glycemic index. This means reduction or elimination of food products made from refined sugars. High intake of glucose and fructose promotes hyperinsulinemia and FFA synthesis, and increases total caloric consumption. In addition, fats should be no more than 30% of total calories and in particular saturated fats should be limited 10% or less.

Pharmacotherapy in children is indicated for treatment of hyperinsulinemia and to protect the liver. Metformin, a biguanide hypoglycemic agent, improves hepatic insulin resistance and is well tolerated in children. It has been shown to improve hepatic steatosis and serum aminotransferase levels in uncontrolled studies and is currently undergoing evaluation in a prospective study in children. Another class of drugs that improves insulin resistance is the thiazolidinediones: pioglitazone and rosiglitazone. These agents have only been used in adults and showed reduction of inflammation, but not fibrosis. Side effects in adults include increased heart disease and fractures.

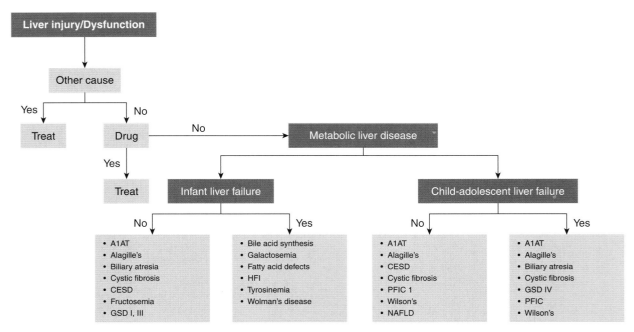

FIGURE 28-6 ■ Algorithm for the evaluation of metabolic-induced liver disease. *Abbreviations:* A1AT = alpha-1-antitrypsin deficiency; CESD = cholesterol ester storage disease; GSD = glycogen storage disease; HFI = hereditary fructose intolerance; NAFLD = nonalcoholic fatty liver disease; PFIC = progressive familial intrahepatic cholestasis.

Vitamin E is an antioxidant and has been used in pediatric NAFLD with normalization of serum aminotransferases, independent of weight change, but with no change in steatosis as measured by ultrasound. As with metformin, vitamin E is currently being studied in a large prospective study.

Course and Prognosis

In a course of only two decades, NAFLD has gone from a rare disorder to the most common cause of liver disease in children. As the obesity epidemic increases, it is fair to conclude NAFLD will also increase in prevalence. Recognition of its association with obesity and in particular with insulin resistance increases the risk for the development of NASH. NAFLD should not be considered a benign disorder but a disease with the potential to progress to cirrhosis. In the adult population NASH is one of the three most common indications for liver transplantation. Data show that early recognition of NAFLD and identification of co-morbidities is essential in not only arresting disease progression, but also for reversal of inflammation and fibrosis. Therapeutic options are currently aimed at treatment of obesity and co-morbidities. Further studies on pathogenesis and treatment are needed.

SUMMARY

With the exception of NAFLD, metabolic-induced liver disease and DILIs are relatively rare conditions whose recognition requires a high degree of suspicion. Treatment to reverse toxic products is often life saving. Many disorders can be treated with dietary elimination or medically. Figure 28–6 provides an algorithmic approach to the evaluation of metabolic-induced liver injury.

REFERENCES

1. Manco M, Bottazzo GT, Devito R, et al. Nonalcoholic fatty liver disease in children. *J Am Coll Nutr.* 2008;27(6): 667–676.
2. Saudubray JM, Nassogne MC, deLonlay P, et al. Clinical approach to inherited metabolic disorders in neonates: an overview. *Semin Neonatal.* 2002;7:3–15.
3. Ghishan FK, Zawaideh M. Inborn errors of carbohydrate metabolism. In: Suchy FJ, Sokol RJ, Balistreri WE, eds. *Liver Disease in Children.* NY: Cambridge University Press; 2007:595.
4. Bosch AM, Bakker HD, Gennip AH, et al. Clinical features of galactokinase deficiency: a review of the literature. *J Inherit Metab Dis.* 2002;25:629–634.
5. Tream WR. Fatty acid oxidation disorders. In: Wylie R, Hyams JS, eds. *Pediatric Gastrointestinal and Liver Disease.* 3rd ed. Philadelphia: Saunder/Elsevier; 2006:883.
6. Sokol RJ. Mitochondrial hepatopathies. In: Suchy FJ, Sokol RJ, Balistreri WF, eds. *Liver Disease in Children.* NY: Cambridge University Press; 2007:803.
7. Stein J, Garly BZ, Dron Y, et al. Successful treatment of Wolman disease by unrelated umbilical cord blood transplantation. *Eur J Pediatr.* 2007;166:663–666.
8. Sundaram SS, Bove KE, Lovell MA, et al. Mechanisms of disease: inborn errors of bile acid synthesis. *Nat Clin Pract.* 2008;5(8):456–468.
9. Davit-Spraul A, Gonzales E, Baussan C, et al. Progressive familial intrahepatic cholestasis. *Orphanet J Rare Dis.* 2009;4:1.
10 Suchy FJ, Schneider BL. Familial hepatocellular cholestasis. In: Suchy FJ, Sokol RJ, Ballistreri WF, eds. *Liver Disease in Children.* NY: Cambridge University Press; 2007:310.
11. Liu C, Aronow BJ, Jegga AG, et al. Novel resequencing chip customized to diagnose mutation in patients with inherited syndromes of intrahepatic cholestasis. *Gastroenterology.* 2007;132:119–126.
12. Roberts EA. Drug induced liver disease. In: Suchy FJ, Sokol RJ, Ballistreri WF, eds. *Liver Disease in Children.* NY: Cambridge University Press; 2007:478.
13. Bonkousky HL, Jones DP, La Brecque DR, et al. Drug induced liver disease. In: Boyer TD, Wright TL, Manns MP, eds. *Zakim and Boyer's Hepatology: A Textbook of Liver Disease.* Philadelphia: Saunders/Elsevier; 2006;503.
14. Sundaram SS, Zeitler P, Nadeau K. The metabolic syndrome and nonalcoholic fatty liver disease. *Curr Opin Pediatr.* 2009;21(4):529–535. Wolters, Kluwer, Health. Lippincott, Williams & Wilkins [Epub ahead of print].
15. Nobili V, Vizzutti F, Arena U, et al. Accuracy and reproducibility of transient elastography for the diagnosis of fibrosis in pediatric nonalcoholic steatohepatitis. *Hepatology.* 2008;48(2):442–448.

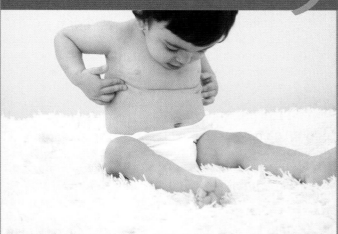

CHAPTER 29

Liver Transplantation

*Yumirle Turmelle and
Ross W. Shepherd*

DEFINITIONS AND EPIDEMIOLOGY

Types of Liver Transplants

Liver transplantation refers to the surgical replacement of a diseased liver with a donor-grafted organ. This is most commonly *orthotopic* (complete removal and replacement), but occasionally *heterotopic*, where the native organ is left in situ. The transplant may be whole liver, a reduced-size liver, or a liver segment, the latter as means of overcoming donor organ scarcity, particularly for pediatric recipients (Figure 29–1). *Reduced-size liver grafts*, such as a left-lateral segment or hemireduction graft, can be derived from either cadaver or living donors, or from *split-liver transplantation*, where two grafts are created from a single donor organ for two recipients, usually an adult and an infant.[1]

MELD and PELD

The United Network for Organ Sharing in the United States has devised the Model for End-stage Liver Disease (*MELD*) and Pediatric End-stage Liver Disease (*PELD*), which are numerical scales that are currently used for liver allocation.[2] Similar systems exist in other countries. These scores are based on a patient's risk of dying while waiting for a liver transplant, derived from objective and verifiable medical outcomes data. The MELD

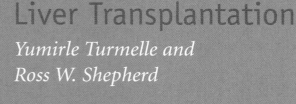

Orthotopic liver transplantation

Whole liver with hepatic and portal veins, hepatic artery and bile duct to be attached to recipient structures

Reduced-size liver transplantation

Standard hemi reduction technique

Recipient : Donor size ratio usually ≤ 4:1

IV II+III → Donor IVC   IV II+III

PV
CBD
CA

"Brisbane" technique

LHV

Recipient : Donor size ratio up to 13:1

II+III → Recipient IVC   II+III

PV
CBD
CA
Donor saphenofemoral junction
Rec. PV
Aortoceliac anastomosis

FIGURE 29–1 ■ Surgical techniques for liver transplantation in children. Orthotopic whole-organ replacement, and reduced-size techniques. Donors are matched for size and blood type.

score, used for patients aged 12 years and older, is based on bilirubin, international normalized ratio (INR), and creatinine. The PELD score is based on bilirubin, INR, albumin, growth failure, and age, factors which better predict mortality in children. These scores do not alone determine the likelihood of getting a transplant. Other factors include matched (blood group and size) organ availability, the occurrence of higher priority exceptions (e.g., those with fulminant hepatic failure), and the distribution of MELD/PELD scores for other patients in a local area or region, and consideration for living donation. The PELD/MELD system also has designated exception scores assigned to specific liver conditions that have preserved liver synthetic function and thus corresponding low allocation scores, such as those children with metabolic liver diseases (e.g., urea cycle disorders) and hepatoblastoma. In addition, a program can request a higher exception score if the calculated score does not truly represent the patient's condition. This is done by submitting an exception score request to their UNOS regional review board for consideration.

Epidemiology

The annualized incidence of liver transplantation in the United States is 10–12 per million total population, that is, 50–60 cases per million children/year (1/16,000 children), or about 600 children, one-third of these being infants. Approximately 55% of these transplants are for end-stage chronic liver disease, the majority of these due to biliary atresia (BA); about 25% are for metabolic liver diseases, 10% for acute liver failure, and 5% for liver tumors (Figure 29–2).[3,4] *BA* (Chapter 23) occurs in about 1/14,000 live births in the United States, but not all cases of BA require transplant (see below). Pediatric acute liver failure (PALF) has estimated annualized incidence of about 2 per million, and about 50% recover

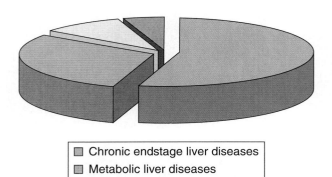

- ☐ Chronic endstage liver diseases
- ☐ Metabolic liver diseases
- ☐ Acute liver failure
- ☐ Liver tumors

FIGURE 29–2 ■ Relative frequency of types of liver disease for which liver transplantation is indicated in children. Of all pediatric liver diseases, biliary atresia is the most common indication (50%).

without transplant.[5] It is notable that the number of long-term survivors of liver transplantation is currently about 10 times these annualized figures. Thus, children who require liver transplantation or are being followed after liver transplantation are likely to be encountered with some frequency in pediatric practice, and the number of these children is expanding.

CLINICAL PRESENTATION AND REASONS FOR REFERRAL

A wide range of chronic liver diseases in children, a number of liver-specific metabolic diseases, some rare tumors of the liver, and presentations of acute liver failure are potentially cured by liver transplantation. These conditions, although individually rare, are collectively not uncommon, and are accompanied by medical and social demands of lifelong aftercare.

Indications

End-stage chronic liver diseases, such as BA, form the commonest indication, accounting for more than half of all pediatric liver transplant recipients, and the majority of infant recipients (Table 29–1). BA has an incidence of 5–7/100,000 live births in the United States and Europe, and 10–15/100,000 in Asia, and in about two-third of cases, the initial attempt at a bile drainage procedure (hepatoportoenterostomy) fails, and the infant/child develops chronic liver failure.[6] Considered together, *liver-specific metabolic diseases* represent approximately 25% of pediatric liver transplants and are the second most common indications for liver transplant after BA. These can be divided into: (1) those that lead to liver injury, with or without other organ involvement, such as alpha-1-antitrypsin deficiency, Wilson's disease, tyrosinemia, familial cholestasis, and cystic fibrosis (CF); and (2) diseases due to a metabolic defect expressed solely or predominantly in the liver but leading to injury to other organ systems, such as the urea cycle disorders, Crigler–Najjar syndrome, and hyperoxaluria. *Acute liver failure* accounts for about 10% of cases. Most cases are of indeterminate cause, followed by acetaminophen toxicity, other drug toxicities, Wilson's disease, autoimmune hepatitis, and perinatal hemochromatosis. Finally, *unresectable liver tumors* such as hepatoblastoma, embryonal sarcomas, and hemangioendotheliomas are rare but important indications for timely liver transplantation.

Contraindications

Some conditions associated with serious liver involvement are not curable by liver transplantation, namely those with life-threatening extrahepatic disease are absolute contraindications to liver transplantation

Table 29–1.

Indications for Liver Transplantation in Children

	Frequency (% of Transplants)
Chronic end-stage liver diseases (60%)	
■ Biliary atresia	55
■ Chronic active hepatitis	4
■ Primary sclerosing cholangitis	1
Liver-specific genetic/metabolic diseases (25%)	
■ Causing chronic liver injury ± other organ involvement	10
■ alpha-1-antitrypsin deficiency	
■ Familial cholestasis	5
■ Cystic fibrosis	2
■ Tyrosinemia	1
■ Glycogen storage diseases	1
■ Alagille syndrome	5
■ Metabolic defect expressed solely or predominantly in the liver but leading to other organ injury/morbidity	
■ Urea cycle disorders	2
■ Hyperoxaluria	1
■ Crigler–Najjar syndrome	<1
■ Maple syrup urine disease	1
■ Ornithine transcarbamylase deficiency	<1
Acute liver failure (10%)	
■ Indeterminate cause	5
■ Acetomenophin toxicity	2
■ Other drug toxicities	<1
■ Wilson's disease	1
■ Perinatal hemochromatosis	1
■ Some fatty acid oxidation defects	<1
■ Viral hepatitis (hepatitis A, B, C, EBV, adeno, CMV, echo, herpes, parvo)	1
■ Autoimmune hepatitis	
Primary unresectable liver tumors (5%)	
■ Hepatoblastoma	2
■ Embryonal sarcoma	<1
■ Hemangioendothelioma	<1

(Table 29–2). Although in the past there have been some technical and management restrictions with regard to age, size, and the occurrence of hepatopulmonary syndrome and portal vein thrombosis, successful liver transplantation is now possible even in the neonatal period, and the various technical issues have been overcome, and these are considered only relative contraindications. There are some conditions in which the transplant should be temporarily deferred, such as acute active infections and recent live virus immunizations.

Reasons for Referral

Those who might benefit from liver transplantation present with a range of clinical problems, some not necessarily with initial obvious links to the liver (Table 29–3). Early referral for evaluation is emphasized in all cases in which transplantation is even remotely an option to allow for timely assessment, full and frank discussion of options, psychological preparation, appropriate pre-transplant aggressive management, and evaluation of donor options.

Presentation

BA is a special case, in which a "failed Kasai procedure" in infancy, manifesting as a failure to clear jaundice within 3–6 weeks, virtually always portends complications of cirrhosis within weeks to a few months. Thus, as soon as a failed Kasai is realized, referral for transplant

Table 29–2.

Contraindications to Liver Transplantation in Children

Absolute
- Curative alternative therapy available
- Uncontrolled systemic sepsis
- Irreversible neurological injury
- Extrahepatic malignancy
- Progressive terminal non-hepatic disease
- Mitochondrial disorders with progressive neurological involvement

Relative
- Severe hepatopulmonary syndrome—actionable management
- Portal vein thrombosis—vein graft availability
- Active primary peritonitis—temporary deferment
- Active viral infection—temporary deferment
- Recent liver virus immunizations—temporary deferment

evaluation should be made. Similarly, recurrent cholangitis, which can be life-threatening and can result in development of acute or chronic synthetic failure, should be a consideration for transplantation. Beyond

that, any presentation with features of end-stage liver disease, such as ascites, portal hypertension, and nutritional growth failure, is a clear indication for referral.

Causes and complications of chronic end-stage liver disease

Any child with chronic liver disease and/or cirrhosis requires regular follow-up, evaluating for signs of end-stage disease, as listed in Table 29–3, the occurrence of which should provoke referral. The complications of chronic liver disease and cirrhosis (listed in Table 29–3) are due to *impaired hepatic function and cholestasis*, which cause nutritional disturbances, jaundice, pruritus, and coagulopathy, and *portal hypertension*, which causes varices, hypersplenism, and hepatorenal or hepatopulmonary syndrome. Encephalopathy and ascites occur as a result of both of these major pathophysiologic events. In addition, impaired immunity with resulting bacterial infection may complicate cirrhosis. Hepatocellular carcinoma can complicate cirrhosis in childhood, particularly in chronic hepatitis B and tyrosinemia type I.

The presentation of some complications can be subtle, such as nutritional growth failure. In some

Table 29–3.

Reasons for Referral for Liver Transplant Evaluation

Chronic end-stage liver diseases

Specific to biliary atresia
- Failed hepatoporoenterostomy (persisting jaundice)
- Recurrent ascending cholangitis
- Any cirrhosis complications listed below

Complications of end-stage liver disease and cirrhosis of any cause
- Nutritional disturbances, growth failure, malabsorption
- Portal hypertension and variceal hemorrhage
- Hypersplenism
- Ascites
- Liver synthetic dysfunction (coagulopathy, hypoalbuminemia)
- Hepatorenal and hepatopulmonary syndromes
- Encephalopathy
- Bacterial infections, spontaneous bacterial peritonitis
- Hepatocellular carcinoma

Liver-specific genetic/metabolic diseases
- Those causing complications of end-stage liver disease listed above ± related morbidities, such as alpha-1-antitrypsin deficiency, familial cholestasis, cystic fibrosis, tyrosinemia, glycogen storage diseases, Alagille syndrome
- Metabolic defects expressed in the liver but leading to other organ injury and/or serious morbidity, and compromised quality of life, such as urea cycle disorders (life-threatening recurrent hyperammonemia and hyperoxaluria (renal failure)), Crigler–Najjar syndrome (brain injury), maple syrup urine disease (brain), ornithine transcarbamylase deficiency

Acute liver failure, presenting as any combination of sudden onset of jaundice, encephalopathy coagulopathy, hypoglycemia, markedly elevated liver transaminases

Primary liver tumors where there is any doubt as to resectability, prior to chemotherapy

Table 29–4.

Stages of Hepatic Encephalopathy in Children

Stage	Clinical	Reflexes	Neurological	EEG
Infant				
Early (I and II)	Inconsolable crying, sleep reversal	Unreliable normal or hyperreflexia	Untestable	
Mid (III)	Somnolence, stupor, combativeness	Unreliable, may be hyperreflexia	Most likely untestable	
Late (IV)	Comatose, arouses with painful stimuli (IVa) or no response (IVb)	Absent	Decerebrate or decorticate	
Older child				
0	Normal	Normal	Psychtesting only	Normal
1	Confused, poor sleep habits, forgetful	Normal	Tremor, apraxia, impaired handwriting	Normal or diffuse slowing
2	Drowsy, decreased inhibitions	Hyperreflexia	Dysarthria, ataxia	Generalized slowing
3	Stuporous, obeys simple commands	Hyperreflexia, up-going toes (+Babinski)	Rigidity	Generalized slowing
4	Comatose, arouses with painful stimuli (IVa) or no response (IVb)	Absent	Decerebrate or decorticate	Abnormal, very slow delta activity

patients, portal hypertension can progress slowly, manifesting only as splenomegaly and hypersplenism (bruising tendency, recurrent epistaxis, and thrombocytopenia). Encephalopathy in children can be very subtle in chronic disease, presenting only as deterioration of school performance, sleep inversion, or intermittent somnolence. In other cases, complications can be dramatic, such as massive ascites and GI bleeding from esophageal varices, and can be the initial presentation of the underlying chronic liver disease.

Metabolic liver diseases causing liver injury are diagnosed following an initial, usually neonatal presentation with cholestasis. Typical of these are alpha-1-antitrypsin deficiency, familial cholestasis, Alagille syndrome, and CF. Metabolic liver diseases in which the defect is expressed in the liver, leading to significant injury of other organs, should also be considered for liver transplantation, as the disease is cured by liver replacement. Each case has to be considered on its merits, in relation to mortality risk, such as in ornithine transcarbamylase deficiency and some urea cycle disorders, risk to the end-organ, such as the brain (in the case of hyperammonemic syndromes and Crigler–Najjar syndrome) and the kidney (as in hyperoxaluria), and the poor quality of life associated with these disorders.

PALF presents most commonly with new-onset jaundice, variable encephalopathy, a coagulopathy, hypoglycemia, and markedly elevated transaminases. By definition, there is no known chronic liver disease, a coagulopathy uncorrected by vitamin K, where the prothrombin time (PT) >15 seconds, and the INR >1.5, and if no encephalopathy, a PT >20 seconds, and INR >2.0 (Figure 29–2). The peak age of onset is in infancy (25% of cases), where jaundice is late feature, early hypoglycemia is common, and most cases are of indeterminate cause.[5] There is another peak of incidence in adolescents, where the etiology is more likely drug toxicity or viral. A good clinical history concerning onset, history of exposures to drugs, viruses, toxins, extrahepatic symptoms, rate of progress of symptoms and signs, and family history may point to an etiology, but at least 50% of cases are idiopathic. Signs of acute hepatic encephalopathy can be staged for monitoring and prognostic purposes, and vary according to age, as listed in Table 29–4. Some metabolic diseases causing ALF can have apparent encephalopathy due to non-hepatic causes, such as hypoglycemia and lactic acidosis. Early referral of suspected cases of PALF to a transplant program is vital, where intensive aggressive supportive therapy can be instituted, urgent attempts at determining the etiology can be instituted, and patients can be listed for a donor search if transplantation is considered an option (Figure 29–3).

Primary liver tumors in children present most commonly as an incidental finding of a painless enlarging

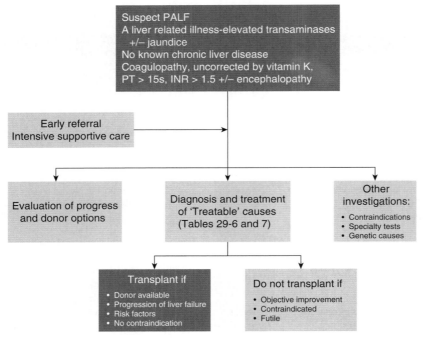

Suspect PALF
A liver related illness-elevated transaminases
+/– jaundice
No known chronic liver disease
Coagulopathy, uncorrected by vitamin K,
PT > 15s, INR > 1.5 +/– encephalopathy

Early referral
Intensive supportive care

Evaluation of progress
and donor options

Diagnosis and treatment
of 'Treatable' causes
(Tables 29-6 and 7)

Other
investigations:
• Contraindications
• Specialty tests
• Genetic causes

Transplant if
• Donor available
• Progression of liver failure
• Risk factors
• No contraindication

Do not transplant if
• Objective improvement
• Contraindicated
• Futile

FIGURE 29–3 ■ Management algorithm of suspected pediatric acute liver failure (PALF).

abdominal mass, or sometimes found on abdominal exam after presentation with abdominal discomfort, pallor, or weight loss, confirmed on imaging studies (Figure 29–4). Total surgical excision and adjunctive chemotherapy are cornerstones of treatment of primary hepatic malignancies in children, and the only option for total surgical excision for unresectable tumors is liver transplantation, which has good long-term outcomes. It is generally recognized that survival after rescue transplantation after incomplete resection is poor, and thus

timely assessment for transplantation in the setting of questionably resectable tumors is indicated.[7] Consultation with a transplantation program at the time of diagnosis and assessment before any chemotherapy should avoid inappropriate attempts at resection and allow appropriate planning of transplantation in relation to chemotherapy.

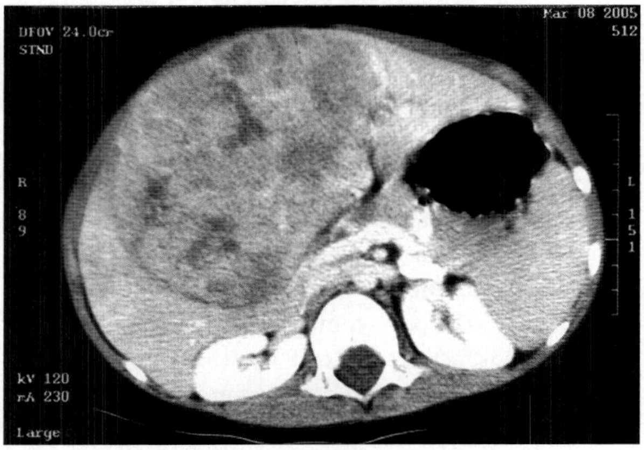

TREATMENT

Liver Transplantation Evaluation and Preparation

The primary goals of the evaluation process (Table 29–5) are to (1) identify the risks versus benefits of transplantation; (2) identify the need for and timing of transplantation; (3) identify technical feasibility and appropriate donor options; (4) establish a pre-transplant management plan; (5) have fully informative, frank discussion of the above with the parents, and patient if possible, to help prepare them to accept and deal with all the issues and possible outcomes of the procedure. The steps taken in this evaluation are detailed in Table 29–5.

Pre-transplant Management

The primary goal of pre-transplant treatment is to keep the patient as well as possible for as long as possible, by a combination of proactive monitoring, active aggressive treatment of complications of liver disease, and multi-

FIGURE 29–4 ■ Computerized tomography of the liver from a child presenting with vague abdominal pains, and a palpable mass on abdominal examination. A central, bilobar tumor without a plane of resection where liver transplant is the only method for complete resection.

Table 29–5.

Pre-transplant Evaluation

1. Establish the need for and urgency for transplantation
2. Assess technical feasiblity. Abdominal ultrasound with Doppler, size of portal vein on US, vascular studies if necessary
3. Consider severity of liver disease (PELD score or exception), based on liver synthetic function, other risk factors, risks, and possible contraindications
4. Assessment of donor options—blood group, size, suitability for reduced-size or split-liver donation
5. Identification of complications of liver disease and extrahepatic conditions
    ■ Nutritional status—global (weight, height, fat folds, mid-am muscle), vitamin, protein, and mineral levels
    ■ Portal hypertension—ascites, varices on endoscopy, hypersplenism
    ■ Cardiac assessment, including echocardiogram
    ■ Repiratory assessment: If cyanosed, perform O_2 saturation, bubble test, ventilation/perfusion, and pulmonary function testing

■ Renal function tests
■ Neurodevelopmental assessment
■ Dental assessment
■ Immunization status, and serology for CMV, EBV, varicella, measles, hepatitis A, B, and C serology
6. Evaluate social systems, issues, and logistic issues
7. Prepare the patient and parents by full, frank discussion
8. Develop a pre-transplant active management plan including
    ■ Immunization update
    ■ Nutritional support
    ■ Ongoing monitoring
    ■ Psychosocial support
    ■ Aggressive management of other complications of liver disease—ascites, coagulopathy, variceal bleeding, encephalopathy, and infections

disciplinary psychosocial support. Good communication systems should be in place between primary physicians and transplant centers to facilitate involvement, set expectations, manage medical and non-medical issues, and provide guidance for both families and all health care professionals toward the common goal of achieving a good outcome for the patient. Because of their long-term relationship with patients and families, primary care physicians/pediatricians are in an advantageous position to detect the early signs of complications, and help families cope with this stressful time.

End-stage chronic liver diseases

The pre-transplant management plan while on the waiting list is developed by the transplant team, in conjunction with the primary care physician, and the family (Table 29–5, item 8). Key features include immunization update, nutritional support, regular monitoring of progress, including active management/notification of intercurrent illness, psychosocial support, and active treatment of complications of liver disease.

Immunization update It is important to ensure that routine immunizations are up to date, and that protection for pneumococcus, *Haemophilus*, and hepatitis A and B be prescribed if possible, and any vaccination requiring live vaccines is administered prior to transplantation.

Nutritional support The liver has a central role in regulating fuel and metabolism, nutrient homeostasis, and absorption of a number of nutrients (Table 29–6).

Table 29–6.

Nutritional Support for End-stage Liver Disease

Vitamin	Received Dose	Preparation
A	5–25,000 IU/day	"Water soluble*" ADEKs[†] Aquasol IV[‡]
D	600–2000 IU 0.02 µg/kg	ADEKs Drisdol[§] 1–250 HD IV**
E	50–100 IU	"Tocopherol polyethylene glycol succinate"
	15–25 IU/kg	Liqui E[††] Aqua E[‡‡] ADEKs
K	2.5–10 mg²/week	Mephyton[§§] Aqua Mephyton injection

Provide adequate absorbed calories—high-energy, semi-elemental supplements, for example, Pregestimil for infants and Peptamen Junior for children. Supplement protein with branched chain amino acids, for example, Tarvil 5 g/20 mL. Avoid fasting and provide calories by nocturnal N/G or G-tube feeding if necessary. Additional fat-soluble vitamins A, D, E, and K.
Also provide minerals: calcium, zinc, and phosphate.
[†]*Axcam.*
[‡]*Mayne.*
[§]*Sanofi Winthrop.*
**Abbott.*
[††]*Twinlab.*
[‡‡]*Yasoo.*
[§§]*Merck.*

These factors result in a catabolic state, particularly during fasting, a deficiency of proteins and calories, which, when combined with anorexia and a poor intake, make

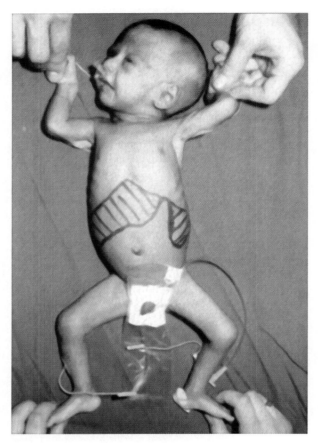

FIGURE 29–5 ■ Malnutrition is a significant potentially modifiable risk factor adversely affecting outcome in children with chronic liver disease, both before and after transplantation, making nutritional support a major focus of pre-transplant management.

malnutrition common in chronic liver disease, particularly if the onset is in infants (Figure 29–5). Malnutrition itself may induce further derangements of liver function because the liver requires energy for a number of synthetic, storage, and detoxification functions. Thus, poor nutritional status is a significant but potentially modifiable risk factor adversely affecting outcome both before and after transplantation, making nutritional support a major focus of pre-transplant management. Efforts to optimize nutritional support by providing adequate protein energy, avoiding fasting, and using specialized amino acid and vitamin formulations including enteral nutritional supplementation can improve nutritional status.

Regular monitoring While on the waiting list, regular medical monitoring is essential. The progression of the liver disease is evaluated by recalculation of the PELD score at intervals, and assessment for development of complications of liver disease, which should be aggressively treated (see below). Any change in mortality risk should prompt re-evaluation of donor options, particularly if cadaver donors via the organ sharing system are likely limited because of size or blood group constraints.

Similarly, any intercurrent illness needs aggressive management, and notification to the transplant center.

Psychosocial support Families and patients find the waiting time very stressful. Mortality on the waiting list, although improved as a result of earlier referral and access to more donor options, is still a possibility. Ongoing counseling and preparation of a fully informed child and family through a multidisciplinary approach, including primary care physicians and family members as part of the team, is essential. The pre-transplant and post-transplant morbidity and mortality and the need for long-term immunosuppression require full, frank discussion, and acceptance of these risks as well as the potential benefits is arguably the most important part of the preparation of a family for liver transplantation.

Treatment of complications of chronic liver disease *Ascites* is a common complication of cirrhosis, and it is a sign of advanced liver disease (Table 29–7). Extravascular fluid accumulation in chronic liver disease represents a breakdown of intravascular volume homeostasis, which is controlled by capillary hydrostatic pressure and plasma colloid osmotic pressure. This process may develop insidiously or be precipitated by events such as gastrointestinal bleeding, infection, or the development of hepatoma. It is manifested by abdominal distension, pitting edema, sometimes pleural effusion, and/or the development of hernias. Treatment includes nutritional support, the judicious use of aldosterone antagonist and thiazide diuretics, and maintenance of plasma oncotic pressure by albumin infusion, but in some cases this becomes refractory. Tense ascites may require large-volume paracentesis and albumin infusion.

Coagulopathy in chronic liver disease is due to a combination of vitamin K malabsorption and deficiency, reduced synthesis of coagulation factors, and thrombocytopenia secondary to hypersplenism. These disturbances are particularly important in prognostic assessment, and in the genesis and management of gastrointestinal bleeding, and may lead to serious complications such as intracerebral bleeding and intravascular consumption coagulopathy. Management is directed at prevention/correction of vitamin K deficiency with oral or parenteral vitamin K supplements. If refractory, or there is active bleeding, or high risk of bleeding or for procedures, fresh frozen plasma infusions, platelet infusions, or the use of desmopressin may achieve temporary hemostasis.

Variceal bleeding, one of the major causes of morbidity and mortality, is a manifestation of portal hypertension, caused by a combination of increased portal blood flow and increased portal resistance. Signs and symptoms of portal hypertension are primarily the result of decompression of this elevated portal blood pressure through portosystemic collaterals, manifest as splenom-

Table 29–7.

Treatment of Complications of Chronic End-stage Liver Diseases

Ascites
Nutritional support
Avoid sodium intakes >2 mmol/kg
Spironolactone ± chlorothiazide, for example, Aldactazide: <3 years 12.5 mg qid, >3 years, up to 50 mg qid
Albumin infusions (if serum albumin >25 g/L) in a dose of 2 g/kg + frusemide 2 mg/kg
If refractory and symptomatic—paracentesis + albumin infusion

Coagulopathy
Vitamin K supplements (see Table 29–5)
Fresh frozen plasma 10 mL/kg—active bleeding, invasive procedures, PT >40 seconds, unresponsive to vitamin K
Platelet infusion—for active bleeding and count <20,000
Desmopressin—for active bleeding with global coagulation protein deficiencies (ii, vii, ix, x)

Variceal bleeding
Secure IV access, and hemostasis with vitamin K and fresh frozen plasma
Treat hypovolemia with blood transfusion and stabilize patient
Administer short-acting splanchnic vasoactive agent, for example, octreotide 25 mg/hour IV
Refer to center experienced in pediatric endoscopy, transcutaneous shunts, and liver transplantation
Prevent recurrence with endoscopic ablation, beta-blockers
Liver transplantation

Encephalopathy
Avoid precipitating factors
Avoid prolonged fasting, ensure nutritional support
Lactulose 0.4 mL/kg/day and PO vancomycin divided into three doses

Bacterial infections
High index of suspicion in biliary atresia (cholangitis) or ascites (primary peritonitis)
Minimize risk by nutritional support, active Rx of ascites, immunization for pneumococcus, hemophilus
Prophylactic antibiotics for invasive procedures, prevention of recurrence
Bacteriological studies and early institution of an extended-spectrum beta-lactam antibiotic

egaly and hypersplenism, the development of ascites, and the occurrence of esophageal, gastric, and rectal varices. Splenomegaly and hypersplenism rarely require specific intervention, and ascites is considered above. Bleeding from esophageal varices may be life-threatening and may precipitate liver failure, and requires prompt diagnosis and treatment (Figure 29–6). Salient points include: a secure intravenous infusion line; urgent blood transfusion; achieving hemostasis via parenteral vitamin K and plasma infusion; consideration for octreotide

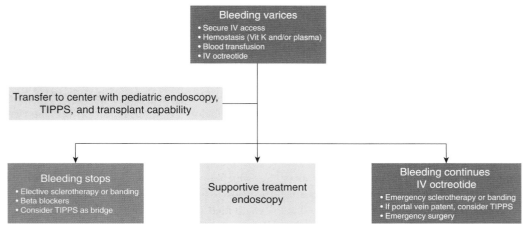

FIGURE 29–6 ■ Management algorithm for upper gastrointestinal bleeding in children with chronic liver disease.

infusion; and referral (when stable) to a tertiary center with experience in endoscopic sclerotherapy or banding, transcutaneous intrahepatic portosystemic shunts (TIPSS), and liver transplantation. Prevention of recurrence with vasoactive pharmacotherapy (e.g., beta-blockers), endoscopic ablation, or TIPSS may be indicated as a bridge to transplantation, but surgical shunts are best avoided in prospective transplant patients.

Encephalopathy in children with chronic liver disease is difficult to recognize, particularly in infants. Pathogenesis is related to four major processes: porto-systemic shunting, hepatocellular dysfunction, interaction of nitrogen metabolites from the intestine with the central nervous system, and altered neurotransmitter function. Early symptoms are subtle and include neurodevelopmental delay, school problems, lethargy, or sleep reversal (somnolent by day and insomnia by night). Intellectual impairment and personality change may occur in older children, while clouding of consciousness, asterixis, ataxia, stupor, and coma are late signs, these tending to develop in conjunction with precipitating events, such as gastrointestinal bleeding or the use of sedatives. It is also common following shunts for portal hypertension. Treatment is directed at removing precipitating factors, avoidance of fasting, and reducing intestinal protein load with lactulose, and broad-spectrum antibiotics (Table 29–7). Protein restriction is not usually necessary, and not recommended in children due to the risk of further nutritional compromise.

Bacterial infections may precipitate other complications, such as encephalopathy, ascites, and hepatorenal syndrome, and are predisposed to liver disease by immune dysfunction, neutropenia, and alterations in mucosal barriers. Portal hypertension makes patients susceptible to bacteremia, perhaps by inducing bacterial translocation of the gut. Spontaneous bacterial peritonitis is a serious complication of ascites and should be considered in all children with ascites who show signs of sepsis. In BA, recurrent cholangitis is a risk factor for death on the waiting list. Urinary and respiratory tract infections are also frequent, and bacteremia commonly results from invasive investigations. Other risk factors for infection are low serum albumin, gastrointestinal bleeding, ascites, intensive care unit admission for any reason, and endoscopy. Certain agents are more virulent and more common in patients with liver disease, including *Klebsiella*, *E. coli*, *Campylobacter*, *Yersinia*, *Plesiomonas*, *Enterococcus*, *Aeromonas*, and *Listeria* species. Preventative measures such as pneumococcal and *Haemophilus* vaccination, prophylactic antibiotics for invasive procedures, nutritional support, and management of ascites may reduce risk. When infection is suspected, immediate bacteriological studies and early institution of antimicrobial therapy with a broad-spectrum antibiotic (e.g.,

Table 29–8.

Medically "Treatable" Causes of PALF

Drugs and toxins
- Acetominophen—*N*-acetyl cysteine (NAC) by continuous infusion
- *Amanita phalloides*—steroids, silibinin, penicillin
- Others—cease/avoid the drug

Immune diseases
- Autoimmune hepatitis—steroids/azathiaprine
- Hemophagocytic (macrophage activation) syndrome—high-dose of steroids, etopaside, cydosporin

Metabolic liver diseases
- Tyrosinemia I—nitisinone (NTBC)
- Wilson's disease—chelation with penicillamine, zinc
- Galactosemia—lactose-free diet
- Neonatal hemochromatosis—antioxidant "cocktail" -IV NAC, selenium 3 mcg/kg/day
- Tocopherol PEG succinate 25 IU/kg/day, vitamin C 25 mg/kg/day

Viral infections
- Herpes viruses—acyclovir
- Enteroviruses—pleconaril
- Other viruses—consider IVIG

an extended-spectrum beta-lactam antibiotic such as tazobactam + piperacillin (Zosyn)) are recommended, while awaiting culture and sensitivities.

Pediatric acute liver failure

Whenever PALF is suspected, as indicated above and in Figure 29–3, early referral to a transplant center is advisable. Key features of management involve simultaneously supporting the patient, evaluating the cause, particularly medically "treatable" causes (Table 29–8), monitoring the progress of the liver failure, and assessing possible donor options in case liver transplant is available.[5] However, 50% of cases recover without transplantation, that is, 50% will die without transplantation, there are some contraindications, and some situations where a transplant becomes futile.

Supportive measures Most cases require intensive care, with aggressive management of coagulopathy and encephalopathy, often requiring ventilatory and hemodynamic support. Hepatorenal syndrome and infection are not uncommon complications that require further aggressive management. Medical treatment for "treatable" causes should be instituted without delay (Table 29–8). *Investigations* are listed in Table 29–9, and are divided into those required for monitoring and supportive treatment, those required to rule out medically "treatable" causes, and those to evaluate other known

Table 29–9.

Investigating Pediatric Acute Liver Failure

Routine patient monitoring

- Hematology—FBC, ESR, reticulocyte count
- Coagulation—PR/INR, APTT, fibrinogen, factor V
- Glucose homeostasis
- Blood gases
- Blood/urine cultures
- Liver bilirubin tests —direct/indirect, ALP, GGT, AST, ALT, total protein, albumin, globulins
- Biochemistry—sodium, potassium, BUN, creatinine, calcium, phosphate, magnesium, chloride, amylase, uric acid, ammonia
- ECG, echocardiogram
- Imaging CXR, abdominal ultrasound and Doppler, head CT if cornatose

"Treatable" causes of PALF

- Infant—neonatal iron storage, tyrosinemia, fructosemia, galactosemia
- Specific investigations—ferritin
- Urine-reducing substances and galactose-1-phosphate uridyltransferase plasma and urine organic acids, amino acids, urine succinylacetone
- Child/adolescent—acetaminophen toxicity, autoimmune hepatitis, Wilson's disease
- Specific investigations—acetaminophen level
- IgG, protein electrophoresis, 24-hour urine copper, split lamp eye exam, liver biopsy

Other diagnostic tests

- Virology HBV, CMV, EBV, HAV, HCV, HSV, HIV, varicella, measles, parvovirus, HHV-6 PCR
- Serology toxoplasmosis, leptospirosis
- Special tests
- Fasting pyruvate/lactate
- Acylcarnitine profile
- Alpha-fetoprotein
- Very-long-chain fatty acids
- Plasma and urine organic acids, amino acids
- Plasma and urine toxicology screen
- Bone marrow
- Skin biopsy
- WBC enzymes
- Muscle biopsy
- Abdominal ultrasound and Doppler
- Liver biopsy

causes, including those where transplant might be contraindicated.

Indications for transplantation Unless there is a contraindication to transplant, most patients are listed for a donor search, and the decision as to whether to proceed is made when a donor becomes available. The decision to go ahead with a transplant at that time is based on rate of progression of liver failure or lack of signs of improvement, and the presence of defined poor prognostic indicators, including age <1 year, progressive encephalopathy, vitamin K-unresponsive PT >40 seconds and INR >4, hypoglycemia with ongoing high dextrose requirement, serum bilirubin >300 μmol/L (17.5 mg/dL), a rapid reduction in liver size clinically (plus precipitous fall in AST), and/or no regenerative features and extensive hepatic necrosis (<20% viable hepatocytes/HPF) on liver biopsy. For acetaminophen liver injury, where specific treatment with *N*-acetyl cysteine should be instituted, consider transplant if pH <7.3, creatinine >0.3 mmol/L, and/or INR >6.5 with no improvement on treatment. While waiting for a donor organ, if there are signs of stabilization or evidence of recovering function (improved coagulation parameters and encephalopathy), transplantation may be deferred. Similarly, if circumstances arise in which a transplant becomes futile, then transplantation is not indicated. Examples include uncontrolled systemic sepsis, irreversible neurological injury, or a diagnosis of underlying non-hepatic disease, such as malignancy or a mitochondrial disorder.

Post-transplant Management

The goals of post-transplant management are to manage and treat postoperative complications, and develop a balanced long-term immunotherapy regimen that minimizes infection and side effects but controls rejection (Figure 29–7). There must be provision for long-term follow-up, with proactive treatment of common problems. As with pre-transplant management, good communication systems should be in place between primary physicians and transplant centers. Because of their accessibility and long-term relationship with patients, primary care physicians are in the best position

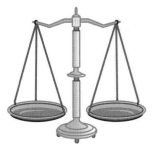

Graft dysfunction
Rejection
Vascular complications
Biliary complications

Immunosuppression
Infection
Side effects
Metabolic effects

FIGURE 29–7 ■ Post-transplant management. The ideal balance in immunotherapy, graft function, and patient well-being.

to detect the early signs of complications, recognize or suspect poor compliance with immunosuppressive therapy, manage common problems, and provide ongoing support to families.

Although most children who have had liver transplants can expect cure of their liver disease and improved quality of life (see the section "Outcomes"), they require indefinite follow-up and often require medical attention for complications or co-morbid conditions related to their immunosuppressive drug therapy. While modern immunosuppressant regimes have reduced rates of graft loss due to rejection, they impart major risks for infection, growth failure, metabolic complications, and malignancy.[4,8,9] Indeed, there is significantly more post-transplant morbidity and mortality from infection than from rejection, particularly in infants. This has led to a trend toward minimization of immunosuppression, which is supported by evidence that some rejection facilitates graft tolerance and thus is not necessarily always harmful in liver transplantation (as distinct from other solid organ transplants).

Complications after liver transplantation

Serious post-transplant complications are divided into those that occur in the first 3–12 months ("early"), and these are relatively common, and those occurring after 12 months ("late"), which are generally uncommon (Table 29–10). In addition, there are many common medical issues, and some specific long-term issues that require medical attention in relation to the long-term use of immunosuppressive medications (Table 29–11). Most "early" complications relate to surgical issues, and/or immunosuppression, most notably infection, vascular complications of the graft, and biliary leaks. Infection (detailed below) is the most common cause of post-transplant mortality.[9] Rejection (see below) does occur but usually responds to treatment with steroid pulse dosing, and appears not to contribute to either graft or patient mortality. "Late" complications include biliary strictures, which are uncommon and generally respond to percutaneous biliary dilatation and stent procedures. Most late complications are primarily related to the effects of long-term immunosuppression, notably infections such as Epstein–Barr virus and associated post-transplant lymphoproliferative disease (PTLD), warts, skin cancers, and side effects of immunosuppression such as renal dysfunction, hypertension, and immune dysregulation. Late or chronic rejection is most often a manifestation of compliance, and late graft losses are most commonly related to this.

Outline of immunosuppression regimens

There is some variability among transplant centers in the details of immunosuppressive therapy. The goals are to avoid rejection and graft injury, to encourage some

Table 29–10.

Post-transplant Complications

'Early': first 12 months
- First month
  - Primary graft non-function
  - Vascular complication
  - Infections/bacterial sepsis
  - Wound and drain issues
  - Biliary leaks
  - Intra-abdominal fluid collections
  - Rejection
- 1–3 months
  - Infections (CMV, EBV)
  - Biliary strictures
  - Hepatic vein stenosis
  - Rejection
- 3–12 months
  - PTLD
  - CMV infections
  - Biliary strictures
  - Rejection
  - Hypertension
  - Poor growth

"Late" >12 months
- PTLD
- Unusual infections
- Renal dysfunction
- Hypertension
- Non-compliance with medications
- Growth failure
- Late biliary strictures

Table 29–11.

Post-transplant Immunization Schedule for Liver Transplant Recipients

Starting 6 months post-transplant	
Hepatitis B	6, 8, 10 months if not previously given
DTP	Resume standard schedule
H. influenzae type b	Resume standard schedule
Polio	Resume standard schedule; patient and siblings must receive inactivated polio vaccine[*]
Measles, mumps, rubella	At 6 months if not previously given, confirmed by vaccine response with titers
Varicella	At 7 months if not previously given, confirmed by vaccine response with titers[†]
Pneumavax	Required for patients with splenectomy or asplenia[‡]
Hepatitis A	At 12 months
Influenza	Yearly

[*]NA live viruses.
[†]Patients may experience low-grade fever and vesicles at injection site.
[‡]Penicillin prophylaxis is also recommended for these patients.

early allorecognition (not necessarily to eliminate rejection altogether), and to minimize immunosuppressive side effects.[4,8,9] Most commonly, the immunotherapy plan is based on initial high-dose steroids, progression to oral steroids, introduction of an oral calcineurin inhibitor (CNI), usually tacrolimus (TAC), and oral mycophenylate mofetil (MMF), with individualized progressive tapering and cessation of steroids over 3–12 months, followed by cessation of MMF. Some centers include induction therapy with monoclonal antibodies to reduce the need for steroids. Most patients achieve low-level TAC monotherapy by 12–24 months post-transplant. The use of cyclosporine, an earlier CNI, is declining because of a higher side-effect profile. TAC, 0.15–0.3 mg/kg/day, is administered orally, with titration of TAC dose to achieve trough levels between 8 and 10 ng/mL on routine monitoring over the first 12 months, beyond which levels of around 5 ng/mL are considered acceptable. If used, MMF is given orally at 150–600 mg/m²/dose and is discontinued after a rejection-free interval of 3–6 months post-transplant. Patients aged <1–2 years, patients with primary liver tumors, or patients who are leukopenic, with white blood count <3000, are not given MMF. Monitoring of kidney function is important in patients on CNIs, assessed by occurrence of systemic hypertension, and serial measurement of serum creatinine. In addition, creatinine clearance studies are done after 1 and 3 years.

Infection prophylaxis and surveillance

Prophylactic antibiotics are given intravenously for 48 hours post-transplant, and then usually discontinued. Any invasive procedure thereafter is usually managed with antibiotic cover, including dental procedures. A prophylactic antifungal agent (such as fluconazole) is administered orally for 2–3 months. Prophylactic antiviral medications are used in all patients. Acyclovir is prescribed for 3 months if both donor and recipient were CMV and EBV negative, and ganciclovir for 6 months if either donor or recipient was positive for either CMV or EBV. CMV and EBV naive patients have surveillance serum CMV and EBV viral load by polymerase chain reaction (PCR), usually on a monthly basis while heavily immunosuppressed, or as indicated if there is presentation with an illness. A post-transplant *immunization schedule* is summarized in Table 29–11. Despite these precautions, serious bacterial infections occur in about one-third of patients, mostly in the first 3 months post-transplantation, and serious viral infections caused by CMV or EBV occur in about 10% of patients.[8,9] Risks for bacterial/fungal infections included young recipient age, Hispanic race, use of donor organ variants, higher bilirubin, prolonged anhepatic time, and use of cyclosporine instead of TAC.[9] Serious viral infection risks include young age (PTLD is 10-fold

higher in infants), donor organ variants, and experiencing rejection episodes causing immunosuppression to be increased. Any illness characterized by fever, respiratory, abdominal, urinary, or gastrointestinal symptoms requires careful evaluation, and, in selected cases, viral, bacterial, and other diagnostic workup. Empiric preemptive therapy should be used as indicated.

The cornerstone of treatment for serious infections is the temporary reduction or cessation of immunosuppression, along with appropriate antiviral or antimicrobial drug therapy. PTLD caused by Epstein–Barr virus is a potentially life-threatening consequence of CNI therapy, resulting in inability of the immune system to control the proliferation of EBV-infected B cells. Presenting features are variable, and include mononucleosis-like symptoms (fatigue, fevers, and lymphadenopathy), or localized or disseminated lymphoproliferation with tumors involving the lymph nodes, liver, lung, kidney, bone marrow, central nervous system, or small intestine. Because increases in EBV viral load in peripheral blood typically precede the development of PTLD, measurement of viral load by quantitative PCR is useful in monitoring. Tissue biopsy of associated tumors shows plasma cell hyperplasia, B-cell hyperplasia, B-cell lymphoma, or immunoblastic lymphoma. Immunostaining can be used to reveal the clonality of the proliferating B cells in these tumors or in circulating leukemic cells. These may be monoclonal, oligoclonal, or polyclonal; patients with polyclonal lesions have the best prognosis. The diagnosis is confirmed by demonstrating EBV proteins in biopsy tissue. Treatment involves cessation or reduction of immunosuppression, surgical removal of local lymphoproliferative lesions, especially in the gastrointestinal tract, ganciclovir, monoclonal-antibody therapy with rituximab, a monoclonal antibody directed against the CD20 B-cell antigen, and in some cases cytotoxic chemotherapy. The latter has been effective for patients with lymphoma or who have had no response to a reduction in the dose of immunosuppressive drugs or to other therapies. Complete cessation of CNIs is used in high-risk patients with low rejection risk (young age and use of cyclosporine or antilymphocyte products).

Monitoring, diagnosis, and treatment of rejection

Routine monitoring of liver biochemistry and CNI trough levels is undertaken frequently during the early post-transplant period, reducing to monthly, unless otherwise indicated. Rises in transaminases without any evidence for biliary or vascular etiology or intercurrent illness are presumptive for acute cellular rejection (ACR) without biopsy. Doubtful cases require diagnostic liver biopsy. Rejection episodes are treated with a 3-day pulse of prednisone (2–5 mg/kg/day) and an increase in TAC to temporarily achieve trough levels of 10–12 ng/mL. If patients do not respond to a 3-day steroid pulse, then other options include higher dose intravenous steroid pulses, and/or addition of other immunosuppressive drugs. As noted above, rejection rarely is a factor in patients of graft losses.[4,8,9] Risks are lowest in infants, higher in adolescents, and highest in those of any age receiving blood type-mismatched organs.[9] Biopsy-proven chronic rejection is uncommon, and is treated with continuation of TAC to achieve levels of 10–12 ng/mL, and the addition of azothioprine at 2 mg/kg/day. In adolescents, this chronic rejection is most commonly related to poor compliance.

Common problems

Patients on long-term immunosuppression are bound to encounter issues related to *common illnesses* such as vomiting, diarrhea, and fevers (Table 29–12). These illnesses should be treated on their merits, but generally always require medical consultation, in case of serious or progressive illness. Missed immunosuppressant medications should not be double dosed, but simply resumed at normal doses as soon as possible. Gastroenteritis illnesses often spuriously result in elevated TAC levels and mild elevations of liver transaminases. *Infection contacts,* particularly with serious viral infections such as *varicella*, require consideration of prophylactic therapy. *Regular dental care* is mandatory, due to the frequency of pre-existing poor dentine, high caries rate and delayed tooth development in patients with liver diseases, and the need for ongoing dental hygiene in immunosuppressed patients. Major dental work requires prophylaxis with antibiotics because of high occurrence of bacteremia during these procedures.[10] *Compliance with medications* is a common issue in adolescents particularly, and poor compliance can have serious consequences. This is suspected when monthly surveillance TAC levels show a large variability, and/or there are unexplained increases in liver transaminases. Systems such as mobile phone reminder, text messages, daily

Table 29–12.

Common Issues in Post-transplant Follow-up

Managing Common Problems	Managing Specific Problems
Vomiting	Compliance
Diarrhea	Liver dysfunction
Fever	Growth
Missed medications	Development
Infection contact	Skin problems—warts, eczema, solar cancers
Dental care	Pregnancy and fertility

diaries, and closer monitoring have been shown to improve compliance.[11] *Unexplained elevations of transaminases* should be evaluated. Although most are temporary due to intercurrent illness or lapses in compliance, persistent changes could indicate late graft dysfunction and require investigation with imaging and/or liver biopsy. Follow-up of growth and development with yearly monitoring is the norm for all pediatric transplant recipients. Deviations require more detailed evaluation and treatment. *Skin conditions* such as eczema and warts are more common in immunosuppressed patients. These often require specialist referral and management. Skin cancers should be minimized with active lifelong solar prophylaxis. Finally, issues of *fertility and pregnancy* are increasingly being raised in long-term survivors of pediatric liver transplantation. Many successful pregnancies have been recorded, and the current evidence suggests that pregnancy is safe after transplant.[12,13] Pregnancy does require close management by a team of experienced physicians. Significant experience has indicated that the use of CNIs, azathioprine, and prednisolone is safe during pregnancy, but few data are available for newer immunosuppressants such as MMF, and thus these agents are not recommended.[13,14]

OUTCOMES

Patient and Graft Outcomes

Current 1-year patient and graft survival rates across pediatric centers of expertise are 90–95% and 80–85%, respectively, and at 3 years approximately 85% and 80%, with only minimal decline after that.[4,8] These overall good outcomes have been achieved by early referral with excellent pre-transplant care (particularly of hepatic complications and nutritional support), the improved donor options mentioned above, and advances in post-transplant management, particularly more targeted and age-specific immunosuppression. Unfortunately, there is still a small but significant risk of dying while on the waiting list. Waiting list mortality risk factors include the infant age group, a high PELD score of ≥20, poor nutrition, and acute liver failure.[4] Early post-transplantation mortality risk factors include infant recipients, poor nutritional status, need for re-transplantation, usually secondary to surgical complications, and acute liver failure.[4] Overall, infection is the single most important cause of death, contributed to by immunosuppression and surgical complications.[9] Early episodes of rejection (<6 months after transplantation) do not contribute to mortality or graft failure. Graft failure risks include poor nutrition, the use of cadaveric reduced-size donor segments, the use of cyclosporine versus TAC, and recurrent/chronic rejection.[4,9]

Functional and Long-term Outcomes

With careful follow-up management and close attention to detail, most pediatric liver transplant recipients can expect an excellent long-term outcome. There is remarkable recovery from the effects of their liver or metabolic disease, an expectation of long-term survival with good graft function, catch-up growth (albeit sometimes incomplete), and a good quality of life.[8,15] In general, in the first 5 years post-transplant, parents report higher emotional stress and disruption of family activities compared to a normal population, although the level of family function appears normal. At 10 years post-transplant, >95% of survivors have normal graft function, and self-report good to excellent quality of life and normal school achievements.[16,17] Non-adherence to the medical regimen is perhaps the most important predictor of late graft dysfunction, and health-related quality of life may independently correlate with non-adherence. As improvements are being realized in long-term immunosuppression regimens, notably minimizing immunosuppression, a diminishing number of patients suffer long-term complications of immunosuppression. These include altered diabetes, decreased renal function, hypertension, cancer, and osteopenia.

Information on Outcomes

In the United States, all transplants and transplant outcomes are monitored by the Organ Procurement and Transplant Network (OPTN), whose primary purposes are to operate and monitor equitable allocation of organs donated for transplantation, maintain a waiting list of potential recipients, match recipients with donor organs according to established criteria, and facilitate the efficient, effective placement of organs for transplantation. Outcome data are available in the public domain, and practitioners and families can view national, regional, and individual center risk-adjusted waiting times, and outcomes by accessing the OPTN website.

REFERENCES

1. Yersiz H, Cameron AM, Carmody I, et al. Split liver transplantation. *Transplant Proc.* 2006;38(2):602–603.
2. Freeman RB Jr, Wiesner RH, Roberts JP, McDiarmid S, Dykstra DM, Merion RM. Improving liver allocation: MELD and PELD. *Am J Transplant.* 2004;4(suppl 9):114–131 [review].
3. Magee JC, Krishnan SM, Benfield MR, Hsu DT, Shneider BL. Pediatric transplantation in the United States, 1997–2006. *Am J Transplant.* 2008;8(4 Pt 2):935–945.
4. Martin SR, Atkison P, Anand R, Lindblad AS, SPLIT Research Group. Studies of Pediatric Liver Transplantation 2002: patient and graft survival and rejection in pediatric recipients of a first liver transplant in the United States and Canada. *Pediatr Transplant.* 2004;8(3):273–283.
5. Squires RH Jr, Shneider BL, Bucuvalas J, et al. Acute liver failure in children: the first 348 patients in the pediatric acute liver failure study group. *J Pediatr.* 2006;148(5):652–658.
6. Bassett MD, Murray KF. Biliary atresia: recent progress. *J Clin Gastroenterol.* 2008;42(6):720–729 [review].
7. Chen LE, Shepherd RW, Nadler ML, Chapman WC, Kotru A, Lowell JA. Liver transplantation and chemotherapy in children with unresectable primary hepatic malignancies: development of a management algorithm. *J Pediatr Gastroenterol Nutr.* 2006;43(4):487–493.
8. Turmelle YP, Nadler ML, Anderson CD, Doyle MB, Lowell JA, Shepherd RW. Towards minimizing immunosuppression in pediatric liver transplant recipients. *Pediatr Transplant.* 2009 Aug;13(5):553–559.
9. Shepherd RW, Turmelle Y, Nadler M, et al., SPLIT Research Group. Risk factors for rejection and infection in pediatric liver transplantation. *Am J Transplant.* 2008;8(2):396–403.
10. Glassman P, Wong C, Gish R. A review of liver transplantation for the dentist and guidelines for dental management. *Spec Care Dent.* 1993;13(2):74–80.
11. De Bleser L, Matteson M, Dobbels F, Russell C, De Geest S. Interventions to improve medication-adherence after transplantation: a systematic review. *Transpl Int.* 2009;22(8):780–797.
12. Surti B, Tan J, Saab S. Pregnancy and liver transplantation. *Liver Int.* 2008;28(9):1200–1206.
13. Coscia LA, Constantinescu S, Moritz MJ, Radomski JS, Gaughan WJ, McGrory CH, Armenti VT; National Transplantation Pregnancy Registry. Report from the National Transplantation Pregnancy Registry (NTPR): outcomes of pregnancy after transplantation. *Clin Transpl.* 2007:29–42.
14. Anderka MT, Lin AE, Abuelo DN, Mitchell AA, Rasmussen SA. Reviewing the evidence for mycophenolate mofetil as a new teratogen: case report and review of the literature. *Am J Med Genet A.* 2009;149A(6):1241–1248.
15. Bucuvalas JC, Campbell KM, Cole CR, Guthery SL. Outcomes after liver transplantation: keep the end in mind. *J Pediatr Gastroenterol Nutr.* 2006;43(suppl 1):S41–S48.
16. Bucuvalas JC, Alonso E, Magee JC, Talwalkar J, Hanto D, Doo E. Improving long-term outcomes after liver transplantation in children. *Am J Transplant.* 2008;8(12):2506–2513.
17. Alonso EM, Neighbors K, Barton FB, et al., Studies of Pediatric Liver Transplant Research Group. Health-related quality of life and family function following pediatric liver transplantation. *Liver Transpl.* 2008;14(4):460–468.

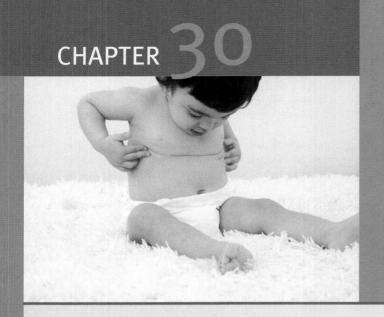

CHAPTER 30

Liver Failure and Portal Hypertension

Elizabeth Mileti and
Philip Rosenthal

DEFINITION AND EPIDEMIOLOGY

Acute liver failure (ALF) is a rare but devastating result of hepatic necrosis in previously healthy individuals. Hepatic function rapidly declines within days to weeks and is often complicated by coagulopathy, hepatic encephalopathy (HE), hypoglycemia, acute renal failure, sepsis, and gastrointestinal bleeding. These complications can lead to death with mortality rates up to 40% in the United States.[1]

Children who develop ALF by definition have no previous history of liver disease. Traditionally, the criteria for defining ALF included the development of HE within 8–12 weeks of the first signs of illness. This definition has since been revised due to the difficultly in assessing HE in infants and younger children and the variability in initial presentation.

In 1999 the Pediatric Acute Liver Failure Study Group (PALFSG) was formed to better understand the pathogenesis and treatment of ALF. An important initial task included defining ALF in childhood and creating a scale to assess encephalopathy in children younger than 4 years of age. The definition of ALF in children included four major criteria: (1) the absence of prior liver disease; (2) serum biochemical markers showing evidence of acute liver injury; (3) coagulopathy not correctable with vitamin K administration; (4) international normalized ratio (INR) ≥1.5 in the setting of HE or ≥2.0 without HE.[2] A scale was created to help assess HE in children under the age of 4 years (Table 30–1).

Table 30–1.

Staging of Hepatic Encephalopathy

Stage	Clinical Presentation	Reflexes/Asterixis	Neurological Signs
Children 3 years and younger			
I	Mood changes, confused	Normal/none	Tremor, apraxia
II	Decreased inhibitions, drowsy, inappropriate behavior	Hyper-reflexic, possible asterixis	Dysarthria, ataxia
III	Stuporous, able to follow simple commands, arousable	Babinski sign/asterixis present	Muscle rigidity
IV	Comatose, arouse to painful stimuli (IV a) or no response to stimuli (IV b)	Absent	Decerebrate or decorticate
Older children			
Early (I and II)	Crying inconsolable, inattention to task, sleep reversal	Normal or hyper-reflexic/unreliable	Untestable
Mid (III)	Somnolence, stupor, combativeness	Hyper-reflexic/unreliable	Most likely untestable
Late (IV)	Comatose, arouse to painful stimuli (IV a) or no response to stimuli (IV b)	Absent	Decerebrate or decorticate

The overall incidence of pediatric ALF is low, but the rate of devastating complications and mortality is high. The primary causes of ALF in children include viral hepatitis, drug-induced liver failure, metabolic causes, autoimmune disease, and idiopathic causes. Approximately 50% of cases of pediatric ALF have no known cause.[2] Regardless of the cause, ALF is a medical emergency and early recognition affects outcome. Prior to liver transplantation becoming an available treatment option, death rates approached 100%.[1] Currently, short-term survival with liver transplantation is >65%.[3]

PATHOGENESIS

The pathologic features of ALF include rapid and massive hepatocyte death, with failure of the remaining hepatocytes to regenerate. The mechanism of this severe hepatic necrosis is unknown. Although approximately 50% of cases of ALF have no identifiable etiology, we know that there is variability with age (Table 30–2).[2,4,5] In neonates, inborn errors of metabolism and infections are often found to be the predominant causes of ALF, while in older children toxins, drugs, and autoimmune disorders are more common causes.[4–7]

Multiple factors must be considered in neonates who develop ALF including maternal exposures, infant exposures, perinatal infections, metabolic disorders, genetic disorders, hypotension/shock, and hematologic disorders.[5] Identifying the cause allows for an improved determination of probable prognosis and treatment options. Neonatal infections can be severe and generalized. Perinatal infections with herpes virus, hepatitis B virus, adenovirus, cytomegalovirus, and echovirus in addition to others have been known to cause ALF in neonates. Herpes simplex virus (HSV), in particular, is the most common viral etiology and a high cause of mortality.[2,5] Skin lesions are not necessarily present, but patients often have a significant serum transaminitis and coagulopathy. Intravenous acyclovir should be instituted immediately if HSV is suspected. Bacterial infections from group B *Streptococcus*, *Escherichia coli*, and *Listeria monocytogenes* are the most frequent causes of sepsis in neonates that can also progress to ALF from hypoperfusion and shock.

Metabolic disorders must be considered in the neonatal period as a cause of ALF and must be investigated promptly since dietary changes and disease-specific treatments can be life saving. Metabolic disorders to consider in this age group include galactosemia, type I tyrosinemia, hereditary fructose intolerance, urea cycle disorders, respiratory chain defects, mitochondrial disorders, and neonatal hemochromatosis (NH). In galactosemia and hereditary fructose intolerance, the treatment is removal of the offending dietary agent that is life saving. Type I tyrosinemia is treated by giving a low-phenylalanine and low-tyrosine diet along with 2(2-nitro-4-trifluoromethylbenzoyl)-1,3-cyclohexenedione (NTBC) that prevents the formation of fumarylacetoacetate, the toxic metabolite of

Table 30–2.

Causes of Acute Liver Failure by Age

Etiology	Disease
Neonates	
Infectious	Herpes simplex virus, cytomegalovirus, hepatitis B, adenovirus, echovirus, coxsackie, syphilis, bacterial infections (leading to sepsis and shock)
Metabolic	Galactosemia, type I tyrosinemia, hereditary fructose intolerance, urea cycle disorders, respiratory chain defects, mitochondrial disorders, neonatal hemochromatosis, Niemann–Pick disease type C, Zellweger syndrome, inborn errors of bile acid synthesis
Vascular/ischemic	Congestive heart failure—as a result of congenital heart disease, hypoperfusion
Hematologic	Hemophagocytic lymphohistiocytosis (HLH)
Older children	
Infectious	Epstein–Barr virus, hepatitis A, B, non-A, non-B, non-C hepatitis, herpes virus, sepsis
Toxins	*Amanita phalloides*, carbon tetrachloride
Drugs	Acetaminophen, halothane, antituberculous medications (isoniazid, rifampicin, pyrazinamide), antimicrobials (beta-lactams, tetracycline, macrolides, sulfonamides), ketoconazole, antiepileptics (carbamazepine, valproate)
Metabolic	Wilson disease
Autoimmune	Types 1 and 2
Vascular/ischemic	Congestive heart failure, Budd–Chiari syndrome
Malignancies	Hepatoblastoma, leukemia, non-Hodgkin lymphoma

tyrosine. Since the introduction of NTBC, patients with type I tyrosinemia have improved survival rates. Patients may still require liver transplantation if they do not respond to NTBC or are at high risk for the development of malignant hepatocellular carcinoma nodules.[8] Mitochondrial disorders have many different clinical presentations, with ALF seen in the context of multiorgan failure. Transmission is through maternal DNA. Liver transplantation is not indicated since the disease is progressive and not localized only to the liver. In NH, ALF occurs at birth. Massive iron deposition is seen both intra- and extrahepatically, but spares the reticuloendothelial system. The exact pathogenesis is unknown but it is thought to be related to maternal alloimmune injury and there is a high recurrence rate in families of affected infants. Diagnosis is made by excluding other causes of liver failure, finding elevated levels of serum ferritin, near complete saturation of iron-binding capacity, MRI demonstration of extrahepatic iron deposition, and biopsy confirmation of elevated iron stores. Treatment with an antioxidant cocktail consisting of vitamin E, N-acetylcysteine (NAC), selenium, desferoxamine, and prostaglandin E1 may be helpful but often NH requires liver transplantation for cure.[9] An article published in 2009 showed newborn infants with NH treated with a combination of high-dose IVIG and exchange transfusion were four times as likely to improve and not require liver transplantation.[10] Additionally, the experimental use of gamma-globulin infusions to pregnant mothers of previously affected infants has had very promising results in preventing recurrence with subsequent pregnancies.[11] Unfortunately, presently there is no way to diagnose NH in a first pregnancy.

In children over the age of 3 years, the most common causes in the United States of pediatric ALF are from acetaminophen ingestion, non-acetaminophen toxins, viral infections, and metabolic derangements. Acetaminophen ingestions, intentional or accidental, account for 21% of pediatric ALF.[2] This is much different from the younger age group where only 2% of ALF in children under the age of 3 years is from acetaminophen overdose. Acetaminophen ingestion fortunately also has the highest rate of spontaneous recovery without the need for liver transplant. Non-acetaminophen, drug-induced liver failure accounts for approximately 7% of PALF in this older age group and is usually caused by antimicrobials, antiepileptics, or antituberculous medications, though multiple drugs can cause hepatotoxicity and can lead to ALF.[12] Ingested toxins from poisonous mushrooms (Amanita phalloides) also referred to as the "death cap" can also cause ALF. Infectious causes of hepatitis, leading to fulminant hepatic failure, occur less frequently and are mostly caused by Epstein–Barr virus. Another major cause of ALF in the older age group is Wilson disease. In Wilson disease, there are low serum copper and serum ceruloplasmin levels; elevated urinary copper excretion and hemolysis are present. Wilson disease can cause chronic liver disease that can be treated with D-penicillamine or triene therapy, but if the presentation is as ALF, liver transplantation is often required for survival (see Chapter 25). Autoimmune hepatitis, which usually presents as a chronic liver disease, can also present as ALF. It causes approximately 6% of all ALF cases and when presenting as ALF often needs liver transplantation for survival. Autoimmune hepatitis is more frequently seen in the older age group, but is also seen in children <3 years old.[2]

CLINICAL PRESENTATION

The characteristic findings in ALF include the abrupt onset of jaundice, encephalopathy, and elevated biochemical markers of liver injury. These include a prolonged prothrombin time (PT) and elevated serum transaminases in a previously healthy child. Initial symptoms of jaundice, abdominal pain, nausea, and vomiting may be non-specific. Clinical presentation may vary with age and etiology of liver failure, so a detailed history is important in determining the next steps in therapy. Symptoms may progress rapidly within days or may take weeks to develop, depending on the etiology of the liver failure.

On physical exam, the child may be jaundiced or may just have scleral icterus. The liver size can be variable. The child may have bleeding gums, bruises, or petechiae. The neurological exam is extremely important and can be difficult to assess, especially in younger children under the age of 4 years (see Table 30–1).

History should focus on immunization status (particularly hepatitis A and B vaccinations), travel history, history of blood transfusions, current medications, recreational drug use, ingestions (intentional or accidental), history of mushroom picking, and family history (Table 30–3). In infants, it is important to ask about history of seizures, hypoglycemic events, or developmental delays that may indicate a metabolic disorder as the cause for the liver failure.

Laboratory findings in ALF include elevated serum aspartate aminotransferase (AST) and alanine aminotransferase (ALT) levels, abnormal coagulation studies (prolonged PT and elevated INR), and increased total and direct-reacting bilirubin levels (Table 30–4). Abnormalities in electrolytes such as hyponatremia, hypokalemia, hypocalcemia, and hypomagnesemia can be present. Hypoglycemia is an important marker of liver failure and an indicator of liver glycogen dysregulation. In patients suspected of having autoimmune hepatitis, a

Table 30–3.

Pertinent History Questions

Any previous history of jaundice or liver disease?

Immunization status: has child had hepatitis A and B vaccinations? Has the child had chicken pox or the vaccine?

Travel history: endemic areas for hepatitis A, E (especially in pregnant women)

Any history of ingestions (accidental or intentional)?

Recent medications: antibiotics, antiepileptics, antituberculous medications, herbal supplements

Acetaminophen history: concentration of acetaminophen preparation (infant drops versus children's elixir)? What amount was given and interval of dosing? Any medications taken with acetaminophen derivative or combination medications with acetaminophen as a component?

Any history of mushroom picking or wild mushroom ingestion?

For infants: any history of developmental delay, seizure history, or hypoglycemia?

Table 30–4.

Initial Laboratory Analysis

Coagulation studies (prothrombin time/INR)

Chemistries (sodium, potassium, chloride, bicarbonate, calcium, magnesium, phosphorus, glucose, blood urea nitrogen, creatinine)

Liver test (AST, ALT, alkaline phosphatase, GGT, total bilirubin, direct bilirubin, albumin, total protein)

Complete blood count with differential

Blood culture

Blood type and screen

Acetaminophen level

Toxicology screen

Ammonia

Amylase

Lipase

Urinalysis and urine culture

Pregnancy test

Viral hepatitis serologies (anti-HAV IgM, HBsAg, anti-HBc IgM, anti-HCV, anti-HEV)

Ceruloplasmin levels

Autoimmune markers (ANA, anti-smooth muscle antibody, anti-LKM, anti-mitochondrial antibody)

HIV

reversed serum albumin to globulin protein ratio is seen. Autoimmune markers are important for diagnosis. These should include antinuclear antibody, anti-smooth muscle antibody, and anti-liver–kidney-microsomal antibody.

Patients with Wilson disease often have a hemolytic anemia that is Coombs-negative. They also tend to have low serum alkaline phosphatase levels, hyperuricemia, and elevated serum copper levels with decreased serum ceruloplasmin levels.

CHRONIC LIVER FAILURE AND PORTAL HYPERTENSION

Chronic Liver Failure

Chronic liver failure is a different disease process than ALF. In chronic liver disease, there is gradual destruction of the liver tissue. This chronic damage causes scar tissue to replace the normal parenchyma that affects hepatic metabolism and leads to decreased hepatic synthesis. The chronic injury can result from many different disease processes such as biliary atresia or prolonged TPN cholestasis.

Chronic liver disease can be either compensated or decompensated. In compensated liver disease, the liver is still able to carry out most or all of its functions. There are no clinical features of liver failure. Compensated liver disease will eventually progress to decompensated liver disease. In decompensated liver disease, the clinical and laboratory findings are consistent with liver synthetic failure. Patients have hepatic dysfunction and cholestasis, leading to malnutrition, coagulopathy, impaired protein synthesis, portal hypertension, ascites, hepatopulmonary syndrome, hepatorenal syndrome, and HE. Treatment is focused on preventing the progression to decompensated liver disease by treating the underlying cause of the liver failure. If this is not successful, the focus becomes treatment of the complications and eventually liver transplantation. With the exception of portal hypertension, treatment of complications in chronic decompensated liver disease is similar to treatment in ALF and this is discussed in the sections that follow.

Portal Hypertension

Portal hypertension is a rare but serious complication of chronic liver disease. The pathophysiology is not completely understood but it is felt to be the result of increased portal venous blood flow or increased portal resistance. Increased portal resistance occurs from disease within the liver. It is thought to be due to a combination of fibrosis, hepatocyte swelling, and vasoactive substances. In portal hypertension, portal pressure increases to levels >10–12 mm Hg, which can result in formation of collateral circulation, hypersplenism, and esophageal varices.[13]

Patients are likely to be asymptomatic until complications ensue. The most dangerous complication is variceal bleeding, characterized by painless, massive upper gastrointestinal hemorrhage. Mortality rates approach 50% in adults but are lower in children.[14,15] Treatment is first focused around fluid resuscitation, stabilizing the patient and then stopping the bleeding. About half the time, bleeding will stop spontaneously. Rebleeding is common and other therapies must be considered. Pharmacotherapy with vasopressin or octreotide causes splanchnic vasoconstriction and should be started emergently to stop bleeding. Vasopressin dosing for gastrointestinal hemorrhage is given as a continuous intravenous infusion. The initial dosing is between 0.002 and 0.005 units/kg/minute and titrated as needed. Maximum dosing is 0.01 units/kg/minute. Once bleeding stops for 12 hours, a taper should be initiated to run over 24–48 hours. Octreotide is more commonly used and similar in that it is given as a continuous infusion. First a bolus of 1–2 mcg/kg is given followed by a 1–2 mcg/kg/hour infusion. The infusion is also titrated to effects. Once hemostasis is obtained, the dosing is tapered by 50% every 12 hours for 24 hours and then stopped.[16] Esophageal variceal obliteration with sclerotherapy or band ligation can be performed once the patient is hemodynamically stable. Multiple treatments need to be repeated to ultimately obliterate the varices. Occasionally, acute variceal bleeds cannot be managed medically and a transjugular intrahepatic portosystemic shunt (TIPS) may be placed by interventional radiology. This decreases portal pressure and decompresses the varices. If TIPS fails, then a surgical shunt may need to be placed to diminish the increased portal hypertension and to control bleeding.

DIAGNOSIS

Diagnosis of ALF depends on the history, clinical presentation, and laboratory findings. There must be no prior history of liver disease and the patient must have biochemical markers consistent with liver disease. These include an INR ≥1.5 and the patient must have signs of HE. There is a long differential diagnosis and determining the etiology of liver failure is important in tailoring the treatment and preventing complications (Table 30–5).

TREATMENT AND MANAGEMENT

Once it has been determined that a patient has ALF, it is important to first stabilize the patient and then work on transferring the patient to a liver transplant center. Stabilization focuses on the management and prevention of the complications of liver failure. (Figure 30–1)

Table 30–5.

Differential Diagnosis/Causes of Liver Failure

Obstruction
Biliary atresia
Choledochal cyst
Inspissated bile
Neonatal sclerosis cholangitis
Spontaneous perforation of bile ducts
Masses/tumors

Genetic disorders
Alagille syndrome
Nonsyndromic paucity of the interlobular bile ducts
Progressive familial intrahepatic cholestasis
Alpha-1-antitrypsin deficiency
Congenital hepatic fibrosis
Cystic fibrosis
Neonatal hemachromatosis

Metabolic disorders
Galactosemia
Hereditary fructose intolerance
Type IV glycogenosis
Tyrosinemia
Wolman
Niemann–Pick
Gaucher
Disorders of bile acid synthesis
Citrin deficiency

Endocrine disorders
Hypopituitarism
Hypothyroidism

Other
Idiopathic neonatal hepatitis
Shock/hypoperfusion
Intestinal obstruction
Neonatal lupus
Infection/sepsis
Autoimmune hepatitis

This consists of careful electrolyte, fluid, and glucose management, hemorrhage prevention, monitoring for cerebral edema and encephalopathy, and use of specific medications such as NAC for acetaminophen overdose or penicillin G and silymarin in poison mushroom intoxication, when appropriate.

Blood glucose should be checked immediately on presentation and the patient should be started on intravenous fluids containing sufficient dextrose, with the goal of keeping blood glucose levels >60 mg/dL. It may be necessary to utilize intravenous fluids with very high concentrations of dextrose to maintain adequate blood glucose levels. It is also important to monitor for coagulopathy and to watch for signs of hemorrhage. Begin by checking the PT and INR. PT is a measure of

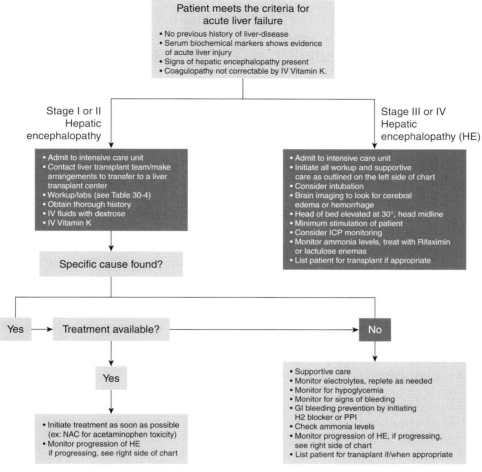

Patient meets the criteria for acute liver failure
- No previous history of liver-disease
- Serum biochemical markers shows evidence of acute liver injury
- Signs of hepatic encephalopathy present
- Coagulopathy not correctable by IV Vitamin K.

Stage I or II Hepatic encephalopathy
- Admit to intensive care unit
- Contact liver transplant team/make arrangements to transfer to a liver transplant center
- Workup/labs (see Table 30-4)
- Obtain thorough history
- IV fluids with dextrose
- IV Vitamin K

Stage III or IV Hepatic encephalopathy (HE)
- Admit to intensive care unit
- Initiate all workup and supportive care as outlined on the left side of chart
- Consider intubation
- Brain imaging to look for cerebral edema or hemorrhage
- Head of bed elevated at 30°, head midline
- Minimum stimulation of patient
- Consider ICP monitoring
- Monitor ammonia levels, treat with Rifaximin or lactulose enemas
- List patient for transplant if appropriate

Specific cause found?

Yes → **Treatment available?** → No

Yes

- Initiate treatment as soon as possible (ex: NAC for acetaminophen toxicity)
- Monitor progression of HE if progressing, see right side of chart

- Supportive care
- Monitor electrolytes, replete as needed
- Monitor for hypoglycemia
- Monitor for signs of bleeding
- GI bleeding prevention by initiating H2 blocker or PPI
- Check ammonia levels
- Monitor progression of HE, if progressing, see right side of chart
- List patient for transplant if/when appropriate

FIGURE 30–1 ■ Algorithm for the evaluation of liver failure in children.

the vitamin K-dependent clotting factors synthesized by the liver and provides the best way to quickly assess hepatic synthetic ability. If the PT is prolonged, administration of vitamin K intravenously once daily for 3 consecutive days is recommended.[17] The use of blood products such as fresh frozen plasma or cryoprecipitate or the use of the recombinant factor VIIa drug, Novo-Seven (Novo Nordisk Health Care A/G), is not proven to be beneficial despite the elevated levels of PT and INR and should be reserved for use when the patient is actively bleeding or prior to invasive procedures. Additionally, giving these products removes the ability to monitor hepatic synthesis.[17] Prevention of gastrointestinal hemorrhage is important and all patients with ALF should be started on intravenous proton pump inhibitors.[18]

Carefully monitoring fluid balance and maintaining renal function are key components in the management of a child with ALF. During ALF, the body is in a hyperdynamic state. There are increased cardiac output, decreased systemic venous resistance, and decreased mean arterial pressure (MAP). Systemic vasodilation

occurs in conjunction with renal vasoconstriction resulting in sodium retention, extracellular fluid retention, and eventually the development of ascites.[13] The goal to appropriate fluid balance is to provide adequate hydration while at the same time maintaining kidney function. Total fluid intake should be calculated to be about 75% of maintenance requirements to prevent fluid overload. Sodium intake should be minimal with no greater than 0.5–1 mmol/kg/day. Patients may have increased potassium and phosphorus requirements and those should be restored as needed. It is important to monitor the patient's urine output and maintain 1–2 mL/kg/hour of urine output. Loop diuretics are initially preferred if needed while sometimes dopamine may be required in order to keep the kidneys perfused and to maintain adequate urine output.

HE and cerebral edema can progress rapidly with ALF. As mentioned previously, encephalopathy is classified by four stages (Table 30–1). The causes of HE are thought to be multifactorial, but the exact mechanism is unknown.[19] Some mechanistic theories suggest an accumulation of neurotoxins or neuroactive substances that the liver cannot sufficiently metabolize that enter the systemic circulation and travel to the brain where they generate their effect. Hyperammonemia is considered to very well reflect the progression of HE. Therapy for progressive HE involves decreasing production of ammonia by the intestinal bacterial flora, eliminating plasma ammonia, and minimizing or avoiding medications that could alter a patient's mental status.[19,20] Protein intake is limited to <1 g/kg/day to decrease ammonia production. In addition, non-absorbable antibiotics or lactulose are used to eliminate ammonia from the gut. Lactulose is a non-digestible disaccharide cathartic that cannot undergo fermentation until it reaches the colon. Once in the colon, intestinal bacteria capable of metabolizing the disaccharide produce gas and short-chain fatty acids as byproducts of anaerobic fermentation in the intestinal lumen. This causes an osmotic shift and diarrhea. The acidification of the luminal contents affects bacterial reproduction and thereby decreases ammonia production. The acidification further rids the body of ammonia by converting ammonia (NH_3) to ammonium (NH_4^+), which is excreted in stool.[19] The intestine effectively becomes a dialysis membrane to rid the body of ammonia in this way. Lactulose can be administered orally, via nasogastric tube, or rectally as an enema. Obviously, a comatose patient should not be administered lactulose orally as there is a risk for aspiration. We do not favor the use of lactulose if a liver transplant is imminent as the byproduct gas that accumulates in the intestines may cause distension and make closure of the abdomen following surgery more difficult. Non-absorbable antibiotics that have been utilized to treat hyperammonemia and HE include rifaximin and neomycin. Neomycin has nephrotoxic and ototoxic properties and should be used with caution in children.

Mental status changes can often be difficult to assess in children. Avoidance of all sedating drugs is important since most of these medications are metabolized in the liver and their administration can affect the mental status exam. Restraints may be necessary in combative patients and should be used to avoid self-injury.

Cerebral edema needs to be treated aggressively.[20] Monitoring for signs of increased intracranial pressure (ICP) such as lethargy, irritability, papilledema, vomiting, and headache is essential. Unfortunately, clinical signs are not always present and can be inconsistent. As a result, it is important to have a high clinical suspicion for cerebral edema. Computed tomography (CT) of the head can demonstrate signs of cerebral edema, but this is not a sensitive method, may not show evidence of cerebral edema early in its course, and up to 30% of patients have no changes on CT.[21] CT scans, however, are useful in detecting intracranial hemorrhage. Treatment includes minimal stimulation, head positioned

midline and elevated at a 30° angle, hyperventilation, maintenance of hemodynamic stability, intravenous mannitol, and hypertonic saline therapy.[19,20] The goal of treatment is to maintain the cerebral perfusion pressure (CPP) about 50 torr. The CPP is calculated by subtracting the ICP from the MAP (CPP = MAP − IP). ICP should be in the normal range and <20 torr. Mannitol infusions have been shown to decrease ICP. Serum osmolality needs to be monitored frequently and maintained in the range of 300–320 mOsm. Mannitol should be held if the serum osmolality is >320 mOsm or renal failure occurs. Hypertonic saline has been shown to improve intracranial hypertension when serum sodium levels are kept between 145 and 155 mmol/L.[22] Newer research studies are showing promising results of moderate hypothermia in decreasing ICPs in patients otherwise refractory to standard medical therapy.[23]

NAC should be administered in any patient suspected of acetaminophen toxicity. The best effect occurs when NAC is administered within 12–36 hours of acetaminophen ingestion. NAC replenishes hepatic glutathione stores. Acetaminophen is metabolized to its *N*-acetyl-*p*-benzoquinoneimine (NAPQI) metabolite. This metabolite is detoxified by hepatic conjugation with glutathione. If glutathione is depleted, as in the case of acetaminophen toxicity, then NADQI binds to cysteine groups on protein and results in hepatotoxic products. NAC replenishes the hepatic glutathione stores and improves outcomes in acetaminophen ingestions by diminishing hepatotoxicity.[24]

Having appropriate central venous access is necessary in order to carry out many of the above treatment regimens. Patients who deteriorate rapidly may require intubation and mechanical ventilation. Arterial lines are important to monitor blood pressure and blood gases. Nasogastric tubes are placed to monitor for gastrointestinal bleeding, gastric decompression, and/or medication administration. Foley catheter placement is often necessary for accurate assessment of urine output. Abdominal ultrasound with Doppler interrogation should be done to assess for anatomic and/or vascular abnormalities. Laboratory testing is performed to assess the rate of hepatic deterioration, manage complications, and help establish the etiology of the fulminant hepatic failure (Table 30–4). Initial laboratory tests include a complete blood count with differential and platelets, chemistry panel with serum electrolytes, blood urea nitrogen, creatinine, glucose, calcium, magnesium, phosphorus, liver panel with AST, ALT, alkaline phosphatase, gamma-glutamyl transferase, total and direct-reacting bilirubins, INR, PT, PTT, amylase, lipase, ammonia, blood culture, and urine and stool cultures. Toxicology screen, acetaminophen, and aspirin levels should be done as appropriate by history. Hepatitis serologies to be obtained include hepatitis A antibody, hepatitis C antibody, hepatitis B surface antigen, and hepatitis B core antibody.

Regardless of the cause of ALF, it is important to recognize it early, stabilize the patient, focus management on prevention of complications, and transfer the patient to a liver transplant center as soon as possible. Referral to a liver transplant center can never be too early when the potential for rapid and significant hepatic failure with subsequent cerebral complications is imminent.

REFERENCES

1. Lee WM. Acute liver failure in the United States. *Semin Liver Dis.* 2003;23:217–226.
2. Squires RHJ, Shneider BL, Bucavalas J, et al. Acute liver failure in children: the first 348 patients in the pediatric acute liver failure study group. *J Pediatr.* 2006;148: 652–658.
3. Organ Procurement and Transplant Network. *Profile of Patient Survival Rates for Liver Transplants.* http://optn. transplant.hrsa.gov/organDatasource/state.htm.
4. Durand P, Debray D, Mandel R, et al. Acute liver failure in infancy: a 14-year experience of a pediatric liver transplant center. *J Pediatr.* 2001;139:871–876.
5. Mieli-Vergani G, Bhaduri B, Dhawan A, et al. Acute liver failure in infancy. *J Hepatol.* 1995;23:A125.
6. Baker A, Alonso ME, Aw MM, et al. Hepatic failure and liver transplant: working group report of the second world congress of pediatric gastroenterology, hepatology, and nutrition. *J Pediatr Gastroenterol Nutr.* 2004;39(suppl 2): S632–S639.
7. Lee WS, McKiernan P, Kelly DA. Etiology, outcome and prognostic indicators of childhood fulminant hepatic failure in the United Kingdom. *J Pediatr Gastroenterol Nutr.* 2005;40:575–581.
8. Kelly DA, Mc Kiernaan PJ. Metabolic liver disease in pediatric patient. *Clin Liver Dis.* 1998;2:1–30.
9. Flynn DM, Mohan N, McKiernan P, et al. Progress in treatment and outcome for children with neonatal haemochromatosis. *Arch Dis Child Fetal Neonatal Ed.* 2003;88:F124.
10. Rand EB, Karpen SJ, Kelly S, Mack CL, Malatack JJ, Sokol RJ, Whitington PF. Treatment of neonatal hemochromatosis with exchange transfusion and intravenous immunoglobulin. *J Pediatr.* 2009 Oct;155(4):566–571.
11. Whitington PF, Hibbard JU. High dose immunoglobulin during pregnancy for recurrent neonatal haemochromatosis. *Lancet.* 2004;364:1690–1698.
12. Murray KF, Hadzic N, Wirth S, Bassett M, Kelly DA. Drug related hepatotoxicity and acute liver failure. *J Pediatr Gastroenterol Nutr.* 2008;47:395–405.
13. Watanabe FD, Rosenthal P. Portal hypertension in children. *Curr Opin Pediatr.* 1995;7:533–538.
14. D'Amico G, Paliaro L, Bosch J. The treatment of portal hypertension: a meta-analytic review. *Hepatology.* 1995;22:332–354.
15. Maksoug JG, Goncalves ME, Porta G, Miura I, Velhote MC. The endoscopic and surgical management of portal hypertension in children: analysis of 123 cases. *J Pediatr Surg.* 1991;26:178–181.
16. Lexi-Comp ONLINE. 2009. http://www.crlonline.com/ crlsql/servlet/crlonline.
17. Polson J, Lee WM. AASLD position paper: the management of acute liver failure. *Hepatology.* 2005;41: 1179–1197.
18. MacDougall BR, Bailey RJ, Williams R. H2-receptor antagonists and antacids in the prevention of acute gastrointestinal haemorrhage in fulminant hepatic failure. Two controlled trials. *Lancet.* 1977;1:617–619.
19. Wendon J, Lee WM. Encephalopathy and cerebral edema in the setting of acute liver failure: pathogenesis and management. *Neurocrit Care.* 2008;9:97–102.
20. Tofteng F, Larsen FS. Management of patients with fulminant hepatic failure and brain edema. *Metab Brain Dis.* 2004;19:207–214.
21. Munoz SJ, Robinson M, Northrup B, et al. Elevated intracranial pressure and computed tomography of the brain in fulminant hepatocellular failure. *Hepatology.* 1991;13: 209–212.
22. Murphy N, Auzinger G, Bernel W, Wendon J. The effect of hypertonic sodium chloride on intracranial pressure in patients with acute liver failure. *Hepatology.* 2004;39: 464–470.
23. Jalan R, Damink SWM, Deutz NEP, Hayes PC, Lee A. Moderate hypothermia in patients with acute liver failure and uncontrolled intracranial hypertension. *Gastroenterology.* 2004;127:1338–1346.
24. Harrison PM, Keyes R, Bray GP, Alexander GJM, Williams R. Late *N*-acetyl cysteine administration improves outcome for patients developing paracetamol-induced fulminant hepatic failure. *Lancet.* 1990;335:1572–1573.

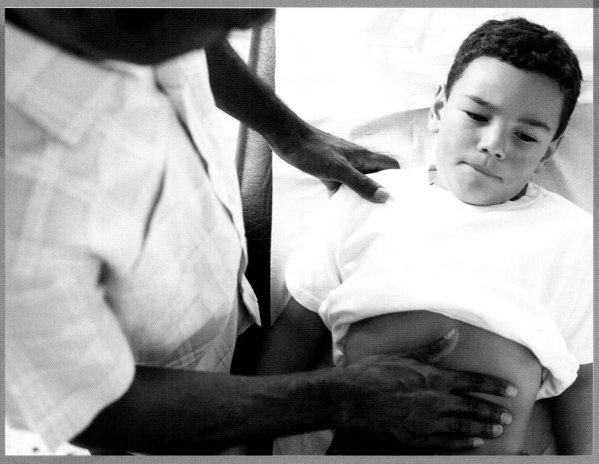

Disorders of the Pancreas

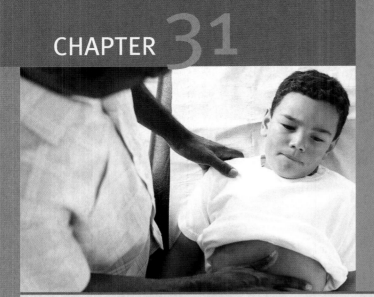

CHAPTER 31

Acute and Chronic Pancreatitis

Mark E. Lowe

DEFINITIONS AND EPIDEMIOLOGY

Inflammatory disorders of the pancreas are classified as acute or chronic. Acute pancreatitis is generally a reversible process with no significant permanent effects on pancreatic histology or function, whereas chronic pancreatitis leads to irreversible changes in the architecture and function of the pancreas. Both are defined clinically. *Acute pancreatitis* is a distinct event requiring two of the following three features for diagnosis: (1) clinical symptoms consistent with acute pancreatitis, (2) serum amylase or lipase levels or both at least three times the upper limit of normal, and (3) findings of acute pancreatitis on transabdominal ultrasonography or on contrast-enhanced computed tomography (CECT). *Chronic pancreatitis* is a progressive disease leading to typical histological and morphological changes in the pancreas, usually identified by radiographic methods, or to loss of digestive function or both.

Acute Pancreatitis

The diagnosis of acute pancreatitis in childhood has increased over the years.[1,2] Currently, the incidence in large children's hospitals may approach 12–15 cases per 100,000 children per year. The reason for the increase remains unsettled, but a recent study suggested that increased awareness of the disease in childhood is the major factor, since increased amylase and lipase testing accounted for the majority of the change at a single institution.

Although a wide range of prevalence in etiologies exists among various reports and the categories often vary among the reports, systemic illness, biliary disease, trauma, and side effects of medications comprise the majority of patients with an identifiable etiology (Table 31–1).[3] A sizable portion of patients have no discerned etiology and are classified as idiopathic. Since there is wide variation in prevalence of etiologies among the available reports, any current compilation of these requires some ambiguity in categorization. The overall variation likely reflects the retrospective nature of the studies, the bias or experience of the clinicians, incomplete investigations for etiologies in many patients, and the recognition of new etiologies over time.

Recurrent episodes of acute pancreatitis occur in about 10% of children. The most common etiologies in these patients are structural abnormalities, genetic pancreatitis, and idiopathic. Some of these patients will eventually develop chronic pancreatitis.

Chronic Pancreatitis

The prevalence of chronic pancreatitis in childhood is unknown, although it is certainly less frequent than acute pancreatitis. Similarly, the frequency of etiologies remains uncertain. As with acute pancreatitis, idiopathic causes comprise a large percentage of the patients with chronic pancreatitis (Table 31–2). Patients with autosomal dominant hereditary pancreatitis or with autosomal recessive familial pancreatitis form another large group.[4–6] There are also toxic or metabolic and obstructive causes.

PATHOGENESIS

Acute Pancreatitis

Acute pancreatitis can be separated into two types, *interstitial edematous*, the most common type, and *necrotizing* pancreatitis. Both result from injury and

Table 31–1.

Etiologies of Acute Pancreatitis

Biliary
- Cholelithiasis
- Choledochal cyst
- Biliary sludge

Anatomic
- Pancreas divisum
- Anomalous junction of the biliary and pancreatic ducts
- Annular pancreas
- Ampullary obstruction
- Crohn disease
- Diverticulum
- Cyst
- Ulcer

Drugs (only the most commonly reported are listed)
- L-Asparaginase
- Valproate
- Metronidazole
- Mercaptopurine
- Azathioprine
- Tetracycline
- Pentamidine
- Didanosine

Systemic disease
- Sepsis
- Hemolytic uremic syndrome
- Diabetic ketoacidosis
- Collagen vascular disease
- Kawasaki disease
- Organ transplantation
- Sickle cell disease
- Anorexia nervosa
- Shock
- Inflammatory bowel disease

Genetic
- *PRSS1* mutations
- *CFTR* mutations

Trauma

Idiopathic

Metabolic
- Hyperlipidemia
- Hypercalcemia
- Glycogen storage disease
- Organic acidemias

Autoimmune pancreatitis

inflammation of the pancreas that may extend to peripancreatic tissues and remote organs.[7] Current models include at least three phases in the development of acute pancreatitis. Initially, an extrapancreatic factor initiates the onset of pancreatitis. In children, systemic illness, medications, trauma, and bile or pancreatic duct

Table 31–2.

Etiologies of Chronic Pancreatitis

Idiopathic

Genetic
- Autosomal dominant
  - *PRSS1* mutations
- Autosomal recessive/modifiers
  - *CFTR* mutations
  - *SPINK1* mutations

Drugs
- See Table 31–1

Metabolic disease
- See Table 31–1

Autoimmune
- Isolated autoimmune pancreatitis
- Syndromic autoimmune pancreatitis

Anatomic
- See Table 31–1

disease secondary to congenital anomalies or gallstones are the common triggers. The mechanism whereby these events cause pancreatitis remains speculative.[8] Early events in experimental pancreatitis include influx of calcium into the acinar cell, the co-localization of pancreatic digestive enzymes and lysosomal enzymes as autophagosomes, and altered secretion of the digestive enzymes, in particular increased basolateral secretion. The early events somehow produce the second phase of pancreatitis, acinar cell injury. Current theories for the mechanism of acinar cell injury center on the premature activation of trypsinogen to trypsin within the acinar cell. Once converted, trypsin activates other proenzymes and the combined action of these enzymes leads to acinar cell injury or autodigestion. Other processes may also contribute to, or even dominate, the early events that damage the acinar cell. These include injury by reactive oxygen species, alterations in the microcirculation of the pancreas producing areas of hypoperfusion, changes in the permeability of the acinar cell plasma membrane, and increased endoplasmic reticulum stress.[8] The resultant acinar damage produces pancreatic edema and a local inflammatory response. The cytokines and chemokines released during this response mediate a systemic inflammatory response, the third phase of acute pancreatitis. The magnitude of the systemic response largely determines the clinical severity of acute pancreatitis.[9] A vigorous response can lead to pancreatic necrosis, inflammation in adjacent tissues and in distant organs, and systemic complications.

Chronic Pancreatitis

Early in their course, patients with chronic pancreatitis may be difficult to distinguish from those with acute pancreatitis.[10] Eventually, the continued inflammation produces enough irreversible morphological change in the gland including fibrosis, acinar cell loss, islet cell loss, and infiltration by inflammatory cells that the diagnosis becomes apparent. The inability to diagnose chronic pancreatitis early in its course and to identify early events has permitted investigators to speculate freely and many theories to explain the pathophysiology of chronic pancreatitis have been proposed over the years. Current knowledge supports the hypothesis that chronic pancreatitis is a progression that begins with an episode of acute pancreatitis followed by ongoing chronic or recurrent inflammation to produce end-stage fibrosis. The sentinel acute pancreatitis event (SAPE) hypothesis was proposed in 1999 and remains the prevailing concept.[11] In this model, a metabolic or oxidative stress initiates the first episode of acute pancreatitis, the sentinel event. Activated lymphocytes, macrophages, and stellate cells increase in number within the pancreas. They produce cytokines and deposit small amounts of collagen. Most patients recover uneventfully and the gland returns to normal. In some, due to the continued presence of stress, inflammatory cells and stellate cells remain active and release cytokines and deposit collagen, eventually producing the fibrotic changes characteristic of chronic pancreatitis). Although the process may be started and perpetuated by environmental factors, other factors must be present for chronic pancreatitis to develop in some individuals and not others. Most recent studies have focused on the role of genetic predisposition to chronic pancreatitis.

CLINICAL PRESENTATION

Acute Pancreatitis

The symptoms and clinical signs of acute pancreatitis are nonspecific and may vary with age (Table 31–3). Upper abdominal pain and vomiting are the most common symptoms. A review of the literature from 1965 to 2000 concluded that abdominal pain is present in 87% of patients.[12] Two subsequent studies reported pain in 95% and 68% of patients.[2,13] Some of the variation in reporting may reflect the age range of the patients in the studies. Only 29% of patients under 3 years of age had abdominal pain reported.[14] Even if irritability was considered a surrogate for pain, the percentage with

Table 31–3.	
Signs and Symptoms	
Acute Pancreatitis	**Chronic Pancreatitis**
Abdominal pain	Abdominal pain
Vomiting	Weight loss
Irritability	Diarrhea/steatorrhea
Abdominal distension	Recurrent acute pancreatitis
Jaundice	Jaundice
Back pain	Upper GI bleeding
Fever	
Feeding intolerance	

abdominal pain was still low, 46%, in this age group. Vomiting occurs in 45–85% of reported cases. It was the most common presenting symptom in patients under 3 years of age. Other less common symptoms and signs include abdominal tenderness, abdominal distention, fever, tachycardia, hypotension, jaundice, and back pain. Blue or green ecchymoses of the flank (Turner's sign) or blue discoloration of the umbilicus (Cullen's sign) from extravasation of blood are rare in childhood. In hospitalized patients, acute pancreatitis may present as a change in clinical status or feeding intolerance.

Chronic Pancreatitis

Recurrent acute pancreatitis may dominate the early course of chronic pancreatitis in many patients (Table 31–3). The signs and symptoms are the same as described for acute pancreatitis. Chronic pancreatitis should be considered in a patient with recurrent attacks of acute pancreatitis. Patients may present with pain as the prominent clinical feature. The pain can range from mild to severe and from intermittent to persistent. Typically, the pain is in the upper abdomen. Many adults describe the pain as deep and penetrating, radiating to the back and worse after meals. Children are often not as descriptive, and the pain may be hard for them to describe. At diagnosis, many have had periodic episodes of pain diagnosed as viral or functional. The cause of the pain is likely mulitfactorial and will vary from patient to patient and depend on the length of the illness. Early in the course, the pain often arises from the acute inflammation of pancreatitis. Later, pain may arise from pancreatic duct hypertension, increased pancreatic tissue pressure, tissue acidosis, or perineural inflammation.

Even though maldigestion is a feature of advanced gland destruction, symptoms of malabsorption may provide the first clue to chronic pancreatitis. These patients usually present with weight loss or fatty stools. Diarrhea may be present, but significant steatorrhea can occur even in patients having a single daily stool. A few may present with extrahepatic biliary obstruction from fibrosis in the head of the pancreas or from a pseudocyst. These patients frequently have jaundice, and may have an unexplained elevation of serum alkaline phosphatase. Rarely, a patient may present with gastrointestinal bleeding secondary to venous thrombosis, often in the splenic vein. Subcutaneous or intramedullary fat necrosis has been described in children as the initial sign of chronic pancreatitis.

Diabetes mellitus may develop late in the course of chronic pancreatitis, and rarely, if ever, do patients present initially with symptoms of diabetes mellitus. Both insulin-producing cells and glucagon-producing cells are destroyed in chronic pancreatitis. Consequently, the diabetes is fragile and blood sugar control is difficult.

DIFFERENTIAL DIAGNOSIS

Acute Pancreatitis

Because the symptoms of acute pancreatitis are quite nonspecific, usually abdominal pain or vomiting or both, the differential diagnosis is broad. In general, there is little in the history or exam that can clearly distinguish acute pancreatitis from these other entities. The most common diagnosis for these symptoms is infectious gastroenteritis, usually viral. Other considerations include celiac disease, peptic ulcer disease, gastritis, gallbladder disease, and Crohn disease. If the presentation is acute, abdominal distension is present, or peritoneal signs are present, then appendicitis and causes of partial or complete bowel obstruction should be considered.

Chronic Pancreatitis

The differential diagnosis of chronic pancreatitis includes recurrent acute pancreatitis and the common causes of chronic pain in childhood. Some patients will have repeated episodes of acute pancreatitis but they do not have irreversible changes in the anatomy of the pancreas or diminished exocrine function. Although many of these patients will eventually meet criteria for a diagnosis of chronic pancreatitis, they are properly classified as recurrent acute pancreatitis until they do not meet the definition of chronic pancreatitis. Peptic ulcers, gastritis, gallbladder disease, and Crohn disease are all considerations as they are for acute pancreatitis. In addition, functional abdominal pain, lactose intolerance, and depression can present with recurrent or constant abdominal pain.

The differential changes if malabsorption dominates the clinical picture. Developmental defects of the pancreas, severe enteropathies, cholestatic liver disease, and isolated enzyme deficiencies should all be considered.

DIAGNOSIS

Acute Pancreatitis

Since the signs and symptoms of acute pancreatitis are nonspecific, the physician must keep acute pancreatitis in mind in any child with gastrointestinal complaints. The accepted clinical definition of acute pancreatitis in adults requires at least two of the following features: (1) abdominal pain consistent with acute pancreatitis; (2) serum amylase or lipase levels (or both) at least three times the upper reference limit; and (3) findings of acute pancreatitis on radiological studies. Although this definition generally holds true in pediatrics, the physician must remember that a number of children may not present with abdominal pain or the pain may be minimal and other symptoms may predominate as discussed above. A suggested algorithm to approaching the diagnosis is given in Figure 31–1.

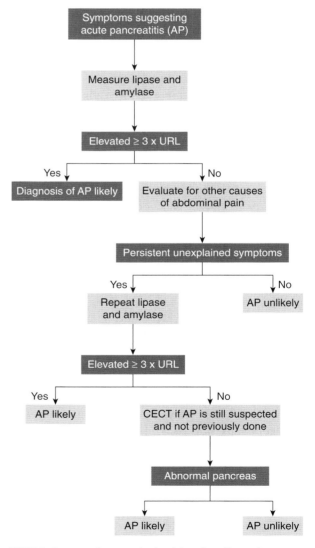

FIGURE 31–1 ▪ Suggested algorithm for diagnosing acute pancreatitis.

Laboratory studies

In practice, the likelihood of acute pancreatitis is generally assessed by measuring the serum levels of lipase and amylase in patients with compatible symptoms.[15] The reliability of these measurements to diagnose acute pancreatitis remains uncertain. All studies to define the sensitivity and specificity of serum amylase and lipase for acute pancreatitis suffer from the lack of a method to separately and definitively diagnose acute pancreatitis. In particular, no studies on the sensitivity and specificity of these enzyme levels in pediatrics are available. Both can be normal when there is clear clinical and radiological evidence of acute pancreatitis. In turn, both can be elevated in other conditions where there is no other evidence for pancreatitis. Importantly, the level of elevation is not diagnostic although the higher the level the more likely there is to be pancreatic inflammation.

In general, other conditions such as renal failure rarely if ever raise levels three times above the upper reference limit. Two exceptions are worth discussion since both can give serum enzyme levels in large excess of three times the upper reference limit. Both are benign and their recognition will prevent unnecessary investigations and therapies. In each case, the patients have elevated pancreatic enzyme levels in their serum at a time when they do not have symptoms. Often the patients present with abdominal pain, have elevated amylase or lipase and normal radiographic studies, and are diagnosed with acute pancreatitis. During follow-up the enzymes remain elevated even though the patient is asymptomatic. Other times the amylase or lipase is part of a test panel and the patient does not have symptoms consistent with pancreatitis.

First, either amylase or lipase or both can exist as a complex with a larger molecule, usually an immunoglobulin, a situation termed *macroamylasemia* or *macrolipasemia*.[16,17] The complex is not cleared from the serum as rapidly as the unbound enzymes, and the enzyme accumulates to higher levels in the serum. At this time, there is a commercially available test for macroamylase but not for macrolipase. Second, some patients have benign elevations of pancreatic enzymes without any clinical or radiographic evidence of pancreatitis.[18,19] Typically, lipase and amylase are detected and followed, but all pancreatic enzymes are also elevated in most subjects. The levels fluctuate with time and may return to normal at times. Other family members may have a similar pattern. The mechanism is not known. Macroenzymes are not present. There is some evidence for alterations in the normal secretory pathways with shunting of more enzymes from apical secretion to basolateral secretion.

Infants present a theoretical, perhaps clinically significant, problem with the use of amylase and lipase to diagnose acute pancreatitis.[3] Pancreatic isoamylase

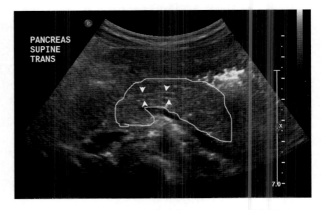

FIGURE 31–2 ■ Ultrasound findings in acute pancreatitis. The pancreas (outlined) is edematous and there are small fluid collections below the pancreas. The pancreatic duct (arrowheads) is dilated.

levels are low at birth and may not reach adult levels until adolescence. Likewise, lipase levels are low at birth and may not reach adult levels until 1 year of age. Some young patients with acute pancreatitis may go undiagnosed because they do not express enough lipase and amylase for the serum levels to increase with acute pancreatitis. Review of the literature reveals that many pediatric patients with acute pancreatitis have a selective elevation of amylase or lipase at presentation. This finding makes it prudent to perform both assays in patients with suspected acute pancreatitis.

Radiology and endoscopy

The utility of imaging studies in investigating children with suspected acute pancreatitis remains uncertain. If the diagnosis is established based on symptoms and increased amylase or lipase activity and there are no systemic signs of severe disease (see the section "Management") or evidence of gallstone pancreatitis, imaging may not be necessary. If the symptoms are suggestive of acute pancreatitis, but the serum enzymes are less than three times the upper reference limit, the diagnosis requires imaging that shows typical findings of pancreatitis. In patients where imaging is indicated, transabdominal ultrasonography presents a reasonable option for the initial radiographic evaluation of children. It is widely available and less expensive than other techniques. Sonographic findings include increased pancreatic size, decreased pancreatic echogenicity, and peripancreatic fluid (Figure 31–2). In addition, gallstones may be seen. The presence of bowel gas may limit the ability to view the pancreas.

Contrast-enhanced CT (CECT) provides another option for imaging and may be the best and most available imaging modality for the overall assessment of the pancreas (Figure 31–3). It can provide information about gallstones as well as additional information about possible etiologies and the presence or absence of necrosis, fluid

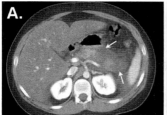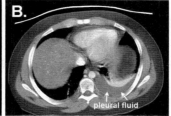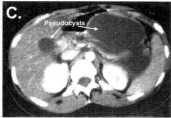

FIGURE 31–3 ■ CECT findings in acute pancreatitis. (A) Necrotizing pancreatitis: areas of low contrast enhancement are present in the tail and body (arrows) of the pancreas indicating low blood flow and the presence of necrosis. (B) Pleural fluid in the left thoracic cavity. (C) Pancreatic pseudocysts.

collections, or other complications. Although intravenous contrast worsened experimental pancreatitis in animals, administration of contrast in humans does not cause clinical deterioration with severe acute pancreatitis.[20]

Increasing evidence of gallstone pancreatitis in childhood provides the best argument for imaging studies early in the course of acute pancreatitis. Elevated serum transaminases (ALT or AST) or bilirubin or both suggest the possibility of gallstone pancreatitis. Of the various imaging studies endoscopic ultrasound (EUS) and magnetic resonance cholangiopancreatography (MRCP) appear superior to transabdominal ultrasound and CECT in adults.[21,22] Similar data are lacking in pediatrics. In addition to gallstones, MRCP can diagnose a variety of pancreatobiliary disorders including choledochal cysts, pancreas divisum, and anomalies of the junction between the pancreatic and biliary ducts. Furthermore, MRCP has been shown to perform well in children of all ages.[23–25] In time, MRCP may supplant CECT as the imaging study of choice in acute pancreatitis, but the need for sedation or general anesthesia in many pediatric patients will limit its routine use in uncomplicated acute pancreatitis. Even so, MRCP has supplanted endoscopic retrograde cholangiopancreatography (ERCP) in the diagnosis of pancreatobiliary disorders. MRCP also has an advantage over CECT and ERCP because it reduces exposure to ionizing radiation.

Secretin-enhanced MRCP may improve visualization of the pancreatic ducts and may improve detection of early changes in chronic pancreatitis. To date, no controlled trials have shown that secretin-enhanced MRCP has any benefit over MRCP alone. Furthermore, the changes reported in many studies have not been correlated with other measures of chronic pancreatitis. Thus, their meaning is uncertain. Currently, there is no evidence that secretin-enhanced MRCP provides any additional, clinically relevant information in childhood.

Experience with endoscopic ultrasound (EUS) in childhood is increasing.[26,27] Still it is not widely employed in pediatrics. Among the current limitations are the size of the endoscopes and the reluctance of trained EUS endoscopists, all adult gastroenterologists, to perform procedures on younger patients. As endoscopists become more comfortable with EUS in pediatric patients, the role of the procedure in acute pancreatitis and management of acute pancreatitis will become better defined. In adults, EUS appears to increase the diagnostic yield for gallstones and microlithiasis.[28]

Chronic Pancreatitis

The diagnosis of chronic pancreatitis requires evidence of irreversible histological or morphological change or a combination of morphological and functional change. The presence of exocrine insufficiency alone is not sufficient evidence for the diagnosis because there are other causes of pancreatic insufficiency aside from chronic pancreatitis such as Shwachman–Diamond syndrome.[29] A suggested algorithm for diagnosing chronic pancreatitis is presented in Figure 31–4.

Radiology and endoscopy

Generally, evidence of morphological change is provided by imaging studies. Five imaging procedures are utilized most often, transabdominal ultrasound, CECT, MRCP, ERCP, and EUS. ERCP has been considered the standard for the diagnosis of changes in the pancreatic ducts. ERCP findings include main pancreatic duct dilation, ductal stones, and changes in main duct branches and small ducts. CECT is reasonably sensitive for detecting advanced chronic pancreatitis with calcification, gland atrophy, fat replacement, and ductal dilatation. CECT has poor sensitivity compared to ERCP, but it has high specificity, around 90%. The test offers the advantage over ERCP in that CECT evaluates the pancreas for other pathology and can detect other abdominal pathology to explain the patient's chronic pain. MRCP is also good at detecting the main ductal changes in advanced chronic pancreatitis. The technique is not yet suitable for detecting subtle side branch abnormalities in early chronic pancreatitis. Still, MRCP has supplanted ERCP as the first diagnostic step in the evaluation of suspected pancreatic disease.

EUS may be more sensitive to changes early in the disease and, in adults, it is rapidly gaining acceptance as the preferred imaging study. EUS is prone to

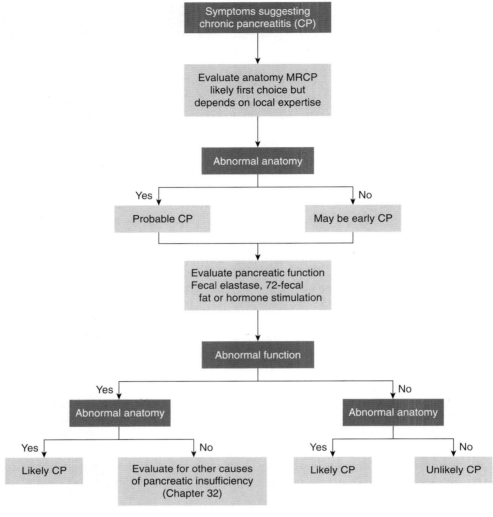

FIGURE 31-4 ■ Suggested algorithm for diagnosing chronic pancreatitis.

false-positives and may be more useful in eliminating the diagnosis of chronic pancreatitis. The reasons for this are many. The technique is highly operator dependent, there are differences in echoendoscopes and imaging techniques that affect the quality of the image, and there is a lack of consensus regarding the endosonographic definition of chronic pancreatitis. A recent consensus conference has proposed EUS standards for the diagnosis of chronic pancreatitis.[30] The recommendations have not been validated, but may provide a framework for future studies. The role of EUS and the other imaging techniques in evaluating children for the morphological changes of chronic pancreatitis has not been systematically investigated.

Pancreatic insufficiency

Pancreatic function testing serves to identify pancreatic insufficiency, to support the diagnosis of chronic pancreatitis and to provide a basis for rationale therapy as chronic pancreatitis progresses in severity.[31] Duodenal intubation with secretin–cerulein stimulation and quantitative collection of secretions is still considered the standard for diagnosis of pancreatic insufficiency. The test can detect intermediate losses of enzyme production before there is detectable maldigestion. The procedure has multiple drawbacks for clinical practice. Only a few centers have the expertise and volume to perform the test reliably. In large part, the lack of availability is because the test is time-consuming and labor-intensive to perform and uncomfortable for the patient. As a result some physicians have collected pancreatic secretions by suctioning duodenal fluid through an endoscope after hormone stimulation. This approach may greatly underestimate pancreatic secretory capacity and misclassify the digestive status of a substantial percentage of patients.[32]

The difficulty with collecting pancreatic secretions quantitatively has led to the development of a number of noninvasive tests of pancreatic function. The alternatives include fecal elastase or chymotrypsin, the pancreolauryl test, the bentiromide test, and breath tests utilizing labeled triglycerides. None of these tests meet clinical needs sufficiently. Each can only detect patients with steatorrhea and advanced chronic pancreatitis. With mild to moderate loss of exocrine function, the sensitivity of these tests is poor. This makes the tests useless in diagnosing chronic pancreatitis in patients with recurrent abdominal pain if they have mild or moderate exocrine dysfunction. Of these tests, fecal elastase is the most readily available. It has the advantage that only a spot stool sample is required and it can be done while the patient is on pancreatic enzyme replacement therapy. Watery stools can dilute the pancreatic elastase and yield a false-positive result.

The 72-hour fecal fat collection remains the best test for steatorrhea. Once it was a routine part of the evaluation for suspected malabsorption, but it has fallen out of favor for multiple reasons. It is nonspecific for pancreatic disease, collection and storage of stool is unpleasant for most patients, adherence to the standard diet for the length of the test may be difficult for some, and the required food diary is unreliable. Some of these difficulties can be overcome by performing the analysis in a metabolic laboratory, but this is impractical for general clinical practice. As with other noninvasive tests, the 72-hour fecal fat collection only reliably detects advanced disease.

MANAGEMENT

Acute Pancreatitis

The management of acute pancreatitis has not changed significantly over the years and incorporates supportive care and evaluation for treatable etiologies (Figure 31–5). Supportive care includes providing analgesia, infusing intravenous fluids, monitoring for complications, and treating complications appropriately.

Pain control

Analgesia generally requires parenteral narcotics. Traditional teaching has been to avoid morphine in acute pancreatitis since it may increase sphincter of Oddi pressure and further inflame the pancreas. Although morphine has been singled out, all narcotics, including meperidine, increase sphincter of Oddi pressure, and no clinical evidence supports the notion that morphine is contraindicated for use in acute pancreatitis.[33] In practice, morphine has been used in patients with pancreatitis because it has a longer half-life and fewer side effects than meperidine. Whatever the choice of analgesia, adequate pain relief should be provided.

Fluid resuscitation

Recently, the role of fluid resuscitation early in the presentation of acute pancreatitis has received considerable attention.[34] Limited data in animal models of acute pancreatitis and retrospective studies in humans

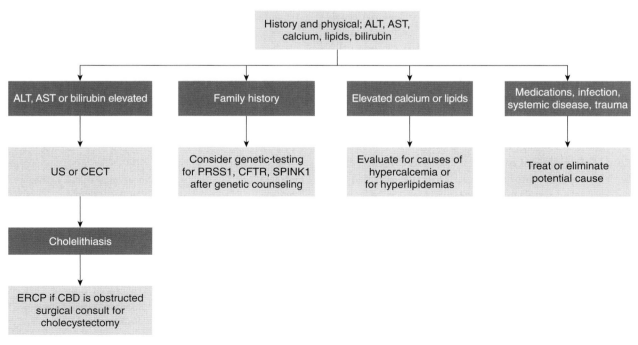

FIGURE 31–5 ■ Suggested algorithm for diagnosing the etiology of acute pancreatitis.

suggest that early fluid resuscitation may improve outcome and prevent progression to more severe disease. The American College of Gastroenterology practice guidelines recommends aggressive IV fluid replacement.[35] However, aggressive is not defined. In the literature on adult patients, recommendations range from 250 to 1000 mL/hour depending on volume status. One recent study in adults suggested that gradually replacing fluid deficits (5–10 mL/kg/hour) resulted in better outcomes than more rapid fluid infusions (10–15 mL/kg/hour).[36] There are no recommendations or studies in pediatrics. In summary, the appropriate method or type of fluid to infuse remains an open question for all ages. At this time, it seems prudent to provide intravenous fluids at a rate that exceeds basal needs and to supply additional fluids as dictated by the patient's hemodynamic status.

Nutritional therapy

Starvation has long been considered part of standard care in patients with acute pancreatitis. Both experimental and clinical evidence has accumulated to suggest that feeding can be started early in the course and may improve outcome.[37] A recent study in adults concluded that patients with mild acute pancreatitis can be safely allowed to eat and drink as tolerated without a period of fasting.[38] Patients allowed immediate oral intake showed no significant differences from the fasted, control group in clinical symptoms, but did advance to solid foods more quickly and had a shorter hospital stay. A second group randomized patients with mild acute pancreatitis to a clear liquid diet or a low-fat solid diet.[39] There was no difference in recurrence of pain or need to stop feeding between the two groups. It appears that patients with mild acute pancreatitis will tolerate oral feeds early in the course and the standard practices of fasting until symptoms resolve or the serum lipase or amylase return to normal are not necessary. No data are available on feeding in children with acute pancreatitis.

Similarly, it is becoming clear that patients with severe pancreatitis can also be orally fed early in the course and that early feedings are beneficial with fewer complications than parenteral nutrition.[37] There is evidence that both nasogastric and nasojejunal feeds are tolerated in patients with severe acute pancreatitis. Delivery of nutrients beyond the ligament of Trietz has several theoretical advantages such as a high prevalence of abnormal gastric emptying, minimal stimulation of the exocrine pancreas, and increased safety due to the ability to deliver nutrients and decompress the stomach. Currently, the choice of route is institution specific. There are also little experimental data to direct the choice of formula. In most studies, so-called semi-elemental formulas containing small peptides and either low-fat content or medium-chain triglycerides are used, although it is unclear if this makes

a difference. Immunomodulating diets supplemented with arginine, glutamine, omega-3 fatty acids, and antioxidants remain controversial in critically ill patients and there use in severe acute pancreatitis is probably not warranted at this time.

Nutritional support is now viewed as an active intervention in patients with acute pancreatitis. Enteral nutrition should begin within 24 hours of admission after an initial period of fluid resuscitation and control of pain. Patients with mild disease can be started on oral feeds; most authors recommend low-fat diets. Nasojejunal feeds are likely the preferred route to start enteral feeds in patients with severe disease.

Complications

A number of complications of acute pancreatitis are recognized (Table 31–4). Most complications are non-life threatening. The development of organ failure, circulatory collapse, or severe metabolic derangements requires the coordinated multispecialty care in an intensive care unit. The development of necrosis does not necessarily require intervention. The development of infected necrosis, a rare event in pediatrics, should be suspected if abdominal pain worsens, fever develops, or there is a leukocytosis. Increasingly, patients with infected necrosis are initially managed with antibiotics to allow the necrosis to liquefy and wall off rather than proceed directly to surgical debridement. Collections of fluid in and around the pancreas are fairly common. They rarely require therapy. Many will resolve spontaneously although time course may be protracted. Asymptomatic pseudocysts can be managed conservatively. If they produce symptoms from obstruction of a surrounding organ such as the stomach, duodenum, or

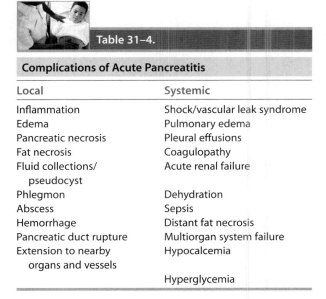

Table 31–4.

Complications of Acute Pancreatitis

Local	Systemic
Inflammation	Shock/vascular leak syndrome
Edema	Pulmonary edema
Pancreatic necrosis	Pleural effusions
Fat necrosis	Coagulopathy
Fluid collections/ pseudocyst	Acute renal failure
Phlegmon	Dehydration
Abscess	Sepsis
Hemorrhage	Distant fat necrosis
Pancreatic duct rupture	Multiorgan system failure
Extension to nearby organs and vessels	Hypocalcemia
	Hyperglycemia

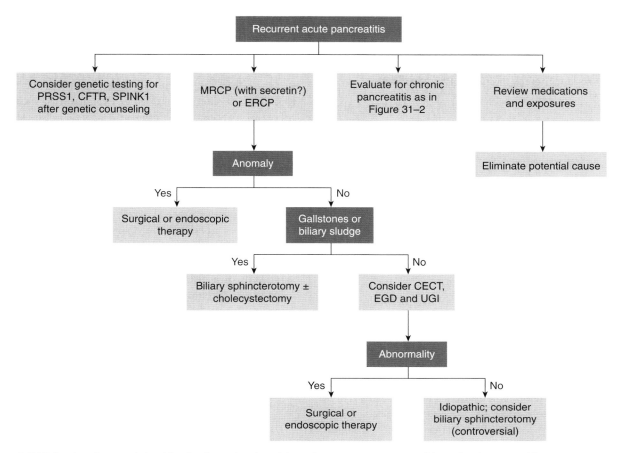

FIGURE 31-6 ■ Suggested algorithm for diagnosing the etiology of recurrent acute pancreatitis or chronic pancreatitis.

bile duct, become infected, rupture, or bleed, then therapy is required. Surgical, radiological, and endoscopic options are available for the management of pseudocysts. The choice depends on the location and size of the pseudocyst and on local expertise.[40]

Chronic Pancreatitis

Treatment of chronic pancreatitis differs with the stage and etiology of the disease. In patients with recurrent episodes of acute pancreatitis, the management of acute attacks is the same as for acute pancreatitis coupled with a systematic search for treatable causes (Figure 31–6). In patients with advancing or advanced disease from an untreatable cause, therapy is directed at the complications, chronic pain, pancreatic insufficiency, or diabetes mellitus, which is usually managed by an endocrinologist and is not covered in this chapter.

Pain relief

Prolonged and persistent pain is the dominating symptom in many patients with chronic pancreatitis. The prevalence of pain likely varies with etiology.[41] Solid prevalence data are not available for pediatric patients.

In all cases, treatment with analgesic medications is the mainstay of pain management. Therapeutic trials of pain management are lacking in both adults and children and practice is guided by local practice and expert opinion. In general, treatment is begun with acetaminophen and advanced to narcotics with patient comfort taking precedence over concerns for addiction. When utilizing chronic narcotics, it is important to remember that they can produce abdominal pain, the so-called narcotic bowel syndrome.

Pancreatic enzyme supplementation is often prescribed based on the theory that they will down-regulate the feedback loop of pancreatic exocrine activation. A handful of trials have examined the effect of pancreatic enzyme supplementation on chronic pain and all have methodological problems. Only two reported efficacy. Both used nonenteric-coated enzyme formulas. Others have argued that each study suggests efficacy in patients who have retained pancreatic function and have predominantly small duct disease.[41] Most physicians will perform a therapeutic trial of pancreatic enzyme supplementation at usual replacement doses (see below) for ages over 1–2 months. If nonenteric-coated enzymes are prescribed, a proton pump inhibitor should be

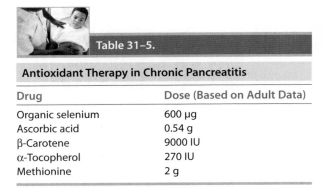

Table 31–5.

Antioxidant Therapy in Chronic Pancreatitis

Drug	Dose (Based on Adult Data)
Organic selenium	600 µg
Ascorbic acid	0.54 g
β-Carotene	9000 IU
α-Tocopherol	270 IU
Methionine	2 g

prescribed as well. There are no data to support the use of octreotide to inhibit pancreatic secretions.

Antioxidant therapy has been evaluated multiple times for efficacy in reducing pain. The results have not been convincing and all studies have methodological issues. A recent study of 183 adults randomized to antioxidant therapy or placebo reported improved pain relief in the treatment group.[42] Further experience is required to demonstrate the utility of this approach. As with pancreatic enzyme replacement therapy, a therapeutic trial is a reasonable approach in empirically treating pain (Table 31–5).

Endoscopic, surgical, and nerve block therapies have all been employed in the treatment of pain.[41] There are no clinical trials supporting the efficacy of any of these treatments. Even so, many therapeutic endoscopists advocate a trial of endoscopic therapy, generally sphincterotomy with stenting, in patients with chronic pain and a dilated duct. Surgical therapy is generally guided by the individual anatomy. Patients with a dilated pancreatic duct are generally treated with operations that aim at drainage and decompression of the duct. Patients who do not have a dilated main duct are treated with various forms of pancreatic resection including total pancreatectomy with islet cell autotransplantation. Interestingly, even these patients have a significant rate of continued pain.[43] Nerve blocks and neurolysis have shown better efficacy for pancreatic cancer than for chronic pancreatitis.

Pancreatic insufficiency

The treatment of pancreatic insufficiency currently depends on the use of pancreatic replacement therapy with extracts or porcine pancreas (see Chapter 32).[44,45]

GENETIC TESTING

The role of genetic testing in the management of patients with recurrent acute pancreatitis or chronic pancreatitis deserves special mention. A major advance in our understanding of pancreatitis took place with the discovery of gene mutations that associate with pancreati-

tis. The first of these were the mutations in the cationic trypsinogen gene, *PRSS1*, associated with hereditary pancreatitis.[4] Although the mutations in *PRSS1* are thought to increase the likelihood of trypsinogen activation within the acinar cell, direct evidence for this mechanism is lacking and other explanations, such as increased protein misfolding leading to endoplasmic reticulum stress, may be responsible. The discovery of the *PRSS1* mutation was followed by descriptions of mutations in the *CFTR* and *SPINK1* genes that increased susceptibility to acute pancreatitis.

Consequently, genetic testing has become an important part of medical care in evaluating recurrent acute pancreatitis and chronic pancreatitis. Genetic testing is done for two general reasons, diagnosis and prediction. Diagnostic testing is done when a patient has symptoms of a disease and the genetic test can determine the underlying cause. Predictive genetic testing is done in subjects without any evidence of pancreatic disease. In general, predictive genetic testing in children is not indicated for *CFTR* or *SPINK1* mutations and is not recommended for *PRSS1* mutations unless there are first-degree relatives with a known *PRSS1* mutation, adequate genetic counseling has been offered, and the child can participate in the decision to undergo testing.

Genetic testing for *PRSS1* mutations is recommended in patients with recurrent attacks of acute pancreatitis for which there is no other explanation, with unexplained chronic pancreatitis, or with a family history of pancreatitis in a first-degree or second-degree relative. Guidelines for testing for *CFTR* and *SPINK1* mutations are less clear. In general, many practitioners consider them a part of the evaluation for patients with unexplained recurrent acute pancreatitis or unexplained chronic pancreatitis. Others would not consider them a part of the evaluation. If proceeding with testing, the physician should order complete sequencing of the *CFTR* gene, since many patients have rare mutations in one or both alleles and these are not included in standard panels designed to diagnose patients with cystic fibrosis. Whereas the presence of a *PRSS1* mutation provides an adequate etiology for pancreatitis, the presence of CFTR or SPINK1 mutant genes should not preclude a careful search for additional etiologies.

Genetic counseling should be provided before ordering gene testing. The patient and family should understand: (1) why the test was suggested; (2) the implications of finding a pancreatitis-related mutation for the health and medical care of the patient; (3) who will communicate the test result and who else has access to the result; (4) will genetic counseling be provided after the test results return; (5) the pancreatic cancer risk and the possible adverse effects on health and life insurance; (6) the implications of a positive test for relatives of the patient.

REFERENCES

1. Nydegger A, Heine RG, Ranuh R, Gegati-Levy R, Crameri J, Oliver MR. Changing incidence of acute pancreatitis: 10-year experience at the Royal Children's Hospital, Melbourne. *J Gastroenterol Hepatol.* 2007;22:1313–1316.

2. Sanchez-Ramirez CA, Larrosa-Haro A, Flores-Martinez S, Sanchez-Corona J, Villa-Gomez A, Macias-Rosales R. Acute and recurrent pancreatitis in children: etiological factors. *Acta Paediatr.* 2007;96:534–537.

3. Lowe ME, Greer JB. Pancreatitis in children and adolescents. *Curr Gastroenterol Rep.* 2008;10:128–135.

4. Kandula L, Whitcomb DC, Lowe ME. Genetic issues in pediatric pancreatitis. *Curr Gastroenterol Rep.* 2006;8: 248–253.

5. Keim V. Role of genetic disorders in acute recurrent pancreatitis. *World J Gastroenterol.* 2008;14:1011–1015.

6. Treiber M, Schlag C, Schmid RM. Genetics of pancreatitis: a guide for clinicians. *Curr Gastroenterol Rep.* 2008;10: 122–127.

7. Pandol SJ, Saluja AK, Imrie CW, Banks PA. Acute pancreatitis: bench to the bedside. *Gastroenterology.* 2007;132: 1127–1151.

8. Thrower E, Husain S, Gorelick F. Molecular basis for pancreatitis. *Curr Opin Gastroenterol.* 2008;24:580–585.

9. Bhatia M. Acute pancreatitis as a model of SIRS. *Front Biosci.* 2009;14:2042–2050.

10. Witt H, Apte MV, Keim V, Wilson JS. Chronic pancreatitis: challenges and advances in pathogenesis, genetics, diagnosis, and therapy. *Gastroenterology.* 2007;132: 1557–1573.

11. Whitcomb DC. Hereditary pancreatitis: new insights into acute and chronic pancreatitis. *Gut.* 1999;45:317–322.

12. Benifla M, Weizman Z. Acute pancreatitis in childhood: analysis of literature data. *J Clin Gastroenterol.* 2003;37: 169–172.

13. Werlin SL, Kugathasan S, Frautschy BC. Pancreatitis in children. *J Pediatr Gastroenterol Nutr.* 2003;37:591–595.

14. Kandula L, Lowe ME. Etiology and outcome of acute pancreatitis in infants and toddlers. *J Pediatr.* 2008 Jan;152(1):106–110

15. Yadav D, Agarwal N, Pitchumoni CS. A critical evaluation of laboratory tests in acute pancreatitis. *Am J Gastroenterol.* 2002;97:1309–1318.

16. Keating JP, Lowe ME. Persistent hyperlipasemia caused by macrolipase in an adolescent. *J Pediatr.* 2002;141: 129–131.

17. Taes YE, Louagie H, Yvergneaux JP, et al. Prolonged hyperlipasemia attributable to a novel type of macrolipase. *Clin Chem.* 2000;46:2008–2013.

18. Gullo L, Lucrezio L, Migliori M, Bassi M, Nestico V, Costa PL. Benign pancreatic hyperenzymemia or Gullo's syndrome. *Adv Med Sci.* 2008;53:1–5.

19. Gullo L, Migliori M. Benign pancreatic hyperenzymemia in children. *Eur J Pediatr.* 2007;166:125–129.

20. Uhl W, Roggo A, Kirschstein T, et al. Influence of contrast-enhanced computed tomography on course and outcome in patients with acute pancreatitis. *Pancreas.* 2002;24:191–197.

21. De Waele E, Op de Beeck B, De Waele B, Delvaux G. Magnetic resonance cholangiopancreatography in the preoperative assessment of patients with biliary pancreatitis. *Pancreatology.* 2007;7:347–351.

22. Levy P, Boruchowicz A, Hastier P, et al. Diagnostic criteria in predicting a biliary origin of acute pancreatitis in the era of endoscopic ultrasound: multicentre prospective evaluation of 213 patients. *Pancreatology.* 2005;5: 450–456.

23. Fitoz S, Erden A, Boruban S. Magnetic resonance cholangiopancreatography of biliary system abnormalities in children. *Clin Imaging.* 2007;31:93–101.

24. Schaefer JF, Kirschner HJ, Lichy M, et al. Highly resolved free-breathing magnetic resonance cholangiopancreatography in the diagnostic workup of pancreaticobiliary diseases in infants and young children—initial experiences. *J Pediatr Surg.* 2006;41:1645–1651.

25. Tipnis NA, Werlin SL. The use of magnetic resonance cholangiopancreatography in children. *Curr Gastroenterol Rep.* 2007;9:225–229.

26. Bjerring OS, Durup J, Qvist N, Mortensen MB. Impact of upper gastrointestinal endoscopic ultrasound in children. *J Pediatr Gastroenterol Nutr.* 2008;47:110–113.

27. Cohen S, Kalinin M, Yaron A, Givony S, Reif S, Santo E. Endoscopic ultrasonography in pediatric patients with gastrointestinal disorders. *J Pediatr Gastroenterol Nutr.* 2008;46:551–554.

28. Morris-Stiff G, Al-Allak A, Frost B, Lewis WG, Puntis MC, Roberts A. Does endoscopic ultrasound have anything to offer in the diagnosis of idiopathic acute pancreatitis? *JOP.* 2009;10:143–146.

29. Stormon MO, Durie PR. Pathophysiologic basis of exocrine pancreatic dysfunction in childhood. *J Pediatr Gastroenterol Nutr.* 2002;35:8–21.

30. Catalano MF, Sahai A, Levy M, Romagnuolo J, Wiersema M, Brugge W, Freeman M, Yamao K, Canto M, Hernandez LV. EUS-based criteria for the diagnosis of chronic pancreatitis: the Rosemont classification. *Gastrointest Endosc.* 2009 Jun; 69(7):1251–1261.

31. Lieb JG 2nd, Draganov PV. Pancreatic function testing: here to stay for the 21st century. *World J Gastroenterol.* 2008;14:3149–3158.

32. Schibli S, Corey M, Gaskin KJ, Ellis L, Durie PR. Towards the ideal quantitative pancreatic function test: analysis of test variables that influence validity. *Clin Gastroenterol Hepatol.* 2006;4:90–97.

33. Thompson DR. Narcotic analgesic effects on the sphincter of Oddi: a review of the data and therapeutic implications in treating pancreatitis. *Am J Gastroenterol.* 2001;96:1266–1272.

34. Gardner TB, Vege SS, Pearson RK, Chari ST. Fluid resuscitation in acute pancreatitis. *Clin Gastroenterol Hepatol.* 2008;6:1070–1076.

35. Banks PA, Freeman ML. Practice guidelines in acute pancreatitis. *Am J Gastroenterol.* 2006;101:2379–2400.

36. Mao EQ, Tang YQ, Fei J, et al. Fluid therapy for severe acute pancreatitis in acute response stage. *Chin Med J (Engl).* 2009;122:169–173.

37. Marik PE. What is the best way to feed patients with pancreatitis? *Curr Opin Crit Care.* 2009;15:131–138.

38. Eckerwall GE, Tingstedt BB, Bergenzaun PE, Andersson RG. Immediate oral feeding in patients with mild acute

pancreatitis is safe and may accelerate recovery—a randomized clinical study. *Clin Nutr.* 2007;26:758–763.

39. Jacobson BC, Vander Vliet MB, Hughes MD, Maurer R, McManus K, Banks PA. A prospective, randomized trial of clear liquids versus low-fat solid diet as the initial meal in mild acute pancreatitis. *Clin Gastroenterol Hepatol.* 2007;5:946–951.

40. Habashi S, Draganov PV. Pancreatic pseudocyst. *World J Gastroenterol.* 2009;15:38–47.

41. Fasanella KE, Davis B, Lyons J, et al. Pain in chronic pancreatitis and pancreatic cancer. *Gastroenterol Clin North Am.* 2007;36:335–364, ix.

42. Bhardwaj P, Garg PK, Maulik SK, Saraya A, Tandon RK, Acharya SK. A randomized controlled trial of antioxidant supplementation for pain relief in patients with chronic pancreatitis. *Gastroenterology.* 2009;136:149–159 e2.

43. Blondet JJ, Carlson AM, Kobayashi T, et al. The role of total pancreatectomy and islet autotransplantation for chronic pancreatitis. *Surg Clin North Am.* 2007;87: 1477–1501, x.

44. Durie P, Kalnins D, Ellis L. Uses and abuses of enzyme therapy in cystic fibrosis. *J R Soc Med.* 1998;91(suppl 34):2–13.

45. Dominguez-Munoz JE, Iglesias-Garcia J, Iglesias-Rey M, Figueiras A, Vilarino-Insua M. Effect of the administration schedule on the therapeutic efficacy of oral pancreatic enzyme supplements in patients with exocrine pancreatic insufficiency: a randomized, three-way crossover study. *Aliment Pharmacol Ther.* 2005;21:993–1000.

CHAPTER 32

Pancreatic Insufficiency and Cystic Fibrosis

Aliye Uc

DEFINITIONS AND EPIDEMIOLOGY

Pancreatic insufficiency (PI) is a term used to define patients who have lost a significant amount (usually >95%) of pancreatic exocrine function and therefore their ability to digest and assimilate nutrients normally.[1] Cystic fibrosis (CF) is by far the most common form of PI in children and the focus of this chapter.

CF is the most common life-threatening autosomal recessive disease in the United States. The prevalence is higher in populations of northern European descent (~1 in 2500 births) compared to people from Hispanic (1 in 4000–10,000), African American (1 in 15,000–20,000), or Asian (1:30,000) ethnic backgrounds. The carrier rate is estimated to be around 3.5% for Caucasians; heterozygotes show no clinically relevant phenotypes.[2]

CF is caused by a mutation in the gene that encodes CF transmembrane conductance regulator (*CFTR*) protein. *CFTR* is expressed in many epithelial cells (sweat duct, airway, pancreatic duct, intestine, biliary tree, and vas deferens) and functions as an apical membrane anion channel, mainly involved in chloride and bicarbonate secretion.[3–5] It is proposed that the lack of *CFTR* leads to acidic, dehydrated, and protein-rich secretions, which then plug the lumen and cause the destruction of the organ.[4] Pulmonary involvement causes the most significant morbidity and mortality in patients with CF. With substantial improvement in the medical care of CF patients, the projected life expectancy has now increased to ~37 years of age.[6]

Although >1500 *CFTR* mutations have been identified, the functional importance is known only for a small number of mutations. *CFTR* mutations can be classified into six types of defects (class I–VI mutations) (Table 32–1)[2]: absence of protein synthesis (class I); defective protein maturation and premature degradation (class II); disordered regulation (class III); defective chloride (Cl⁻) conductance or channel gating (class IV); a reduced number of *CFTR* transcripts due to a promoter or splicing abnormality (class V); and accelerated turnover from the cell surface (class VI) (Figure 32–1).[4,7,8] *CFTR* function is virtually absent with class I–III and VI mutations while class IV and V mutations allow some residual *CFTR* function.[6] Pancreatic function appears to correlate well with the gene mutations at the *CFTR* locus. Exocrine pancreatic dysfunction is seen almost exclusively in association with class I–III and VI mutations.[7] Patients with at least one mutation belonging to class IV or V generally present with symptoms in late childhood or adulthood.

The absence of phenylalanine at position 508 (ΔF508, a class II mutation) constitutes two-thirds of *CFTR* mutations in northern European and North American populations. No other single mutation accounts for >5% of *CFTR* mutations worldwide.[2] Among the various gastrointestinal organs affected by CF, the exocrine pancreas shows the strongest association between genotype and phenotype. In most cases, considerable destruction of the pancreas starts in utero and functional loss of the exocrine pancreas develops at birth or in early infancy.[2]

The pancreas is commonly involved in patients with CF, and CF is the most frequent cause of exocrine PI in childhood. Eighty-five percent of CF patients have PI; 50–65% have PI at birth, and 20–30% of pancreatic sufficient (PS) patients become rapidly insufficient during the first few months and years of life.[9] The 15% of CF patients who are PS have a markedly improved prognosis and lung disease of later onset.

Table 32–1.

Classes of *CFTR* Mutations That Cause CF

Class	Defect	Examples	%
I	Protein production (no *CFTR* made)	G542X	2.4
		3905 insT	2.1
		621 + G–T	1.3
II	Processing (defect in protein trafficking leads to degradation)	ΔI507	0.5
		ΔF508	67.2
		S549R	0.3
		N1303K	1.3
III	Regulation (*CFTR* not activated by ATP or cyclic AMP)	G551 D	1.6
		G551S	Rare
		G1349D	Rare
IV	Conduction (reduced anion transport through *CFTR*)	R117H	0.8
		R334W	0.4
		R347P	0.5
V	Splicing defect (reduced production of normal *CFTR*)	3849 + 10 kb C → T	
		1811 + 1 · 6 kb A → G	
		IVS8-5T, 2789 + 5G → A	

Although it has "sufficient" function, pancreas is never normal in CF patients with PS. Pancreas does not manifest failure until >95% of its exocrine portion is lost.

PATHOGENESIS

There are four potential mechanisms that could explain pancreatic damage and PI in CF: (1) obstruction of pancreatic ducts by inspissated plugs, (2) inhibition of endocytosis in acinar cells, (3) inflammation, and (4) imbalance in membrane lipids. Any of these abnormalities alone or in combination may explain the development of pancreatic lesions in CF.[10]

Obstruction of Pancreatic Ducts by Inspissated Plugs

In healthy mammals, pancreatic juice is first secreted as protein and pancreatic enzyme-rich fluid by acinar cells. As it passes through the pancreatic ducts, the fluid composition is changed by the secretion of fluid and HCO_3^- into the lumen, a function regulated mainly by *CFTR* in the ductal epithelial cells. Patients with CF have low-flow pancreatic secretions with a high protein concentration that presumably precipitates in the duct lumen causing obstruction, damage, and atrophy. Inspissated secretions may also be due to increased mucus production and alterations of proteins through proteolysis or modification of the milieu in which these proteins reside.

Inhibition of Endocytosis in Acinar Cells

It appears that blunted ductal bicarbonate (HCO_3^-) secretion is the initiating event in CF pancreatic disease. Acidification of the acinar and duct lumen may cause defective endocytosis of the zymogen granule membranes and decreases solubilization of the pancreatic secretory proteins, resulting in precipitation and formation of lamellar plugs.

Inflammation

It is possible that inflammation plays an important role in the development and progression of pancreatic lesions in CF. Recurrent acute and chronic pancreatitis are known complications of CF, and they may occur in ~ 20% of patients with the PS phenotype.[4,11] It is not known why a subgroup of patients with CF develops pancreatitis, but preservation of acinar cells seems to be a prerequisite for this complication.

Imbalance in Membrane Lipids

Essential fatty acid deficiency is well described in CF patients, even in the absence of other nutritional deficiencies. Plasma eicosatrienoic acid levels are high, whereas linoleic and docosahexaenoic acid levels are low in patients with CF. Docosahexaenoic acid is an important regulator of membrane fluidity and transport systems and it also down-regulates arachidonic acid incorporation into the membrane phospholipids.

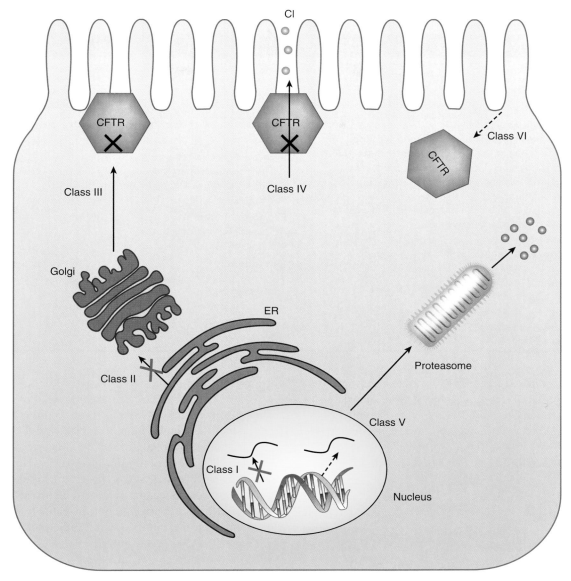

FIGURE 32–1 ■ Classes of *CFTR* mutations. Classes of defects in the *CFTR* gene are: absence of protein synthesis (class I); defective protein maturation and premature degradation (class II); disordered regulation, such as diminished ATP binding and hydrolysis (class III); defective Cl⁻ conductance or channel gating (class IV); a reduced number of *CFTR* transcripts due to a promoter or splicing abnormality (class V); and accelerated turnover from the cell surface (class VI).

The imbalance between docosahexaenoic acid and arachidonic acid in CF can potentially explain the observed mucin hypersecretion, alterations in the acinar cell endocytosis, and pancreatic inflammation observed in CF. Studies are ongoing to understand the mechanisms by which mutations in *CFTR* lead to this membrane lipid abnormality.[10]

CLINICAL PRESENTATION

CF involves many organ systems (Table 32–2), but the pulmonary disease is the major cause of morbidity and mortality.[2] This chapter focuses only on the pancreatic findings

in CF (Table 32–3).[12] Other causes of PI (see the section "Differential Diagnosis") present with similar findings.

Pancreatic Insufficiency

More than half of infants with CF are pancreatic insufficient at birth; 20–30% of infants with normal pancreatic function at birth become rapidly insufficient during the first few months and years of life. The major consequences of PI are fat malabsorption secondary to decreased production of pancreatic enzymes. Fat malabsorption is defined by a fecal fat >7% of oral fat intake in a 3–5-day fat balance studies. Fat malabsorption, steatorrhea, and malnutrition are the hallmarks of CF patients with PI.

Table 32–2.

Clinical Manifestations of Cystic Fibrosis

Pulmonary
- Persistent, productive cough
- Obstructive airway disease
- Chronic bronchitis with or without bronchiectasis
- Acute exacerbations of lung disease (increased cough, tachypnea, dyspnea, increased sputum production, malaise, anorexia, and weight loss)
- Digital clubbing
- Colonization of the airway with pathogenic bacteria (*Staphylococcus aureus, Haemophilus influenzae, Pseudomonas aeruginosa*)
- Predisposition to lung infections

Pancreas
- Diarrhea
- Steatorrhea
- Malnutrition
- Fat-soluble vitamin deficiencies
- Pancreatitis

Intestine
- Meconium ileus (newborn period)
- Distal intestinal obstruction syndrome (older children)

Liver
- Focal biliary cirrhosis
- Cholestasis (rare in infancy)
- Cirrhosis and portal hypertension
- End-stage liver disease (in older children, rare)

Ear, nose, and throat
- Chronic rhinosinusitis
- Nasal polyps

Genitourinary
- Male infertility most commonly due to absence of vas deferens
- Female infertility due to chronic lung disease and malnutrition

Insufficient secretion of pancreatic enzymes (proteases, amylase, lipase, and colipase) leads to malabsorption of fat and protein. Patients with CF and PI have frequent, bulky, foul-smelling, sometimes oily stools. The subsequent calorie and protein losses are usually associated with diarrhea and lead to a decrease in fat

Table 32–3.

Pertinent History and Physical Exam Findings in CF Pancreatic Disease

History
- Poor weight gain or weight loss
- Diarrhea
- Frequent, bulky, foul-smelling, sometimes greasy stools
- Bloating
- Flatulence
- Rectal prolapse
- Abdominal pain (if pancreatitis is present)
- Bleeding tendencies (if vitamin K is deficient)
- Bone fractures (if vitamin D is deficient)
- Night blindness (if vitamin A is deficient)
- Diabetes

Physical examination
- Loss of subcutaneous fat
- Decreased muscle mass
- Digital clubbing
- Edema (if hypoproteinemia is present)
- Abdominal tenderness (if pancreatitis is present)
- Acrodermatitis (if vitamin A is deficient)
- Neuropathy (if vitamin E is deficient)

stores with loss of subcutaneous fat, decreased muscle mass, and failure to thrive within the first few months of life. In severe cases, fat malabsorption can lead to deficiencies of fat-soluble vitamins A, D, E, and K. Routine vitamin supplementation has made clinical evidence of vitamin deficiency uncommon. Nevertheless, vitamin K and D deficiencies may still occur despite supplementation. Decreased bone mineral density, increased fracture rates, and kyphosis are common in patients with CF, even among those with pancreatic sufficiency. The risk for bone disease increases with advancing age and severity of lung disease and malnutrition.

Malnutrition and poor growth are commonly found in infants with CF at the time of diagnosis, and they are more prevalent if PI is present. Among children with CF, ~15% are below the fifth percentile for weight and height. Growth parameters improve after diagnosis and appropriate treatment, but growth delay continues to be a problem in CF. Although the etiology of malnutrition is multifactorial (inadequate intake, increased losses, lung disease, and increased energy needs), PI seems to have a major impact on growth and nutrition. Infants identified with PI at diagnosis are more malnourished as evidenced by poor weight gain, depressed fat stores, low serum albumin, and BUN. These findings are noted despite an increased dietary intake in these patients.

Chronic progressive lung disease is the most prominent cause of morbidity and mortality in patients with CF. Good nutritional status has a positive impact on lung disease and patient survival, whereas malnutrition and PI are associated with more rapid decline of the pulmonary function. Patients with PS have normal growth, develop lung disease at a later age, and are less likely to have lung colonization with *Pseudomonas*.

Rectal prolapse and digital clubbing are common in children with CF, associated with PI and malnutrition. In older children, pulmonary symptoms dominate the picture and PI symptoms may not be elucidated unless directly asked by the examiner or investigated by laboratory testing.

Loss of pancreatic function can ultimately lead to glucose intolerance and CF-related diabetes (CFRD). The risk of developing CFRD increases with advancing age (25% by age 20 years), the presence of PI, ΔF508 homozygous genotype, and female gender.[4] CFRD has the features of both type I and type II diabetes, including both decreased insulin production and insulin resistance. Patients with CF-related pancreatic disease usually have decreased insulin secretion, but glucose tolerance may be either normal or decreased. Some have normal glucose tolerance because of the unusual combination of increased hepatic glucose production and increased peripheral glucose utilization. When impaired glucose tolerance or overt diabetes develops, peripheral glucose utilization and hepatic insulin sensitivity are decreased.

PS patients have adequate endogenous pancreatic function to ensure normal fat absorption. The functional capacity of the exocrine pancreas in PS patients varies widely, from borderline normal values to values within the normal range for healthy controls. Patients with PS usually have normal growth parameters and the diagnosis of CF may be delayed until the second or third decade of life.

Pancreatitis

Pancreatitis occurs in 2–4% of all CF patients and 15–20% of PS patients with mild *CFTR* mutations during adolescence or later in life.[13,14] Pancreatitis is rare in most CF patients, presumably because the pancreas loses its acinar cell mass early in life. Nevertheless, pancreatitis may be the presenting symptom in some patients, and in a small group it may precede the diagnosis of CF by several years.[11] Recurrent attacks of pancreatitis may lead to PI several years after the initial diagnosis. Pancreatitis may go undetected in pancreatic insufficient individuals.[4] CF patients with significantly reduced acinar cell mass may not show a marked pancreatic amylase and lipase elevations; therefore, diagnosis may be difficult.[14]

Patients with idiopathic chronic pancreatitis (ICP) carry a higher frequency of *CFTR* mutations than the general population and a subset of these patients have CF. *CFTR* mutations may also contribute to the development of chronic pancreatitis in patients who have additional risk factors for chronic pancreatitis. Most commercially available genetic screening tests only

identify the most severe *CFTR* mutations; therefore, "milder" mutations may be missed in patients with ICP. In fact, almost half of patients with ICP have at least one abnormal allele when complete DNA analysis is performed looking for >1000 known mutations in *CFTR*.

DIFFERENTIAL DIAGNOSIS

CF is the most frequent cause of exocrine PI in childhood. Other etiologies include: Shwachman–Diamond syndrome (SDS), Pearson marrow–pancreas syndrome, Johanson–Blizzard syndrome, and isolated enzyme deficiencies (lipase, colipase, trypsinogen, amylase, lipase–colipase, and enterokinase) (Table 32–4).

Shwachman–Diamond syndrome

SDS is the second most common cause of exocrine PI in children after CF.[15] It is characterized by PI, neutropenia, which may be cyclic, and skeletal defects, with abnormal development of the growth plate and metaphysis (Figure 32–2), failure to thrive, and short stature. In 90% of affected patients, mutations can be detected in the Shwachman–Bodian–Diamond syndrome (SBDS) gene located on chromosome 7. Patients typically present in infancy with poor growth and greasy, foul-smelling stools, characteristic of PI. Contrary to children with CF, these children have normal sweat Cl⁻, no *CFTR* mutations, typical metaphyseal lesions, and fatty pancreas on computerized tomography. Short stature does not usually improve despite adequate pancreatic replacement therapy. PI is often transient, and steatorrhea may spontaneously improve over time. Recurrent suppurative infections (otitis media, pneumonia, osteomyelitis, dermatitis, and sepsis) are common and a frequent cause of death. Diagnosis of SDS is usually made by characteristic clinical findings. Genetic testing may be used to confirm the diagnosis. A negative test for SBDS gene mutations does not exclude the diagnosis because 10% of patients clinically diagnosed with SDS lack these mutations.

Table 32–4.

Causes of Pancreatic Insufficiency in Childhood

Cystic fibrosis
Shwachman–Diamond syndrome
Pearson marrow–pancreas syndrome
Johanson–Blizzard syndrome
Isolated enzyme deficiencies (lipase, colipase, trypsinogen, amylase, enterokinase)

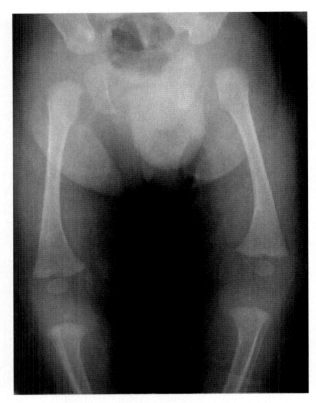

FIGURE 32-2 ■ Skeletal abnormalities in Shwachman–Diamond syndrome. Dysplasia of the metaphyses of the long bones is evident in this radiograph of a 2-year-old male with pancreatic insufficiency, neutropenia, and linear growth failure, typical clinical features of SDS. Note the flared widening of the distal femoral metaphyses with lucencies and calcific foci.

Pearson Marrow–Pancreas Syndrome

Pearson marrow–pancreas syndrome is caused by defects in oxidative phosphorylation due to sporadic mutations in the mitochondrial DNA.[16] Affected infants have severe macrocytic anemia and variable thrombocytopenia. It is distinguished from SDS by the presence of sideroblastic anemia, bone marrow changes (cell vacuolization and ringed sideroblasts), pancreatic fibrosis rather than lipomatosis, and the absence of bone lesions. Children with Pearson marrow–pancreas syndrome have PI and growth failure.

Johanson–Blizzard syndrome

This syndrome is characterized by pancreatic exocrine deficiency, aplasia or hypoplasia of the alae nasi, congenital deafness, hypothyroidism, developmental delay, microcephaly, midline ectodermal scalp defects, absence of permanent teeth, urogenital malformations, and imperforate anus.[1] In contrast to SDS, children with Johanson–Blizzard syndrome do not have bone marrow and skeletal abnormalities.

Isolated Enzyme Deficiencies

Isolated deficiencies of trypsinogen (protein malabsorption), lipase and colipase (fat malabsorption), and enterokinase have been reported. Enterokinase is a brush border enzyme that activates pancreatic proteases (trypsinogen, chymotrypsinogen, etc.); therefore, its deficiency will lead to protein malabsorption. Deficiencies of trypsinogen or enterokinase present with failure to thrive, hypoproteinemia, and edema. Isolated amylase deficiency is developmental and resolves by 2–3 years of age.[1]

DIAGNOSIS

Tests to Diagnose CF

The diagnosis of CF is made if: (1) typical clinical features of the disease are present; (2) sweat Cl^- ≥60 mmol/L; (3) sweat Cl^- is intermediate (30–59 mmol/L for infants <6 months of age and 40–59 mmol/L for older individuals) plus two disease-causing *CFTR* mutations are identified (Figure 32–3).[17]

Newborn screen (NBS)

Patients with CF are now diagnosed in almost all 50 states via NBS. NBS identifies infants with high values of immunoreactive trypsinogen (IRT). IRT is elevated because the enzyme escapes to the blood stream from a damaged pancreas. A specific cutoff value defines an elevated IRT. It has to be kept in mind that normal IRT reference values vary slightly from state to state. After an abnormal IRT value is identified, most NBS programs perform DNA testing to identify known *CFTR* gene mutations (IRT/DNA strategy), while other programs repeat the IRT measurement in a second blood sample obtained from the infant at age approximately 2 weeks (IRT/IRT strategy). Both strategies provide ~90–95% sensitivity and identify newborns at risk for CF.[17]

Sweat chloride

Sweat is traditionally collected onto gauze or filter paper, under an occlusive dressing to prevent evaporation, following stimulation of sweat gland secretion with pilocarpine. Avoidance of evaporation is critically important, as it may cause falsely elevated chloride levels. Some newer commercial sweat-collection devices use capillary tubing to collect sweat with greater reliability (Figure 32–4). To increase the likelihood of collecting an adequate sweat specimen, it is recommended that sweat Cl^- first be performed when the infant is at least 2 weeks of age and weighs at least 2 kg. Sweat Cl^- reference ranges for infants up to age 6 months: ≤29 mmol/L, CF

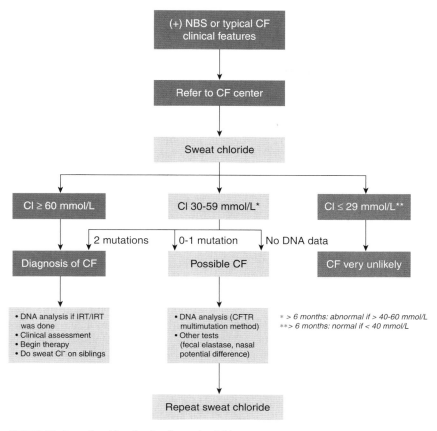

FIGURE 32–3 ■ Algorithm for the diagnosis of CF.

unlikely; 30–59 mmol/L, intermediate; ≥60 mmol/L, indicative of CF. Individuals with intermediate results should undergo repeat sweat Cl⁻ testing and referred to a CF center with expertise in diagnosing CF in infancy.

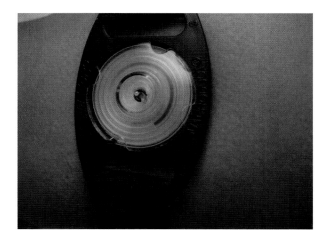

FIGURE 32–4 ■ Capillary sweat-collection device. Sweat is collected as it forms into a coiled plastic capillary tube in this commercially marketed device. A blue dye in the tubing facilitates visualization of the quantity obtained, and risk of evaporative concentration of the sweat is minimized, compared to older methods using an absorptive pad.

For children older than 6 months, reference ranges are slightly different: individuals over age 6 months: ±39 mmol/L, CF unlikely; 40–59 mmol/L, intermediate; ≥60 mmol/L, indicative of CF.[2,17] Individuals with intermediate results should undergo repeat sweat Cl⁻ testing and further evaluation, including detailed clinical assessment and more extensive *CFTR* gene mutation analysis.

DNA analysis

For children with intermediate sweat Cl⁻ values, DNA analysis can help establish the diagnosis of CF. Genetic testing for CF may not be straightforward. Although currently available mutation screening panels can identify 90% of *CFTR* mutations, 9.7% of genotyped individuals in the Cystic Fibrosis Foundation Patient Registry have at least one unidentified mutation. Even if the genotype is identified, the consequences of the vast majority of *CFTR* mutations remain unknown. Fifteen percent of *CFTR* mutations are designated as sequence variants with no resulting clinical effect. Only 1% of *CFTR* mutations have been shown to cause sufficient loss of *CFTR*. These mutations are found in ~85% of the CF population and cause PI and pulmonary complications.[17]

Table 32–5.

Tests to Determine Pancreatic Insufficiency in Childhood

Fecal fat excretion
Fecal elastase
Pancreatic stimulation tests
C^{13} triglyceride breath test

Tests to Assess Pancreatic Exocrine Function

Pancreatic function tests (PFTs) are classified as direct or indirect (Table 32–5).[18] Direct PFTs involve the stimulation of the pancreas with pancreatic secretagogues followed by collection of duodenal fluid and analysis of its contents (i.e., enzymes, Cl^-, and HCO_3^-). Direct PFTs are more sensitive and specific to measure the exocrine pancreatic function. However, they are not easy to perform and only available at a few centers. Indirect tests measure the consequences of PI, but lack sensitivity and specificity. These tests are more widely available and easier to perform than the direct pancreatic testing. In this section, we will focus on the most commonly used tests to diagnose PI.

Indirect tests

Fecal fat excretion Steatorrhea of pancreatic origin implies a loss of >90% of normal enzyme secretory output. Steatorrhea can be measured by a 72-hour stool collection and calculation of coefficient of fat absorption (CFA = (grams of fat ingested − grams of fat excreted)/(grams of fat ingested) × 100). In children younger than 6 months of age, a fecal fat >15% of fat intake is considered abnormal; this value is 7% for children over 6 months of age. When performed correctly, CFA is very useful to determine the degree of fat malabsorption and evaluate response to enzyme therapy.[19] Collection of stools for this technique is very difficult in young children who are still wearing diapers. Qualitative measurement (Sudan stain) of a single stool specimen is much easier to perform but less reliable than a quantitative 72-hour collection. Fecal fat excretion does not discriminate among hepatobiliary, mucosal, or pancreatic causes of fat malabsorption. Other problems with this test are the lack of precision and reproducibility. This test is not well accepted by patients/parents; sample and data collection are not always accurate.

Stool enzyme excretion Measurement of fecal trypsin and chymotrypsin tests may be inaccurate due to intraluminal degradation and cross-reactivity with ingested enzymes. Fecal elastase is resistant to degradation and it is the preferred test to measure PI.

Fecal elastase-1 (FE1). Because it is easy to use and relatively inexpensive, this ELISA-based method is now the most preferred test to diagnose PI in CF (Figure 32–5). FE1 can also be used to monitor PS CF patients for the development of PI. A value of <100 µg/g is considered indicative of PI. Intermediate values of fecal elastase (100–200 µg/g) may be due to loss of pancreatic function, but not severe enough to cause clinical PI. FE1 may be used for screening pancreatic function in CF patients after 2 weeks of age. The use of a monoclonal antibody for ELISA testing is generally preferred over the polyclonal antibody tests, because reference values for the polyclonal antibody test have not been established, and there is possibility for some cross-reactivity with ingested porcine pancreatic enzyme supplements with the polyclonal testing. The sensitivity of FE1 to diagnose moderate and severe PI is close to 100%. In patients with mild loss of pancreatic function, the test sensitivity is ~25% with a specificity of 96%.[20] Therefore, the value of FE1 to determine patients with mild PI or borderline normal pancreatic function is limited. Because monoclonal FE1 antibodies do not cross-react with porcine pancreatic elastase-1, monoclonal ELISA can reliably detect PI in patients who take pancreatic enzyme supplements. Unlike fecal fat analysis and C^{13} triglyceride breath tests (see below), FE1 cannot be used to assess response to pancreatic enzyme therapy. FE1 may be falsely low when the stool is diluted as a result of infectious diarrhea, severe enteropathies, and short gut, or if it is collected from an ileostomy.

C^{13} triglyceride breath test C^{13} triglyceride is given in a test meal to measure pancreatic exocrine function.[19] It is hydrolyzed within the intestinal lumen in proportion to the amount of pancreatic lipase activity. The hydrolyzed products are absorbed, metabolized, and released to the breath as $^{13}CO_2$. Measurement of $^{13}CO_2$ by mass spectrometry or infrared analysis gives an accurate assessment of PI. Numerous factors such as rate of gastric emptying, degree of solubilization by bile acids, mucosal absorption, endogenous CO_2 production, and pulmonary excretion may influence the test results. This test is nonspecific and inaccurate for the diagnosis of mild PI. The C^{13} triglyceride breath test can be used to quantify steatorrhea, avoiding the need for cumbersome stool collections.

Direct tests

Pancreatic stimulation tests These tests involve the collection of pancreatic fluid secreted into the intestine and measurement of enzymes, fluid volume, and

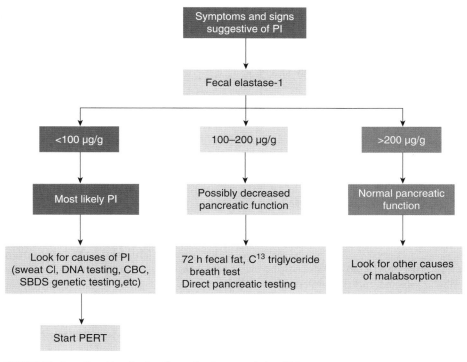

FIGURE 32-5 ■ Algorithm for the diagnosis of pancreatic insufficiency.

electrolytes (mainly Cl^- and HCO_3^-).[18,19] In patients with CF and pancreatic involvement, fluid volume, Cl^- and HCO_3^- concentrations, and total enzyme output are low. Duodenal intubation is performed, with concomitant aspiration of gastric contents, and collection of duodenal fluid before and after stimulation with pancreatic secretagogues (cholecystokinin and secretin) is the "gold standard" to quantify pancreatic function directly. The invasiveness and cost of the test discourage its routine clinical use. Direct PFTs are invasive: they involve placement of nasogastric and nasoduodenal catheters, IV cannulation, sedation, and radiographs to ensure the correct placement of the tube. Reference values have not been well established in individuals with CF. Pancreatic stimulation tests are not routinely used for the assessment of pancreatic function in CF.

TREATMENT

Currently the only treatment of PI is pancreatic enzyme replacement therapy (PERT), and all commercially available enzyme preparations are of porcine origin.[5] A recombinant pancreatic enzyme preparation will most likely be available soon. Because pancreatic enzyme preparations can be easily inactivated by gastric acid and pepsin, formulations with HCO_3^- and enteric-coated enzymes have been developed. Currently, there is no evidence that HCO_3^- offers an advantage over enteric-coated formulations. Unfortunately, PERT does not completely correct maldigestion in the majority of patients with PI or effectively treat the growth delay and nutritional deficiencies associated with PI.

Quality and consistency of the pancreatic enzyme products has always been a problem. These products have never received Food and Drug Administration (FDA) approval because they predate the 1938 passage of the FDA approval act. The FDA has allowed these products to be "grandfathered" and to remain on the market because of their lifesaving benefits for patients. In April 2004, FDA issued a statement to pancreatic enzyme manufacturers to get their drugs approved by the FDA within 4 years, requiring clinical trials in people with pancreatic diseases. It is expected that the clinical trials and the FDA approval will enhance the effectiveness and the safety of the pancreatic enzyme products.

PERT is based on number of lipase units administered per meal. Children <4 years of age require 1000 lipase units/kg per meal, 500 lipase units/kg per meal are used for those >4 years of age, and 25,000–40,000 units/meal are used for adults. Fewer enzymes per kilogram of body weight are recommended in older children because they eat less fat per kilogram of body weight. For snacks half the dose is recommended. Infants may be given 2000–4000 units per 120 mL of infant formula or per breastfeeding (Table 32–6). The daily dose for most patients is <10,000 units of lipase/kg/day or 6000 units of lipase/kg per meal to prevent fibrosing colonopathy.[21] For children who cannot swallow capsules, delayed

Table 32–6.

Pancreatic Enzyme Therapy for Patients with CF and PI

Infants
- 2000–4000 units per 120 mL of infant formula or per breastfeeding

<4 years of age
- 1000 lipase units/kg per meal and 500 lipase units/kg per snacks

>4 years of age
- 500 lipase units/kg per meal and 250 lipase units/kg per snacks

release capsules containing enteric-coated microspheres or microtablets may be opened and the contents sprinkled on soft food that does not require chewing and has a low pH (applesauce, gelatins, pureed apricot, banana, or sweet potatoes). Foods having a pH >7.3, such as milk, custard, or ice cream, should be avoided as a vehicle for the sprinkled enzymes because the protective enteric coating can dissolve in these foods, leaving the enzymes vulnerable to inactivation by gastric acid. For infants who are breastfeeding or bottle feeding, the enzyme beads from the capsule can be mixed in a very small amount of applesauce or another acidic baby food. Parents can "dip" their finger in applesauce and sprinkle the beads on the applesauce and have baby suck their finger or use a small baby spoon to feed applesauce and beads. Parents have to make sure that there are no beads left in the babies' mouth at the end of the feed or on mom's breast as the beads can cause ulcers if left on the breast or baby's mouth. The infant's mouth should be swept after administration to prevent ulceration. Powdered formulations (which are not enteric-coated) can cause ulcerations in the gut; therefore, they are not preferred. Pancrelipase tablets or capsules should not be crushed or chewed. Concurrent administration with H_2 antagonists or proton pump inhibitors may enhance enzyme efficacy.

Nutritional Therapy

Patients with CF and poor nutritional status are more prone to lung infections than those who have good nutritional status, and children with normal pancreatic function have a better pulmonary prognosis than those who do not. Because poor nutritional status is associated with the worse outcome in CF, nutritional issues must be managed aggressively to maintain normal weight and growth in children with CF. Fat-soluble vitamin supplementation is mandatory in all patients with PI. Patients' height and weight should be measured and

their body mass index (BMI) calculated every 3–4 months. A careful dietary history should be obtained at each clinical visit.[2]

Breastfeeding is recommended for infants with CF until 12 months of age. For older children, a balanced diet enhanced with high-fat snacks and supplements is necessary to meet the high-energy needs. Heavy cream, full-fat cheese, sour cream, butter or margarine, heavy syrup, gravy, and powdered milk can be added to foods in order to enrich their caloric contents. Children are encouraged to eat three meals and two snacks per day and pick foods that are high in fat and protein rather than sugar. Nutritional supplements with higher calories can be substituted for milk and their calorie contents may be increased by adding yogurt or ice cream. Children with mild pulmonary disease require only a 5–10% increase over the recommended daily caloric intake versus children with more severe lung disease and PI may need up to 20–50% increase over the recommended daily allowance. Nutritional supplementation via nasogastric tube or gastrostomy may be needed if children are unable to gain weight with oral intake.[22]

Vitamin Supplementation

Fat malabsorption may lead to deficiencies of the fat-soluble vitamins A, D, E, and K. Thus, all patients with CF should receive supplementation of these vitamins (Table 32–7). Vitamin levels should be checked yearly to monitor for adequate or excessive supplementation.

Table 32–7.

Fat-soluble Vitamin Supplementation for Patients with CF and PI

Vitamin A
- <3 years: 1500 IU/day
- 1–3 years: 5000 IU/day
- 4–8 years: 5000–10,000 IU/day
- >8 years: 10,000 IU/day

Vitamin D
- <1 year: 400 IU/day
- >1 year: 400–800 IU/day

Vitamin E
- 0–12 months: 40–50 IU/day
- 1–3 years: 80–150 IU/day
- 4–8 years: 100–200 IU/day
- >8 years: 200–400 IU/day

Vitamin K
- 300–500 mcg/day

REFERENCES

1. Durie PR. Inherited causes of exocrine pancreatic dysfunction. *Can J Gastroenterol.* 1997;11(2):145–152.

2. O'Sullivan BP, Freedman SD. Cystic fibrosis. *Lancet.* 2009;373(9678):1891–1904.

3. Quinton PM. Too much salt, too little soda: cystic fibrosis. *Sheng Li Xue Bao.* 2007;59(4):397–415.

4. Wilschanski M, Durie PR. Patterns of GI disease in adulthood associated with mutations in the CFTR gene. *Gut.* 2007;56(8):1153–1163.

5. Borowitz D, Durie PR, Clarke LL, et al. Gastrointestinal outcomes and confounders in cystic fibrosis. *J Pediatr Gastroenterol Nutr.* 2005;41(3):273–285.

6. Wolfenden LL, Schechter MS. Genetic and non-genetic determinants of outcomes in cystic fibrosis. *Paediatr Respir Rev.* 2009;10(1):32–36.

7. Welsh MJ, Smith AE. Molecular mechanisms of CFTR chloride channel dysfunction in cystic fibrosis. *Cell.* 1993;73(7):1251–1254.

8. Rowe SM, Miller S, Sorscher EJ. Cystic fibrosis. *N Engl J Med.* 2005;352(19):1992–2001.

9. Couper RT, Corey M, Durie PR, Forstner GG, Moore DJ. Longitudinal evaluation of serum trypsinogen measurement in pancreatic-insufficient and pancreatic-sufficient patients with cystic fibrosis. *J Pediatr.* 1995;127(3):408–413.

10. Freedman SD, Blanco P, Shea JC, Alvarez JG. Mechanisms to explain pancreatic dysfunction in cystic fibrosis. *Med Clin North Am.* 2000;84(3):657–664, x.

11. Walkowiak J, Lisowska A, Blaszczynski M. The changing face of the exocrine pancreas in cystic fibrosis: pancreatic sufficiency, pancreatitis and genotype. *Eur J Gastroenterol Hepatol.* 2008;20(3):157–160.

12. Durie PR, Forstner GG. Pathophysiology of the exocrine pancreas in cystic fibrosis. *J R Soc Med.* 1989;82 (suppl 16):2–10.

13. Durno C, Corey M, Zielenski J, Tullis E, Tsui LC, Durie P. Genotype and phenotype correlations in patients with cystic fibrosis and pancreatitis. *Gastroenterology.* 2002;123(6):1857–1864.

14. Gooding I, Bradley E, Puleston J, Gyi KM, Hodson M, Westaby D. Symptomatic pancreatitis in patients with cystic fibrosis. *Am J Gastroenterol.* 2009;104(6):1519–1523.

15. Burroughs L, Woolfrey A, Shimamura A. Shwachman–Diamond syndrome: a review of the clinical presentation, molecular pathogenesis, diagnosis, and treatment. *Hematol Oncol Clin North Am.* 2009;23(2):233–248.

16. Cormier V, Rotig A, Quartino AR, et al. Widespread multitissue deletions of the mitochondrial genome in the Pearson marrow–pancreas syndrome. *J Pediatr.* 1990;117(4):599–602.

17. Farrell PM, Rosenstein BJ, White TB, et al. Guidelines for diagnosis of cystic fibrosis in newborns through older adults: Cystic Fibrosis Foundation consensus report. *J Pediatr.* 2008;153(2):S4–S14.

18. Schibli S, Corey M, Gaskin KJ, Ellis L, Durie PR. Towards the ideal quantitative pancreatic function test: analysis of test variables that influence validity. *Clin Gastroenterol Hepatol.* 2006;4(1):90–97.

19. Leus J, Van Biervliet S, Robberecht E. Detection and follow up of exocrine pancreatic insufficiency in cystic fibrosis: a review. *Eur J Pediatr.* 2000;159(8):563–568.

20. Daftary A, Acton J, Heubi J, Amin R. Fecal elastase-1: utility in pancreatic function in cystic fibrosis. *J Cyst Fibros.* 2006;5(2):71–76.

21. Baker SS. Delayed release pancrelipase for the treatment of pancreatic exocrine insufficiency associated with cystic fibrosis. *Ther Clin Risk Manag.* 2008;4(5):1079–1084.

22. Pitts J, Flack J, Goodfellow J. Improving nutrition in the cystic fibrosis patient. *J Pediatr Health Care.* 2008;22(2):137–140.

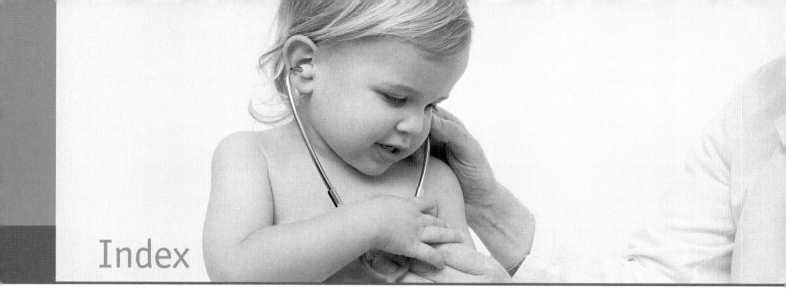

Index

	DATE DUE		